PRIMARY CARE
OF THE
POSTERIOR SEGMENT

SECOND EDITION

PRIMARY CARE
OF THE
POSTERIOR SEGMENT

SECOND EDITION

Larry J. Alexander, OD
Professor
UAB School of Optometry/The Medical Center
University of Alabama at Birmingham
Birmingham, Alabama

APPLETON & LANGE
Norwalk, Connecticut

Notice: The author and the publisher of this volume have taken care that the
information and recommendations contained herein are accurate and compatible
with the standards generally accepted at the time of publication. Nevertheless,
it is difficult to ensure that all the information given is entirely accurate
for all circumstances. The publisher disclaims any liability, loss, or damage
incurred as a consequence, directly or indirectly, of the use and application
of any of the contents of this volume.

Copyright © 1994 by Appleton & Lange
Paramount Publishing Business and Professional Group
Copyright © 1989 by Appleton & Lange

96 97 98 / 10 9 8 7 6 5 4 3 2

Prentice Hall International (UK) Limited, *London*
Prentice Hall of Australia Pty. Limited, *Sydney*
Prentice Hall Canada, Inc., *Toronto*
Prentice Hall Hispanoamericana, S.A., *Mexico*
Prentice Hall of India Private Limited, *New Delhi*
Prentice Hall of Japan, Inc., *Tokyo*
Simon & Schuster Asia Pte. Ltd., *Singapore*
Editora Prentice Hall do Brasil Ltda., *Rio de Janeiro*
Prentice Hall, *Englewood Cliffs, New Jersey*

Library of Congress Cataloging-in-Publication Data

Alexander, Larry J.
    Primary care of the posterior segment / Larry J. Alexander—2nd
ed.
      p.   cm.
    Includes bibliographical references and index.
    ISBN 0-8385-7970-1
    1. Posterior segment (Eye)—Diseases.   I. Title.
    [DNLM: 1. Eye Diseases—therapy.   2. Eye Diseases—diagnosis.
3. Diagnosis, Differential.   WW 140 A376p 1994]
RE475.A44   1994
617.7'3—dc20
DNLM/DLC
for Library of Congress   93-35782

Acquisitions Editor: Cheryl L. Mehalik
Senior Managing Editor, Production: John Williams
Production Assistants: Jennifer Szakonyi; Todd Miller
Designer: Janice Bielawa

PRINTED IN THE UNITED STATES OF AMERICA

ISBN 0-8385-7970-1
90000

9 780838 579701

Dedicated
to my family and friends for their support
and to the doctors who strive to help their patients, for their inspiration.

Living by Grace
Grace is doing for another being kindnesses he
doesn't deserve, hasn't earned, could not ask for,
and can't repay.
Its main facets are beauty, kindness, gratitude, charm,
favor and thankfulness.
Grace offers man what he cannot do for himself.
The unwritten creed of many is that God is under
obligation to them, but grace suggests that
we are under obligation to God.
To live in that consciousness is to live by grace.
Living by grace is costly; it means sharing.
It has no meaning apart from a spirit of self-sacrifice
that prompts the soul to think more of giving
than of receiving, of caring for others
rather than for one's self.

McElroy

Contents

Clinical Pearls

■ ■ ■ ■ ■ ■

*I*ntroduction

In today's health care environment of gatekeepers, patient ID numbers, and the overall depersonalization in our society, much patient care involves handholding and patients' perceptions of how much the clinician actually cares about them.

Unfortunately, there co-exists an information overload. More and more knowledge regarding health conditions is being found and published daily. Instrumentation appears almost more rapidly than we can pay for the now-obsolete piece of equipment. This combination makes "keeping up" a most difficult task. I wrote *Primary Care of the Posterior Segment*, second edition, to help simplify the information overload to give you more time to care.

The first edition of *Primary Care of the Posterior Segment* had as its theme a simplification of diagnosis and management of most disorders of the posterior segment. My approach was that of explaining the complexities of the underlying disease process in "down to earth" terms to allow the overloaded intern and resident, as well as the busy practitioner, the opportunity to quickly diagnose a condition and render a reasonable management plan. The information existed in various texts, but no single reference/teaching text put it all together. According to most practitioners, interns, and residents, I succeeded in my goal for the first edition.

As with anything that we do in life, after reflecting on the job done, we often see ways for improvement the next time around. In this second edition, I attempt to rectify most criticism of the first edition and improve on both the teaching and reference aspects of the text. Material has been added, re-arranged, and updated, a more comprehensive reference section has been added, photographs have been improved, numerous figures have been added, the color photographs have been enlarged, the number of color photos has been increased, the layout has been improved, and the index has been significantly expanded and improved. Color has been added in the text to highlight the Pearls and Clinical Examples.

The main thrust of the second edition is an embellishment of the management section. Instead of calling for a complete medical workup as was done in the first edition, the specifics of that workup are outlined in detail in this second edition. This has been done to improve intraprofessional communications and to ensure the proper differential diagnostic testing of a patient asked to consult another physician. This improvement in management recommendations is readily apparent in the Pearls.

To support the expansion of the management discussion for each disorder, a new Chapter 2 was added on specific testing procedures to assist in differential diagnosis. This chapter lays the groundwork for some of the basic diagnostic testing procedures, visual field testing, diagnostic B-scan ultrasonography, and physical diagnostic testing as it relates to primary eye care, as well as some of the basics of clinical laboratory testing.

Another major change in the text is the addition of Chapter 1 on clinical decision making in primary eye care. This has been added to enforce the fact that much of health care involves the cognitive process (or art) of differential diagnosis. The remainder of the text involves facts, whereas this chapter addresses how to apply these facts in the diagnosis and subsequent management of the patient. This chapter is intended to encourage the intern, resident, and practitioner to think about differential diagnosis in a slightly different manner. It is also intended to familiarize the health care provider with the basic concept of justification of the performance of diagnostic testing that will soon permeate the health care industry. This justification of actions will be forced by managed care, either nationalized or privatized.

Chapter 3 on congenital and acquired anomalies of the optic nerve head has been totally rewritten to update much of the information as well as to add glaucomatous optic neuropathy, thyroid eye disease, and orbital inflammatory pseudotumor and to significantly improve the section on optic nerve head and optic nerve tumors. All Pearls were expanded and updated.

Chapter 4 on retinal vascular disorders has also been heavily revised with an update on all subjects and a significant embellishment of the management sections. The changes regarding recommendations for management can readily be seen by referring to the Pearls on branch or central retinal vein occlusion. Sections have been added on hypertensive retinopathy, the relationship of retinal vaso-occlusive disease to cerebrovascular disease, radiation retinopathy, and acute retinal necrosis syndrome. A significant change has been made in the section on diabetic retinal disease.

Chapter 5 on exudative and nonexudative macular disorders has been updated and sections on birdshot retinochoroidopathy and ocular manifestations of Lyme disease have been added. The greatest improvement in this chapter is associated with a much-improved section on age-related macular degeneration, including a discussion of the value of antioxidants in its management. The Pearls have also been expanded, updated, and improved.

Chapter 6 on anomalies of the vitreous peripheral retina has also been updated, especially in the areas of management including potential complications. In addition, a section has been added on the hereditary vitreoretinal dystrophies and degenerations. A glance at the Pearls on rhegmatogenous retinal detachment will give you a sense of how each and every Pearl has been improved.

Significant changes have been made in Chapter 7 on hereditary retinal–choroidal dystrophies. Each topic has been updated, photographs added, and Pearls improved. Sections on pigmented paravenous retinochoroidal atrophy, syphilitic chorioretinitis, rubella retinopathy, and retinal dystrophies associated with storage disease have been clarified.

The second edition has been written to improve the quality of the first edition and to expand the knowledge it presents. My goals have been the improvement in the understanding of the clinicopathology of ocular disease and the ocular manifestations of systemic disease, as well as the enhancement of the management of each of the disease processes. Through my attempts at simplifying and expanding the knowledge presented, I hope that each of you can improve patient care. Remember that Chapter 1 intends to stimulate the clinical thought process, Chapter 2 provides some of the basics of differential diagnostic testing, and Chapters 3 through 7 provide all of the information to plug into the diagnostic equation. Your job is to make the observation on the patient, understand what you are seeing from a clinicopathological standpoint, consider the differential diagnostic possibilities, apply sensitive and specific diagnostic testing, arrive at a reasonable diagnosis, and then develop an effective management plan. All the while, continue to hold the patient's hand and make them feel that you care.

Larry J. Alexander

Color Plates

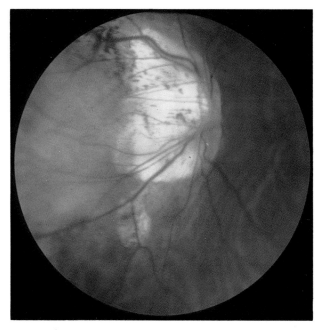

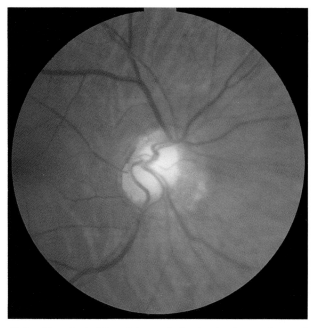

Color Plate 1. Posterior staphyloma involving the optic nerve head with severe reduction in visual acuity.

Color Plate 2. A tilting of the vertical axis of a disc and a small staphylomatous area adjacent to the disc.

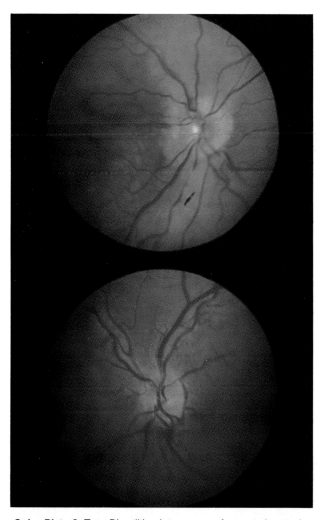

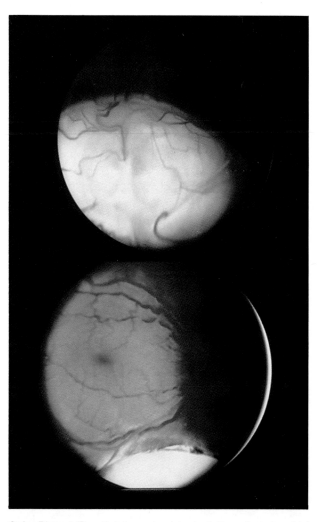

Color Plate 3. Top. Disc tilting into a zone of a posterior staphyloma. When compared to the "normal" fellow disc (**bottom**), it is easy to establish that the affected disc is larger, which implies a congenital variation.

Color Plate 4. Top. Coloboma involving both the retinal choroidal area and the optic nerve head (*arrow*). **Bottom.** The fellow eye has only a retinal choroidal coloboma, but both eyes are at great risk for the development of a retinal detachment.

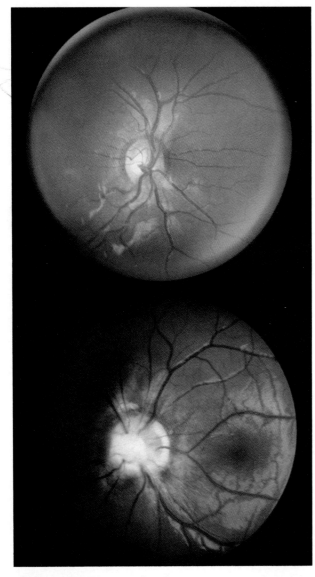

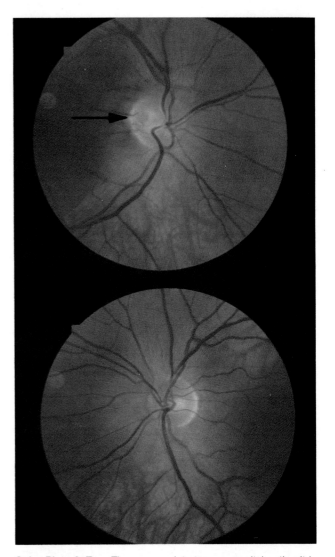

Color Plate 5. Top. "Normal" optical nerve head in an eye with 20/20 vision. Bottom. The fellow eye is amblyopic with a morning glory disc anomaly. Note the size difference between the two discs, implying a congenital variation.

Color Plate 6. Top. The arrow points to a congenital optic pit in the temporal aspect of the right eye. This eye is at risk for a nonrhegmatogenous macular detachment. When compared to the fellow disc (bottom), it becomes apparent that the affected disc is larger, implying a congenital variation.

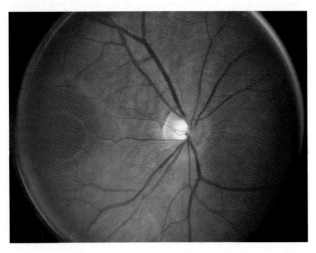

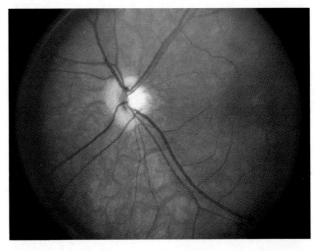

Color Plate 7. "Normal" optic nerve head in a 20/20 eye. Note reflections from the nerve fiber layer, especially around the macular area. Contrast this nerve head with the fellow nerve head shown in Color Plate 8.

Color Plate 8. This nerve head is smaller than the nerve head in Color Plate 7 and represents a congenital optic nerve hypoplasia with 20/200 vision. Note the absence of the nerve fiber layer reflection and that there is a surround of atrophy corresponding to the "expected" size of the nerve head.

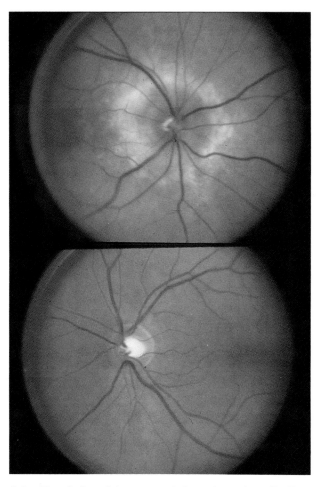

Color Plate 9. One of the many variations of megalopapilla. **Top.** The nerve head is large but flat, with 20/20 acuity. The fellow nerve head (**bottom**) is "normal" with 20/10 vision. Note the nerve head size difference, implying a congenital variation.

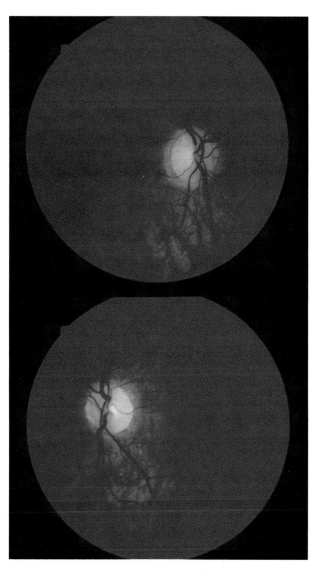

Color Plate 10. Temporal sector optic atrophy is apparent in this pair of photographs. The patient had vision reduced to 20/70 OU and a color vision defect. The discs can appear the same in cases of toxic optic neuropathy (Color Plate 21).

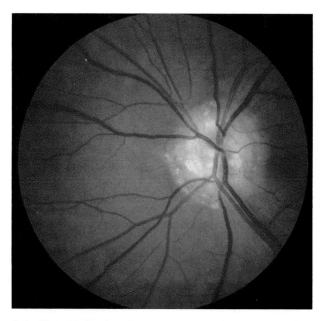

Color Plate 11. Glowing globules representing buried drusen of the optic nerve head have a tendency to become more visible with age. Visual field defects are usually present by this stage.

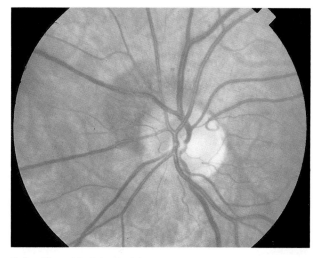

Color Plate 12. Subretinal hemorrhage at the superior nasal aspect of the optic nerve head associated with buried drusen of the nerve head confirmed by B-scan ultrasonography. The hemorrhage cleared on its own in four weeks.

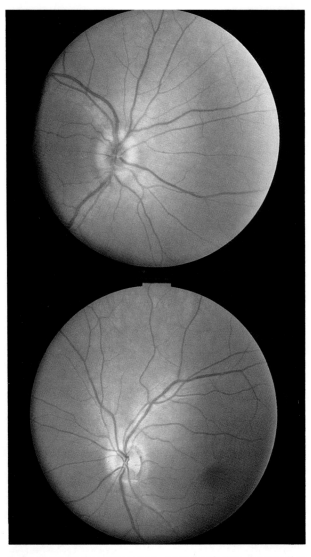

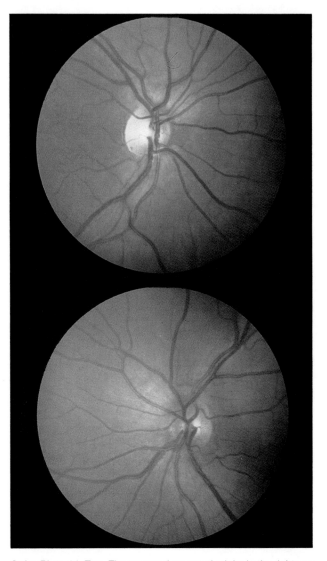

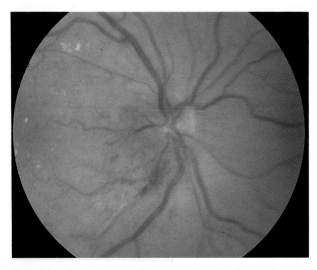

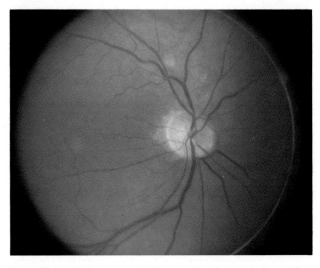

Color Plate 13. Top. Edematous nerve head when compared to the fellow nerve head (**bottom**). Vision was reduced in the right eye of this young person, implicating inflammatory optic neuropathy, which is often referred to as papillitis.

Color Plate 14. Top. The temporal neuroretinal rim in the right eye is atrophic when compared to the left eye (**bottom**). This occurred in a patient with other signs of demyelinizing disease and was suspected to be secondary to demyelinizing optic neuropathy in the right eye.

Color Plate 15. Ischemic optic neuropathy with disc swelling and flame-shaped hemorrhages. This patient has diabetes and presented with decreased visual acuity.

Color Plate 16. Non-excavated temporal optic atrophy in a patient with diabetes and an altitudinal visual field defect. This is characteristic of ischemic optic neuropathy that has run its course.

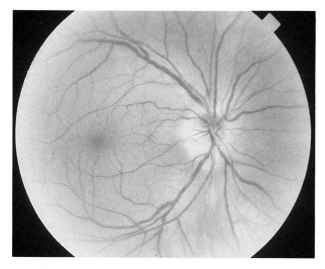

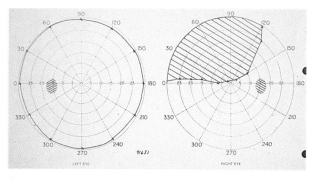

Color Plate 18. Visual field defect corresponding to the ischemic optic neuropathy in Color Plate 17. The defect is characteristic, with the scotoma respecting the horizontal raphe.

Color Plate 17. Active ischemic optic neuropathy characterized by optic disc swelling. Color Plate 18 demonstrates the associated visual field defect.

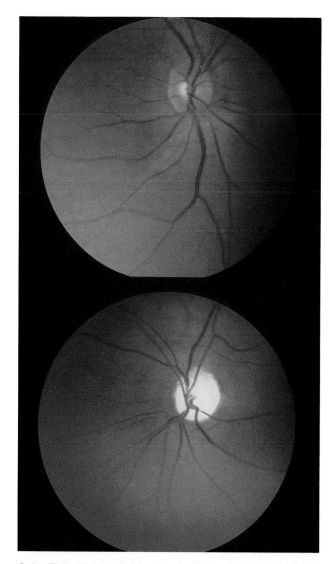

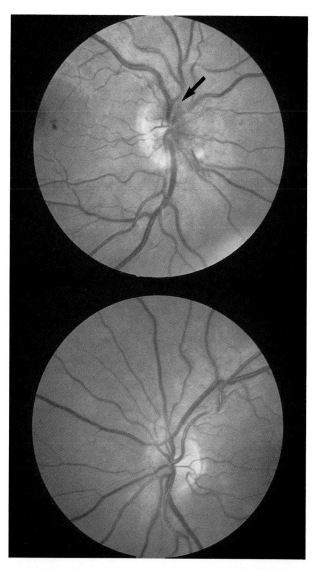

Color Plate 19. Top. Total optic atrophy of the right nerve head secondary to temporal arteritic ischemic optic neuropathy. **Bottom.** The fellow disc is normal in this photography, but soon after became involved in spite of aggressive steroid therapy.

Color Plate 20. Top. "Normal" optic nerve head in a 19-year-old diabetic patient. The fellow optic nerve head (**bottom**) is edematous (*arrow*) secondary to diabetic papillopathy.

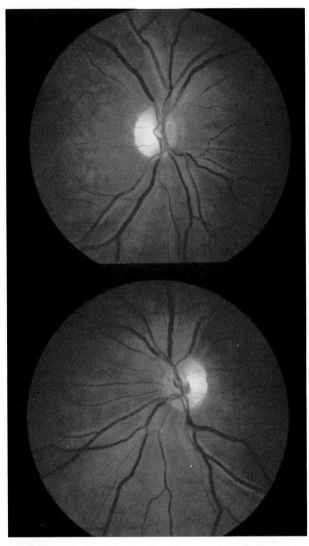

Color Plate 21. Example of toxic optic neuropathy. Temporal optic atrophy with significantly reduced visual acuity secondary to alcohol abuse.

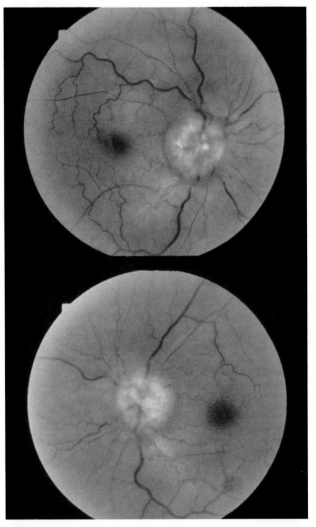

Color Plate 22. Chronic compensated papilledema secondary to benign intracranial hypertension. Note the gross swelling, venous dilation and tortuosity, and the conspicuous absence of flame-shaped hemorrhages and cotton-wool spots.

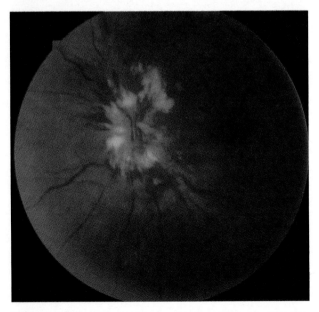

Color Plate 23. Acute noncompensated papilledema characterized by gross swelling, flame-shaped hemorrhages, and cotton-wool spots. This patient was treated surgically the next day.

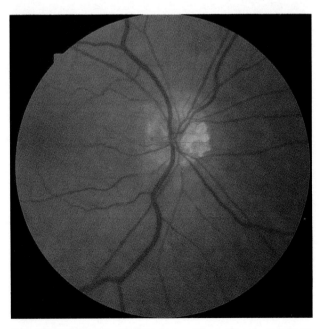

Color Plate 24. Astrocytic hamartoma of the optic nerve head with a mulberry-like lesion resembling buried drusen.

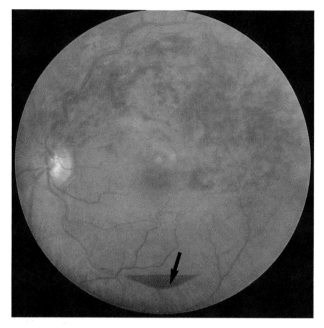

Color Plate 25. Example of a preretinal hemorrhage (*arrow*) associated with a hemicentral retinal vein occlusion.

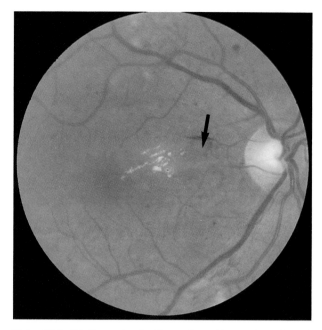

Color Plate 26. Example of a flame-shaped hemorrhage (*arrow*) near a zone of hard exudates encroaching into the macular area in a diabetic patient. The flame hemorrhage is an indication of hypoxia in this patient.

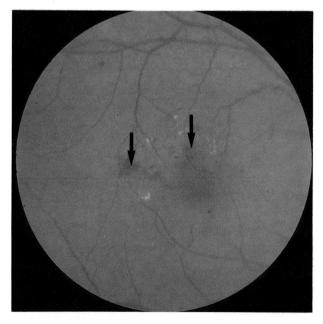

Color Plate 27. Arrows point to dot/blot hemorrhages within an area of intraretinal edema in a diabetic patient. Another sign of the intraretinal edema is the presence of hard exudates.

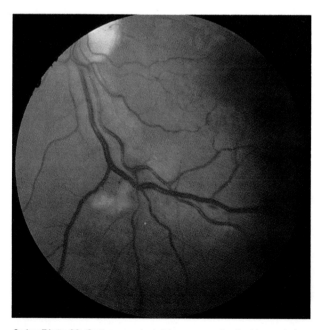

Color Plate 28. Cotton-wool spot in an area of retinal hypoxia in a diabetic patient. This is a sign of oxygen starvation, the immediate precursor to the development of proliferative diabetic retinopathy.

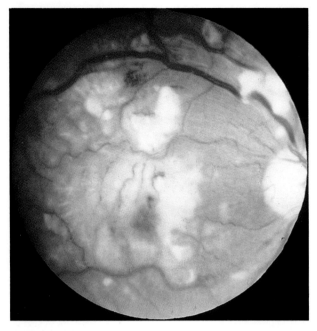

Color Plate 29. Example of cotton-wool spot formation in sytemic lupus erythematosus. The significant formation in this case was associated with end-stage disease.

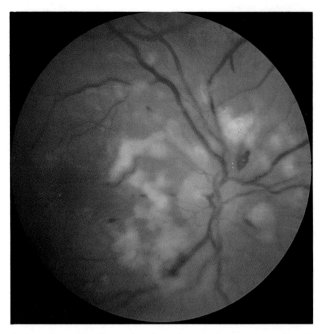

Color Plate 30. Example of cotton-wool spot formation in Purtcher's retinopathy associated with truncal trauma. These spots clear on their own with no compromise to acuity. *(Courtesy of C. Amos)*

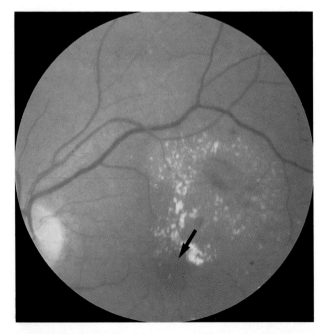

Color Plate 31. Hard exudates surround an area of intraretinal edema and encroach into the macular area *(arrow)*, representing a direct threat to vision.

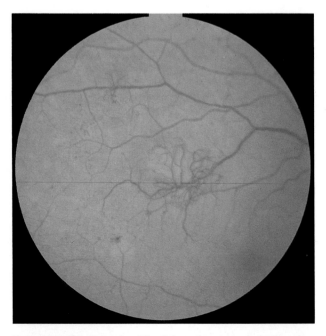

Color Plate 32. Example of 2 patches of neovascularization elsewhere in a diabetic patient. These patches leaked profusely with fluorescein angiography.

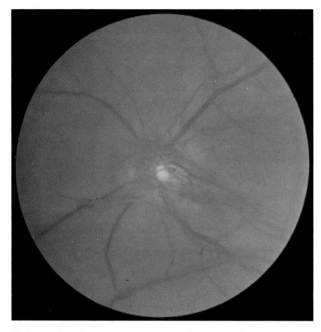

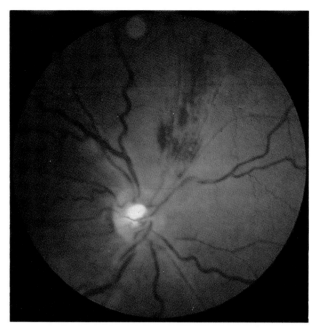

Color Plate 33. Example of significant neovascularization of the optic nerve head in a diabetic patient. Leakage is evidenced by the haze over the disc and was confirmed with fluorescein angiography.

Color Plate 34. Example of acquired venous tortuosity indicating retinal hypoxia. There is also an area of dot/blot hemorrhages, representing a small superior nasal branch retinal vein occlusion.

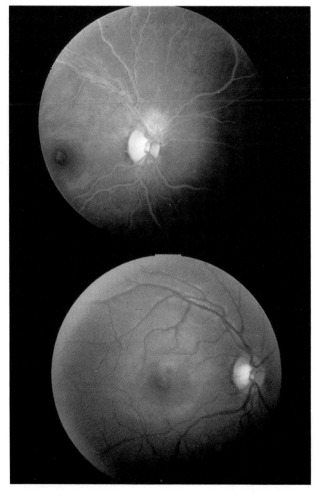

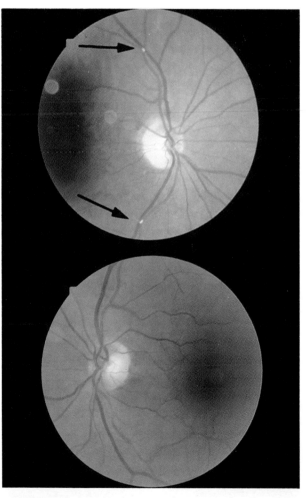

Color Plate 35. Top. Lipemic arteries and veins are indistinguishable in this case of severely elevated serum triglyceride levels. **Bottom.** The same patient with controlled triglyceride levels.

Color Plate 36. Top. Arterial emboli (*arrows*) secondary to severe cardiovascular and internal carotid disease. When compared to the bottom photograph, the top optic nerve head demonstrates relative atrophy secondary to ischemic optic neuropathy.

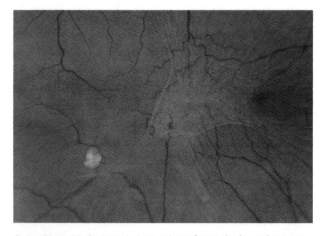

Color Plate 37. Gathered pleat variety of preretinal membrane surrounding the macula. Note the acquired vascular tortuosity and vitreous condensation.

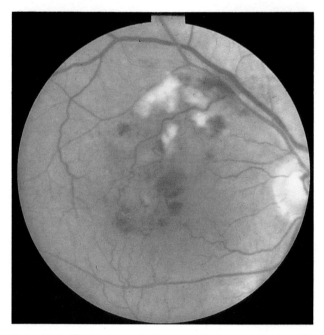

Color Plate 38. Example of a branch retinal vein occlusion with dot/blot hemorrhages and cotton-wool spots impacting on macular function.

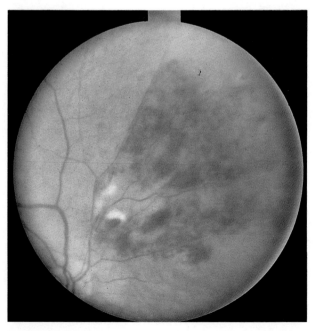

Color Plate 39. Example of a branch retinal vein occlusion in the nasal retina that is no threat to macular function, but is a threat to the development of disc, retinal, and iris neovascularization.

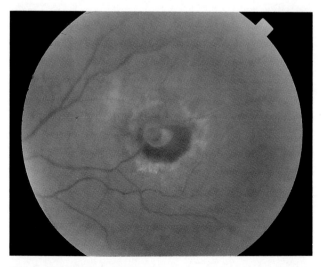

Color Plate 40. Example of a retinal macroaneurysm secondary to long-standing systemic hypertension. The aneurysm was pulsating and had already hemorrhaged into the retina. Note the ingress and egress vessels.

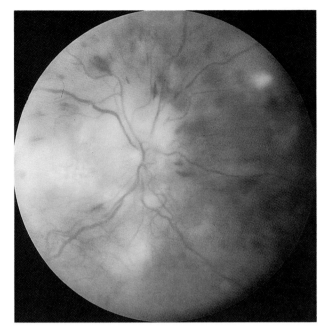

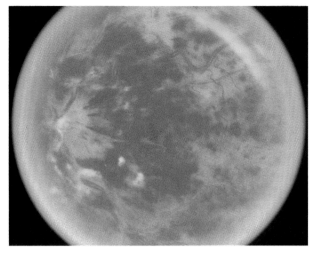

Color Plate 42. Example of severe hemorrhagic intrusion into the macular area in central retinal vein occlusion.

Color Plate 41. Example of disc swelling and hemorrhage in central retinal vein occlusion.

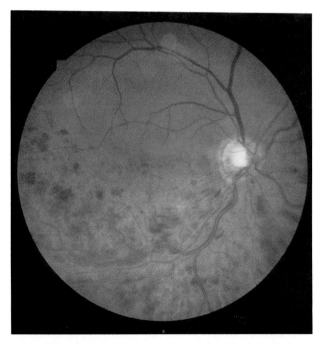

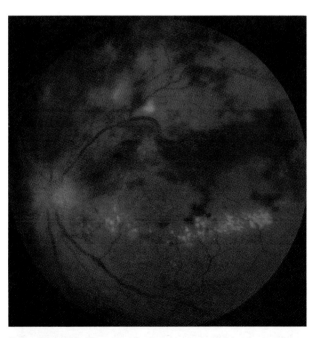

Color Plate 43. Example of a hemicentral retinal vein occlusion in the inferior retina. Note the photocoagulation scars applied in an attempt to minimize retinal hypoxia.

Color Plate 44. Example of a hemicentral retinal vein occlusion. Note the significant intrusion into the macula by edema and hard exudates, and the development of disc neovascularization secondary to significant hypoxia.

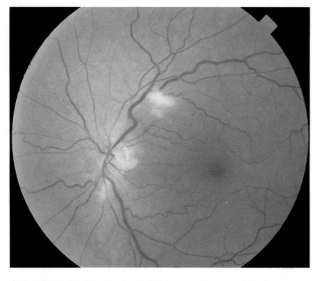

Color Plate 45. Zones of retinal infarct (white areas) that occurred as a result of arteriography for assessment of the internal carotid system. There are both cotton-wool spots and branch retinal artery occlusions.

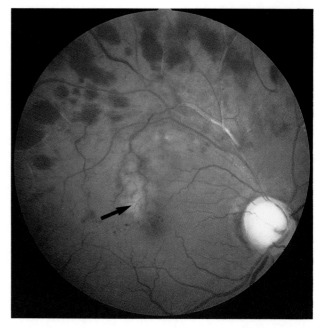

Color Plate 46. Zone of opaque retina (*arrow*) created by a branch retinal artery occlusion within a branch retinal vein occlusion. Vision was significantly reduced. Note the coincidental glaucomatous optic atrophy.

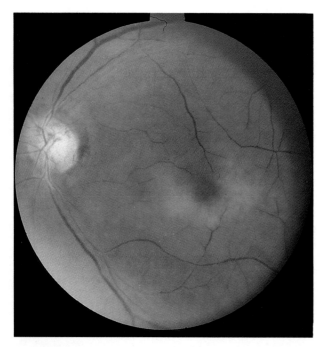

Color Plate 47. Central retinal artery occlusion. Vision is reduced; there is a "cherry red spot" in the macula and segmentation of venous flow.

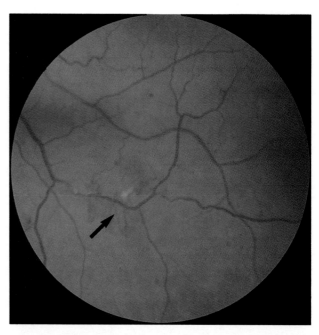

Color Plate 48. Intraretinal microvascular abnormalities (IRMA) (*arrow*) near an area of cotton-wool spot formation in a diabetic patient. Both signs indicate retinal hypoxia and require a retinal consult.

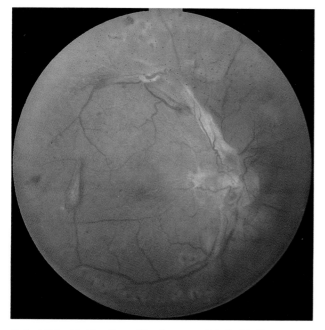

Color Plate 49. Fibrotic proliferation associated with disc neovascularization in severe proliferative diabetic retinopathy.

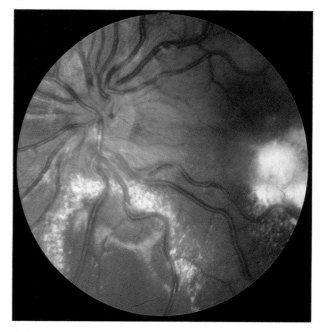

Color Plate 50. Example of severe hard exudative response in a retinal capillary hemangioma.

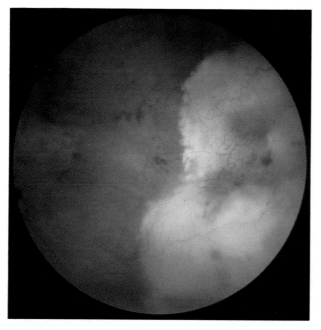

Color Plate 51. Example of a temporal periphery severe hard exudative response in a case of a retinal capillary hemangioma (angiomatosis retinae).

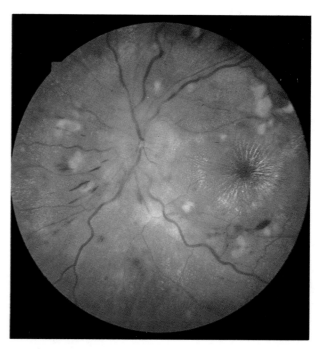

Color Plate 52. Severe disc edema, hemorrhaging, and stellate exudate formation in a case of malignant hypertension.

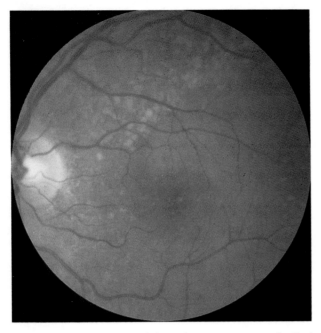

Color Plate 53. Examples of the various appearances of retinal drusen.

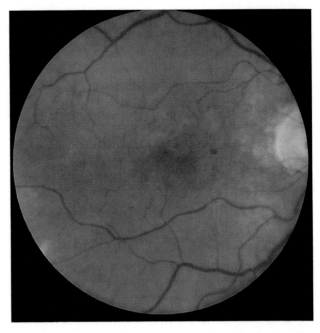

Color Plate 54. Variation of dry age-related macular degeneration (ARM) demonstrating disorganization and migration of the retinal pigment epithelium.

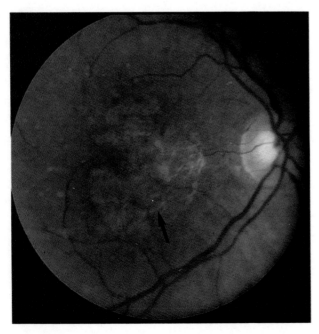

Color Plate 55. Variation of dry ARM demonstrating a more geographic alteration (*arrow*) of the retinal pigment epithelium.

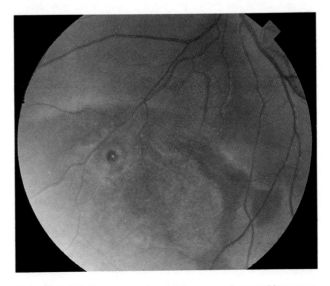

Color Plate 56. Gray-green choroidal neovascular net with an overlying subretinal hemorrhage in a patient with coincidental dark without pressure.

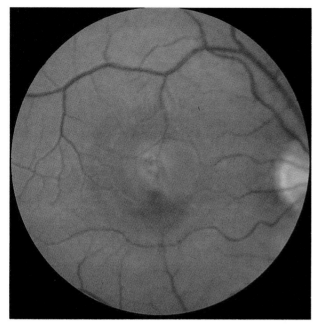

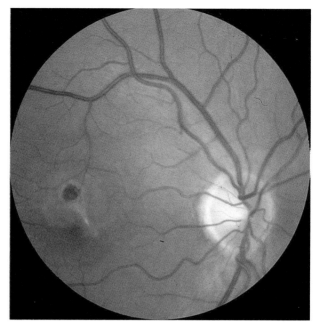

Color Plate 57. Gray-green choroidal neovascular net with a surrounding sensory non-rhegmatogenous retinal detachment. Note the inferior notch in the sensory detachment, corresponding to the tightly bound foveal area resisting intrusion of fluid.

Color Plate 58. Same eye as shown in Color Plate 57, one year later with retinal pigment epithelium (RPE) hyperplasia and spontaneous resolution without treatment. Vision also improved with resolution of some of the sensory detachment.

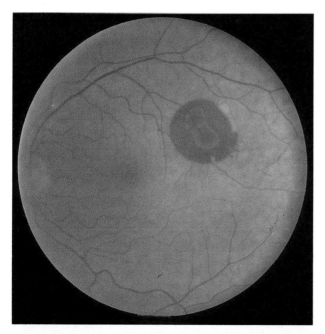

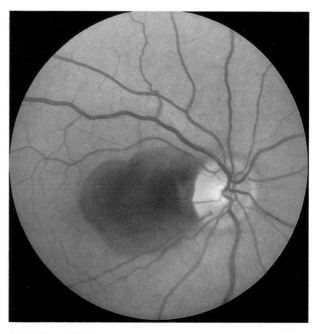

Color Plate 59. Gray-green hemorrhage under the RPE with an overlying subretinal hemorrhage. Remember that the sensory retina to RPE attachment is much looser than the attachment of the RPE to Bruchs' membrane, allowing for the larger subretinal hemorrhage.

Color Plate 60. A large subretinal hemorrhage associated with a choroidal neovascular net near the edge of the optic nerve head.

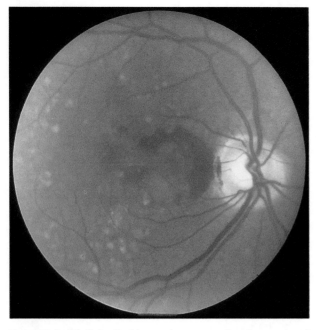

Color Plate 61. Subretinal hemorrhage secondary to a ruptured choroidal neovascular net near the edge of the disc. The outcome is shown in Color Plate 62.

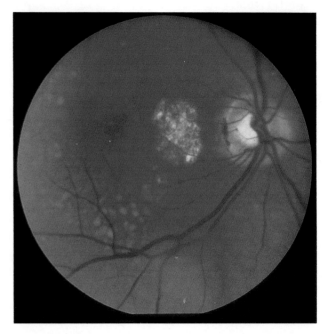

Color Plate 62. Postphotocoagulative scarring of the lesion shown in Color Plate 61. Note the "soft drusen" in the posterior pole.

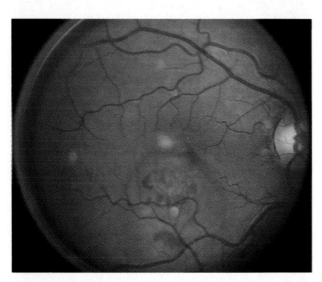

Color Plate 63. The subtleties of choroidal neovascularization: sensory non-rhegmatogenous retinal detachment with an underlying gray-green neovascular net.

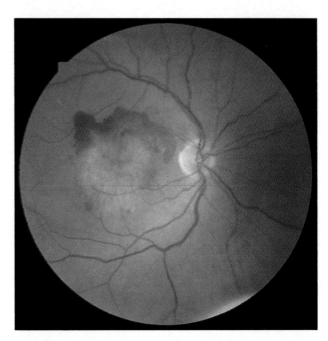

Color Plate 64. Example of wet ARM with an RPE detachment, a gray-green neovascular net, and retinal hemorrhaging surrounding the lesion.

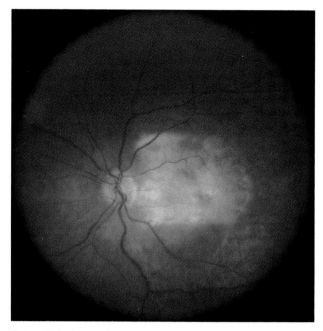

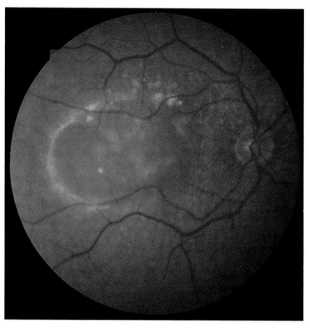

Color Plate 65. Example of wet ARM with a very significant RPE detachment in the posterior pole.

Color Plate 66. Example of a variation of wet ARM with an RPE detachment and a surround of hard exudates (Coats' response).

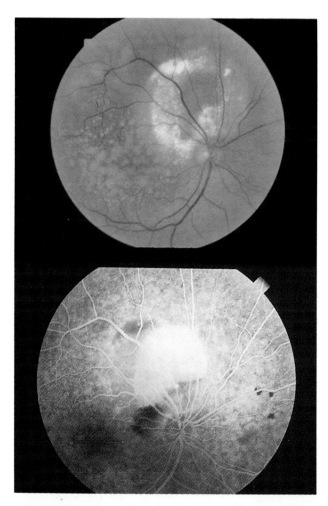

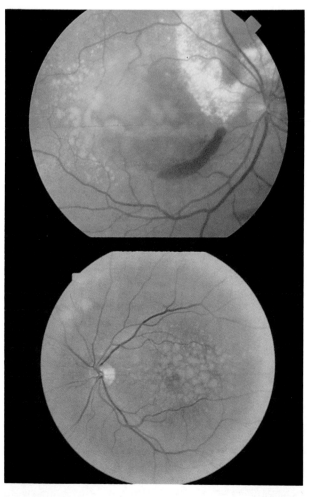

Color Plate 67. Top. The macula is characterized by soft drusen. Above the disc is a zone of hard exudates (Coats' response) surrounding a gray-green zone. The zone proved to leak on fluorescein angiography (**bottom**), but was confined, indicating an RPE detachment.

Color Plate 68. The neovascular disease shown in Color Plate 67 progressed to severe hemorrhagic disease (**top**). The fellow eye (**bottom**) has numerous soft drusen thought to be RPE disease or a detachment that is very conducive to the development of choroidal neovascular disease.

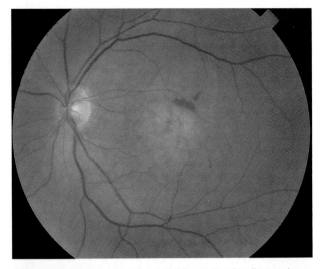

Color Plate 69. Example of choroidal neovascular disease (gray-green) in the macular area characteristic of wet ARM.

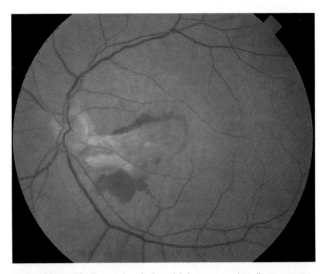

Color Plate 70. Example of choroidal neovascular disease emanating from the edge of the optic nerve head. Note hemorrhage, exudates, and the gray-green appearance.

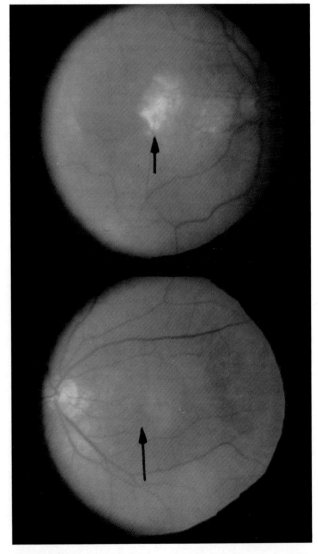

Color Plate 71. Wet ARM. The arrow in the top photograph points to a disciform scar, while the arrow in the bottom photograph points to an obscure evolving choroidal neovascular net. If there is a disciform scar in one eye and reduced vision or metamorphopsia in the fellow eye, it is imperative to assume that a net is evolving until proven otherwise.

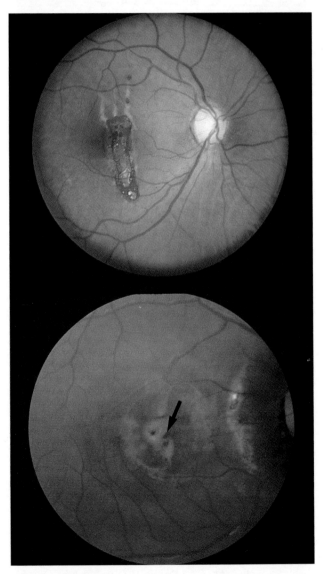

Color Plate 72. Top. Choroidal rupture following the contour of the optic nerve head with considerable reactive RPE hyperplasia. **Bottom.** An eye with multiple choroidal ruptures and a developing choroidal neovascular net (*arrow*) confirmed by fluorescein angiography. The lesion was untreatable.

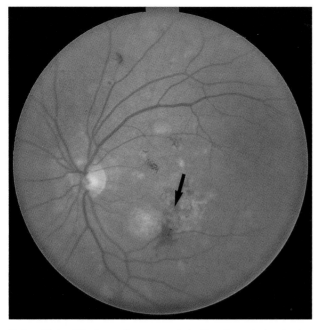

Color Plate 73. Area of neovascularization (*arrow*) developing within a photocoagulative scar. The patient has diabetes and other eye signs of retinal vascular disease.

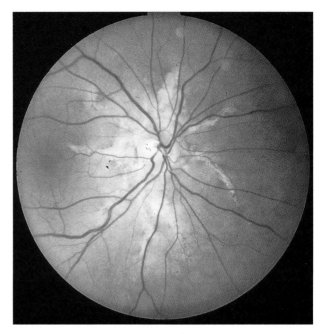

Color Plate 74. Classic presentation of angioid streaks radiating from a circumpapillary hub.

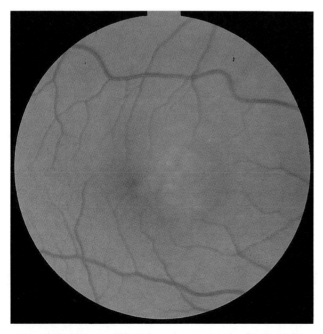

Color Plate 75. Area of RPE disorganization in a patient with idiopathic central serous chorioretinopathy (ICSC). This discolored zone was elevated creating metamorphopsia. Color Plate 76 shows the fluorescein angiography of this lesion.

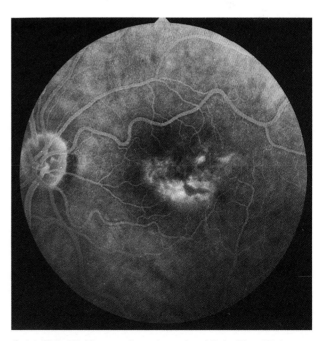

Color Plate 76. Fluorescein angiography of Color Plate 75 demonstrating several areas of focal leakage associated with ICSC. This stage represents the "sick retinal pigment epithelium syndrome."

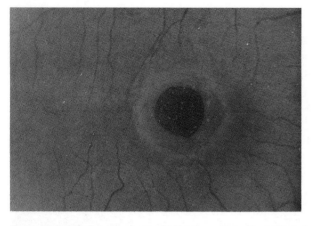

Color Plate 77. Stage 3 macular hole with a surround of retinal elevation and the presence of pathological drusen at the base.

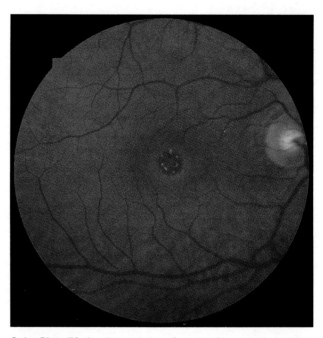

Color Plate 78. Another variation of a stage 3 macular hole with a surround of retinal elevation and very dramatic pathological drusen at the base.

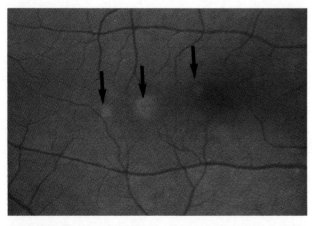

Color Plate 79. Choroidal infiltrates (*arrows*) in a case of presumed ocular histoplasmosis. These areas are very conducive to the development of choroidal neovascular nets.

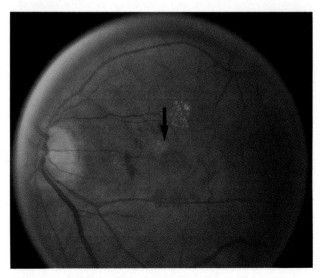

Color Plate 80. Choroidal neovascularization (*arrow*) in the macular area in presumed ocular histoplasmosis. Hemorrhages and exudates surround the area of leakage.

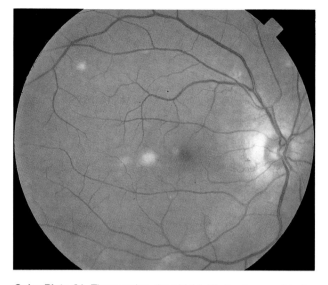

Color Plate 81. Three active choroidal infiltrates temporal to the macula in a case of presumed ocular histoplasmosis. Note also the circumpapillary scarring and peripheral histoplasmosis spots.

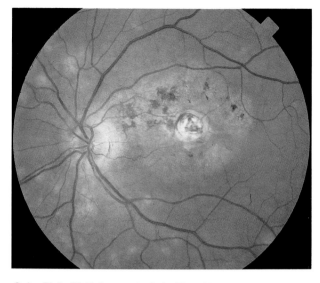

Color Plate 82. Fellow eye to Color Plate 81 demonstrating significant macular scarring, circumpapillary scarring, and peripheral histoplasmosis spots.

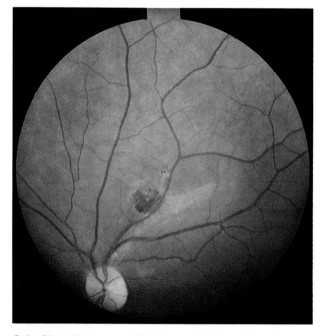

Color Plate 83. An area of RPE hyperplasia above the optic nerve head associated with an inactive toxoplasmosis scar.

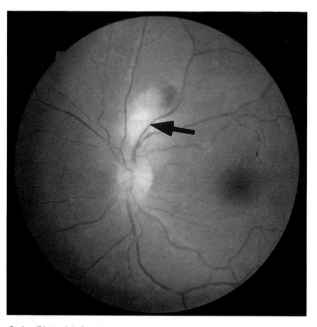

Color Plate 84. Same patient shown in Color Plate 83, 5 years later, with indications of reactivation of the toxoplasmosis scar (*arrow*). The reactivation occurred during pregnancy.

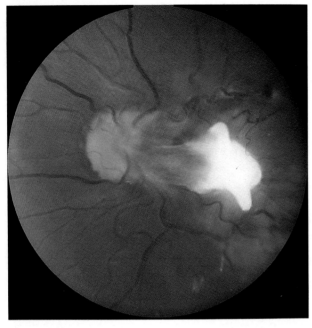

Color Plate 85. Dense white elevated toxocara granuloma creating significant reduction in visual acuity. *(Courtesy of R. Coshatt.)*

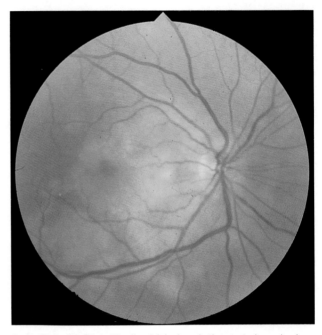

Color Plate 86. Placoid yellowish lesions in the posterior pole characteristic of acute posterior multifocal placoid pigment epitheliopathy (APMPPE). *(Courtesy of P. Ajamian.)*

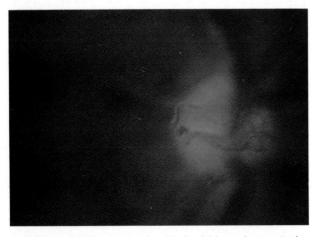

Color Plate 87. The annular ring (the hyaloid membrane attachment to the optic nerve head) associated with a posterior vitreous detachment.

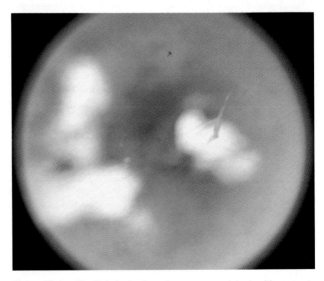

Color Plate 88. Debris in the vitreous associated with a postinflammatory chorioretinal scar.

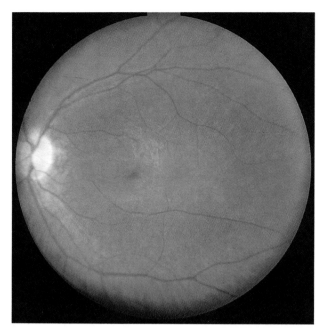

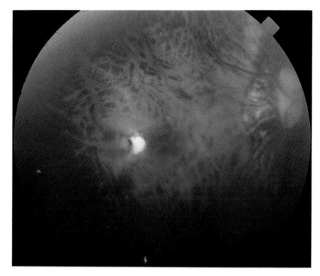

Color Plate 90. Eye with Wagner's hereditary vitreoretinal degeneration.

Color Plate 89. Congenital hereditary retinoschisis showing minimal rippling in the macular area. The rippling effect is secondary to the schisis of the retinal layers.

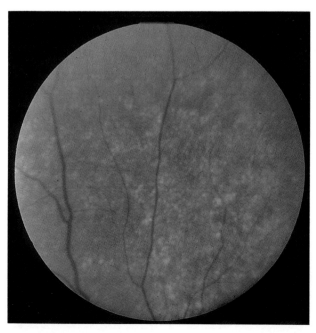

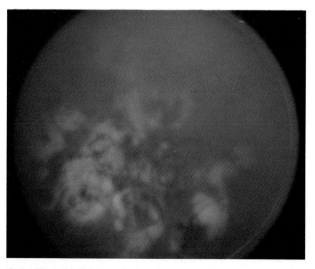

Color Plate 91. Peripheral RPE disorganization associated with aging. The pigment often migrates and takes on a bone-spicule appearance similar to the "look" of retinitis pigmentosa.

Color Plate 92. Primary chorioretinal atrophy (pavingstone or cobblestone) in the inferior equatorial zone of the retina associated with aging.

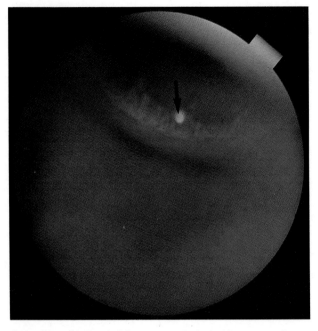

Color Plate 93. Pearl of the ora serratta (*arrow*) in an area of grayish-appearing peripheral cystoid degeneration. *(Courtesy of W. Townsend.)*

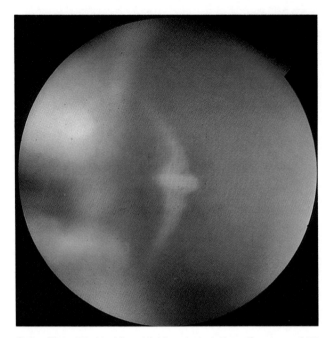

Color Plate 94. Meridional fold on indentation. *(Courtesy of W. Townsend.)*

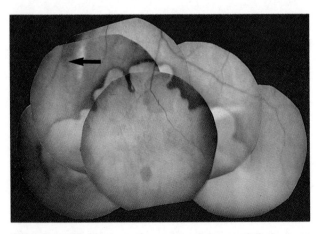

Color Plate 95. Montage of an extremely large, relatively young congenital hypertrophy of the retinal pigment epithelium. For orientation, the arrow points to a short posterior ciliary nerve.

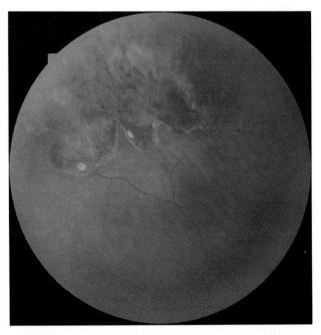

Color Plate 96. Variation of a congenital hypertrophy of the RPE with internal areas of choroidal atrophy indicating aging of the lesion.

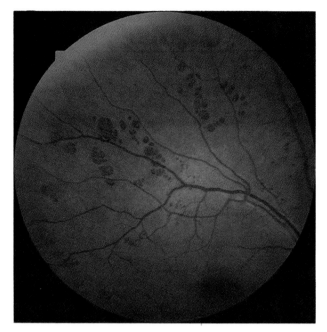

Color Plate 97. Bear tracks of the retina representing a histopathological variation of congenital hypertrophy of the RPE.

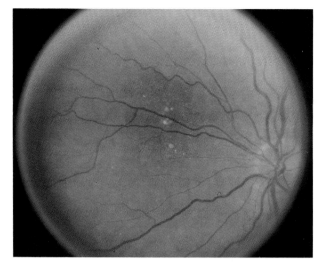

Color Plate 98. Benign choroidal melanoma (nevus) with overlying drusen.

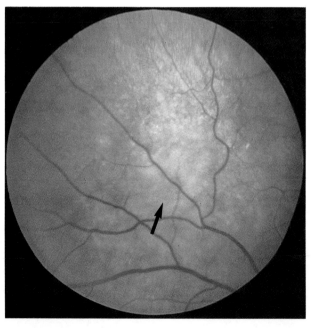

Color Plate 99. A very suspicious lesion with elevation, drusen, and orange lipofuscin pigmentation (*arrow*). This lesion should be considered malignant until proven otherwise.

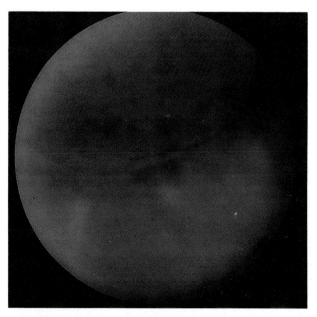

Color Plate 100. Non-rhegmatogenous retinal detachment secondary to an underlying malignant choroidal melanoma.

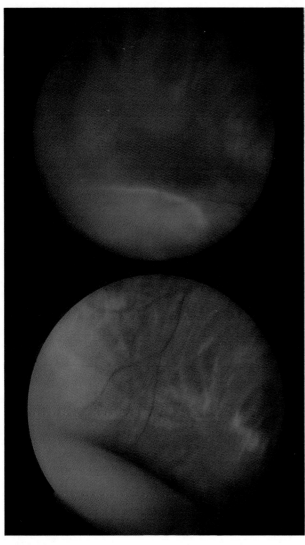

Color Plate 101. Top. Retinal white without pressure not indented. **Bottom.** Indentation of the lesion shown in the top picture. *(Courtesy of W. Townsend.)*

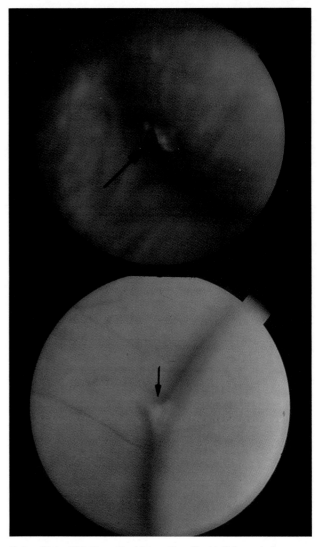

Color Plate 102. Top. Double cystic retinal tuft *(arrow)* shown on indentation. **Bottom.** Zonular traction tuft *(arrow)* shown on indentation. *(Courtesy of W. Townsend.)*

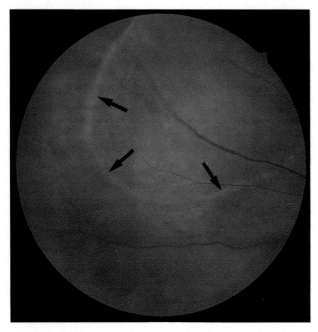

Color Plate 103. Arrows delineate the borders of a retinoschisis.

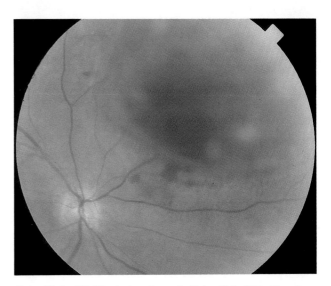

Color Plate 104. The lesion shown in Color Plate 103 with subsequent retinal detachment and bleeding into the cavity.

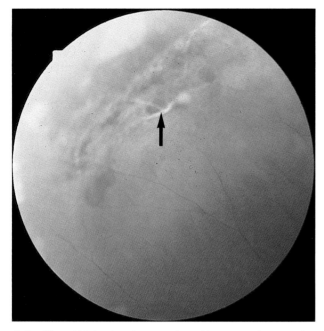

Color Plate 105. Lattice degeneration with tears at the posterior border (*arrow*).

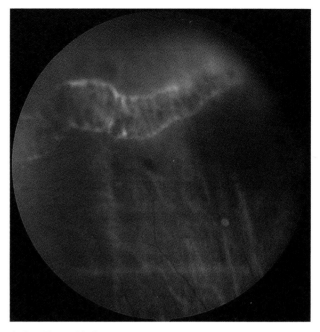

Color Plate 106. Snail track degeneration, a variant of lattice degeneration. *(Courtesy of M. Taroyan.)*

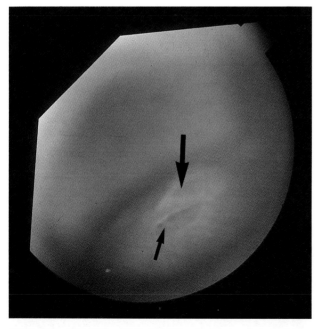

Color Plate 107. Three small, atrophic retinal holes on indentation (*small arrow*) with an overlying retinal cyst (*larger arrow*). *(Courtesy of W. Townsend.)*

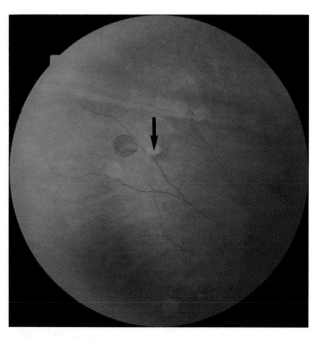

Color Plate 108. Operculated retinal tear in the temporal periphery. The arrow points to the operculum (the overlying plug of tissue).

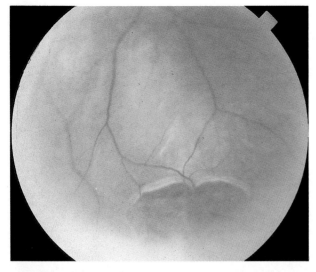

Color Plate 109. Retinal tear representing an area that once surrounded lattice degeneration. The tear occurred in association with a posterior vitreous detachment.

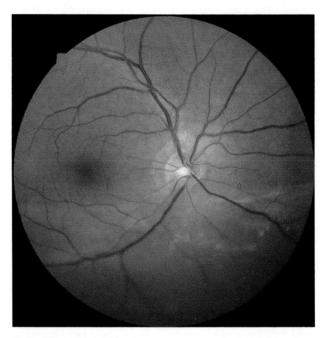

Color Plate 110. Inferior rhegmatogenous retinal detachment approaching the macular zone. Note the loss of choroidal detail in the inferior retina.

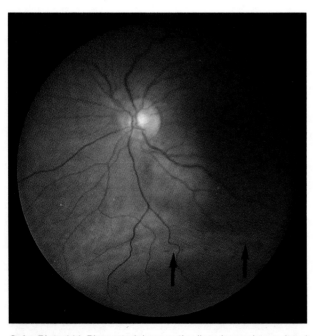

Color Plate 111. Pigmented demarcation lines (*arrows*) associated with a progressive yet long-standing rhegmatogenous retinal detachment.

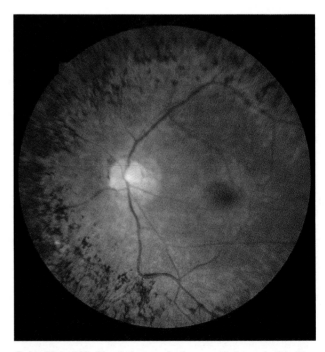

Color Plate 112. Classic bone spicule presentation, arterial attenuation, and optic atrophy present in retinitis pigmentosa.

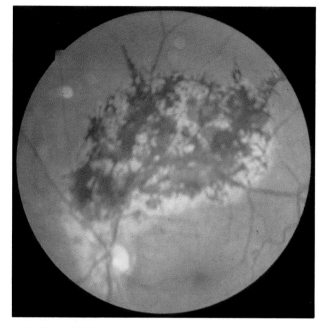

Color Plate 113. Sectoral pseudoretinitis pigmentosa, which is often secondary to trauma.

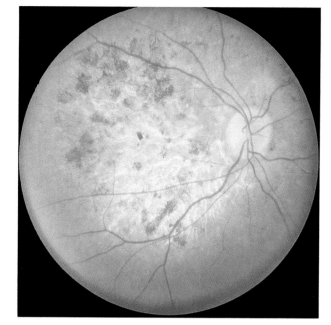

Color Plate 114. Central or inverse retinitis pigmentosa with severe reduction in visual acuity.

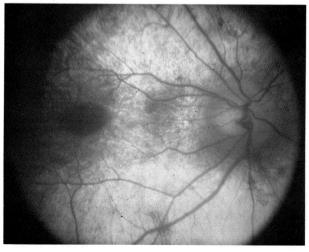

Color Plate 115. An advanced case of choroideremia.

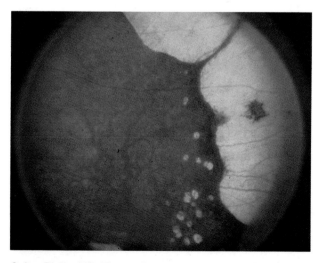

Color Plate 116. The scalloped borders and severe retinal/choroidal destruction associated with gyrate dystrophy. *(Courtesy of R. Nowakowski.)*

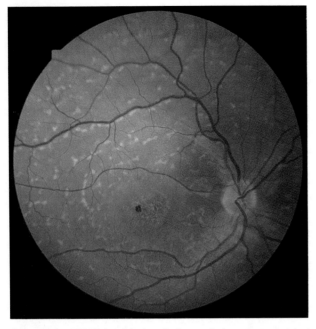

Color Plate 117. Fish-tail lesions in the posterior pole associated with fundus flavimaculatus. Also note early macular changes that place this in a pattern of Stargardt's dystrophy.

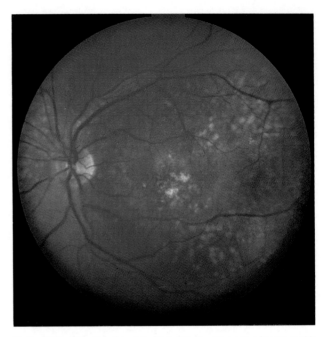

Color Plate 118. Dominant drusen affecting the macular area with resultant early reduction in visual acuity.

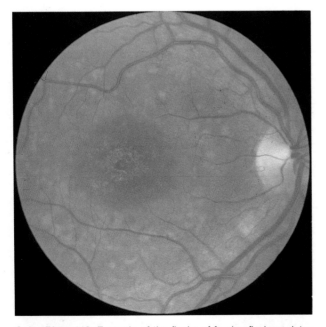

Color Plate 119. Example of the flecks of fundus flavimaculatus with grayish yellow pigmentary alteration surrounding a normal appearing fovea.

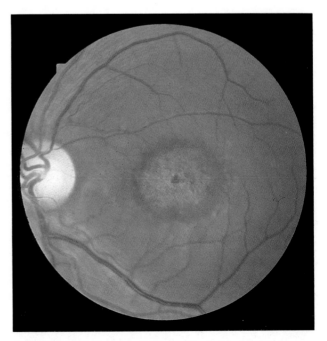

Color Plate 120. Example of Stargardt's dystrophy with pigmentary alteration in the macular area.

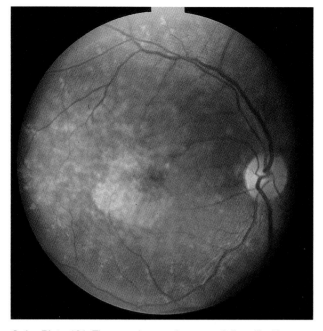

Color Plate 121. The macular area becomes "slimed" with a surround of fish-tail lesions in Stargardt's disease.

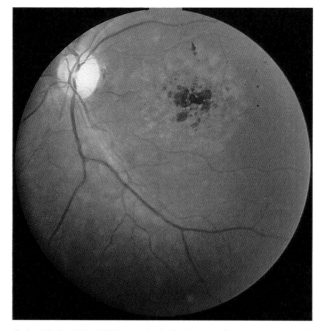

Color Plate 122. RPE hyperplasia in the macular area associated with Stargardt's disease.

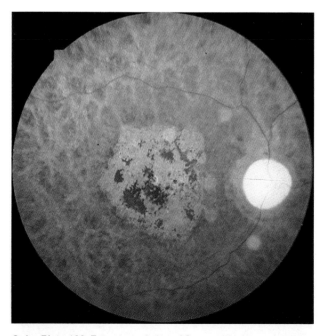

Color Plate 123. Extreme variation of Stargardt's dystrophy with a moth-eaten appearance to the retina, macular disease, and significant optic atrophy. Variations of hereditary disorders complicate diagnosis.

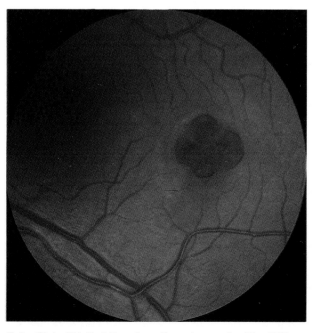

Color Plate 124. Variation of a patterned anomaly of the RPE.

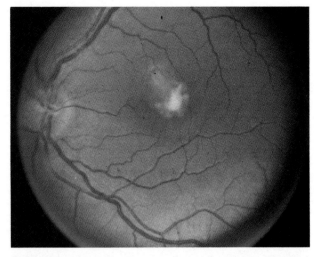

Color Plate 125. Egg yolk pattern in the macula with mild vision reduction in a case of vitelliform dystrophy.

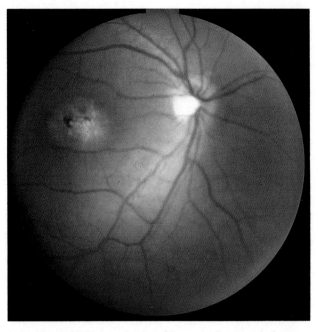

Color Plate 126. Disorganization of the egg yolk pattern in the macula in a case of vitelliform dystrophy. In this case, there was associated severe visual acuity reduction.

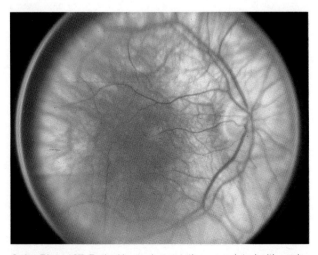

Color Plate 127. Retinal hypopigmentation associated with oculocutaneous albinism and ocular albinism. There was also foveal hypoplasia and nystagmus.

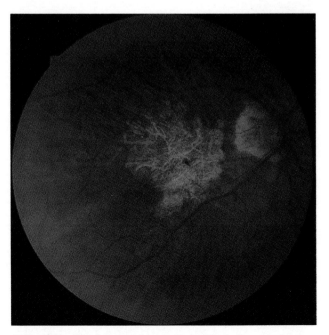

Color Plate 128. An area of excavated retina in the macular area secondary to central areolar choroidal dystrophy.

Chapter One ■ ■ ■ ■ ■ ■

C linical Decision Making in Primary Eyecare

The primary eyecare practitioner must have a bank of facts (a knowledge base) to effectively carry out the diagnostic and management process. The present book is intended to provide the source for that data base of facts for the more commonly encountered conditions of the optic nerve, retina, and choroid. This text is an accumulation of facts concerning different diagnostic tests applicable to disorders of the posterior segment of the eye, in addition to facts about various disorders of the posterior segment of the eye. This is the bank of knowledge from which the primary care practitioner must draw the basics for differential diagnosis. Each presentation of the disorder is organized into the epidemiology of the condition; the clinical, ethnic, age, and gender characteristics of the patients; a clinical description of the condition; recommendations for differential diagnostic procedures and tests; and recommended management of the disorder. Specific emphasis is placed on the relationship of the ocular condition to associated systemic diseases and disorders.

Armed with the knowledge base, the practitioner must then face the problems of the patient in the everyday primary care practice. The data base is, however, only the foundation on which to build the diagnosis. The cognitive process of differential diagnosis uses this base of facts but also relies on the "art" of understanding patient complaints and applying differential diagnostic tests to assist in the diagnosis. Once the diagnosis is accomplished, and only then, can effective management procedures be applied. In fact, the management process is often so straightforward that it is simply a matter of looking up the current standard protocol and modifying the approach according to the patient's response. Management is the technical process of health care, and is usually carried out well by the majority of practitioners. Differential diagnosis is the cognitive process of health care, which is difficult to teach and difficult to learn.

EVOLUTION OF CLINICAL HYPOTHESES: THE CLINICAL ALGORITHM

A clinical hypothesis must evolve from the bank of facts, but the differential diagnosis of conditions must evolve in a cognitive process that is difficult to teach. Without proper differential diagnosis, proper management is impossible. The following recent clinical example can offer a set of limited guidelines for the thought process of differential diagnosis.

■ ■ ■ ■ ■ ■

Clinical Example: Difficulties in Making a Differential Diagnosis

A 45-year-old white female enters the office complaining of a sudden onset (this morning) of loss of vision in the lower left area of her left eye. She is corrected to 20/20 OU, is currently taking no medication, has no allergies, has a positive family history of glaucoma, and has intraocular pressures of 12 mm Hg OU at 1:30 PM. Her pupils are reactive and her extraocular muscles are functional. There are no other systemic signs or symptoms noted. What must be done to differentially diagnose and manage this patient? Why would some practitioners choose one direction to proceed while others choose another direction? What is the basis for the cognitive process of medical decision making?

In this example there are several directions that one could pursue. What are the possibilities that can produce a left inferior temporal visual field defect perceived in the left eye? Some of the possibilities include the following:

- Branch retinal artery occlusion OS
- Branch retinal vein occlusion OS
- Ischemic optic neuropathy OS
- Demyelinizing optic neuropathy OS
- Retinal detachment OS
- Reactivated chorioretinitis OS

As a practitioner, I would immediately eliminate all of the above even before examining the patient, in spite of the fact that many practitioners would pursue all or some of these options. I would discount them all because a patient will typically not readily perceive a loss of visual function in a sector of only one eye unless accompanied by other symptoms such as flashes and floaters of sudden onset. Patients usually perceive quadrantic or hemianopic defects only if the defects are present in both eyes. My immediate response after a case history and basic visual function tests would be to investigate visual fields at threshold levels, strongly suspecting a neurological cause. The practitioner must learn to effectively construct a differential diagnostic algorithm (a step-by-step method for solving a problem) to solve the clinical problem and to provide proper management. In this example, the algorithm could look like the following.

Problem: Loss of Inferior Temporal Vision in the Left Eye

↓	↓	↓	↓
Answer: BRAO (branch retinal artery occlusion)	Answer: BRVO (branch retinal vein occlusion)	Answer: retinal detachment	Diagnostic test: threshold visual fields showing incongruous left inferior quadrantanopsia
↓	↓	↓	↓
Ophthal-moscopy normal	Ophthal-moscopy normal	Ophthal-moscopy normal	Right superior and anterior lobe lesion
↓	↓	↓	↓
Start over	Start over	Start over	Immediate neurological consultation

In this clinical case, the patient had a left inferior quadrantanopsia that was fairly incongruous with absolutely no retinal changes or optic nerve head abnormalities. The management of this patient was a neurological consultation for magnetic resonance imaging (MRI) and computerized tomography (CT) studies.

In order to minimize wasted time in the clinical decision-making process, how should this process evolve? There are several basic concepts to avoid and basic principles to follow. Initially, the practitioner must analyze each problem as a single diagnostic dilemma. As we will see later, the rule of parsimony dictates that it is highly unlikely that two separate conditions will create the same sign or symptom complex. The least desirable approach is to look at the complexity of multiple answers and the action required for each answer.

Dilemma

↓	↓	↓	↓
Answer 1	Answer 2	Answer 3	Answer N
↓	↓	↓	↓
Action 1	Action 2	Action 3	Action N

The dilemma is the patient's sign or symptom, whereas each answer represents a diagnostic hypothesis. As we will see, the number of answers (diagnostic hypotheses) is often excessive and must be pared down to a workable number to improve diagnostic efficiency. The actions represent either interventive diagnostic tests or management protocol.

Our initial case example would plot as such:

Loss of Inferior Temporal Vision in the Left Eye

↓	↓	↓	↓
BRAO	BRVO	Retinal detach-ment	Visual field defect
↓	↓	↓	↓
Ophthal-moscopy	Ophthal-moscopy	Ophthal-moscopy	Visual field

The most desirable approach would be a binomial construction with two certain outcomes, to minimize the difficulty of differential diagnosis:

Dilemma

↓	↓
Answer 1	Answer 2
↓	↓
Yes	No

Unfortunately, the clinical situation is not quite so simple, so there must be an uncertain outcome inserted into the thought process algorithm. The insertion of the "maybe" into the process would plot as such:

Dilemma

↓	↓	↓
Answer 1	Answer 2	Answer 3
↓	↓	↓
Yes	Maybe	No
↓	↓	↓
Action 1	Action 2	Action 3

To minimize the necessary actions, the action options may be grouped according to severity of the yes, maybe, and no diagnoses:

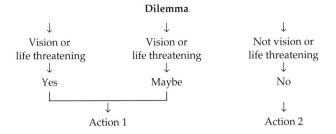

Our example could be plotted as such:

Loss of Inferior Temporal Vision in the Left Eye

↓	↓	↓
Retinal detachment	BRAO	Demyelinizing optic neuropathy

Immediate consult — Consult within 2 weeks

Using a construction including the uncertain outcome would create a situation where the number of actions could be minimized. The basics of the algorithm construction can be applied to any diagnostic dilemma. These basics need not be written down for each patient to be effective, but should serve as a methodology for the cognitive diagnostic process.

In the development of the diagnostic algorithm, certain factors become crucially important in the determination of the effectiveness and efficiency of the diagnostic outcome. Initially it is important to have a list of sound answers (diagnostic hypotheses) to the dilemma (the signs or symptoms). This list must be prioritized according to expected prevalence. The list must also be bundled according to degree of severity, so that vision- or life-threatening conditions are addressed as top priority. Additionally, the action plan must be sound. The use of diagnostic tests must be carefully planned, with consideration of the abilities of the various tests to assist in the differential diagnosis. Performance of a threshold central visual field analysis in the case of a macular subretinal hemorrhage adds little to the differential diagnosis of the process, whereas the performance of fluorescein angiography is of tremendous value. The ability of a diagnostic test to discriminate disease from normalcy—the sensitivity and specificity of the test—also become important in the determination of the diagnosis.

Understanding the importance of the ability of the diagnostic test to determine the diagnostic outcome is essential in the determination of outcome.

PERFORMANCE OF PROPER DIFFERENTIAL DIAGNOSTIC TESTS

Performance of proper differential diagnostic tests is imperative in assisting in the elimination of the

"maybe" from the algorithm. It has been suggested that three questions should be addressed before ordering any laboratory test or diagnostic procedure:

1. Will the results of this test potentially benefit the patient by altering the diagnosis, prognosis, or therapy?
2. Will these results contribute to understanding the patient's condition or to the body of medical knowledge?
3. Is there potential that something will be discovered by performing the tests?

I would add one more question:

4. Is the test potentially harmful to the patient when considering the relative sensitivity and specificity of the test as it applies to the diagnostic outcome?

Although the criteria seem straightforward, in differential diagnostic testing there are always caveats created by the error rates of even the best tests. An illustration of the fallacy of laboratory diagnostic testing is presented at the end of this chapter regarding a patient with giant cell arteritic optic neuropathy. From a laboratory-testing standpoint, there are considerable complexities, best illustrated by the issue of diagnosing Lyme disease, which can be both visually and systemically devastating. The testing protocol can actually confuse the differential diagnosis. The laboratory testing for Lyme disease (the next greatest mimicker of a number of diseases to syphilis) consists of (1) the Lyme immunofluorescent antibody (IFA) test, which has a cross-reactivity of 22 to 54 percent with the fluorescent treponemal antibody-absorption (FTA-ABS) test; or (2) the Lyme enzyme-linked immunosorbent assay (ELISA), which has a cross-reactivity of 32 percent with the FTA-ABS. If both the FTA-ABS and the Lyme serology are positive, a negative microhemagglutination assay–*Treponema pallidum* (MHA-TP) test and rapid plasma reagin (RPR) test for syphilis would strongly suggest a diagnosis of Lyme disease. Sensitivities of the Lyme ELISA and the IFA tests have been reported to be as low as 0.24 in the initial stages of the disease. Sensitivities this low actually minimize the predictive values in differential diagnosis. Nevertheless, the tests must be ordered. Fortunately, the western blot test is affording improved specificity and sensitivity in the differential diagnosis of Lyme disease.

Sensitivity and Specificity

Statistical probability must also figure into the algorithm or decision-making process. The probabilities may be applied to laboratory tests (Lyme IFA), diagnostic procedures (threshold visual fields), differential diagnostic options (retinal detachment versus branch retinal vein occlusion), and ophthalmoscopic signs (the cause of retinal hard exudates). The "ideal" diagnostic or laboratory test would be able to distinguish disease from health in every instance. This ideal test would always be negative in a healthy patient and positive in a diseased patient. The probabilities of tests are stated in the terms "sensitivity" and "specificity." *Sensitivity* applies to the ability of a test to give a positive result when the test is applied to a patient known to have the disease. An example would be a threshold visual field performed on 100 patients known to have glaucoma and glaucomatous field loss based on a "gold standard." Performance of the chosen test demonstrates field loss in only 65 of the known diseased patients. This would indicate a sensitivity of 0.65, meaning that the test will only discover the field loss in 65 of 100 patients known to have glaucoma (65 percent). This test would miss 35 patients with glaucomatous field defects (false negatives).

Specificity applies to the ability of a test to give a negative result when given to a person known to not have the disease (a normal). When the above threshold field was performed on 100 patients known to not have either glaucoma or glaucomatous field loss based on a "gold standard," it demonstrated field loss in 35 patients (false positives) and a normal field in 65 of the patients. This represents a rate of 0.65 specificity, or the ability to give a negative result when given to normal patients. Stated another way, the test will correctly diagnose a normal field 65 percent of the time in a normal patient. The false-positive rate is 1 minus the specificity, which in this case is 0.35. Stated another way, the test will incorrectly diagnose a glaucomatous field loss in 35 of 100 normal patients, or 35 percent of the time.

The ideal diagnostic test will have 100 percent sensitivity and specificity, always discovering the diseased state and never calling a healthy person diseased. An example of some specificities and sensitivities for diagnostic tests used in keratoconjunctivitis sicca (KCS) are given in Table 1–1. The conclusions that can be drawn by analysis of the sensitivities and specificities outlined in Table 1–1 are that a well-designed case history is one of the most effective procedures for the diagnosis of KCS, and that expensive, invasive procedures are not any more effective than more conventional procedures in assisting in the differential diagnosis.

DEVELOPMENT OF PREDICTIVE VALUES

To carry the evolution of differential diagnosis one step further, the practitioner must be able to apply sensitivity and specificity to clinical situations to determine predictive values of tests and clinical decisions. The predictive values (positive or negative) are determined in part by the prevalence of each condition being considered. The more prevalent the condition, the higher the sensitivity; the higher the specificity of a particular diagnostic test, the higher the positive predictive value of the test.

The practitioner must apply probabilities in the decision-making process to develop positive predictive values for tests and diagnoses. *Probability* refers to the likelihood of an occurrence. If it is said that there is a 0.70 probability of an occurrence, it means that the situation will occur 70 percent of the time, or in 70 out of 100 patients with the demographic characteristics of your patient. A scale of the likelihood of an event is illustrated below.

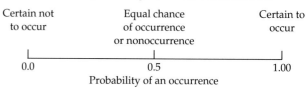

Scale for Representing the Likelihood of an Event

In our example of a 70 percent likelihood, the plot would appear as follows:

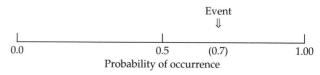

Plot of a 70-percent Likelihood of Occurrence of an Event

This represents our initial level of certainty without the advantages of differential diagnostic testing. Correct diagnosis is achieved by approaching 1.0 probability, or a 100 percent chance of being correct. Improving probability is often attained by application of additional appropriate diagnostic testing. A measure of probability of the initial diagnosis being correct can then be attained through application of Bayes' theorem. Bayes' theorem allows the practitioner to adjust the probability of a disease accounting for new diagnostic information. The probability of a disease before new diagnostic information is called *prior probability*. The probability after new information is called the *posterior probability*. Prior probability can

TABLE 1–1. SENSITIVITIES AND SPECIFICITIES IN DIFFERENTIAL DIAGNOSTIC TESTS USED IN KCS

Test	Sensitivity	Specificity
Tear breakup time	0.82 (82%)	0.86 (86%)
Rose Bengal staining	0.58 (58%)	1.00 (100%)
Schirmer tear test	0.10 (10%)	1.00 (100%)
Lactoferrin tear immunoassay	0.54 (54%)	0.94 (94%)
Conjunctival impression cytology	1.00 (100%)	0.87 (87%)
Case history	0.98 (98%)	0.97 (97%)

also be equated to the prevalence of the disease in a particular patient population. This concept is illustrated below, using a prior probability of 0.4 or a prevalence of 40 percent in the patient population. The application of the diagnostic testing in this instance improved our predictive value for our diagnostic hypothesis to 70 percent.

Prior Probability Versus Posterior Probability After Application of Differential Diagnostic Testing

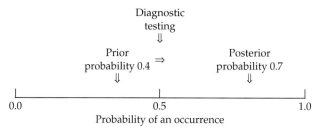

Bayes' Theorem

The components of Bayes' theorem include (1) the prior probability of the disease (prevalence), (2) the probability of a test result conditional on the patient's having the disease (sensitivity), and (3) the probability of the test result conditional on the patient's not having the disease (specificity and false positives). Application of Bayes' theorem can determine a positive predictive value (PPV), which is the probability that the patient does have the disease. Conversely, the theorem can be applied to discern the negative predictive value (NPV), which is the probability that the patient with a negative result really does not have the disease. Bayes' theorem can be written as such:

Positive Predictive Value (PPV) =
$$\frac{(Prevalence)(Sensitivity)}{(Prevalence)(Sensitivity) + [(1 - Prevalence)(1 - Specificity)]}$$

where

$$sensitivity = true\text{-}positive\ rate = \frac{number\ of\ diseased\ patients\ with\ positive\ tests}{number\ of\ diseased\ patients}$$

$$(1 - specificity) = false\text{-}positive\ rate = \frac{number\ of\ nondiseased\ patients\ with\ positive\ tests}{number\ of\ nondiseased\ patients}$$

$$likelihood\ ratio = \frac{true\text{-}positive\ rate}{false\text{-}positive\ rate}$$

Because sensitivity is the same as the true-positive rate (TPR), prevalence is the probability of disease, (1 − prevalence) is the probability of no disease, and (1 − specificity) is the false-positive rate (FPR), the equation may be rewritten as:

PPV =
$$\frac{(Prevalence\ of\ Disease)(TPR)}{(Prevalence\ of\ Disease)(TPR) + (Prevalence\ of\ No\ Disease)(FPR)}$$

Table 1–2 illustrates the effect of prevalence of a condition or a disease on the positive predictive value

TABLE 1–2. EFFECT OF RISING PREVALENCE ON POSITIVE PREDICTIVE VALUE OF A TEST WITH 90 PERCENT SENSITIVITY AND 95 PERCENT SPECIFICITY

Prevalence	Sensitivity	Specificity	Positive Predictive Value
0.0002 (0.02%)	0.90	0.95	0.00358 (0.4%)
0.002 (0.2%)	0.90	0.95	0.03482 (3.5%)
0.02 (2%)	0.90	0.95	0.26866 (26.9%)
0.20 (20%)	0.90	0.95	0.81818 (81.8%)

when the test has a sensitivity of 90 percent and a specificity of 95 percent.

Let us now apply sensitivity, specificity, and prevalence to a diagnostic challenge and manipulate specificities, sensitivities, and prevalence estimations to illustrate the strength of choosing a good diagnostic test as opposed to a poor diagnostic test.

■ ■ ■ ■ ■ ■

Clinical Example: A Good Diagnostic Test versus A Poor Diagnostic Test

A 37-year-old black female enters the office for a routine eye examination. She is correctable to 20/20 in each eye. She has type 2 (non–insulin-dependent) diabetes mellitus and is taking oral hypoglycemic agents. She also has hypertension and is taking a calcium channel blocker. The patient has a positive family history of primary open-angle glaucoma (POAG). Her 10:00 AM intraocular pressures are 22/23 mm HG and she has asymmetrical optic nerve heads. The retina is clear to the periphery, showing no signs of diabetic retinopathy. The angles are open by gonioscopy. You choose to perform a threshold visual field test, which shows good patient reliability and demonstrates cluster visual field defects inferiorly and nasally in both eyes. Your field tester is known to have a 0.5 sensitivity and a 0.6 specificity. You *estimate* that the prevalence of POAG in this particular population is 2 percent (0.02). What is the positive predictive value of your positive automated visual field test findings?

PPV =
$$\frac{(Prevalence)(Sensitivity)}{(Prevalence)(Sensitivity) = [(1 - Prevalence)(1 - Specificity)]}$$

$$PPV = \frac{(0.02)(0.5)}{(0.02)(0.5) + [(1 - 0.02)(1 - 0.6)]}$$

PPV = 0.0248

PPV = 2.48%

In this case there is only a 2.48 percent chance that this patient actually has POAG visual field loss in spite of a positive test result. The prior predictive value was 2.0 percent (the prevalence in the population), and has only been improved to a 2.48 percent likelihood with the application of this diagnostic test.

By changing the field-testing apparatus in your office, you now have a machine that has a sensitivity of 0.95 and a specificity of 0.95. The field test reveals inferior nasal clustering of visual field defects in both eyes. Just with this simple modification, the posterior predictive value is altered as demonstrated:

$$PPV = \frac{(Prevalence)(Sensitivity)}{(Prevalence)(Sensitivity) \; = \; [(1 - Prevalence)(1 - Specificity)]}$$

$$PPV = \frac{(0.02)(0.95)}{(0.02)(0.95) + [(1 - 0.02)(1 - 0.95)]}$$

$$PPV = 0.279$$

$$PPV = 27.9\%$$

In this case there is a 27.9 percent chance that this patient has POAG visual field loss with the positive results from the visual field testing device. The prior predictive value of 2% has now increased to a posterior predictive value of 27.9%.

Prevalence also has a significant effect on the positive predictive value in this example. Were this patient a 75-year-old black female with all of the prior characteristics, the prevalence of POAG probably approaches the 5 to 6 percent range. Using the instrument with 95 percent sensitivity and 95 percent specificity, the positive predictive value becomes:

$$PPV = \frac{(Prevalence)(Sensitivity)}{(Prevalence)(Sensitivity) \; = \; [(1 - Prevalence)(1 - Specificity)]}$$

$$PPV = \frac{(0.05)(0.95)}{(0.05)(0.95) + [(1 - 0.05)(1 - 0.95)]}$$

$$PPV = 0.50$$

$$PPV = 50\%$$

In this case the patient has a 50 percent chance of having a POAG visual field loss associated with a positive test. Prevalence of the disease, especially within the demographic characteristics of the patient, has a very strong effect on the development of the posterior predictive value, and thus a strong influence on the ability to confirm a diagnostic hypothesis.

It becomes apparent that to improve the chances of making the correct differential diagnosis, the practitioner must consider prevalence in addition to the sensitivity and specificity of tests performed on the patient. Although it is not realistic to get specific data on each of these variables, the clinician can use the proper knowledge base regarding epidemiological characteristics of the diseases as presented in many examples in the text to improve probability of a correct diagnosis. In addition, diagnostic tests with higher sensitivity and specificity will also improve the chances of pursuing the proper line of action on the algorithm.

PROCESS OF DIFFERENTIAL DIAGNOSIS

Algorithms, specificity, sensitivity, probability, and positive predictive values all fit into the differential diagnostic scenario. A diagnosis is typically achieved through a step-by-step process starting with the patient's presenting complaint (symptom) or a particular clinical physical finding (sign). In the case of primary eye care, often the sign is a retinal or optic nerve alteration that is discovered with or without accompanying symptomatology.

Chief Complaint

Unfortunately, the chief complaint can often reflect multiple potential diagnoses. Without modification of the thought process, the practitioner faces the problem of multiple independent answers with multiple independent actions before making the proper diagnosis. To minimize the problem of multiple independent answers (diagnostic hypotheses), the practitioner must initially consider many factors to create a better diagnostic climate, including (1) patient personal, family, and medical history, (2) age, (3) race, (4) sex, and (5) current medications. Taking such factors into account can reduce the number of potential differential diagnostic possibilities. Basic eye tests such as best corrected vision, pupillary responses, and binocular vision status can further reduce the possible differential diagnostic options. After reaching this point in the examination, specific differential diagnostic procedures or tests with a high positive predictive value may be used to further improve the posterior probability of a correct diagnosis. Figure 1–1 illustrates the reduction in the number of potential diagnoses with each of the above steps.

The starting point for the differential diagnostic process is the chief complaint. From the chief com-

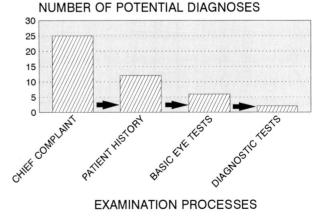

NUMBER OF POTENTIAL DIAGNOSES

EXAMINATION PROCESSES

Figure 1–1. The effect of the evolution of diagnostic hypotheses on reducing potential diagnoses.

TABLE 1–3. SOME REASONS FOR SUDDEN UNILATERAL REDUCTION OF VISION

Retinal detachment	Central retinal artery occlusion
Central retinal vein occlusion	Branch retinal artery occlusion
Branch retinal vein occlusion	Ischemic optic neuropathy
Demyelinizing optic neuropathy	Presumed ocular histoplasmosis
Idiopathic central serous choroidopathy (ICSC)	Multiple evanescent white dot syndrome (MEWDS)
Acute multifocal choroidopathy	Acute retinal necrosis syndrome
Exudative macular degeneration	Macular hole
Transient monocular blindness	HIV retinopathy
Inflammatory optic neuropathy	Coats' disease
Papillophlebitis	Preretinal hemorrhages
Geographical helicoid peripapillary choroidopathy	Hemicentral retinal vein occlusion
Trauma	Vitreous hemorrhage
Ocular parasititis	Acute posterior multifocal placoid pigment epitheliopathy (APMPPE)
Toxoplasmosis	Giant-cell arteritic optic neuropathy

plaint, the practitioner should develop a mental hypothesis for the diagnosis starting with the most common or prevalent disease condition for the specific age, race, and sex characteristics of the patient. Recall that the higher the prevalence of the condition, the higher the positive predictive value (PPV) of each differential diagnostic test applied.

An excellent illustration of the concept is the complaint of unilateral, abrupt reduction of vision. Sudden unilateral reduction of vision can occur from a number of conditions. Some of these are listed in Table 1–3. As the list of potential causes for acute onset of vision loss is exhaustive, that particular chief complaint creates an unmanageable diagnostic challenge without modification of the entire list. The list of answers in the algorithm is impossible to handle efficiently and effectively. In the case of sudden unilateral reduction of vision, a clinical example will illustrate the elimination of many diagnostic hypotheses by simple application of patient characteristics. In addition, the clinical example will illustrate the efficacy of prioritizing diagnostic hypotheses by utilization of prevalence rates within the characteristics of the patient's demographic base.

■ ■ ■ ■ ■ ■

Clinical Example: Prioritizing Diagnostic Hypotheses Using Patient Characteristics

Our patient is a 35-year-old healthy white female with no recent history of trauma and no admitted intravenous drug use. Her best corrected vision is OD 20/50 and OS

TABLE 1–4. SOME REASONS FOR SUDDEN UNILATERAL REDUCTION OF VISION IN A 35-YEAR-OLD HEALTHY WHITE FEMALE

Retinal detachment	Acute multifocal choroidopathy
Papillophlebitis	Acute posterior multifocal placoid pigment epitheliopathy (APMPPE)
Coats' disease	Multiple evanescent white dot syndrome (MEWDS)
Demyelinizing optic neuropathy	Presumed ocular histoplasmosis
Idiopathic central serous choroidopathy (ICSC)	Toxoplasmosis

20/20. She has no family history of eye disease and no contributing family history of systemic disease. She works as an accountant. Our differential diagnostic hypotheses list is suddenly reduced to the more likely hypotheses listed in Table 1–4. If the factor of prevalence is added to the equation, the list in Table 1–4 can be rearranged from most to least prevalent, as it appears in Table 1–5.

In this clinical example, the practitioner is faced with a difficult differential diagnosis using just ophthalmoscopy, as the top two likely differential diagnostic candidates are often subtle in their clinical presentation, requiring additional differential diagnostic tests such as fluorescein angiography and perhaps MRI. Diagnostic exclusions can, however, be accomplished by the simple performance of binocular indirect ophthalmoscopy and fundus lens evaluation. Diagnosis is a two-way street in that as a clinician you are both determining what it can be and what it cannot be. A normal ophthalmoscopic examination can reduce the likelihood of the diagnostic hypotheses to those listed in Table 1–6. It suddenly becomes apparent how important the simple in-office neurological tests, visual fields, and fluorescein angiography become in this case. It is also important to realize that the performance of ophthalmoscopy under dilation has all but eliminated the diagnostic hypotheses that are of immediate threat to severe loss of vision.

TABLE 1–5. SOME REASONS FOR SUDDEN UNILATERAL REDUCTION OF VISION IN A 35-YEAR-OLD HEALTHY WHITE FEMALE RANKED FROM MOST PREVALENT TO LEAST PREVALENT

MOST PREVALENT	ICSC
	Demyelinizing optic neuropathy
	Retinal detachment
	Presumed ocular histoplasmosis
	Toxoplasmosis
	Papillophlebitis
	APMPPE
	Acute multifocal choroidopathy
	MEWDS
LEAST PREVALENT	Coats' disease

TABLE 1–6. SOME REASONS FOR SUDDEN UNILATERAL REDUCTION OF VISION IN A 35-YEAR-OLD HEALTHY WHITE FEMALE WITH RELATIVELY NORMAL OPHTHALMOSCOPIC AND FUNDUS LENS FINDINGS RANKED FROM MOST PREVALENT TO LEAST PREVALENT

MOST PREVALENT	Idiopathic central serous choroidopathy (ICSC)
	Demyelinizing optic neuropathy
	Acute posterior multifocal placoid pigment epitheliopathy (APMPPE)
	Acute multifocal choroidopathy
LEAST PREVALENT	Multiple evanescent white dot syndrome (MEWDS)

TABLE 1–8. SOME REASONS FOR UNILATERAL HARD EXUDATES IN THE POSTERIOR POLE IN A 75-YEAR-OLD MALE WITH SYSTEMIC HYPERTENSION

Retinal macroaneurysms	Wet age-related macular degeneration
Hemicentral retinal vein occlusion	Idiopathic juxtafoveal telangiectasia
Branch retinal vein occlusion	Central retinal vein occlusion
Hypertensive retinopathy	Macular hole (in the center of the hole)
Angiomatosis retinae	

Using Ocular Signs

Like chief complaints, ocular signs can often reflect multiple potential diagnoses. Again, patient characteristics and basic eye tests can reduce the number of potential differential diagnostic possibilities. An excellent illustration of the multiple diagnostic possibilities associated with a particular ocular sign is the presentation of hard exudates in the posterior pole of one eye. Some of the conditions associated with unilateral presentation of hard exudates in the posterior pole are illustrated in Table 1–7. Again, the list of answers in the algorithm is impossible to handle efficiently and effectively. In the case of unilateral hard exudates in the posterior pole, a clinical example will illustrate the efficacy of prioritizing diagnostic hypotheses by utilization of the prevalence rates within the characteristics of the patient's demographic base.

■ ■ ■ ■ ■ ■

Clinical Example: Prioritizing Diagnostic Hypotheses Using Ocular Signs

A 75-year-old white male enters your office complaining of a reduction in visual acuity in the right eye starting about 1 month ago. He did not come in sooner because he thought it was just a floater like one that occurred 2 years ago in the other eye. Entrance acuity is OD 20/70 and OS 20/25. He is hypertensive, taking an angiotensin converting enzyme (ACE) inhibitor, and has no strong family history of ocular or systemic disease. He had a physical examination 2 months ago including a complete blood count (CBC), cholesterol evaluation, and a fasting blood glucose level. Refraction and pinhole tests do not improve acuity. All other ocular findings are normal. The differential diagnostic list is reduced to that given in Table 1–8. Prioritized according to estimated relative prevalence in this aged population, the list becomes that shown in Table 1–9.

On dilated fundus examination, a partial arc of hard exudates lie temporal to the macula in the right eye. The macular area is somewhat dulled and gray-green in appearance, while the remainder of the retina demonstrates only pavingstone degeneration. The retina in the left eye shows only pavingstone degeneration and a few isolated macular drusen. The differential diagnostic list is now reduced to age-related macular degeneration because of the significant absence of other retinal vascular signs such as hemorrhage and cotton wool spots and the pathognomonic feature of a dull gray-green membrane in the macular area.

TABLE 1–7. SOME REASONS FOR UNILATERAL HARD EXUDATES IN THE POSTERIOR POLE

Diabetic retinopathy	Wet age-related macular degeneration
Coats' disease	
Branch retinal vein occlusion	Idiopathic juxtafoveal telangiectasia
Presumed ocular histoplasmosis	Central retinal vein occlusion
Inflammatory optic neuropathy–papillitis	Macular hole (in the center of the hole)
Hemicentral retinal vein occlusion	Papillophlebitis
	Toxoplasmosis
Angiomatosis retinae	Hypertensive retinopathy
Retinal macroaneurysms	Papilledema

TABLE 1–9. SOME REASONS FOR UNILATERAL HARD EXUDATES IN THE POSTERIOR POLE IN A 75-YEAR-OLD MALE WITH SYSTEMIC HYPERTENSION RANKED FROM MOST PREVALENT TO LEAST PREVALENT

MOST PREVALENT	Wet age-related macular degeneration
	Branch retinal vein occlusion
	Macular hole
	Hemicentral retinal vein occlusion
	Central retinal vein occlusion
	Hypertensive retinopathy
	Idiopathic juxtafoveal telangiectasia
	Retinal macroaneurysm
LEAST PREVALENT	Angiomatosis retinae

Medical Interview

The chief complaint is the springboard for the medical interview. The interview should serve many functions. A casual yet professional approach to the patient interaction will often establish trust and reveal data crucial to the differential diagnosis. The interview should begin as the patient enters the office to sit in the chair. If the doctor does not observe the entrance of the patient, the nurse or technician who moves the patient should do so and notify the doctor of any departure from normalcy. Mannerisms, gait, and general appearance, among other characteristics, must be carefully observed and noted. The interview should also be effective in reducing the list of possible diagnoses without the questions leading toward the diagnosis expected by the practitioner. The interview should create specific diagnostic hypotheses, which may each then be considered independently. The cyclic process of differential diagnosis is demonstrated in Figure 1–2.

When looking at the algorithm shown in Figure 1–2, it is easy to see that testing each hypothesis can be very exhaustive. The practitioner must always test the most prevalent or common diagnostic hypothesis first. In our example of the complaint of sudden unilateral vision reduction in a 35-year-old white female, consider the fact that MEWDS is very rare and ICSC far more common. Always initiate the differential diagnostic process with the more common conditions, but do not automatically exclude the more esoteric ones.

When cross-examining the specific complaint to gather more data, several strategies are available. In what is called *screening and branching*, the practitioner asks about a specific finding that usually accompanies the specific diagnostic hypothesis (screening). If this finding is not present, another hypothesis is pursued (branching). Screening and branching in our example for idiopathic central serous choroidopathy (ICSC) would evolve as such:

Doctor: Do you feel that you are a type A personality? That is, do you feel that you are high strung or do you feel under stress of late?

Patient: No! (Patient acts offended.)

Doctor: Did you see flashes of light or floaters with this occurrence of vision reduction?

Patient: No.

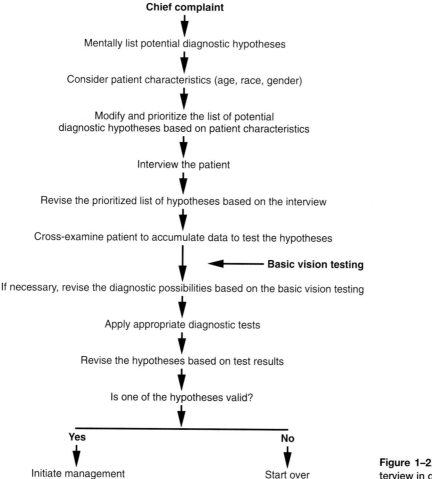

Chief complaint

↓

Mentally list potential diagnostic hypotheses

↓

Consider patient characteristics (age, race, gender)

↓

Modify and prioritize the list of potential diagnostic hypotheses based on patient characteristics

↓

Interview the patient

↓

Revise the prioritized list of hypotheses based on the interview

↓

Cross-examine patient to accumulate data to test the hypotheses

↓ ←——— **Basic vision testing**

If necessary, revise the diagnostic possibilities based on the basic vision testing

↓

Apply appropriate diagnostic tests

↓

Revise the hypotheses based on test results

↓

Is one of the hypotheses valid?

↓

Yes   **No**

Initiate management   Start over

Figure 1–2. The cyclic process of the interview in differential diagnosis.

This process can be misleading, because in differential diagnosis "always" and "never" do not exist. In addition, the practitioner is leading the patient's symptoms with the perceived question regarding the patient's personality. By offending the patient, the doctor got the wrong answer to the right question and automatically branched to the symptom associated with retinal detachment. The first question could be rephrased in this way: "Could you please describe your personality and how you react to life's problems." Should screening and branching be used on a highly prevalent hypothesis, several screening questions should be pursued. The above patient should be asked:

> **Doctor:** Do you notice any wavy or distorted vision in the eye?
> **Patient:** Yes.
> **Doctor:** Has this ever happened before?
> **Patient:** Yes. Four years ago when I was working in New York City. The retinal specialist said I had a blister under my retina.
> **Doctor:** Could you please describe your personality and how you react to problems in life.
> **Patient:** Well, I sort of overreact. I can see it right now in my new job. I think that I take everything too seriously.

By actively pursuing the most prevalent condition with a few more insightful questions, the diagnostic dilemma is minimized.

Another strategy involved in cross-examination is the use of pathognomonic findings that occur in only one disease. Unfortunately, very few truly pathognomonic findings actually exist in eyecare. In our example, if investigating the possibility of retinal detachment, the symptom of flashes of light and multiple gnat-like floaters is the closest feature that we have to pathognomonic of this particular disease process. Unfortunately, a posterior vitreous detachment with a small-vessel break and bleed can likewise present that same symptomatology, and an occipital lobe migraine can present the same symptoms only with bilaterality.

Other methods involved in the cross-examination during the interview are the following.

1. Weighing of the risks and costs of gathering the information against the potential value of the information. Outcome studies coupled with the pressures of the evolving health care system will dictate the evolution of these methods.
2. Obtaining more data than are necessary to test a hypothesis. This is very intimately tied to the problems of weighing risks and costs, and will soon be better controlled through specification of standards of care and the development of management protocol. Assessing the specificity and sensitivity of all diagnostic tests will also minimize the likelihood of obtaining useless data, as the fiscal constraints of health care will eventually curtail these problems.
3. Avoiding testing a hypothesis that would not affect the chosen management techniques. There is little to be gained from exhaustive differential diagnostic tests for distinguishing between diabetic maculopathy or the possibility of whether the maculopathy in diabetes is secondary to an associated branch retinal vein occlusion.

In addition to cross-examination, there are other methods available to reduce the potential list of hypotheses. After ranking the hypotheses according to prevalence, cross-examination, basic vision testing procedures, and mentally listing the evidence for each hypothesis, proceed with special procedures to test the hypothesis. Remember the rule of parsimony, that the likelihood of two independent, unrelated diseases causing a complaint is the product of the probabilities of each independent event. This means that it is highly unlikely that two independent diseases that could create the chief complaint would present at the same time. In addition, it is sometimes useful to bundle hypotheses with similar characteristics that can be differentially diagnosed with similar testing procedures. In our initial example, demyelinizing optic neuropathy and a shallow retinal detachment could be bundled and tested by a threshold visual field.

Armed with the above principles, the practitioner should then become familiar with the characteristics of the several different ocular conditions. An example of this would be the fact that a unilateral altitudinal visual field loss carefully respecting the horizontal meridian is probably the result of (1) normotensive glaucoma, (2) ischemic optic neuropathy, or (3) branch retinal artery occlusion. In employing this concept, the practitioner need remember that this visual field defect can only be the result of some process destroying the nerve fiber layer that terminates at the horizontal raphe. Conditions such as a branch retinal vein occlusion creating intraretinal edema will easily cross over the horizontal raphe. Understanding retinal and optic nerve head anatomy is crucial to differential diagnosis and management. Similarly, the practitioner can bundle hypotheses when facing a patient with bilateral constriction of visual fields. The bilateral constriction of visual fields is secondary to (1) vertebral basilar insufficiency, (2) buried drusen of the optic nerve head, (3) retinitis pigmentosa, (4) syphilitic optic neuropathy, or (5) hysteria (conversion reaction). Again, we are employing an understanding of retinal and optic nerve anatomy, anatomy of the visual pathway, and patient psychology.

Often in eyecare, the hypothesis can be easily tested just by looking with the slit lamp biomicroscope or variations of fundus evaluation techniques and adding the information so obtained to the decision-making process. It is imperative to remember, however, that there are precious few ocular diseases. The majority of ocular conditions are related to systemic processes. In addition to the ocular presentation, the practitioner must always consider and investigate the possibility of associated systemic diseases. The procedures necessary to diagnose both the ocular condition as well as the underlying systemic condition can become very complex.

An excellent example of the complexity of ocular processes is illustrated by the pearls on hemicentral retinal vein occlusion.

RULES OF DIFFERENTIAL DIAGNOSIS

In differential diagnosis, keep the following rules in mind at all times:

1. Always pursue the most prevalent hypothesis first. Rare manifestations of common diseases are far more likely than common manifestations of rare diseases. If it smells like a fish, looks like a fish, and tastes like a fish—it probably is a fish.
2. Do not get caught pursuing just one possible hypothesis. If you see a black chorioretinal scar in the temporal periphery with a moderate amount of vitreous traction, do not assume that it could only be an inactive toxoplasmosis scar. In a black patient this could be a sunburst scar associated with undiagnosed sickle cell anemia.
3. If you perform a test for differential diagnosis and the results are equivocal, repeat the test to improve the positive predictive value before either initiating treatment or abandoning the hypothesis. The best example in primary eyecare is threshold visual field testing, in which poor patient reliability actually invalidates the test altogether.

Pearls

Hemicentral Retinal Vein Occlusion

Characteristics
Δ Strong association with systemic disease
Δ Occlusion at lamina cribrosa in one branch of the central retinal vein
Δ Maximal threat to neovascularization of disc and retina in the ischemic form

Nonischemic variety (1/2 of retina involved)
Δ Dot-blot hemorrhages to the periphery
Δ Variable macular edema
Δ Dilated tortuous veins
Δ Optic disc edema possible
Δ Minimal threat to neovascular glaucoma (NVG) and retinal/disc neovascularization
Δ Management
   Ascertain underlying cause
   Rule out glaucoma
   Possible use of intraocular-pressure-lowering drugs
   Possible need for anticoagulation
   Fluorescein angiography
   Retinal consult to determine degree of ischemia. Follow every 4 weeks for conversion to ischemia

Ischemic variety (1/2 of retina involved)
Δ Dot-blot hemorrhages to the periphery
Δ Dilated tortuous veins
Δ Variable macular edema
Δ Cotton wool spots and flame-shaped hemorrhages
Δ Arterial changes
Δ Optic disc edema possible

Δ Strong tendency for disc/retinal neovascularization and threat for neovascular glaucoma (NVG)
Δ Management
   Ascertain underlying cause
   Rule out glaucoma
   Possible use of IOP lowering drugs
   Possible need for anticoagulation
   Fluorescein angiography
   Retinal consult for possible photocoagulation of affected area
   Follow every 3 to 4 weeks for 6 months for development of NVG or retinal/disc neovascularization

Primary workup
Δ Blood pressure and pulse evaluation
Δ Fasting blood glucose
Δ Complete blood count with differential and platelets
Δ Serum protein electrophoresis in younger patients
Δ FTA-ABS
Δ Antinuclear antibodies
Δ Carotid palpation and auscultation—ODM (ophthalmodynamometry)?

Secondary workup
Δ Hemoglobin electrophoresis
Δ Prothrombin and partial thromboplastin times
Δ Erythrocyte sedimentation rate
Δ Cryoglobulins
Δ Chest X-ray
Δ Carotid screening—Duplex ultrasound
Δ Consider a cardiovascular workup

TABLE 1–10. SOME REASONS FOR SUDDEN UNILATERAL REDUCTION OF VISION IN A 67-YEAR-OLD WHITE FEMALE

Retinal detachment	Vitreous hemorrhage
Central retinal vein occlusion	**Central retinal artery occlusion**
Branch retinal vein occlusion	Branch retinal artery occlusion
Exudative macular degeneration	Ischemic optic neuropathy
	Macular hole
Transient monocular blindness	Preretinal hemorrhages
Giant-cell arteritic optic neuropathy	Hemicentral retinal vein occlusion

4. In spite of prevalence, cross-examination, testing, and so forth, *never* dismiss any diagnostic hypothesis that could be an immediate threat to the patient's life or vision without compelling results from specific diagnostic testing procedures. Never let the diagnostic test, or artificial intelligence, overrule your better diagnostic judgment.

A recent case reported by another physician comes to mind in which a 67-year-old white female presented to the emergency room with the complaint of reduced vision in the left eye (20/40). A number of hypotheses could cause the problem (refer back to Table 1–3). Considering the patient's age, however, the possibilities can be reduced to those listed in Table 1–10. The diagnostic hypotheses that would be considered an ocular medical emergency are in bold type. The patient experienced pain in the jaw especially with mastication, and an accompanying headache, both of which strongly implicate giant-cell arteritic optic neuropathy. With fundus lens evaluation, mild optic disc edema was present in the left eye, further implicating giant-cell arteritic optic neuropathy. A Westergren sedimentation rate test was ordered; it demonstrated 25 mm (normal for women = [Age + 10]/2]). The patient was neither medicated nor biopsied. The patient returned the following day with light perception in the left eye and a Westergren sedimentation rate of 32 mm, still within normal limits. The optic disc edema was still present. She was again not medicated and developed light perception in the right eye within the week. At that point a temporal artery biopsy confirmed giant-cell arteritis, and the patient was placed on intravenous steroids. The major mistake in this case was the reliance on the Westergren sedimentation rate test as having 100 percent sensitivity and 100 percent specificity when clinical observations and clinical judgment dictated the immediate institution of intravenous or at least oral steroid treatment. Obviously, this was a costly error for the patient.

SUMMARY

The remainder of this text is concerned with identifying the clinical testing procedures and the characteristics of specific ocular conditions. Included in the description of the ocular conditions will be the characteristics of the patients with these conditions, the signs and symptoms of the conditions, and the specific management techniques for each of the conditions. It is important to remember the lessons of this chapter when using the knowledge base that follows to formulate diagnostic hypotheses and management protocol. Pursuing the wrong branch of the algorithm by not considering prevalence, omission of key questions in the interview and cross-examination, and misutilization of diagnostic tests and utilization of diagnostic tests without realizing their sensitivity and specificity, can lead you very quickly to the improper diagnosis, and likewise to the improper management plan.

REFERENCES

Cebul RD, Beck LH. *Teaching Clinical Decision Making.* New York: Praeger; 1985.

Nowakowski R. A review of theoretical and practical aspects of clinical laboratory testing. *Optom Clin.* 1992;2:1–14.

Shortliffe EH, Perreault LE. *Medical Informatics: Computer Applications in Health Care.* Reading, MA: Addison-Wesley; 1990.

Sox HC, et al. *Medical Decision Making.* Boston: Butterworths; 1988.

Weinstein MC, Fineberg HV. *Clinical Decision Analysis.* Philadelphia: Saunders; 1980.

Chapter Two ■ ■ ■ ■ ■ ■

S pecific Testing Procedures to Assist in Differential Diagnosis

A number of tests are currently available to the eyecare practitioner to assist in differential diagnosis of ocular anomalies and ocular manifestations of systemic diseases. The tests are varied and new variations are being developed daily. This section will be limited to a discussion of the generalities rather than the specifics.

CASE HISTORY AND CHIEF COMPLAINT

Doctors are doctors because of their deductive reasoning. They are trained to help the patient by listening to the patient and by performing tests to determine the cause of the complaint. Case history and complaint will often give the best clue regarding the answer to a perplexing clinical question.

Should there be a particular complaint, the clinician should establish a temporal profile or a history of the complaint as it unfolds over time. The temporal profile establishes how, when, and where the symptoms first occurred. It establishes the duration of the complaint, what followed the first symptom, whether or not it recurred, circumstances surrounding the incident, and if there were associated signs or symptoms, such as headache or loss of mobility.

In addition to the temporal profile, the clinician should consider the age and sex of the patient, the family history (pedigree), medical and medicine history, history of alcohol abuse, and history of environmental exposure. Figure 2–1 demonstrates the flow pattern of generating a good case history. Table 2–1 gives examples of symptoms that assist in diagnosis.

After determination of the complaint and case history, testing may be performed. One of the most crucial tests is visual acuity.

VISUAL ACUITY TESTING

Certainly, visual performance analysis is the bottom line in the assessment of any eye disease. The clinician must remember that any and all tests of visual performance must be carried out through the best refractive prescription available. A significant aspect of any acuity assessment is the refraction to best visual acuity or a multiple pinhole test over the current prescription.

Visual acuity may be tested in many ways (Snellen acuities, illiterate Es, potential acuity assessment, visually evoked potentials, contrast sensitivity) depending on the situation. In testing for diseased conditions, one also must consider assessment of functional acuities. Functional acuity can be defined as the ability to perform a vision task, such as reading. A patient with a right homonymous hemianopsia might very well be able to recognize isolated letters but would have noticeable difficulty reading a line of print. Monocular functional acuities would act as an effective means of detecting subtle ocular disease conditions. Monocular acuities are crucial, as many pa-

---

Abbreviated Example of Case History and Complaint

Complaint: Lost vision in both eyes for 20 minutes this past weekend
Age: 35. Nurse
Sex: Female. No reported medications; no family history that would contribute to diagnosis
What time of the day? 11:00 AM
Where? A local mall. I was just walking along.
Was vision lost in both eyes or just one? Both eyes for 20 minutes
Did it come back normally? Yes
Did anything else happen during this time? Yes, I lost function of my legs.
What do you mean? I couldn't walk for about a half-hour.
Did you get a headache with this? Yes. One of my migraines.
But you told me you didn't have headaches. I forgot.
Did you forget to tell me anything else, like medications? Does a new experimental injectable birth control system count as medication?

Further investigation revealed a history of migraine headaches exacerbated by the injectable birth control system. Vasospasm in the vertebrobasilar area had precipitated the attacks.

Figure 2–1. Example of generation of a case history as related to a specific complaint.

TABLE 2–1. EXAMPLES OF TEMPORAL PROFILE SYMPTOMATOLOGY

Symptom	Probable Cause
Loss of vision overnight	Common in thrombosis
5- to 15-second losses or blurs of vision	Transient obscurations of papilledema or impending central retinal vein occlusion
Abrupt loss of vision, getting progressively worse	Hemorrhage
Loss of vision for a few days, with a partial return	Demyelinizing disease
5- to 15- (up to 60-) minute losses of vision, returning to normal	Transient monocular blindness of internal carotid stenosis
Slowly progressive loss of vision	Neoplasm
Sudden bilateral contraction of fields (tubular)	Vertebrobasilar stroke sparing macular fibers
Sudden hemianopic field loss	Contralateral postchiasmal interruption of blood flow
Sudden fading of vision with postural change	Hypotensive attack; may also occur with mitral valve prolapse

tients with vision loss are unaware of their condition until one of their eyes is covered.

Another consideration in visual function examination is contrast sensitivity. Tests for contrast sensitivity range from the simplest available in hand–held card form or projectable form to those generated by a computer with bracketed response curves. Temporal contrast sensitivity, or the threshold determination of sensitivity to flicker, may also be of some value, especially when attempting to assess visual function through an opacity such as a cataract. As tests vary considerably, the clinician should refer to the specific guidelines from each manufacturer for performance of the test. In general, because of the variability found in the results of the tests, contrast sensitivity has yet to become a routine test in the clinical environment.

PUPILLARY TESTING

Proper pupillary testing is a crucial adjunct in testing for optic nerve disease. The swinging flashlight test or assessment for an afferent pupillary defect (APD) is the most specific test for optic nerve disease. This is

■ How To Do It ■
Swinging Flashlight Test

This example demonstrates a case of reduced acuity secondary to optic neuropathy in the left eye. The same result would occur if the left macula were significantly compromised.

1. Penlight on OD: OD constricts, OS constricts
2. Swing penlight to OS: OD dilates, OS dilates
3. Swing penlight to OD: OD constricts, OS constricts
4. Conclusion: OS optic nerve dysfunction or severe macular problem OS

■ When To Do It ■
What To Do With the Answers

Indications	Test	Conclusions
• Reduced vision	• Swinging flashlight	• Negative Marcus-Gunn test indicates reduced visual acuity secondary to a macular lesion • Positive Marcus-Gunn test indicates reduced visual acuity secondary to optic nerve disease or a severe macular lesion

also known as the Marcus–Gunn pupil test. This is a test of nerve conduction defects.

Should you want to enhance the view of the consensual or near response, you may darken the room and hold a Burton ultraviolet lamp about a foot from the patient to illuminate the eyes. The natural accumulation of fluorogens with age within the crystalline lens will glow when stimulated with the ultraviolet light without constricting the pupil. This provides an illuminated or backlit pupil on which to view the actions of the iris. The near response now becomes very easy to view.

COLOR VISION TESTING

The clinician realizes that when photoreceptors are affected in a disease process, there is a reduction or loss of function. When the cones or nerve fibers associated with the cones are involved, this will appear as some degree of color loss or desaturation. Lesions of the retina that can reduce visual acuity do not necessarily cause a proportionate reduction in color perception. Often, in–depth testing will demonstrate only mild defects. Defects in the optic nerve will, however, create faulty conduction of the nerve impulse, leading to a reduction in color perception (Table 2–2). The concept of optic nerve defects has been described as a barrier to impulse conduction within the optic nerve and to which the nerve fibers associated with cone function are preferentially sensitive. This barrier concept can be used to illustrate light comparison testing, con-

TABLE 2–2. TYPICAL DEFECTS PRODUCED BY SPECIFIC CONDITIONS

Disease	Color Defect
Optic Nerve	
Glaucoma	B–Y
Dominant optic atrophy	B–Y
Alcohol optic atrophy	B–Y
Nicotine optic atrophy	R–G
Leber's optic atrophy	R–G
Optic nerve and pathway disease	R–G
Optic neuropathy	R–G
Drusen	R–G/B–Y
Papilledema	R–G/B–Y
Macula	
Idiopathic central serous choroidopathy	B–Y
Chorioretinitis	B–Y
Diabetic maculopathy	B–Y
Hypertensive retinopathy	B–Y
Age-related maculopathy	B–Y
Stargardt's dystrophy	R–G
Vitelliform dystrophy	R–G
Central areolar dystrophy	R–G

B, blue; G, green; R, red; Y, yellow.

■ How To Do It ■
Color Vision Assessment

Must be performed monocularly

1. The easiest and most effective method is the standard pseudoisochromatic plates from Igaku–Shoin, Tokyo. These plates effectively reveal blue–yellow defects
   a. Part 1 for congenital vision defects
   b. Part 2 for acquired vision defects
2. AO HRR: Very good if you still have an old set around the office; they are no longer manufactured. AO HRR can diagnose red–green versus blue–yellow defects
3. Dvorine plates cannot diagnose tritan defects; therefore are of questionable value in acquired defects and are designed primarily to detect congenital defects
4. D–15: Hue discrimination
   a. Mild color defectives can pass
   b. Does not distinguish between mild and moderate color deficiency
5. 100 Hue: Hue discrimination
   a. Separates normal color vision into superior, average, and low discrimination
   b. Measures zones of color confusion in congenital or acquired defects
   c. Most definitive but longest to administer
6. Desaturated D–15: Hue discrimination. Same as D–15 but requires better hue discrimination; therefore, thought to be more sensitive

■ When To Do It ■
What To Do With the Answers

Characteristics of Congenital Versus Acquired Color Defects

Congenital	Acquired Color Defects
Usually no compromise to vision function	Often altered vision function
Symmetrical loss	May be asymmetrical loss
No change in defect over time	Defect may change with status of disease
Test repeatable	Often poor reproducibility

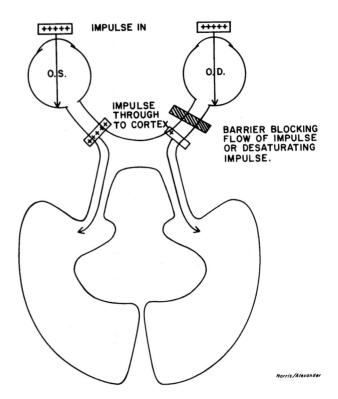

Figure 2–2. Schematic illustration of the barrier to an impulse created by an optic nerve conduction defect. *(Modified from Alexander LJ. Diseases of the optic nerve. In: Bartlett JD, Jaanus SD, eds. Clinical Ocular Pharmacology. Boston: Butterworth; 1989.)*

trast sensitivity testing, Pulfrich stereo phenomenon testing, neutral density filter testing, and evoked potential testing. In all cases, the patient presents a delayed or diminished response to stimulation. Figure 2–2 illustrates this barrier concept.

Standardized color vision tests definitely have value in the assessment of diseases of the optic nerve and macula. However, a test of color comparison provides a quick appraisal of the general status of color vision. After the patient's eyes have been equally light adapted, the clinician can present a red colored target, such as a red Mydriacyl bottle cap, to each eye alternately. The patient is asked to compare the intensity or quality of the color. The patient with a lesion of the optic nerve will report that the color is washed-out or grayish in the affected eye when the bottle cap is held in the area of the defect. This test also can be used to investigate quadrantic optic nerve defects by moving the test object around in the visual field. Should a field defect be present, the patient will report a color change in the cap in that part of the field.

Color vision testing has recently taken on a new dimension with the addition of colored target options in some of the automated perimeters. Macular integrity testing can be enhanced with certain autoperimeters by using the colored target function. Blue and blue-green can be of benefit in the early detection of diabetic macular defects as well as macular degenerative changes. Age-related standards have yet to be developed to allow broad use of these techniques diagnostically, but they do offer an excellent method for monitoring patients with known ocular conditions that affect macular function.

LIGHT COMPARISON TEST

A method of evaluating optic nerve conduction is the light comparison test. This test is a subjective evaluation of nerve conduction quality. It is similar to color comparison in that the patient is alternately presented a bright light and asked to compare his or her perception of the intensity or quality of the light. A patient with an optic nerve conduction defect may perceive a lower-intensity light on the affected side.

The clinician typically presents the light first to the good eye and states, "This light is worth a dollar." The light is then moved to the suspect eye, and the patient is asked, "How much is the light worth now?" I have noted, however, that patient response to this test is at best equivocal. Responses can be very misleading, and as a result the test should be used only as an adjunct to other diagnostic procedures.

NEUTRAL DENSITY FILTER TEST

If you have a 2-log-unit neutral density (2ND) filter around your office, you can use it to assist in the diagnosis of an eye with an optic nerve conduction defect. Table 2–3 illustrates the effect on visual acuity of placing a 2ND filter over a normal eye, an eye with functional amblyopia, and an eye with an optic nerve conduction defect. This test is not routinely performed in the clinical setting.

PULFRICH STEREO PHENOMENON

Although I would not actively advocate this test, it is a good illustration of optic nerve conduction defects. Patients who have optic nerve disease may report that moving objects appear to look odd to them or that they are having trouble with depth perception while driving. Historically, it has been reported in patients with demyelinizing optic neuropathy having difficulty while riding on a train. The Pulfrich phenomenon induced in this situation actually creates significant motion sickness.

The Pulfrich stereo phenomenon is the binocular perception of a pendulum swinging in an elliptical path when, in fact, it is swinging in a straight path. The patient is asked to look straight ahead beyond the swinging pendulum while the pendulum bob is swung from side to side in a straight line. This illusion is created by a latency in visual signal to the cortex. This can be created artificially by placing a 2ND filter in front of one eye or by dilating one eye. It can also be created by an optic nerve conduction defect, such as that occurring in optic neuropathy or optic atrophy.

MACULAR PHOTOSTRESS RECOVERY TEST

Macular photostress testing provides the clinician a noninvasive method of evaluating macular physiologic function. It is important to employ tests for macular function to differentiate vision loss secondary to optic nerve disease or to macular disease.

The photostress test has been defined as a dynamic test of macular performance that is based on precisely measuring the time required for an eye to

---

■ How To Do It ■
Macular Photostress
Recovery Test (MPSRT)

1. Determine the best refractive correction and place it in a trial frame
2. Use a darkened room and dark adapt 1 minute
3. Occlude one eye and project the line of best acuity
4. Bleach the patient's macula for 10 seconds by projecting the fixation target of the direct ophthalmoscope on the fovea.
5. After bleaching, time the recovery to reading one line above best visual acuity
6. Repeat the procedure on the other eye after an equal time of dark adaptation
7. The average normal recovery time using this technique is 50 seconds

■ When To Do It ■
What To Do With the Answers

Indications	Test	Conclusion
Reduced vision	MPSRT	If MPSRT is elevated, it may indicate edema in macula
Differentiating macular disease from optic nerve disease		If one eye is elevated relative to the other, the eye with elevated MPSRT may have edema. If no elevated MPSRT, probable optic nerve dysfunction

---

TABLE 2–3. NEUTRAL DENSITY FILTER TEST

Condition	Response When Filter Placed Over Eye
Normal eye	Two- to three-line reduction in acuity
Functionally amblyopic eye	Minimal if any reduction in acuity
Eye with optic nerve conduction defect	Severe reduction in acuity

recover sufficient visual function to perform a defined visual task after it has been dazzled with an intense flash of light. A prolonged photostress recovery time is thought to be secondary to altered retinal adaptation. Several studies have proven that the efficiency of retinal adaptability to stress depends not only on the photochemical mechanism of vision but also on the anatomic relationship of the photoreceptors to the retinal pigment epithelium. The photostress test serves as a reasonably sensitive discriminator between subtle maculopathy and optic neuropathy, but should not be used alone as a differential diagnostic test.

This test can also be performed using a commercially available instrument such as the brightness acuity tester (BAT), which is normally employed to assess the effect of glare on acuity in patients with cataracts.

AMSLER GRID TEST

The Amsler grid is used as a test of visual integrity of the macular area. The test can be sensitive if performed properly or if variations on the theme are applied effectively. Figure 2–3 illustrates the retinal area covered by Amsler grid testing. This test can be used to evaluate for retinal elevations and depressions as well as for scotomas. The Potter–Wild variation is the first significant improvement in this testing technique in years (Fig. 2–4). The author has employed the "calling-card variety" of grid illustrated in Figure 2–5. A variation using a red central fixation target may also be of value in that both metamorphopsia and central

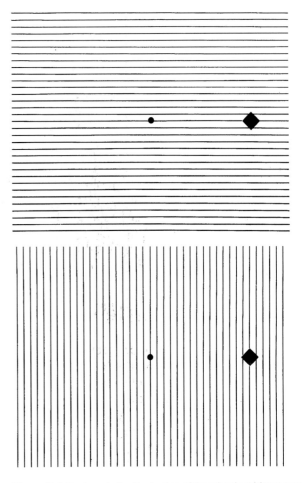

Figure 2–4. Reduced-size illustration of the macula grid test as proposed by Potter and Wild.

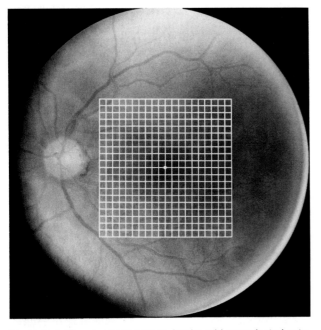

Figure 2–3. The area tested by an Amsler grid as projected onto the retinal area.

■ How To Do It ■
Standard Amsler Grid

1. Seven different charts are in the Amsler grid manual that test for macular integrity and metamorphopsia within a 20-degree diameter field
2. Test at 30 cm where each 5 mm square corresponds to a 1-degree visual angle
3. Use even illumination that is repeatable from time to time
4. Use the patient's correction at 30 cm
5. Ask the patient to
   a. Look at the central fixation spot
   b. Tell you if he or she sees all four corners
   c. Tell you if there are any halos or blurry spots on the chart
   d. Tell you if there are any wavy lines
   e. Draw defects on a recording grid

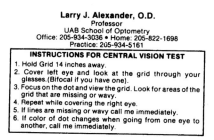

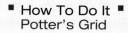

Figure 2–5. Reduced-size illustration of the calling card used by the author.

▪ How To Do It ▪
Potter's Grid

1. The diamond and fixation targets are red. The diamond is always temporal, that is, right side for OD testing, left side for OS testing. The diamond serves as a control of test distance
2. The patient holds the horizontal chart at arm's length with one eye closed and pulls the chart inward until the red diamond disappears in the blind spot. This is usually about 40 cm
3. The patient is asked to look for waviness or areas missing on the grid
4. The patient now repeats the test with the vertical chart

▪ When To Do It ▪
What To Do With the Answers

Indications	Test	Conclusion
Reduced vision	Amsler grid	Scotoma with no apparent macular disease indicates optic nerve dysfunction
Complaints of metamorphopsia		Metamorphopsia indicates active or resolved macular dysfunction. Scotoma with macular disease apparent indicates that the lesion is probably inactive

color vision may be evaluated simultaneously.

The home Amsler grid is often advocated for patients suspected of having the early signs of macular diseases such as age-related macular degeneration. Unfortunately the patient is often noncompliant or does not understand the significance of the test, and often misses the early development of the wet phases of the disease process. However, the home Amsler grid is still an important adjunct in our battle with macular degenerative diseases. The nonspecificity and often insensitivity of Amsler grid testing dictates that it is not effective when used alone.

POTENTIAL ACUITY/ INTERFEROMETRY TESTING

The assessment of vision function is essential prior to making decisions about cataract surgery or regarding potential for recovery if other media opacities are present. Several methods are available, but most rely on coherent light creating a Maxwellian view being directed toward the macular area. Either letters or interference patterns are projected directly on the retina. The test must be performed through a dilated pupil in order to direct the beam around the media opacities as the beam cannot actually "burn through" the haze. The refractive error is irrelevant in the interferometry systems but must be compensated in the systems relying on Snellen acuity equivalents. The clinician should consult the specific directions available from individual manufacturers.

There are interferometers that actually use a laser as a source of illumination, but other varieties use incandescent light sources. Clinical experience has shown that each variety has benefits but neither seems superior. Experience has also shown that the test is not infallible and that not all patients can perform the test. It is, however, a test that can provide some insight into the retinal status with a compromised cornea or media.

STEREOSCOPIC VIEWING TECHNIQUES

Several instruments are available for examination of the retina anterior to the equator. Monocular indirect ophthalmoscopy can get the job done but suffers from (1) a lack of stereo examination ability, (2) a relatively poor light source, (3) no method of adjusting magnification, (4) lower resolution capabilities than binocular indirect ophthalmoscopy, and (5) inability to effectively perform scleral indentation.

Examination of the peripheral retina with a three-mirror lens has the advantage of variable magnification, variable illumination, availability of filters, and stereopsis. One can perform scleral indentation with specially adapted three-mirror lenses. The primary disadvantage of this technique is the reduction in observable field of view accompanied by a reduced resolution ability. The view is similar to looking at a grainy photograph at a close distance. This technique is useful as an adjunct to binocular indirect ophthalmoscopy.

The binocular indirect ophthalmoscope and the currently available variety of fundus lenses all offer an excellent view of the posterior pole. The panfundus lens varieties also open a new dimension for stereoscopic evaluation of the posterior pole and equatorial zone. The new technology in digitized imagery offers both a superb recordable view of the optic nerve head and the potential of stereoscopic fluorescein angiography, opening the doors for incredible diagnostic latitude. Elevations, depressions, color variations, and size differences all are key factors in diagnosing optic nerve and retinal disease. Stereoscopic viewing techniques are indispensable for proper ocular diagnoses. Regardless of the new technology, the best tools that the practitioner has available are the binocular indirect ophthalmoscope with scleral indentation, the fundus lenses, and the three-mirror lenses for observation of the peripheral retina.

The binocular indirect ophthalmoscope is an absolute necessity for effective evaluation of vitreoretinal diseases, especially those anterior to the equator. The binocular indirect ophthalmoscope offers (1) variable field of view and variable magnification, (2) access to the farthest peripheral regions of the retina, (3) a bright light source and improved resolution, (4) excellent stereopsis, and (5) the ability to add scleral indentation for more complete fundus evaluation. The disadvantages to binocular indirect ophthalmoscopy involve adaptation to the inverted reversed image as well as the difficulty of adaptation to the instrument.

Binocular Indirect Ophthalmoscopy

Binocular indirect ophthalmoscopy provides a method for evaluation of the entire fundus under dilation. Adjunctive procedures such as scleral indentation allow for the dynamic evaluation of the peripheral retina. The optics of the situation and the resolution capacity allow for viewing through hazy media or around central opacities of the lens with relative disregard for the degree of refractive error. This system also has the ability to uncover lesions with poor resolution such as benign choroidal melanoma and cotton-wool spots. The most important aspect of the binocular indirect ophthalmoscope is the fact that stereopsis becomes reality and most disease is manifest as elevation or depression and color change. The type of scope used is an individual preference, but the key to a good scope is the light source. It must be uniform in intensity and defocused—that is, the filament should not be seen. The position of the light source is also crucial. When viewing the posterior pole, the source should be directed in the upper half of the field to minimize corneal reflections. When viewing the periphery, the view is enhanced by moving the source more centrally in the field, as the pupil becomes elliptical when the eye is positioned for peripheral viewing.

The condensing lens is also an important aspect of the binocular indirect examination. The standard +20D lens produces 2.5× magnification and a 35-degree or 8 disc diameter field. The direct scope on the other hand produces a 2 disc diameter field and 15× magnification. With a reduction in condensing lens power the field decreases and the magnification increases, whereas an increase in power increases the field and reduces the magnification. A +14D lens gives 3.5× magnification, and a +28D lens gives 1.5× magnification. One other variation on the condensing lens is the optional amber tint, which increases patient comfort as well as reducing phototoxic risk from the short blue wavelengths of light. With increasing evidence of the negative effects of short blue wavelengths of light precipitating degenerative conditions of the retinal pigment epithelium and retina, it is advisable to minimize these wavelengths whenever possible.

Technique is crucial for success with binocular indirect ophthalmoscopy. After adjusting the scope and setting the light source, turn the most convex surface of the condensing lens toward you, and stand at about arm's length from the patient. A perpendicular line should run from the intersection of the light source and the condensing lens to the oculars of the scope. Alteration of this alignment will compromise the view. After introducing the light into the dilated pupil, introduce the condensing lens near the eye and move it toward you until the lens is filled with the fundus image. Remember that you always stand opposite the area that is to be viewed, and that all images are upside-down and reversed. The examination of the entire fundus is accomplished by having the patient alter fixation combined with movements of the examiner into the different fields. The total examination is very difficult; I advise that if the clinician is totally comfortable during the examination, it is probably not a thorough examination. Binocular indirect ophthalmoscopy is a dynamic procedure; the clinician must keep moving. It should also be remembered that when viewing the extreme periphery, it is impossible to fill the condensing lens, and stereoscopic viewing is minimized.

Scleral Indentation

The anterior portion of the retina is difficult at best to see even with maximal dilation. Stereoscopic viewing is minimized, as is resolution in an area that can be critical in the symptomatic patient.

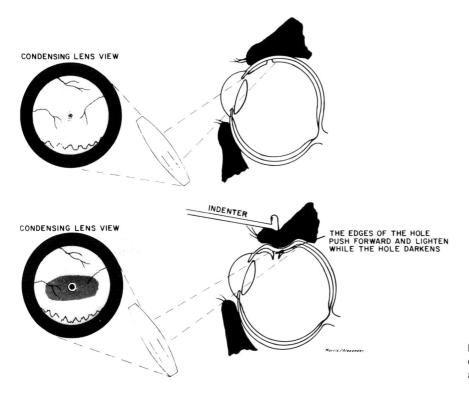

CONDENSING LENS VIEW

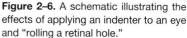
INDENTER

CONDENSING LENS VIEW

THE EDGES OF THE HOLE
PUSH FORWARD AND LIGHTEN
WHILE THE HOLE DARKENS

Figure 2–6. A schematic illustrating the effects of applying an indenter to an eye and "rolling a retinal hole."

Mastering scleral indentation elevates the clinician to the highest level of diagnostic skill in peripheral retinal evaluation. In reality, it is close to impossible to discern subtleties of the retina near the ora without the benefit of scleral indentation. Not only does scleral indentation push retinal structural alterations into view but it increases the contrast between intact retina and retinal breaks (Fig. 2–6). The indented retinal–choroidal structure is darker than the surrounding retina, which increases the contrast. It is also important to realize that there is decreased retinal translucency with indentation because the examiner is viewing the retina at a more oblique angle. Scleral indentation is a kinetic procedure as well, which enhances the discovery of subtle changes. It is far easier to see changes when the retinal structures are moving. The discovery of retinal tears and holes is facilitated with indentation, as the edges roll upward and lighten while the hole darkens. The rolling of holes is illustrated in Figure 2–6.

It is important to orient oneself to retinal structure prior to the performance of scleral indentation. Figure 2–7 gives the basic ocular dimensions from the corneal limbus to facilitate orientation with common retinal landmarks. It is important to realize that to indent the equator, it is only necessary to place the indenter 13 mm or about ½ inch posterior to the limbus. The distance back from the limbus to most structures that need to be viewed is almost always less than 13 mm.

Scleral indentation can be performed safely in most patients. Patients with active glaucoma or intraocular lenses should be indented with great care. Patients with recent intraocular surgery or those suspected of having penetrating trauma should not be indented. Choice of the type of indenter is at the discretion of the practitioner.

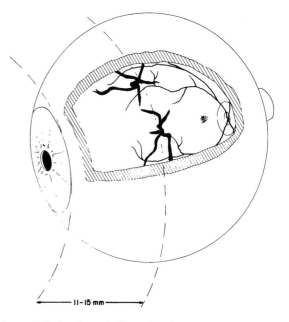

11–15 mm

Figure 2–7. A schematic illustrating the relatively short distance from the limbus to the equator.

Technique for Scleral Indentation

1. Topical anesthesia may be applied to the eye prior to indentation, but remember that this may cause mild corneal edema and sloughing. This will obviously compromise the view. Most of the time indentation is performed through the lids, which eliminates the need for anesthesia.
2. Maximal dilation is an absolute necessity. This often necessitates a combination of 1% tropicamide plus 2.5% phenylephrine.
3. Educate the patient as to the mild discomfort (pressure) experienced during the procedure.
4. Recline the patient and tilt the head forward, backward, and side to side to maximize the view. An example of this would be tilting the head back (chin up) to facilitate the view of the superior retina.
5. To view the 12 o'clock position (the easiest zone to view), ask the patient to gently close the eyes and to look down. Place the tip of the indenter on the upper lid at the margin of the tarsal plate (do not attempt to indent through the tarsal plate as this will be painful to the patient).
6. While maintaining the position of the indentor, have the patient slowly look up—the practitioner must move the indentor tip back as the eye rolls upward.
7. Remember that the indenter tip should always be tangential to the globe—not perpendicular, as this would be painful. Also remember to keep line of sight, condensing lens, and shaft of the indenter aligned. Figure 2–8 illustrates proper alignment. If any factor is out of alignment the retinal orientation is quickly lost.
8. When all factors are aligned, exert gentle pressure and view the mound created by the indentation.

The necessary pressure can only be attained through practice.

9. Remember that indentation is intended to be a kinetic procedure. Move the indenter gently, remembering to keep the entire observation system aligned. Also recall that the indenter must be moved opposite to what appears to be necessary when viewing through the condensing lens. Said another way, move the indenter toward the cornea to view the retina inferior in the condensing lens. Once the accessible area has been examined, move to the next quadrant.
10. To depress the 3 o'clock and 9 o'clock quadrants, it may be necessary to drag the lids up or down into position. If there is not enough laxity of the lids, it may be necessary to anesthetize and depress directly on the bulbar conjunctiva.

There is no magic to performing scleral indentation. Just remember that it is like rubbing one's stomach and patting one's head at the same time. Keep the tip tangential to the globe, exert gentle pressure, move the tip, and keep line of sight, condensing lens, and shaft of the indenter aligned.

Fundus Lens Examination

Stereoscopic examination of the posterior pole has reached new heights with the introduction of fundus lens evaluation. The fundus lens, like the condensing lens, creates an inverted reversed image that takes some getting used to, but the view is incredible. Several lenses are available including +60D, +78D, and +90D, with the option of a lens holder for the +90D and spacing rings for the other lenses as well that rest on the patient's lids. Now included in the list are the

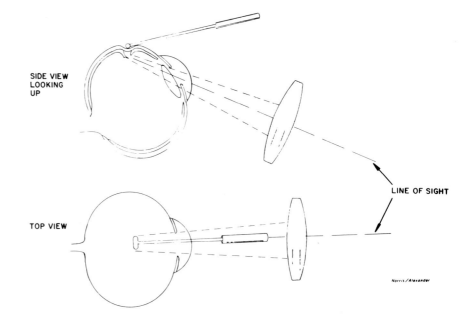

SIDE VIEW LOOKING UP

TOP VIEW

LINE OF SIGHT

Norris/Alexander

Figure 2–8. A schematic illustrating the proper alignment of the scleral indenter, condensing lens, and line of sight.

variations of the panfundus lenses. The lenses vary in the degree of magnification—the lowest power with the highest magnification—and the field of view. The amber tint is also available to improve patient comfort and to minimize the risk from the short wavelengths.

After dilation, the patient is placed in the slit lamp at low magnification and a 2 to 3 mm width beam perpendicular to the cornea. The lamp is then moved close to the cornea to create a retroilluminated red pupillary reflex. The lens is then introduced near the cornea and moved toward the practitioner until the fundus is viewed. Manipulations of the lens, the lamp, the patient's eyes, and the practitioner are necessary to maximize effectiveness of the examination. The magnification of the lamp may be increased to facilitate more extensive examination of a specific area, remembering that rapid eye movements will be enhanced and will compromise the view. Although it is possible to examine a reasonable portion of the retina with fundus lenses, the technique is not a replacement for binocular indirect ophthalmoscopy.

FLUORESCEIN ANGIOGRAPHY

Fluorescein angiography is a crucial test for the differential diagnosis of retinal vascular disease and acquired serous macular disease. The technique has recently gained favor for assisting in the differential diagnosis of optic nerve disease. This is logical, because the majority of acquired optic nerve diseases would manifest delayed filling from infarcted vessels or leakage from neovascularization or inflamed discs.

The Basics of Fluorescein Studies

Fluorescein angiography and oral fluorography are gaining importance as diagnostic tools now that new developments are being made in laser treatment of retinal vascular disease. Laser modifications and a better understanding of ocular vasculopathy are allowing for earlier therapeutic intervention, treatment closer to the macula (foveal avascular zone, or FAZ), and better visual results. All recent studies point to the importance of early diagnosis of retinal and choroidal vascular disease. In general, the earlier a disease process is discovered and treated, the better the clinical results.

Fluorescein has been used in vision care for over 100 years. The use of fluorescein by the oral route of administration to study the retinal vasculature was attempted in 1910. The first use of intravenous fluorescein was reported in 1930, and several other reports followed over the next 30 years. The most significant work, however, came in 1961, with photodocumentation of fluorescein studies. The photographs allowed a more detailed logical approach to understanding fluorescein angiography. The first comprehensive text on fluorescein studies was published in 1977 and was soon followed by other works.

The concept of oral fluorography was resurrected in 1979 to conduct fluorescein studies without the potential systemic side effects. Further studies in oral fluorography established the technique as a viable alternative in diagnosis of retinal vascular diseases. The Oral Fluorescein Study Group was formed in 1984 to further evaluate the orally administered fluorescein technique. The report in 1985 concluded that oral fluorography was not a substitute for the diagnostic capabilities of intravenous fluorescein angiography but was a significant diagnostic tool, especially for fundus disorders that demonstrated fluorescein leakage. It was concluded that minimal side effects occurred with oral administration, whereas it is known that intravenous fluorescein administration carries risks.

Why Perform Fluorescein Angiography?

There must be justification for any diagnostic procedure that has an inherent risk to the patient. Is it safe to assume that a careful dilated fundus examination with state-of-the-art instrumentation is sufficient for maximal patient care? Unfortunately, this assumption is not always valid. It is reasonable to assume that the more diagnostic input that is available, the more efficient and effective is patient management.

Fluorescein angiography is especially useful in detection of subclinical retinal changes in diabetic patients. One study reported that of 272 eyes of 166 patients with no ophthalmoscopically visible vascular changes, fluorescein angiography demonstrated diabetic vascular changes in 66.5 percent. Other reports cite angiographic changes in diabetic children that were not observed by ophthalmoscopy alone. Fluorescein studies have demonstrated significant vascular changes in the midperiphery that were overlooked previously. Prudent clinical judgment would dictate that fluorescein studies should be performed in diabetic patients with any unexplained reduction in macular function, with encroachment of diabetic retinopathy into the macular area, with any sign of proliferative retinopathy, with the appearance of intraretinal microvascular abnormalities (IRMA), and with the appearance of three or more signs of preproliferative diabetic retinopathy. Table 2–4 outlines some ocular disease processes that indicate the need for fluorescein angiography to assist in the differential diagnosis.

The one fact that the clinician must always remember is that a very high percentage of vision-threatening ocular disease has associated leaking retinal or choroidal vessels. Leaking retinal and choroidal vessels are best seen with fluorescein angiography. Edema is most difficult, if not impossible at times, to see with ophthalmoscopy alone.

TABLE 2–4. COMMON OCULAR DISEASE CONDITIONS INDICATING THE NEED FOR FLUORESCEIN ANGIOGRAPHY

Acute posterior multifocal placoid pigment epitheliopathy (APMPPE)
Angiomatosis retinae
Anterior ischemic optic neuropathy
Behçet's disease
Branch retinal vein occlusion
Cavernous hemangioma of the retina
Choroidal rupture (when developing choroidal neovascularization)
Coats' disease (retinal telangiectasia)
Cystoid maculopathy (Irvine–Gass syndrome)
Diabetic retinopathy: If near macula, if proliferative, if intraretinal microvascular abnormalities
Eales disease
Fuch's spot (degenerative myopia)
Hemicentral retinal vein occlusion
Idiopathic central serous choroidopathy
Iris neovascularization
Maculopathy of angioid streaks
Malignant choroidal melanoma
Preretinal macular fibrosis
Presumed ocular histoplasmosis (macular changes)
Proliferative peripheral retinal disease
Retinal capillary hemangioma
Retinal macroaneurysm
Retinal pigment epithelial dystrophies (central)
Retinal pigment epithelial detachment
Retinal tumors
Sensory retinal detachments
Tumors of iris and ciliary body

Technique of Intravenous Fluorescein Angiography

Fluorescein studies may be performed with or without an appropriate fundus camera. If performed with a binocular indirect ophthalmoscopy, the technique is known as fluorescein angioscopy. To successfully perform fluorescein angioscopy, the binocular indirect ophthalmoscope must be equipped with a high-intensity light source and appropriate filters. Most currently available binocular indirect ophthalmoscopes are not equipped to perform fluorescein angioscopy.

If fluorescein photographic studies are desired, it is necessary to use an appropriately equipped fundus camera. This camera must have a high-intensity flash system with a rapid recycle time as well as appropriate blue excitation and yellow–green barrier filters. The excitation filter should be either the Baird Atomic B4 470 or Kodak Wratten 47 to create a light to stimulate fluorescence. The standard cobalt blue filter is ineffectual. The barrier filter should be either an Ilford 109 Delta Chromatic 3 or Kodak Wratten G15 to block the exciting light from the film plane, allowing only visualization of the fluorescing blood. It should be noted that both barrier and excitation filters lose specificity (fade) with age and should be replaced according to manufacturer's guidelines. It is advisable to fit the camera back with a power winder, because the early phases of fluorescein studies necessitate rapid-fire photography.

Several films and developing processes are available to enhance the results of the studies. Although it is easy to advise the use of any high-speed 200 to 400 ASA black-and-white film, it is difficult to advise on processing. It is probably best to contact a local film-processing laboratory or someone else in the community who routinely performs fluorescein studies regarding the optimal processing and film usage. There are some studies that advocate color film because of the ability of the studies to eliminate autofluorescence, but adoption of this technique has met with resistance.

Although other dyes have been tried, sodium fluorescein is still the accepted standard. Sodium fluorescein for intravenous injection is available in 5, 10, and 25% concentrations. Generic brands are available at considerably reduced prices and may be used without fear. One study, however, reports the presence of a toxic substance, dimethyl formamide, an industrial solvent, in commercially prepared sodium fluorescein for injection. Outdated fluorescein carries the potential for side effects, such as an increase in the incidence of nausea.

Sodium fluorescein is considered pharmacologically inert and fluoresces when stimulated by an excited light source. Fluorescein is injected into a suitable vein in the antecubital space or on the hand. It reaches ocular circulation bound to serum albumin and in a free unbound state. This then fluoresces, allowing for easy visualization of vascular alterations and leakage out of altered vasculature. Factors affecting the quality of the results include clarity of the media, maximal dilation of the patient, and most of all the concentration of sodium fluorescein reaching the retinal–choroidal vascular system. Improper injection is the most significant factor contributing to decreased retinal–choroidal concentration. The injection must be into the vein and performed in a 10 to 15 second time frame.

A crash cart (cardiopulmonary resuscitation unit) must be available on site to handle any potential side effects. Before the procedure, the clinician must ensure that (1) a release form has been read and signed, (2) the patient is aware of what is about to transpire, (3) the patient is maximally dilated, (4) color photographs of the fundus have been taken, (5) red-free photographs of the fundus have been taken on the black-and-white angiographic film, (6) the fundus camera and patient are adjusted to appropriate comfortable height, (7) the filters are placed in the camera, (8) the proper flash settings are made, and (9) an appropriate intravenous line has been established and maintained with heparinized saline. Then, with 5 mL of 10% sodium fluorescein ready in a syringe to replace the heparinized saline, situate the patient in front of the camera and have an assistant attach the syringe of fluorescein. When behind the camera with the appropriate area of the patient's fundus in focus and the filters in place, have the assistant rapidly (over 10 to 15 seconds) inject the bolus of fluorescein. The photography usually begins within about 15 seconds, which is the choroidal flush phase, before which nothing can be seen in the fundus. Rapid-sequence photographs are taken within the first few minutes, then intermittently for the next 10 to 20 minutes. Late-phase photographs will pick up leakage problems, such as sensory retinal detachments associated with choroidal neovascular nets. Specific timing sequences depend on the suspected disease being investigated.

Complications of Intravenous Fluorescein Angiography

Complications are inherent in any procedure such as fluorescein angiography. Fortunately, the more common complications can be managed easily without aborting the diagnostic procedure. One study reported adverse reactions in 4.82 percent of 5000 procedures. Of these, nausea was most frequent (2.24 percent), followed by vomiting (1.78 percent) and urticaria or pruritus (0.34 percent). It was also found that there was no higher rate of side effects when 25% sodium fluorescein was used than when 10% sodium fluorescein was used. The itching and hives are thought to be associated with a change in the plasma complement level associated with a rise in the histamine level. In another study of 2631 procedures, it was found that males and young patients experienced side effects at a higher rate. In this study, a single life-threatening situation, acute pulmonary edema, was reported. Attempts have been made to provide prophylaxis against the histaminic side effects of fluorescein angiography, but statistically significant positive results were not achieved. The author has found that the primary side effect of nausea or warm flush occurs within the first 30 seconds after injection and is very transient in nature. Advising the patient of this potential side effect and assuring the patient that it is very quick to leave has allowed me to take the patient through the problem without aborting the procedure. It is wise to advise patients that their skin and urine will be discolored for a few days after the procedure.

Technique of Oral Fluorography

Oral fluorography can give results similar to those obtained with intravenous fluorescein angiography without the potential side effects. Oral fluorography is especially useful in cases where late dye leakage is expected. It can be performed using either USP bulk and powder sodium fluorescein or commercially available 5-mL vials of 10% injectable sodium fluorescein. The powdered form is difficult to obtain, but using two to three 5-mL vials of 10% fluorescein is usually sufficient to obtain good results. The fluorescein is mixed with a powdered flavored citrus drink and allowed to cool in crushed ice. The patient fasts about 8 hours before the test. The patient is then asked to remove any dentures, because the solution will discolor these devices. Before the procedure it must be ensured that (1) a release form has been read and signed, (2) the patient is aware of what is about to transpire, (3) the patient is maximally dilated, (4) color photographs of the fundus have been taken, (5) red-free photographs have been taken, (6) the fundus camera has been adjusted, and (7) the proper film has been loaded, filters put in place, and flash settings set. The patient is then asked to drink the solution rapidly through a straw to prevent staining of the lips.

Photography begins at the first sign of retinal circulation (15 to 30 minutes), with the late phase showing in about 1 hour. As with intravenous studies, the skin and urine will be slightly discolored for a few days.

Reported complications of oral fluorography are few and minor. It has been suggested that it would take ingestion of 90 g of fluorescein by a 100-pound person to produce a toxic effect.

The technique has been reported useful in children and certainly has potential in patients with cardiovascular compromise who may be at risk for an intravenous procedure.

Interpretation of Fluorescein Angiography

A good basic understanding of retinal–choroidal anatomy and vasculature is crucial for interpretation of fluorescein angiography. Some basic features of the retinal and choroidal system create the diagnostic capabilities of fluorescein angiography:

1. Healthy retinal vessels do not leak fluorescein because the vessel walls are not fenestrated.
2. Healthy choriocapillaris vessels are fenestrated and freely leak, creating a spongelike tissue.
3. In a healthy retina, the fluid in the choriocapillaris is kept away from the sensory retina by an intact RPE–Bruch's membrane barrier. The RPE (retinal pigment epithelium) also serves as a filter to allow only part of the choroidal glow to show through. If the RPE is absent, more glow (hyperfluorescence) will be visible; if there is an excess of RPE, less glow (hypofluorescence) will be visible. Dense RPE and xanthophyl mask the choroidal flush in a healthy macula.

In addition to the basic anatomic characteristics, there is the consideration of the time-related stages of the angiogram. The stages are classically described as the choroidal flush (prearterial phase), the arterio-venous phase, and the late phase. The choroidal flush occurs within seconds postinjection. The posterior ciliary arteries supply the choroidal system in a patchy pattern that is quickly masked by the fluorescein leaking into the choroidal swamp through fenestrated vasculature. With RPE retention disease and some choroidal dystrophies, the choroidal flush is silent. This fluorescein will stay within the swamp if the RPE–Bruch's membrane barrier is healthy. Observation of the choroidal flush stage is especially useful in the determination of diseases of the choroidal vasculature or the RPE–Bruch's membrane barrier, such as the choroidal neovascularization in age-related maculopathy.

Within a few more seconds, the retinal arteries start to fill in a laminar flow pattern. The central core of the artery glows first, followed by filling to the limits of the walls. The capillaries then fill, followed by the laminar filling of the veins. With the veins, the area of the blood column near the walls glows first, followed by filling to the center. The walls of the arteries, capillaries, and veins in the healthy retina are not fenestrated, and as such should demonstrate no leakage. Any disease condition that creates breakdown of vessel walls with subsequent leakage or neovascularization would be most apparent in this stage. An example of a breakdown in the vessel walls is the leaking of microaneurysms in diabetic retinopathy.

The late stages of fluorescein angiography usually occur about 10 minutes postinjection. During this stage, the arteries and veins have almost emptied of fluorescein, and the underlying choroidal flush is minimized. The optic nerve remains hyperfluorescent as the dye adheres to the nerve tissue. During this stage, leakage of choroidal and retinal vessels becomes more apparent by the diffusely spreading staining pattern overlying the vascular lesion. Late staining also occurs in sensory retinal detachments and RPE detachments because of leakage through Bruch's membrane from underlying choroidal structures.

Application of the time stages of fluorescein angiography and the basic retinal–choroidal anatomy allows for effective fluorescein angiogram interpretation. Two basic situations occur in diseased conditions: (1) hypofluorescence, or a blockage of the glow where you would normally expect it; and (2) hyperfluorescence, or an excessive glow where you would not normally expect it.

Disease Conditions That Create Hypofluorescence and Hyperfluorescence

Fluorescein angiography is an invaluable tool for the differential diagnosis of retinal vascular disease. Table 2–5 outlines conditions that create hypofluorescence or hyperfluorescence.

TABLE 2–5. COMMON OCULAR CONDITIONS CREATING HYPOFLUORESCENCE OR HYPERFLUORESCENCE

Site	Hypofluorescence	Hyperfluorescence
Retinal pigment epithelium (RPE)–Bruch's membrane	APMPPE, Early Congenital hypertrophy of RPE RPE hyperplasia	Age-related maculopathy, dry Angioid streaks APMPPE, late Choroidal folds Choroioretinal scars Drusen ICSC (cystoid maculopathy) Retinal hole RPE detachment RPE window defects Serous sensory RD
Choroid	Benign choroidal melanoma with no overlying serous detachment	Choroidal neovascularization Malignant choroidal melanoma
Retina	Branch retinal artery occlusion Central retinal artery occlusion Cotton wool spots Preretinal hemorrhages Retinal exudates Subretinal hemorrhages	Angiomatosis retinae Capillary hemangioma Cavernous hemangioma, stasis Leaking compromised veins Macroaneurysms Microaneurysms Neovascularization, retina Periphlebitis Telangiectasia
Optic nerve		Anterior–ischemic optic neuropathy Neovascularization, disc Papilledema

APMPPE, acute posterior multifocal placoid pigment epitheliopathy; ICSC, idiopathic central serous choroidopathy; RD, retinal detachment.

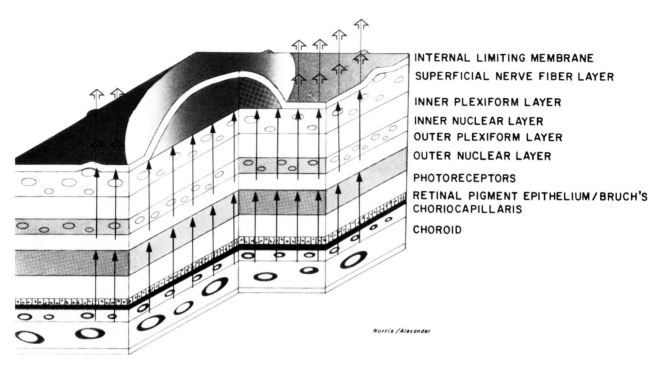

INTERNAL LIMITING MEMBRANE
SUPERFICIAL NERVE FIBER LAYER

INNER PLEXIFORM LAYER
INNER NUCLEAR LAYER
OUTER PLEXIFORM LAYER
OUTER NUCLEAR LAYER

PHOTORECEPTORS
RETINAL PIGMENT EPITHELIUM/BRUCH'S
CHORIOCAPILLARIS

CHOROID

Norris/Alexander

Figure 2–9. A clinicopathologic cross section of the retina with a preretinal hemorrhage. *(Reprinted with permission from Alexander LJ. How to perform and interpret fluorescein angiography. Rev Optom. 1988;125:72–82.)*

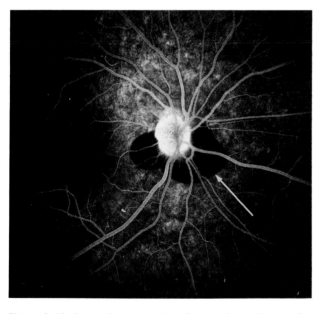

Figure 2–10. An arteriovenous-stage fluorescein angiogram of a subretinal hemorrhage *(arrow)*.

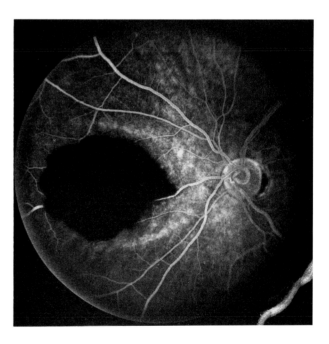

Figure 2–11. An arteriovenous-stage fluorescein angiogram of a preretinal hemorrhage.

■ ■ ■ ■ ■ ■

Clinical Example: Hypofluorescence (I)

Preretinal hemorrhages lie on top of the retina, blocking the view of both the choroid and retinal structure. A scotoma is created in this area. Figure 2–9 shows a clinico-pathologic cross section of the retina with a preretinal hemorrhage. The dark arrows represent the fluorescein pattern of the choroidal flush coming toward the observer, and the open arrows represent the choroidal flush that is actually seen. The preretinal hemorrhage blocks the choroidal flush. Figure 2–10 shows an arteriovenous-

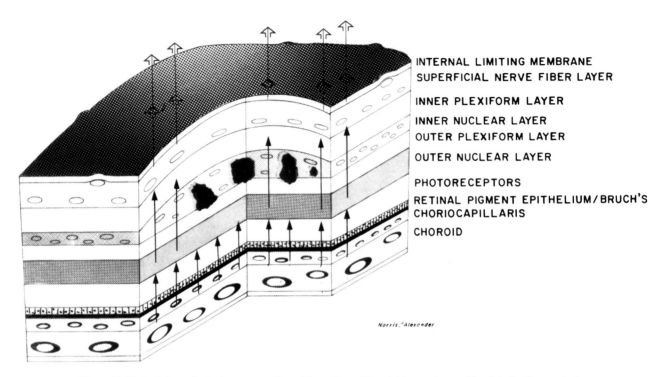

INTERNAL LIMITING MEMBRANE
SUPERFICIAL NERVE FIBER LAYER

INNER PLEXIFORM LAYER

INNER NUCLEAR LAYER

OUTER PLEXIFORM LAYER

OUTER NUCLEAR LAYER

PHOTORECEPTORS

RETINAL PIGMENT EPITHELIUM/BRUCH'S

CHORIOCAPILLARIS

CHOROID

Norris/Alexander

Figure 2–12. A clinicopathologic cross section of the retina with a dot hemorrhage. *(Reprinted with permission from Alexander LJ. How to perform and interpret fluorescein angiography. Rev Optom. 1988;125:72–82.)*

stage fluorescein angiogram demonstrating a hemorrhage around the disc that blocks choroidal fluorescence but does not block retinal vessel fluorescence. This means that the hemorrhage is between the retinal vessels and the choriocapillaris, or subretinal. Figure 2–11 shows an arteriovenous-stage fluorescein angiogram demonstrating a hemorrhage that blocks both choroidal and retinal vessel fluorescence. This is interpreted as the hemorrhage being above the choroid and the retinal vessels, or a preretinal hemorrhage.

◼ ◼ ◼ ◼ ◼ ◼
Clinical Example: Hypofluorescence (II)

Dot-blot hemorrhages lie within the retina near the inner nuclear layer blocking the photoreceptors and the underlying choroid but not the retinal vessels. Figure 2–12 illustrates dot-blot hemorrhages in a clinicopathologic cross section. The dark arrows represent the fluorescein pattern of the underlying choroidal flush coming toward the observer, and the open arrows represent the choroidal flush that is actually seen. The dot-blot hemorrhage blocks the choroidal flush. Figure 2–13 shows an arteriovenous-phase angiogram demonstrating an isolated area of blockage of the choroidal flush secondary to a dot-blot hemorrhage.

◼ ◼ ◼ ◼ ◼ ◼
Clinical Example: Hypofluorescence (III)

Cotton-wool spots represent areas of ischemia in the superficial nerve fiber layer. As such they lie above retinal and choroidal structures. Figure 2–14 illustrates a clinicopathologic cross section of a cotton-wool spot. The dark arrows represent the fluorescein pattern of the underlying choroidal flush, and the open arrows represent

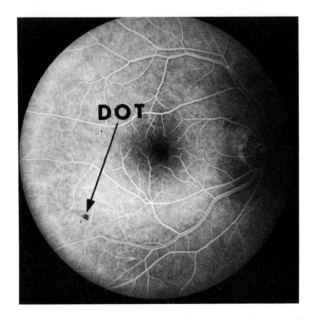

Figure 2–13. An arteriovenous-stage fluorescein angiogram of a dot hemorrhage.

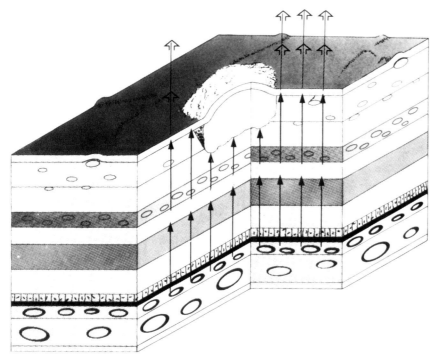

INTERNAL LIMITING MEMBRANE
SUPERFICIAL NERVE FIBER LAYER

INNER PLEXIFORM LAYER

INNER NUCLEAR LAYER
OUTER PLEXIFORM LAYER
OUTER NUCLEAR LAYER

PHOTORECEPTORS

RETINAL PIGMENT EPITHELIUM/BRUCH'S
CHORIOCAPILLARIS
CHOROID

Figure 2–14. A clinicopathologic cross section of the retina with a cotton-wool spot. *(Reprinted with permission from Alexander LJ. How to perform and interpret fluorescein angiography. Rev Optom. 1988;125:72–82.)*

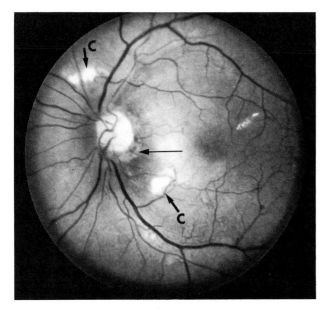

Figure 2–15. Photograph demonstrating areas of cotton-wool spots and disc neovascularization.

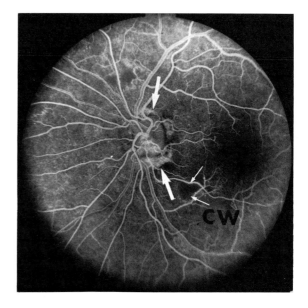

Figure 2–16. Fluorescein angiogram of cotton-wool spots and disc neovascularization shown in Figure 2–15. Large arrows point to leaking disc neovascularization and small arrows to hypofluorescence created by cotton-wool spots.

the choroidal flush that actually is seen. The cotton-wool spot blocks the choroidal flush and retinal vessel glow. Figure 2–15 is a photograph of cotton-wool spots (small arrows) and disc neovascularization (large arrows). Figure 2–16 shows the venous phase, with the large arrows pointing to the enlarging disc neovascularization and the small arrows to the area of blockage of background choroidal fluorescence secondary to a cotton-wool spot. It should be noted that the vessels surrounding the cotton-wool spot are compromised and leaking.

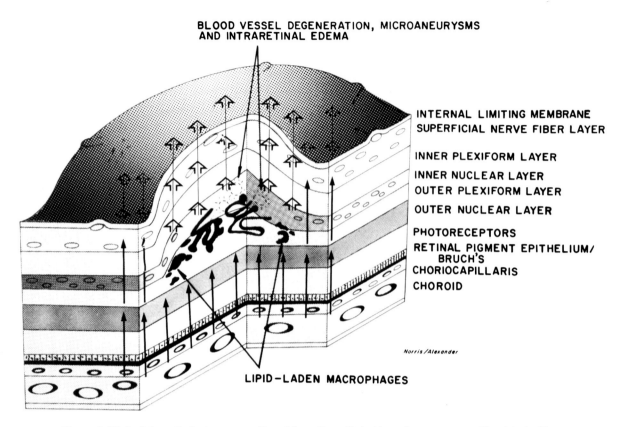

BLOOD VESSEL DEGENERATION, MICROANEURYSMS
AND INTRARETINAL EDEMA

INTERNAL LIMITING MEMBRANE
SUPERFICIAL NERVE FIBER LAYER

INNER PLEXIFORM LAYER
INNER NUCLEAR LAYER
OUTER PLEXIFORM LAYER
OUTER NUCLEAR LAYER

PHOTORECEPTORS
RETINAL PIGMENT EPITHELIUM/
BRUCH'S
CHORIOCAPILLARIS
CHOROID

Norris/Alexander

LIPID–LADEN MACROPHAGES

Figure 2–17. A clinicopathologic cross section of the retina with leaking microaneurysms. *(Reprinted with permission from Alexander LJ. How to perform and interpret fluorescein angiography. Rev Optom. 1988;125:72–82.)*

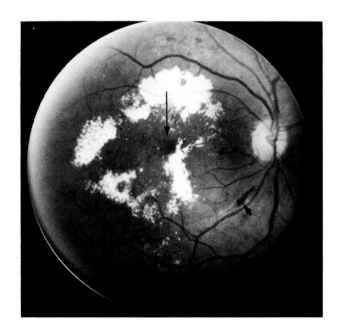

Figure 2–18. Photograph of hard exudates surrounding the macula *(long arrow)*. The short arrow points to a flame-shaped hemorrhage.

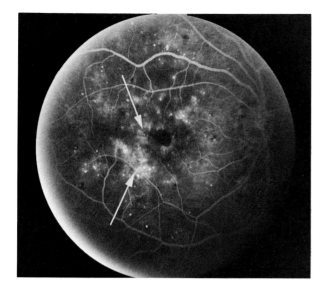

Figure 2–19. Fluorescein angiogram of patient in Figure 2–18, demonstrating areas of significant edema *(arrows)* secondary to leaking microaneurysms.

■ ■ ■ ■ ■ ■
Clinical Example: Hyperfluorescence (I)

Hard exudate formation occurs secondary to a breakdown in retinal tissue and blood vessels. This breakdown occurs when microaneurysms leak, creating intraretinal edema in which a lipid soup is cooked. Figure 2–17 illustrates a clinicopathologic cross section of the retina in which microaneurysms are leaking. The dark arrows represent the fluorescein pattern of the underlying choroidal flush, and the open arrows represent the flush that actually is seen. Hard exudates lie deep within the retina, blocking underlying choroidal fluorescence. The leaking microaneurysms that contribute to the problem will hyperfluoresce. Figures 2–18 and 2–19 show a patient with hard exudates in the macula secondary to leaking microaneurysms. The ensuing edema compromises the retina, creating reduced visual acuity.

With this basic description of the clinicopathologic process, further case presentations will enhance the understanding of fluorescein angiogram interpretation.

■ ■ ■ ■ ■ ■
Clinical Example: Hyperfluorescence (II)

Figures 2–20 to 2–23 illustrate the differentiation of benign drusen and/or RPE window defects from microaneurysms. Figures 2–20 and 2–21 show different patients with RPE window defects, Figure 2–20 being an early phase (note that the vein is just starting laminar filling) and Figure 2–21 a later phase. In both instances, the macular area pigment blocks background choroidal fluorescence, but isolated areas of glow occur within the hypofluorescence (black arrows). These isolated areas of glow do not spread with time, implying no leakage. When there is hyperfluorescence that does not enlarge over time, it is safe to assume that there is a benign defect in the RPE, such as a drusen or an RPE window defect. Figure 2–22 demonstrates hyperfluorescence at the early stages of the angiogram, with an enlargement of the area of hyperfluorescence over time (Fig. 2–23). When this occurs, there is spread of edema, with a resultant direct threat to vision.

■ ■ ■ ■ ■ ■
Clinical Example: Hyperfluorescence (III)

Another situation that can create edema with a threat to vision is idiopathic central serous choroidopathy (ICSC). ICSC results from a break in the RPE–Bruch's membrane barrier, allowing for seepage of the choriocapillaris fluid into the retina. Figure 2–24 illustrates an area of hyperfluorescence in the normally dark macular area that enlarges slightly and becomes more diffuse in the later stages (Fig. 2–25). This is a case of ICSC in a 45-year-old man. Figures 2–26 and 2–27 demonstrate the progression of this case over a 5-year period. Metamorphopsia increased significantly over the years.

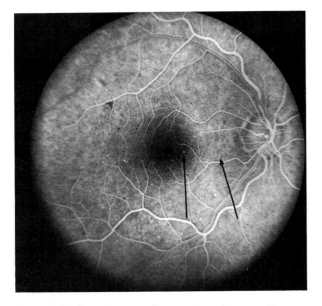

Figure 2–20. An early-stage fluorescein angiogram with arrows pointing to hyperfluorescence.

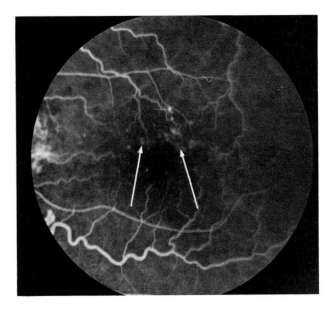

Figure 2–22. An early-stage angiogram demonstrating areas of focal hyperfluorescence *(arrows)*.

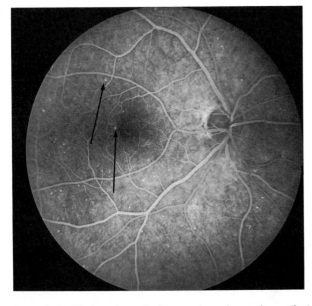

Figure 2–21. The late stage of a fluorescein angiogram in a patient with a benign defect in the RPE with no spread of hyperfluorescence.

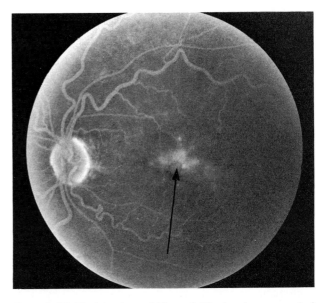

Figure 2–23. The late stage of Figure 2–22, showing a spread of hyperfluorescence. In this case, it is indicative of leaking microaneurysms.

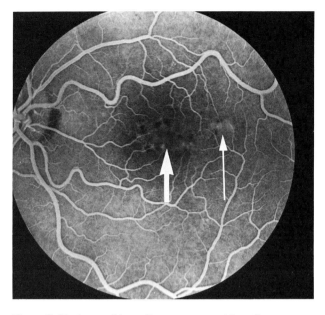

Figure 2–24. Areas of hyperfluorescence and hypofluorescence in the macular area characteristic of idiopathic central serous choroidopathy.

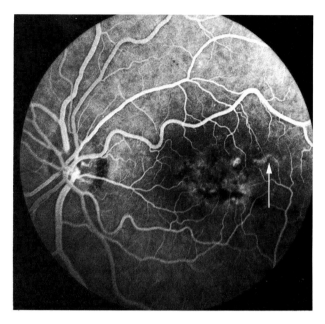

Figure 2–26. An early-stage angiogram of the patient shown in Figure 2–24 only 5 years later.

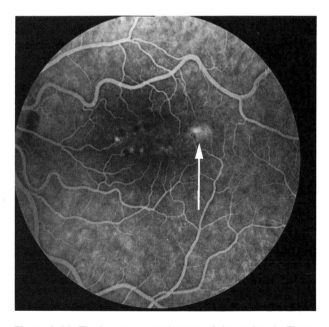

Figure 2–25. The late-stage angiogram of the patient in Figure 2–24, demonstrating the actively leaking zone *(long arrow)* characterized by a spread of hyperfluorescence.

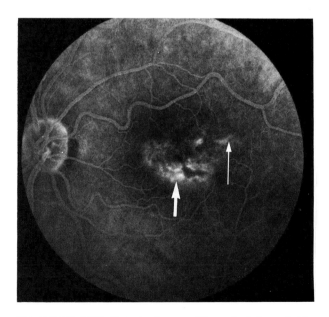

Figure 2–27. A late-stage angiogram of the patient shown in Figure 2–26, demonstrating the degree of destruction that can occur over time in idiopathic central serous choroidopathy.

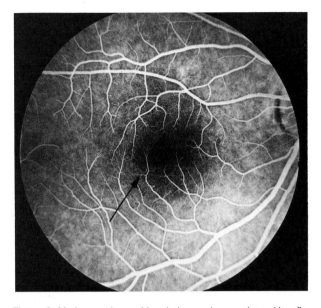

Figure 2–28. A normal eye with a dark macular area *(arrow)* in a fluorescein study.

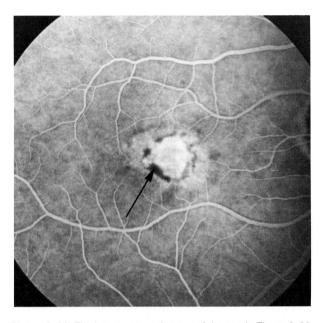

Figure 2–30. The late-stage angiogram of the eye in Figure 2–29, showing a spread of hyperfluorescence secondary to a neovascular net.

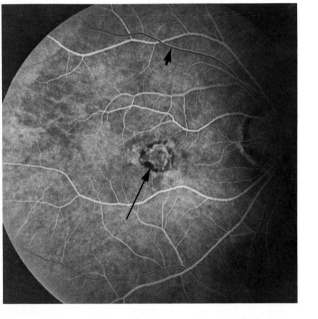

Figure 2–29. An area of hyperfluorescence in a normally dark macular area in an early-stage angiogram. The small arrow points to laminar flow in the vein.

■ ■ ■ ■ ■ ■

Clinical Example: Hyperfluorescence (IV)

One of the most dangerous ocular conditions that can develop is a choroidal neovascular net in the macular area. It can be devastating to vision because of the possibility of hemorrhage or scar formation. The neovascularization develops because of a combination of a break in the RPE–Bruch's membrane barrier and the presence of

oxygen starvation (hypoxia). This condition can occur in age-related maculopathy, angioid streaks, degenerative myopia, and presumed ocular histoplasmosis, among other conditions. The factor that makes this condition so dangerous is that these developing nets are extremely difficult to see ophthalmoscopically in the early stages of development. If patients are elderly, or if they have other conditions lending to the development of choroidal neovascular nets and they report with reduced vision or metamorphopsia, it is prudent to assume the presence of a neovascular net until proven otherwise. Order fluorescein angiography!

Figure 2–28 illustrates a healthy eye, with the arrow pointing to the normally dark macular area in a fluorescein study. Figures 2–29 and 2–30 represent early and later fluorescein studies, respectively, with hyperfluorescence in the normally dark macular area. Figure 2–29 shows the early venous phase (small arrow pointing to laminar venous flow), with the large arrow pointing to a choroidal neovascular net. All neovascularization leaks, as is demonstrated by the expanding area of edema in the late stage of Figure 2–30 (large arrow). This patient had presumed ocular histoplasmosis (20/200).

It is extremely important to diagnose choroidal neovascular nets as soon as possible, because laser photocoagulation may be able to seal the nets and abort progressive vision loss.

■ ■ ■ ■ ■ ■

Clinical Example: Hyperfluorescence (V)

Retinal and disc neovascularization can also be diagnosed earlier by fluorescein angiography than by ophthalmoscopic observation. Disc and retinal neovascularization is very fine and may be difficult to observe with

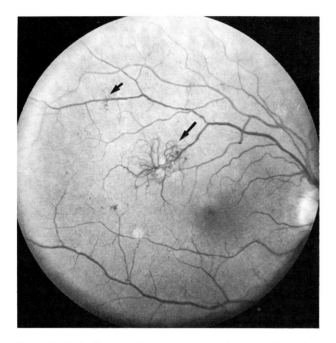

Figure 2–31. A photograph of two patches of neovascularization elsewhere in the retina *(arrows)*.

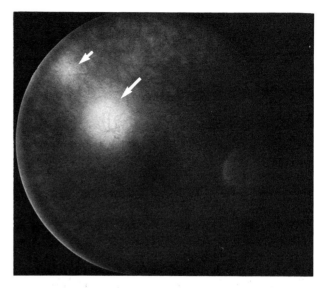

Figure 2–33. Late-phase angiogram of the neovascularization shown in Figure 2–31.

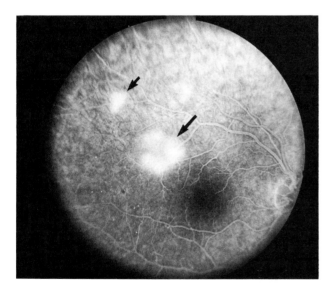

Figure 2–32. Early-phase angiogram of the neovascularization shown in Figure 2–31.

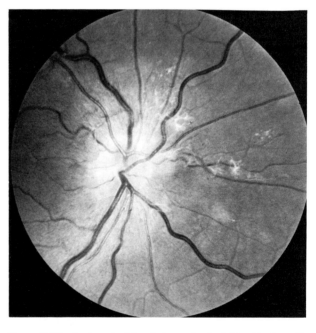

Figure 2–34. Black-and-white photograph of a right optic disc with subtle disc neovascularization.

ophthalmoscopy. The staining pattern with fluorescein angiography is, however, classic.

Figure 2–31 is a black-and-white photograph of neovascularization of the retina (arrows). The large net is easily observable, but the small net offers a challenge. Figure 2–32 shows an early-phase angiogram of this area, demonstrating the characteristic leakage from the nets (arrows). Figure 2–33 illustrates the late-stage staining pattern (arrows).

Figures 2–34 to 2–39 illustrate the right and left eyes of a person with diabetes who had no observable diabetic retinopathy by ophthalmoscopy. Black-and-white photographs of both optic nerves show areas of suspicion (white arrows) that are confirmed as neovascularization of the disc by fluorescein angiography. The time-sequenced angiogram of the right eye demonstrates a spreading of the staining pattern characteristic of neovascularization of the disc (white arrows). The left eye an-

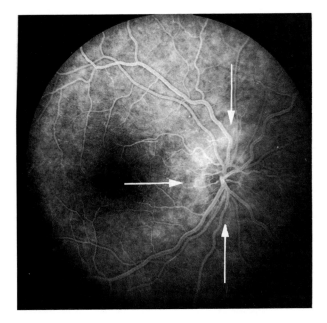

Figure 2–35. Early-phase angiogram of the eye in Figure 2–34, showing leakage *(arrows)* from the disc neovascularization.

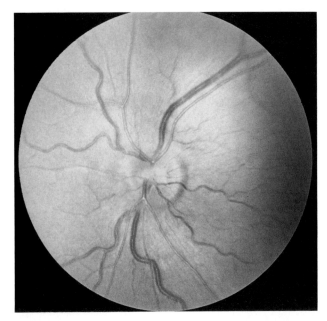

Figure 2–37. Black-and-white photograph of very subtle disc neovascularization in the fellow left eye to that in Figure 2–34.

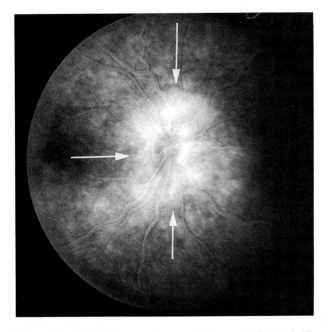

Figure 2–36. Late-phase angiogram of the eye in Figure 2–35, showing considerable new leakage.

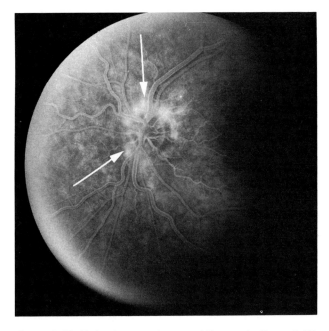

Figure 2–38. Early-phase angiogram of the eye in Figure 2–37, showing leakage *(arrows)*.

giograms demonstrated a similar pattern.

Figures 2–40 and 2–41 give another example of hyperfluorescence of the disc (arrow), but in this case the condition was anterior ischemic optic neuropathy (AION) in an insulin-dependent diabetic patient.

Early diagnosis of neovascularization is extremely important because of the imminent threat to vision. The earlier the diagnosis, the better the cure rate.

■ ■ ■ ■ ■ ■

Clinical Example: Hyperfluorescence (VI)

Disc neovascularization can occur in other conditions that create a hypoxic stimulus in the retina. Figure 2–42 is a photograph of a hemicentral retinal vein occlusion (hemi-CRVO). This is characterized by retinal vascular

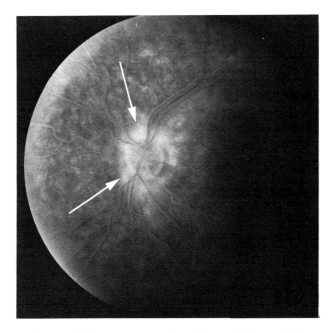

Figure 2–39. Late-stage staining of the eye in Figure 2–37.

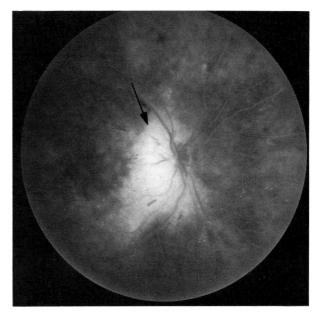

Figure 2–41. The late-stage angiogram of the disc area in Figure 2–40, demonstrating leakage associated with active anterior ischemic optic neuropathy.

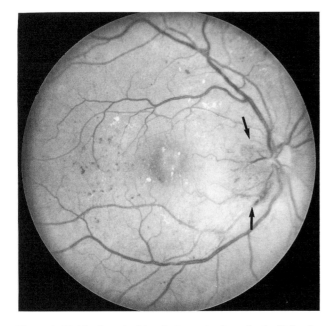

Figure 2–40. Black-and-white photograph of a patient with background diabetic retinopathy and active anterior ischemic optic neuropathy (arrows). The affected disc area is elevated.

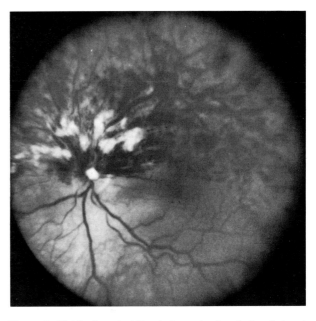

Figure 2–42. Black-and-white photograph of an ischemic hemicentral retinal vein occlusion. The cotton-wool spots indicate severe hypoxia.

changes in either the superior or inferior portion of the retina. Figures 2–43 and 2–44 show another patient, illustrating the potential sequela to a hemi-CRVO, disc neovascularization. Figure 2–43 shows the early stage, illustrating the frilly net on the nerve head, and Figure 2–44 demonstrates the late-stage leaking of that neovascularization. This is of particular significance because of the likelihood of vitreous hemorrhage.

■ ■ ■ ■ ■ ■

Clinical Example: Hyper- and Hypofluorescence

Branch retinal artery occlusion (BRAO) and branch retinal vein occlusion (BRVO) also create classic fluorescein angiography patterns. Figures 2–45 and 2–46 illustrate a combined BRAO and BRVO. Figure 2–45 is a photo-

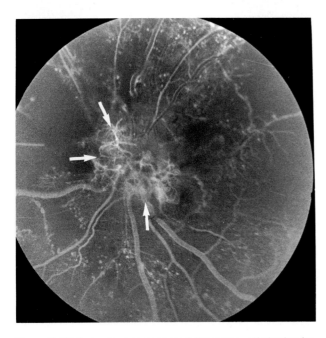

Figure 2–43. Early-stage angiogram of disc neovascularization *(arrows)* secondary to the hypoxia of hemicentral retinal vein occlusion.

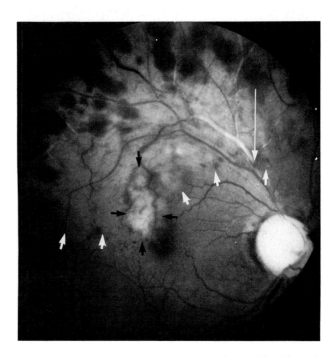

Figure 2–45. Black-and-white photograph of a combined branch retinal artery occlusion (BRAO) and branch retinal vein occlusion (BRVO). The white arrows point to the effects of the BRVO, the long white arrow points to the site of the occlusion, and the black arrows outline the zone of arterial infarct.

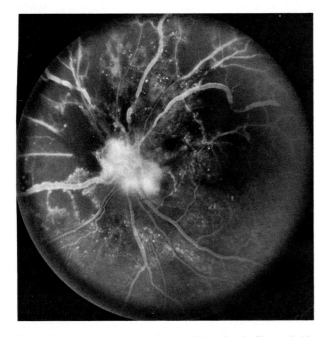

Figure 2–44. Late-stage angiogram of the disc in Figure 2–43, demonstrating significant spread of hyperfluorescence from the disc neovascularization.

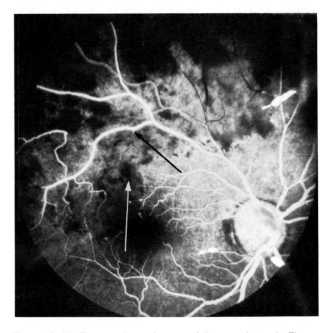

Figure 2–46. Fluorescein angiogram of the eye shown in Figure 2–45. The black arrow points to the site of arterial occlusion, and the white arrow to the zone of infarct. The zone of the branch retinal vein occlusion dims the background choroidal fluorescence.

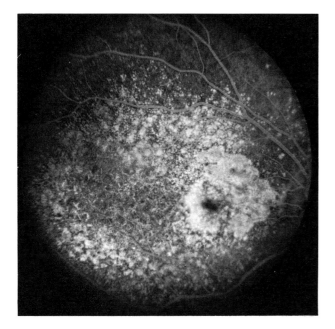

Figure 2–47. Fluorescein angiogram of right eye of an approximately 30-year-old patient with dominant drusen.

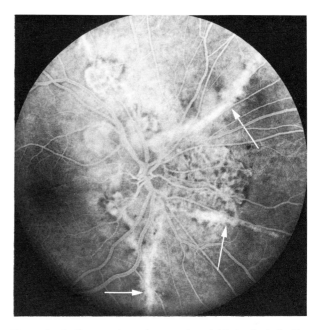

Figure 2–49. Fluorescein angiogram of angioid streaks indicating severe retinal pigment epithelium dropout in the circumpapillary region, with spokes *(arrows)* radiating outward.

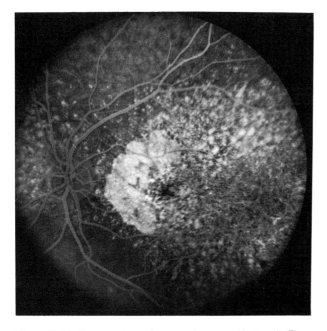

Figure 2–48. Fluorescein angiogram of same patient as in Figure 2–47. The characteristic feature is widespread hyperfluorescence.

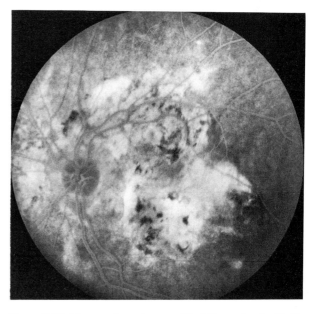

Figure 2–50. Fluorescein angiogram of the left eye of patient in Figure 2–49. The angioid streaks in this eye allowed for choroidal neovascularization, with the development of the massive disciform scar.

graph of the combination, with white arrows pointing to the area of BRVO and black arrows outlining the retinal infarct of the BRAO. Large intraretinal hemorrhages appear superiorly as black spots, and a long white arrow pinpoints the site of the vein occlusion. The long white arrow in Figure 2–46 points to the hypofluorescent area created by the BRAO. The site of the BRAO is pinpointed in Figure 2–46 by the black arrow. In most cases of BRVO,

the area of stasis is characterized by leaking microaneurysms and intraretinal edema.

■ ■ ■ ■ ■ ■

Clinical Example: Hyperfluorescence (VII)

RPE–Bruch's membrane barrier changes can also influence the angiogram pattern. Figures 2–47 to 2–50 show examples of these alterations. Figures 2–47 and 2–48 illustrate dominant drusen (Doyne's honeycomb choroidopathy) and the effect on the macular area. Hyperfluorescence is the characteristic feature. Figure 2–49 shows angioid streaks in the right eye (arrows). Figure 2–50 is a fluorescein angiogram of the left eye of the same patient, with an exudative macular scar secondary to trauma. Fluorescein angiography is invaluable in diagnosing RPE–Bruch's membrane disorders.

Illustrations and examples of the benefits of fluorescein angiography are endless. The technique of fluorescein angiography gives an added dimension to differential diagnosis. Often, fluorescein angiography is the only diagnostic technique that will reveal an underlying smoldering disease process. The technique is easy to understand if the doctor visualizes the clinicopathologic process as disease that is nothing more than an alteration of retinal structure at specific layers. Fluorescein angiography enhances and often pinpoints the specific clinicopathologic alteration. The more tools, the better the understanding; the better the understanding, the better the patient management.

DIAGNOSTIC ULTRASONOGRAPHY

Ocular diagnostic ultrasonography is an excellent tool for the assessment of elevations, depressions, hyperreflective situations such as buried drusen, and calcified tumors. Ultrasonography is also invaluable when retinal assessment is crucial in the presence of media opacification. The technique is especially valuable when there are no other means of assessing retinal status prior to cataract surgery. The ultrasonographic test may be of value in suspect neoplasia or thyroid eye disease, but neurologic studies are infinitely more helpful. In addition, ultrasonography is used to determine the length of the eyeball for determination of intraocular lens (IOL) power in psuedophakic surgery.

A-scan ultrasonography, also known as biometry, is used to measure the length of the eye. The transducer is usually placed on the corneal surface after topical anesthesia. The probe emits sound waves to create a time–amplitude recording, which is then displayed on an oscilloscope screen. The technique uses spikes on the screen that represent strongly reflective surfaces in the ocular tissue. Cursors or gates are then placed near these spikes and the machine electronically measures the distance between the cursors. The instruments also have averaging programs to facilitate the calculations necessary when performing the recommended multiple measurements. Some instruments automatically place the gates in a preset position. In a phakic eye, the typical spikes occur at the

cornea, the anterior and posterior lens surface, and the retina. In addition to the generation of the measurements, most biometers include programs to actually calculate the necessary power for the IOL when the operator enters the keratometry readings, the "constant for the IOL," and the desired postsurgical correction. Most machines also include a program that locks in when all parameters are met to consider the scan an effective measurement. The technique requires practice to achieve proper perpendicularity to the corneal plane to achieve effective readings. Figures 2–51 and 2–52 represent the A-scan reading and an IOL calculation. The A-scan technique can also be used in the evaluation of pathologic conditions, as the spikes will occur associated with media debris, elevations, and depressions.

B-scan ultrasonography is far more effective for the assessment of disease conditions of the eye and orbit because it provides a two-dimensional cross section of the eye. The classical use comes when the clinician is faced with media opacification to the point that evaluation of the retina and optic nerve becomes impossible. B-scan ultrasonography is a series of focused short-wavelength sound waves with frequencies of about 10 MHz. The probe is different than the A-scan probe in design, and is usually placed on the closed lid after the application of a conducting paste. It is best to attempt to not "shoot" through the crystalline lens to eliminate the possibility of the added reflections from the lens surfaces and at the edges of the lens—the Baum's bumps. The test can also be performed directly on the surface of the globe and cornea after topical anesthesia to the eye and methylcellulose on the probe. The probe can usually be focused selectively to allow for anterior enhancement or orbit enhancement (referred to as the time variable gain, or TVG). The

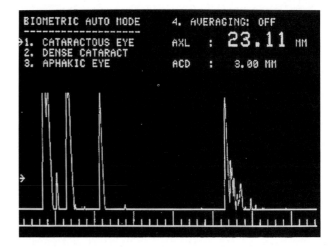

Figure 2–51. An A-scan demonstrating the necessary four peaks, corneal surface, anterior capsule, posterior lens surface, and retinal spike. The eyeball length is registered as 23.11 mm.

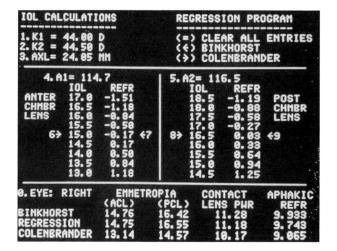

Figure 2–52. An example of the IOL-calculating capacity of the A-scan. Numerous variations are available on this theme.

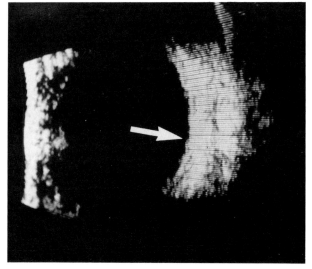

A

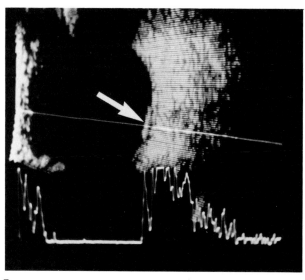

B

Figure 2–53. A. A normal B-scan. **B.** A B-scan with the arrow pointing to an elevated optic nerve head. The elevation in this case was secondary to buried drusen.

sound waves transverse the ocular contents and are reflected back at surface interfaces. The reflected waves are then recorded by the probe and passed back to the processor to be displayed on the video screen. The test is dynamic and may be recorded directly on attached video recorders, or it may be recorded in stop action by built-in printers or by polaroid photos of the video screen. The dynamic feature is especially important when viewing freely moving structures such as detached retinas.

Another interesting feature is the ability to reduce the gain or reflectivity of the sound waves. This becomes especially valuable in the differentiation of soft tissue problems such as papilledema versus infiltrations such as buried drusen of the optic nerve head (Fig. 2–53). When reducing the gain on an elevated structure, the detail of the soft tissue structure will disappear; but when the cause of the elevation is a highly reflective body such as a buried drusen, the echo will remain. Running the cursor through the orbital fat and evaluating the spike amplitude (Fig. 2–54A), and then running the cursor through the suspected drusen and evaluating the spike amplitude (Fig. 2–54B), will demonstrate increased reflectivity of the buried drusen. Conditions creating high reflectivity include buried drusen of the optic nerve head, retinoblastoma and other calcium-containing tumors, and a pthisical globe. Less reflectivity occurs in other tumors and cysts. Instruments vary considerably in their added features requiring that the clinician consult each owner's manual to ascertain the latitude of the abilities of each instrument. Figures 2–55 to 2–72 illustrate the value of B-scan ultrasonography in the diagnosis of ocular and orbital conditions. Table 2–6 outlines the uses of A- and B-scan ultrasonography. Ultrasonography is invaluable when needed, but does require some practice for performance and interpretation.

TABLE 2–6. SOME USES OF A- AND B-SCAN ULTRASONOGRAPHY

- Axial length measurements, both relative and precise
- Determination of posterior staphylomas
- Determination of colobomas
- Assessment of the degree of optic nerve head cupping in glaucoma
- Evaluation of retina through hazy or opaque media
- Evaluation of suspected ocular and orbital tumors
- Evaluation for suspected intraocular foreign bodies
- Evaluation of extraocular muscles
- Differential diagnosis of optic disc edema from buried drusen of the optic nerve head
- Precise measurement of ocular lesions—available on most instruments
- Early determination of ocular status in trauma but not if there is the threat of globe penetration
- Determination of retinal detachment versus retinoschisis

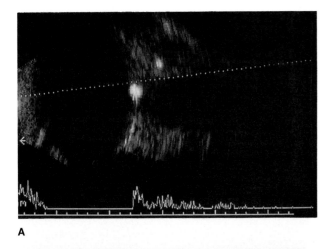

A

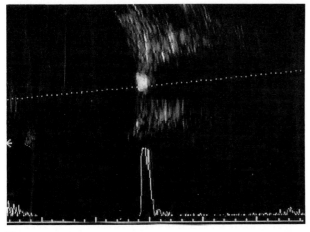

B

Figure 2–54. The concomitant use of B and A-scan. **A.** The cursor is running next to a buried drusen in the optic nerve head. The corresponding A-scan spike is low. **B.** The cursor is running through the highly reflective drusen creating a marked spike in the A-scan tracing below.

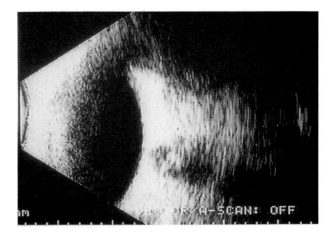

A

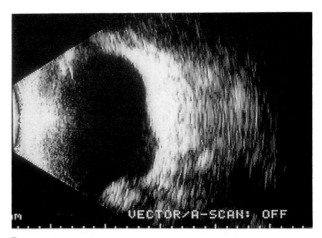

B

Figure 2–56. A. An eye without a posterior staphyloma. **B.** The fellow eye with a posterior staphyloma.

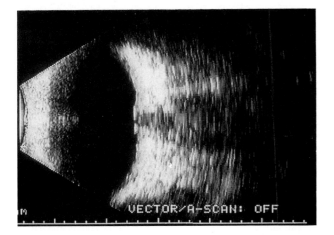

Figure 2–55. A B-scan of papilledema demonstrating the elevated optic nerve head and a grossly expanded retrolaminar optic nerve.

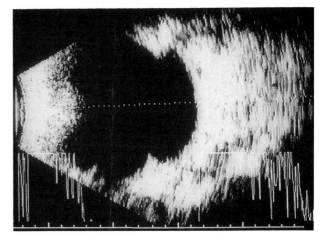

Figure 2–57. Another variation of a posterior staphyloma as demonstrated on B-scan ultrasonography.

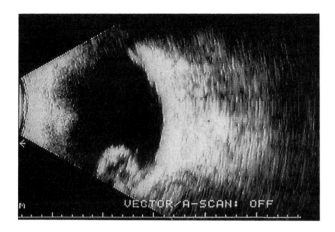

Figure 2–58. In the lower aspect of this B-scan, the clinician can see a traumatically dislocated crystalline lens.

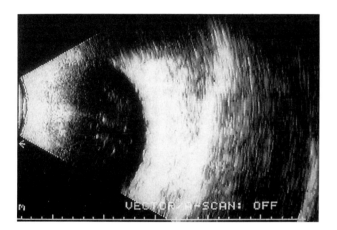

Figure 2–59. B-scan ultrasonography can also demonstrate vitreous opacities such as the dense asteroid hyalosis in this photograph.

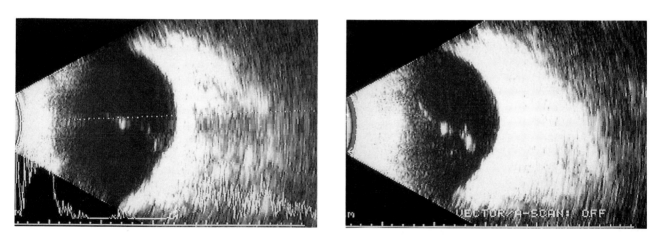

Figure 2–60. B-scan ultrasonography is invaluable in the evaluation of the status of the retina and vitreous behind a dense cataract. In this case the practitioner can observe the presence of persistent hyperplastic vitreous coursing from the optic nerve head forward to the posterior surface of the cataract in both scans of the same eye.

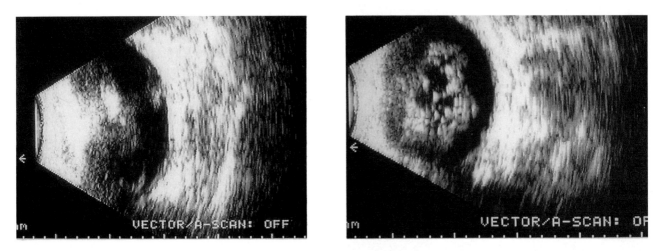

Figure 2–61. Examples of the appearance of a vitreous hemorrhage behind a dense cataract. These B-scans were performed prior to cataract surgery to ensure the retinal status.

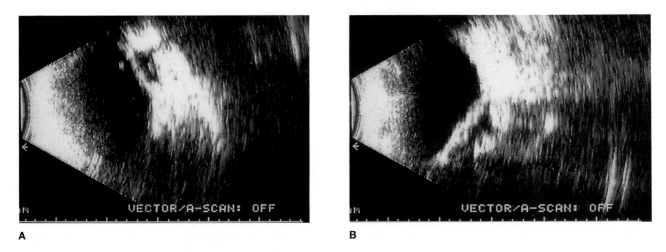

A   B

Figure 2–62. These B-scans demonstrate the appearance of an encircling scleral buckle. In **A** the buckle is shown above, while in **B** the buckle appears inferiorly.

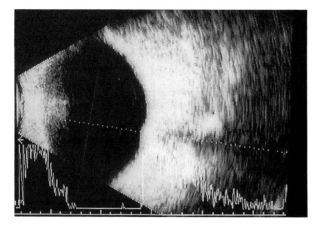

Figure 2–63. This B-scan has the cursor running through a long-standing metallic retinal foreign body. Notice the shadow cast behind the foreign body in the orbital fat area.

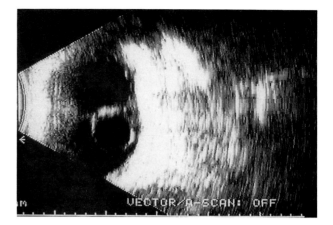

Figure 2–65. B-scan showing retinal cyst-like formations indicative of a long-standing detachment.

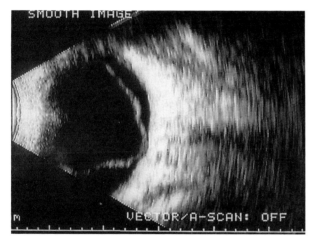

A

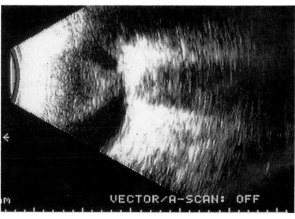

B

Figure 2–64. Two scans demonstrating different variations of retinal detachments. **A.** B-scan demonstrating a retinal detachment discovered behind a dense cataract prior to cataract surgery. **B.** B-scan representing a funnel retinal detachment with the retina still attached at the optic nerve head.

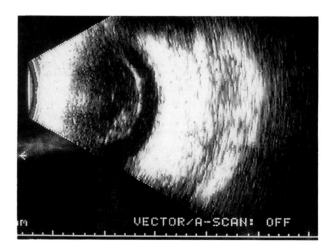

Figure 2–66. B-scan demonstrating a complete vitreous detachment associated with an intravitreal hemorrhage blocking the view of the underlying retina even with a binocular indirect ophthalmoscope.

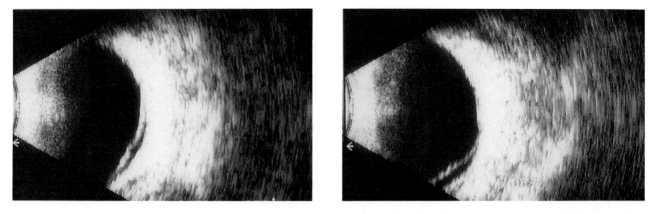

Figure 2–67. These two scans demonstrate two different views of a shallow retinal detachment associated with a 4-month (gleaned from a history of trauma) duration retinal dialysis.

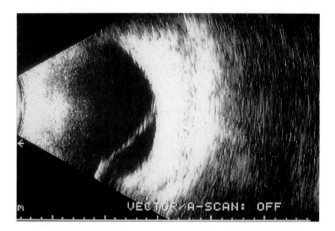

Figure 2–68. A retinal detachment involving the entire lower half of the retina and encroaching on the macula.

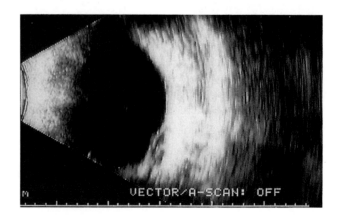

Figure 2–69. A retinal detachment in the inferior retina associated with a posterior vitreous detachment occurring 5 weeks prior. The PVD created a significant tear in an area of lattice, allowing ingress of liquefied vitreous.

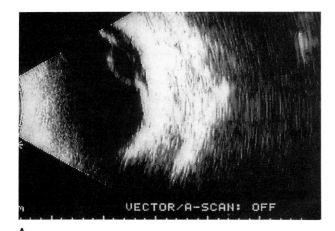

A

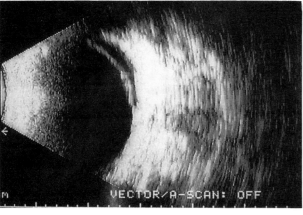

B

Figure 2–70. B-scans of a patient being followed for retinoschisis who developed a significant underlying retinal detachment. The schisis appears as a blister lying over the detachment in **A. B** is another B-scan angle taken on the underlying detachment.

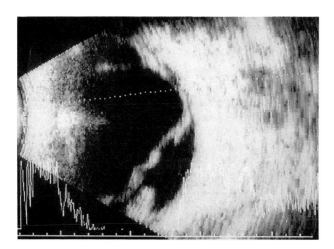

Figure 2–71. A long-standing retinal detachment demonstrating thickening of the detached retina and underlying scarification.

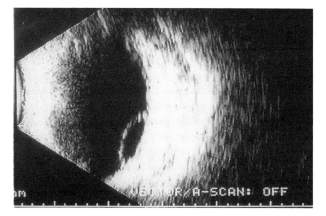

Figure 2–72. A classical presentation of a retinoschisis with the "blister" appearing on B-scan ultrasonography.

VISUAL FIELD TESTING

Screening Visual Field Testing

Brief mention must be made of screening visual field testing. Screening fields are just that. The screening field test will uncover a number of field defects, but the disparity between the diagnostic capability of the screening field and subsequent threshold field tests is often very dramatic. However, some patients just cannot handle a full threshold visual field test. Perhaps a major flaw in screening fields is the test design.

Comer and associates (1988) report a screening strategy yielding 90.9 percent sensitivity and 100 percent specificity in uncovering visual field defects. The strategy involves a single intensity stimulus of 24 dB presented at 40 points within the central 30 degrees (Central 40 Test on Allergan Humphrey). The criteria for abnormality include (1) two or more missed points adjacent to one another and repeated misses on retest, (2) one or more misses within the central 20 degrees of fixation and repeated misses on retest, and (3) a central reference level of 26 dB or less on threshold phase. The major benefit of this test beyond excellent specificity and sensitivity is the fact that each eye is tested in less than 2 minutes average for the normal group and under 3 minutes average for the abnormal group. Another report using 120 screening test points in the 60 degree field gave a 96 percent sensitivity and an 84 percent specificity using 17 or more defects occurring anywhere. The test points were specifically skewed for glaucoma suspects. If the clinician is interested in performing screening visual field testing with some value, the fields must be initiated with a specific central reference level that is consistent with the age of the patient (Table 2–7). Some of the newer screening programs require the patient's age as part of the patient information, to facilitate age-matched normal comparisons.

TABLE 2–7. CENTRAL REFERENCE LEVELS BY AGE FOR EFFECTIVE VISION SCREENING FIELD RESULTS

Age	Appropriate Central Reference Levels (dB)
<40	36–37
40–45	35
46–50	34
51–55	33
56–60	32
61–75	31

Threshold Visual Field Testing

Visual field testing is a very important factor in the analysis of the glaucoma suspect as well as in patients suspected of neurologic, optic nerve, and retinal diseases. In fact, visual fields are often the primary clue as to the appropriate diagnosis. In the past, glaucoma was defined as visual field loss in the presence of optic nerve head changes and elevated IOP. We now know that visual field changes can occur at "nonglaucomatous" IOP levels, and we also realize how difficult it is to evaluate glaucomatous optic atrophy. Visual fields are often the key factor in making your decision regarding the diagnosis of glaucoma.

Unfortunately, visual field testing carries all of the problems inherent in any subjective test. The majority of the problems involve patient reliability. Some patients are unable to give reliable results. In addition to patient problems, the clinician must deal with which visual field test to perform. Confrontation fields are useless in the patient suspected of having glaucoma. The tangent screen test is close to useless unless the patient has fairly advanced glaucoma and the clinician is especially adept at performing the test. However, the tangent screen test becomes the definitive diagnostic test in patients suspected of having hysterical problems or conversion reactions. In this instance the clinician should test the patient at 1 meter with a 3- to 5-mm target, expecting to get tubular fields in the 5-degree range; and then back the patient to 2 meters and retest with a doubled target size of 6 to 10 mm. At the retest distance, the tubular fields should overlap the original fields in the case of a conversion reaction (hysterical visual fields). This is then diagnostic of the conversion reaction and cannot occur with any form of organic disease. The author has also found the tangent screen to be invaluable in testing vertebral basilar stroke patients and traumatic brain injury patients, who often have difficulty responding to the automated field tests.

Kinetic Goldmann perimetry has value in some patients with neurologic lesions, but the test is so labor-intensive and requires a superbly trained technician or doctor to detect the subtle changes secondary to early axonal death that it becomes only an acceptable test for glaucoma. In fact, glaucomatous visual fields rarely respect the classical definitions of arcuate scotomas, Bjerrum scotomas, and classical nasal steps. The defects are instead regions of variable decreased sensitivity with ill-defined borders. These defects are often so subtle that they may be missed in automated perimeter testing employing suprathreshold and modified suprathreshold techniques. If you want to play in the game of diagnosis and management, you must use static or static–kinetic threshold testing, or both. Even at that, you must realize that loss of disc tissue in conditions such as glaucoma often precedes the creation of visual field defects.

Visual Field Defects in Glaucoma

Visual field defects associated with glaucoma can vary considerably, but certain classical characteristics have been described in the literature. Small paracentral scotomas within the central 20 degrees of the field are often considered the earliest defects in glaucoma. It has been suggested that this is true in up to 80 percent of the cases. These scotomas appear most often superiorly. A nasal step is a bite taken out of the nasal field limited by the horizontal raphe. The defect takes many forms. The nasal step is thought to occur in 6 to 18 percent of patients with glaucoma. One other classically described visual field defect in glaucoma is temporal constriction. The constriction is above or below the horizontal in the temporal visual field. Temporal constriction has been described as being sectoral-shaped, but may take many forms. The temporal constriction has been considered to occur in 3 to 6 percent of glaucoma patients.

Unfortunately, the classical descriptions often do not fit the reality of the clinical environment. Often a glaucomatous visual field is nondescript and clinicians find themselves trying to fit the defect to the classically described pattern. Current thoughts regarding visual field defects in glaucoma are more consistent with the results of automated threshold testing. One of the more important recent realizations is that glaucoma and ocular hypertension can cause a *diffuse visual field loss or an overall decrease in threshold values across the visual field (a depression of the hill of vision)*. This diffuse reduction or depression of the field becomes even more diagnostic when it is asymmetrical in presentation. Asymmetry in psychophysical testing and optic nerve head appearance is a very important factor in the diagnosis of glaucoma. Although IOPs may be the same at the time of testing, it is common to have asymmetry in other tests and observations in patients with glaucoma.

It stands to reason that central vision is also affected early in the course of open-angle glaucoma, but we have yet to create tests sensitive enough to discover this reduction in the clinical setting. As a clinician, you should look at the central threshold values that straddle fixation on the visual field printout. Often you will notice a reduction of these central threshold values in patients with glaucoma. This can also commonly occur if the patient is not corrected for the working distance of the field test. Start making this observation! The central foveal threshold test can also give you some information regarding depressed central sensitivity. Macular threshold testing, especially using blue targets, is also showing some promise in the early detection of depressed central sensitivity in glaucoma and may be of value in retinal conditions such as diabetic macular edema and age-related macular degeneration.

Another factor that must be considered in field analysis is how much glaucoma is being missed by not testing beyond the central 30 degrees. Most visual field programs concentrate on the 30-degree central field while some of the new devices only cover the central 24 to 26 degrees. Certainly, as a clinician you have the ability to test beyond the central 30 degree test zone with certain automated perimeter tests, but you also sacrifice time to perform this function. The switch to testing just the central 30 degrees has created some degree of controversy, but it still has a 93 to 96 percent positive hit rate. When we compare this to our batting average before automated threshold perimetry testing existed, it is easy to see the positive effect that this technology has had on glaucoma diagnosis and management.

One of the more important concepts that has recently evolved in field testing is the analysis of hemifield sensitivity. It should be noted that there is a difference between this loss of sensitivity in POAG as compared to normotensive glaucoma. The loss in normotensive glaucoma almost approaches the appearance of a visual field defect associated with ischemic optic neuropathy. This is a logical approach to visual field analysis when you realize that the technique is based on neuroretinal anatomy and the sequence of glaucomatous optic atrophy. The nerve fiber bundles in the temporal retina stop at the horizontal raphe. Damage to these fibers secondary to glaucoma runs to the horizontal raphe. This demarcation corresponds well with the classical nasal step. It has been shown that visual field defects are limited to one or the other altitudinal hemifield, and the corresponding hemifield may remain unaffected for up to 10 years.

Cluster point analysis carries the hemifield analysis one step further. Threshold field testing has established that early loss in glaucoma consists of clusters of depressed points. Cluster point comparison, or mirror image analysis, compares thresholds of clusters of test points above and below the horizontal. The comparison is an internal comparison rather than an analysis based on age-matched normal controls. The sensitivity for this strategy is reported at 97 percent and the specificity is 87 percent. Statpac (Humphrey/Zeiss), on comparison, reportedly yields 93 percent sensitivity and 84 to 90 percent specificity. Sensitivity is the degree to which abnormal fields are shown as being abnormal, and specificity is the degree to which normal visual fields are found to be normal. A perfect test would have 100 percent sensitivity and specificity.

Visual Field Defects in Optic Nerve and Retinal Diseases

Optic nerve defects can create a variety of visual field defects. Although these are not hard and fast rules, Table 2–8 summarizes the more common defects associated with optic nerve disorders.

Disorders of the retina usually create variable defects according to the extent of the process and the layers involved. A choroidal disorder such as presumed ocular histoplasmosis will create a localized defect with the field loss approximating the size of the lesion. Disorders such as toxoplasmosis involve the nerve fiber layer and can create much more extensive defects than expected by just looking at the lesion. Hereditary retinal–choroidal defects may create defects in special lighting situations such as mesopic levels and are crucial in the determination of the disease. Subtle macular defects such as diabetic macular edema may require testing at threshold with colored targets to detect the earliest of changes.

TABLE 2–8. VISUAL FIELD DEFECTS ASSOCIATED WITH OPTIC NERVE HEAD DISORDERS

Disorder	Expected Defect
Optic atrophy	Variable defect
Optic pit	Loss corresponding to area of pit that is often arcuate
Demyelinizing optic neuropathy	Variable from central loss to peripheral constriction
Buried drusen	Variable scotomas to full peripheral constrictions
Ischemic optic neuropathy	Usually an altitudinal field approaching fixation
Papillitis	Central scotoma
Papilledema	Enlarged blind spot that progresses toward the fovea with time
Papillophlebitis	Grossly enlarged blind spot
Optic nerve head colobomas	Variable depending on extent of coloboma

TABLE 2–9. INTERPRETATION OF UNIOCULAR VISUAL FIELD DEFECTS[a]

Type of Defect	Probable Location	Possibilities	Type of Defect	Probable Location	Possibilities
Hemifield defects that do not cross horizontals and must affect nerve fiber layer	Optic nerve or retinal lesion	1. Primary open-angle glaucoma 2. Normotensive glaucoma 3. Ischemic optic neuropathy 4. Branch retinal artery occlusion 5. Localized retinal inflammatory or dystrophic lesion 6. Optic pit 7. Buried drusen of the optic nerve head	Scotoma elsewhere	Retinal or choroidal disease	1. Any retinal or choroidal inflammatory or dystrophic disease 2. Myelinated nerve fibers
Enlarged blind spot	Optic nerve	1. Congenital disc anomalies 2. Papilledema (asymmetry)	Centrocecal scotoma	Optic nerve or retinal vascular	1. Papilledema (asymmetrical) 2. Leber's hereditary optic neuropathy 3. Toxic optic neuropathy 4. Cilioretinal artery occlusion (rare)
Central scotoma with a normal-appearing macula	Optic nerve lesion	1. Demyelinizing optic neuropathy 2. Papillitis 3. Optic atrophy 4. Optic nerve compressive disease	Peripheral contraction or constriction— may be in the form of ring scotomas	Optic nerve or retina	1. Retinal detachment 2. Retinoschisis 3. Glaucoma 4. Tilted discs, colobomas, staphylomas 5. Optic nerve head drusen 6. Compressive optic nerve lesion 7. Optic atrophy 8. Unilateral generalized retinal disease (e.g., rare unilateral retinitis pigmentosa) 9. Remote possibility of conversion reaction
Central scotoma	Macular, retinal, or choroidal disease	1. Idiopathic central serous choroidopathy 2. Choroidal neovascularization 3. Any inflammatory or dystrophic retinal or choroidal lesion 4. Any RPE inflammatory disease			

[a]Implies a prechiasmal lesion or defect and will give associated optic nerve conduction defects on comparison of the two eyes.

The true value of visual field testing lies in the ability to detect the silent neurologic lesions such as the pituitary tumors. Table 2–9 illustrates the associations of unilateral visual field defects while Tables 2–10 and 2–11 illustrate the associations of bilateral visual field defects. Unfortunately the patterns are usually not quite as precise as the figures indicate, but the end result is still the same. The practitioner should ask for a neurologic consultation on the majority of bilateral field defects after they have been repeated and confirmed. Understanding the visual pathway and the defects created in differing parts of this pathway can be of tremendous assistance to the neurologic specialist in pinpointing the location of lesions.

Concepts of Automated Perimetry

Although controversy exists as to the value of automated perimetry, it is currently the standard of care in the diagnosis of glaucoma and is also of tremendous value in retinal and visual pathway disorders. It is also recognized that the comparison of threshold visual fields obtained by two different instruments is an apples-to-oranges comparison. Certainly, a part of the comparison problem can be attributed to different testing protocols and different background intensities. Nevertheless, it is imperative that the clinician understand automated threshold perimetry. To understand perimetry, each component will be dissected and reintegrated to understand the implications of the results. The parameters of automated perimetry include size of target, luminance of background, luminance of target, duration of target exposure, and testing strategies. The method of thresholding varies from instrument to instrument and the details can be found in the owner's manuals.

Stimulus size is usually related to the equivalent Goldmann notations. The standard target size (default

TABLE 2–10. INTERPRETATION OF BINOCULAR VISUAL DEFECTS—NONHOMONYMOUS

Type of Defect	Possibilities
Generalized binocular constriction	1. In young, a conversion reaction 2. Vertebrobasilar insufficiency 3. Buried drusen of the optic nerve head 4. Syphilitic optic atrophy 5. Variations of retinitis pigmentosa
Enlarged blind spots	1. Congenital nerve head variations 2. Papilledema
Bitemporal hemianopsias respecting the verticals	1. Chiasmal lesion
Bitemporal hemianopsias crossing the verticals	1. Tilted disc syndromes 2. Posterior circumpapillary staphylomas
Binasal hemianopsias	1. Asymmetrical glaucoma 2. Chiasmal disease 3. Buried drusen of the optic nerve head 4. Chronic papilledema 5. Congenital optic nerve head variations
Altitudinal hemianopsias	1. Buried drusen of the optic nerve head 2. Occipital cortex lesions

TABLE 2–11. INTERPRETATION OF BINOCULAR VISUAL FIELD DEFECTS—HOMONYMOUS OR SAME-SIDED DEFECTS

- Must be postchiasmal
- Implies lesion in the contralateral visual pathway
- The more congruous (the more alike) the defects, the more posterior the location in the visual pathway
- Macular sparing occurs in occipital pole lesions

Characteristics of Defects	Possibilities
Very incongruous	Contralateral lesions in the anterior optic tract
Very congruous	Contralateral lesions in the posterior optic tract
Inferior quadrantic defects	Contralateral parietal lobe optic radiation lesion
Superior quadrantic defects	Contralateral temporal lobe optic radiation lesion
Quadrantic defects along the horizontal meridian	Contralateral lateral geniculate area lesion
Macular hemicentral (macular splitting) defects	Contralateral occipital cortex lesion
Isolated temporal crescent defects	Contralateral lesion of the anterior lip of the calcarine cortex

target size) used in automated perimetry is size III, which subtends 0.43 degrees of arc. This represents a compromise that is supposed to be only minimally affected by refractive error. Most perimeters allow the clinician to vary this target size, although the standard has been found to be effective in detecting even the smallest scotoma.

Background luminance varies between perimetry units. The Humphrey/Zeiss unit and most other units use a background luminance of 31.5 apostilbs, which is the standard for Goldmann perimetry. The Interzeag system uses a background luminance of 4 apostilbs. This variability makes comparison of results between instruments difficult if not impossible.

The stimulus intensity is also measured in apostilbs but is converted to decibels (dB). The higher the decibel reading for threshold, the more sensitive the retinal receptor field at that point. In suprathreshold testing there is a defined level of light stimulus presented in all testing locations and the patient either sees or does not see the stimulus. Suprathreshold testing is not always age-related and as such has the potential to "miss" field defects if the hill of vision is established at a low level. In threshold testing, the patient reports the light seen at different levels of presentation and the unit calculates the level at which, in theory, there is a 50 percent chance of perception. A 5 dB difference in the expected threshold level and that found by testing is considered significant. This 5 dB difference is the equivalent of a half log unit change

in brightness, which corresponds to an intensity twice as bright as expected. It is important to recognize that this sensitivity may vary 2 to 4 dB in nondiseased eyes, and that some studies have shown that most normals have one point or more that is 5 dB less sensitive than surrounding points. Another study reported 27 percent of eyes had over ten points depressed at least 6 dB. This variability has also been substantiated by others. It should also be remembered that sensitivity to differential stimuli declines naturally toward the periphery (hill of vision) and declines naturally with advancing age.

The duration of the stimulus is a variable in automated perimetry. Most devices use a stimulus duration of 0.1 to 0.2 seconds, which is usually too short for the patient to make an eye movement toward the target. Beyond 0.5 seconds duration, there is no effect of sensitivity (Bloch's law).

Testing strategies vary considerably, but the standard threshold test used at this point in time is a variation of a 76-point pattern within the central 30 degrees spaced at 6-degree intervals. Numerous screening strategies exist from suprathreshold to modified suprathreshold. To definitively diagnose glaucoma, or to follow a glaucoma patient, threshold testing must be performed. However, screening strategies do serve the purpose of (1) getting a field on inattentive patients because of reduced testing time and (2) obtaining a training field for the future performance of a threshold field test.

Performing Automated Visual Field Tests

The concepts and complexity of automated visual field testing aside, field tests are still a wonderful clinical tool. The practitioner must, however, realize that the field test is only a single diagnostic tool with variable sensitivity and specificity and the diagnostic value is strongly dependent on the prevalence of the disease being investigated. To perform automated field testing the practitioner must first decide whether it will be with or without dilation, and must stay with that decision for each subsequent performance of the field test. The pupil should be 3 mm or greater in all situations and should be specified each time the test is performed. The use of the proper refractive correction is critical. There is about 1 dB of threshold increase with 1 diopter of refractive error and about 3 dB of increase with 2 diopters of refractive error. If there is a significant central depression in an automated visual field test, the first thing to suspect is the use of an improper correction for the visual field. It is also important to add plus power to compensate for the 33-centimeter test distance in patients with reduced amplitude of accommodation or in patients who have some degree of cycloplegia from dilation. When incorporating the prescription for the test, use only large-aperture trial lenses. Remember, if the proper prescription is not used, you can expect depressed threshold levels centrally but not peripherally. Media opacities and reduced visual acuity will both cloud the results when performing threshold perimetry. Take care to record acuity and make your notations regarding opacities on the visual field printout.

Attempt to match the testing strategy to your expectations from the patient. Often an older or debilitated patient will not have the patience or faculties to perform a full threshold visual field test. Start with a simpler or faster strategy when in doubt.

The results attained on visual field tests are a direct reflection of the perimetrist's interest in and interaction with the patient during the test. Patient reliability can improve dramatically when using a video monitoring system rather than a periscope monitoring system. The perimetrist must constantly monitor the patient's fixation, false-positive errors, and false-negative errors. It has even been recommended that the test be stopped when the patient starts displaying excessive errors. The patient should then be reinstructed and the test restarted. Patient fatigue is another important factor to consider. Should the patient require more than 20 minutes to perform a field test, it is best to abort the test for the second eye and reschedule for another visit. In fact, a two office visit plan is not a bad idea for many patients who require a full threshold visual field test. *Never forget that a field test performed with poor reliability factors is useless.* Taking time during the testing session will pay off with good patient reliability factors. Interaction with the patient during the test can also improve reliability, and some field testing systems have built-in voice interaction for their instructional system. A moving fixation target has also been advocated to improve patient interest and reliability. Also remember that on the equivocal cases of glaucoma where IOP is low or borderline and the optic nerve heads are only questionable, one positive visual field is not a strong case for initiation of therapy. The clinician should rarely base a decision in equivocal cases on just one field in any clinical circumstance. Repeatable psychometric testing is necessary for proper diagnosis. Threshold visual field testing requires a careful explanation so that patients will understand that the process may require multiple visits.

Interpreting Automated Visual Field Tests

Let us now assume that we have threshold visual field test results in our hands. How do we interpret the fields? One important fact to realize is that automated visual field testing without a statistical analysis package is virtually useless when following glaucoma or neurologic patients. The statistical analysis package allows comparison of the patient's field result to a composite of age-matched nondiseased patients. Threshold decreases with advancing age. This decrease correlates with a depression in the hill of vision. If the visual field testing software does not correct for this normal aging change, the resultant visual fields will be of limited clinical use. This is especially important when you realize that a 5 to 6 dB decrease in sensitivity is considered a significant field loss. The majority of the literature and clinical experience supports the fact that currently the two most used automated devices are the Humphrey field tester and the Interzeag/Octopus device, with the Dicon device gaining acceptance.

HUMPHREY/ZEISS STATPAC VISUAL FIELD TESTS: THE 30-2 ANALYSIS

Humphrey/Zeiss visual field testing can be broken down into three distinct analyses: (1) patient reliability data, (2) printout of the visual fields, and (3) global indices. A fourth feature, a written analysis of the field, is also available but is self-explanatory.

Patient Reliability Factors

Patient reliability factors include the number of fixation losses, number of false-positive errors, number of false-negative errors, and short-term fluctuation. Fixation losses, false-positive errors, and false-negative errors are printed in the upper left hand corner with the duration of the test in minutes. The short-term fluctuation is printed in the lower right hand corner. The duration of the test in minutes may be considered a patient reliability indicator, as tests running over 20 minutes in the full field program are considered suspicious. The Fast Pac feature has greatly improved the test time, reducing elapsed time by 40 percent. However, there may be some sacrifice in the ability to accurately follow the visual field in the patient with the Fast Pac feature.

Fixation Losses. Fixation checks are obtained by periodically projecting into the blind spot. A report of seeing the spot when projecting into the blind spot is recorded as a fixation loss. Fixation losses exceeding 20 percent are flagged (XX) indicating poor patient reliability.

False-Positive Errors. False-positive errors are obtained by not projecting a light in the normal sequence to check to see if the patient is responding to a rhythm rather than a target. If there is an abnormally high number of false positives, it may indicate that the patient is consistently reporting prior to presentation, with the result that decibel threshold levels will be greater than expected for that population. If the patient indicates that they see the light when it is not presented (false-positive error) greater than 33 percent of the time, it is flagged (XX) as poor patient reliability.

False-Negative Errors. False negatives are obtained by projecting a stimulus of maximum intensity into a previously determined "known" seeing point. This is a gross determination of short-term fluctuation. Unfortunately, a diseased retina or nerve fiber layer that has been tested once may become "desensitized" and unable to respond properly when restimulated. It is therefore possible to have a high false-negative error in a diseased eye and still have reliable data. Some clinicians consider high false-negative errors to be indicative of a diseased ocular situation. If the patient reports that they do not see the light when projected at maximum intensity (false negative) greater than 33 percent of the time, it is flagged (XX) as poor patient reliability.

Short-term Fluctuation. Short-term fluctuation (SF) is determined by retesting threshold twice at 10 preselected locations. These are represented as threshold levels stacked on one another with the retest in parentheses. This is a broader assessment of internal consistency than false negatives with the average short-term fluctuation being represented in the global

indices. To the right of the numerical value is a probability figure indicating the significance of this level of internal consistency fluctuation. As with false-negative errors, short-term fluctuation may be high in the diseased eye because of the poor recovery of affected fibers. All patient reliability factors can be improved by diligence on the part of the perimetrist. *If fixation losses or false-positive errors are poor, or if false-negative errors or short-term fluctuation figures are excessive, the field is questionable. If patient reliability is poor, do not proceed to the analysis of the visual field.*

Long-term Fluctuation. One other factor that should be considered in the area of patient reliability is long-term patient fluctuation. There is no specific indication of this on the printout, but long-term fluctuation refers to variations that occur on two successive tests. Normal fluctuations occur as there is day-to-day variability in any subjective test. The average long-term fluctuation for a "normal" visual field is about 1 dB. These fluctuations may be greater in patients with glaucoma even if the disease is considered to be controlled. It has also been shown that long-term fluctuation is usually lower in the central part of the field and greatest in the peripheral areas. Certainly, a part of this effect can be attributed to the fact that the ganglion cell receptive fields are larger in the periphery.

Another important consideration regarding the patient reliability factors is the learning curve. The automated field is a learnable test and reliability factors may improve with retest. Other studies point out that there is little if any learning effect on the retest of visual fields. It is certain that some patients will never learn the test regardless of the number of retakes.

Visual Field Printouts

Upper Left—Raw Data. If patient reliability factors are acceptable, you may now proceed to the array of visual field printouts. The Humphrey/Zeiss device gives six separate fields to analyze. The upper left field (raw data) displays the true resultant threshold decibel levels at each of the tested points. In addition, there is a display of the decibel levels in retest areas in parentheses under the original findings. This raw data is difficult if not impossible to interpret especially if you are trying to compare to age-matched "normals."

Upper Right—Gray Scale. The upper right field is a display of the gray scale. The gray scale is a substitute for the isopter display of the Goldmann-type perimetry. The gray tone assigned to each decibel level is demonstrated at the bottom of the printout. The gray scale is a direct representation of the absolute threshold levels in the raw data field. The darker the tone, the less sensitive the area; the lower the decibel level, the higher the apostilb level needed to see the target. Remember that the decibel level is the inverse of the apostilb level. Gray scale printouts are dangerous! Areas between test points are shaded in spite of the fact that they were not tested. The most dangerous aspect of the gray scale is the fact that it does not represent an age-matched comparison. It is entirely possible that the gray scale may appear normal but the corresponding threshold levels would be inappropriate for the patient's age. The only benefit of the gray scale is that you can demonstrate the visual field loss to the patient. The picture of the visual field loss is often more effective in helping the patient to understand the problem than an attempt at an explanation.

Middle Left—Total Deviation. The third display is located in the middle left portion of the printout and is entitled the total deviation. This display has significance from the standpoint that it is a display of the deviation from "normal" expecteds in an age-matched population. Normal values are based on visual acuity of at least 20/25 for patients under age 50 years and 20/30 for patients over age 50 years. The actual values for each point are subtracted from expected values with the difference being displayed. This display is of tremendous value as it is a comparison to age-matched "normals" and as such reflects alterations in the hill of vision with age. This plot reflects the degree of depression of the hill of vision.

Lower Left—Probability Plot of Total Deviation. Unfortunately, the clinician still does not know the significance of each numerical display. The display located directly below the numerical total deviation solves the problem of determining the significance of the numerical data. This display in the lower left hand corner is a plot of the probability of significance of the degree of loss for each numerical display. It tells you, for example, if a 7-dB difference is significant and tells the level of significance. A probability of 5 percent means that fewer than 5 percent of the population in this age category had a drift of decibel levels this high. A probability symbol of 0.5 percent means that

TABLE 2–12. PRINTOUT SUMMARY FOR THE HUMPHREY/ZEISS DEVICE

Top left: Display of true decibel values (inverse of apostilb)

Top right: Gray scale approximation of true decibel levels

Middle left: Total deviation or decibel difference between patient and expected normals

Middle right: Pattern deviation or decibel difference corrected for overall depression of the hill of vision

Lower left: Probability display of total deviation

Lower right: Probability display of pattern deviation

TABLE 2–13. GENERAL RULES FOR USE OF THE HUMPHREY/ZEISS PRINTOUT

- Use lower left display when there are no media opacities or if the pupil is larger than 3 mm
- Use lower right display when there are media opacities or small pupils. This also graphically represents deep scotomas

fewer than 0.5 percent of the population had a drift of decibel levels this high. A 0.5 percent probability is very significant when compared to a 5 percent probability.

Middle Right—Pattern Deviation. The middle right display is a plot referred to as pattern deviation. This plot represents a correction of the numerical values in the total deviation. This correction is an adjustment for overall changes in the height of the hill of vision. The instrument assumes that an overall depression in the hill of vision is secondary to media opacities or small pupils. Unfortunately, this is *artificial intelligence* in action. The machine does not know if the patient has media opacities, and it is entirely possible that a patient with severe reduction in threshold at all points will show a totally normal field in the pattern deviation mode. You *cannot* look at this for your final analysis but must use it in combination with the other factors. The pattern deviation is actually a plot of the smoothness of the hill of vision. The pattern standard deviation plot is an excellent determinant of the depth of scotomatous areas. The primary value in the pattern deviation plot lies in following patients over the years as media opacities, such as cataracts, develop. The instrument will factor out the depression caused by the cataract. The lower right pattern is a probability plot of the pattern deviation numerical values. This probability plot serves the same function as the plot for total deviation. Table 2–12 represents a summary of the printout and Table 2–13 gives some general rules for its use.

Global Indices

The final components of the Humphrey/Zeiss Statpac field analysis are the global indices. These are printed on the right side of the form. The global indices are provided as overall guidelines for the visual fields. Each of the indices is calculated from the age-matched values in the total deviation and pattern deviation. Each global index also has a corresponding probability value to the right.

Mean Deviation. The mean deviation (MD) is a numerical representation of the overall depression (−) or elevation (+) of the visual field with scotomas or depressions as compared to age-matched normals. This representation is not particularly sensitive to scotomas. The mean deviation is a numerical equivalent to the total deviation pattern. If the total deviation pattern of the middle and lower left is high, the mean deviation value will be high. Again, the probability factors indicate the significance of the numerical value. If $p < 2$ percent, it indicates that less than 2 percent of the normal age-matched population has an MD larger than that found on this patient. The MD is not specific; it can refer to overall depressions or deep scotomas.

Pattern Standard Deviation.

The pattern standard deviation (PSD) is a measure of the smoothness of the hill of vision. A high PSD indicates isolated depressions in the "normal" overall hill of vision (rough hill) or variability in patient responses. The PSD is a numerical equivalent of the pattern deviation field representations. If the pattern deviation fields are high, the PSD will be high. Probability values also accompany the PSD.

Short-term Fluctuation and Corrected Pattern Standard Deviation.

The short-term fluctuation (SF) has been addressed in the section on patient reliability factors. The corrected pattern standard deviation (CPSD) is a modification of the PSD. It is supposed to represent the deviation from the normal smooth hill of vision corrected for by the SF, or the internal variability of the patient. This is the one global index that adjusts for the patient reliability. If SF is high, the

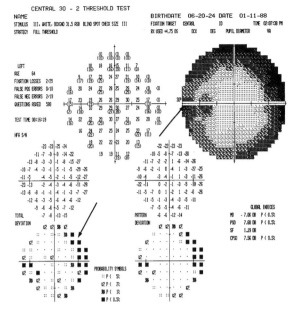

Figure 2–73. A visual field illustrating a classical spectacle ring scotoma resulting from either a narrow-aperture trial lens or from having the patient sitting too far from the trial lens.

CPSD will be significantly lower than the PSD. If the SF is low, the CPSD will be similar to the PSD.

All global indices are of value when used in conjunction with the field printouts but none are of any value in and of themselves. The Humphrey/Zeiss unit has many other functions that are of use in eval-

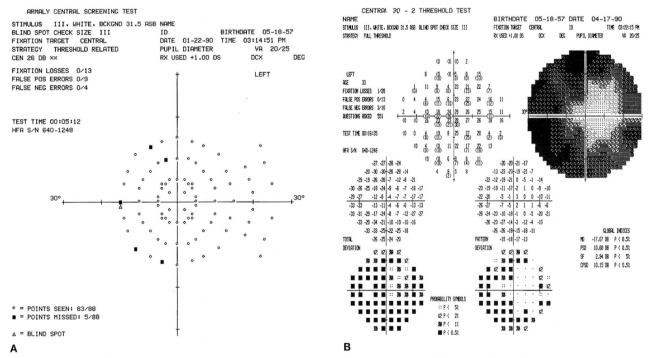

Figure 2–74. An illustration of the danger of using a nonage-related visual field screening test. In **A,** there are apparently 4 absolute visual field defects on this 33-year-old patient. The central decibel level is flagged as being too low. When comparing to the field shown in **B** for the same patient only using age-matched reference levels, the total deviation probability plot shows the true severity of the defect.

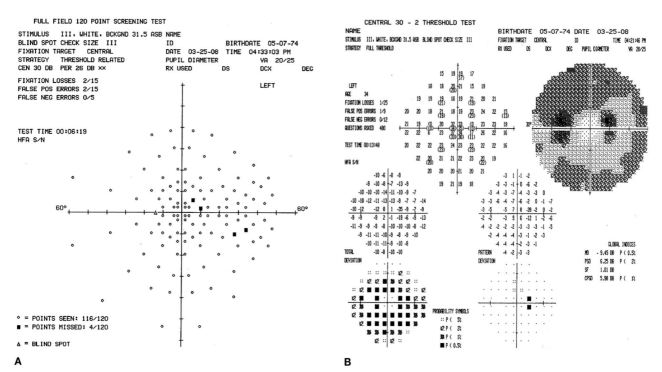

Figure 2–75. Another illustration of the dangers of not using age-related parameters in visual field testing. The screening field **(A)** for this 34-year-old does not reflect the totality of the visual field defect present in the age-related total deviation probability plot **(B).**

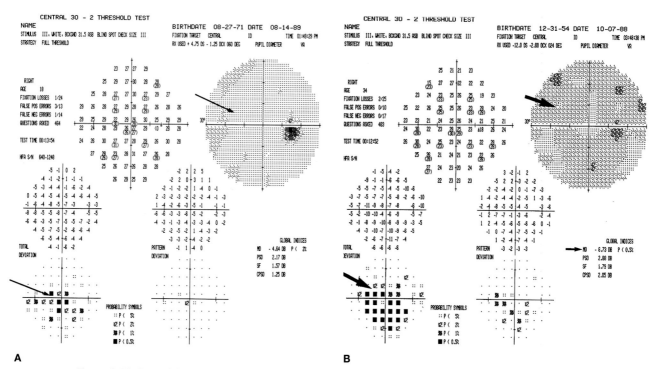

Figure 2–76. Potential misinformation that may be deduced from using the gray-scale printouts of visual field testers. In **A,** the gray scale appears "normal" because the figure is no more than a graphical representation of the decibel levels. The total deviation probability plot, however, demonstrates the actual losses in an 18-year-old patient with buried drusen of the optic nerve head when compared to age-matched normals. **B** illustrates an apparent normal gray scale in a 34-year-old patient with IOPs of 32 mm Hg, whereas the total deviation probability plot represents the true loss of function.

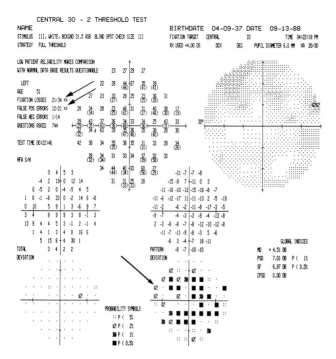

Figure 2–77. Example of very poor patient compliance. She had 21 of 34 fixation losses and 12 of 21 false-positive errors. The false-positive errors meant that she was pressing the button before the target appeared and created the classical losses in the pattern deviation probability plot with no losses in the total deviation probability plot.

uation of the patient but are beyond the boundaries of this discussion. Figures 2–73 to 2–91 illustrate many of the variations encountered in visual field testing.

INTERZEAG/OCTOPUS VISUAL FIELD ANALYSIS

Interzeag/Octopus visual field analysis is similar to the Humphrey/Zeiss analysis but uses different terminology and different field printouts. When applicable, a comparison will be made to avoid replication of explanation.

Interzeag/Octopus visual fields may be broken into distinct analyses including (1) patient reliability factors, (2) assorted field printouts, and (3) indices of fluctuation. As with the Humphrey/Zeiss unit, corrections in the hill of vision are automatically made when related to the age of the patient. Slightly different thresholding and a reduced background intensity are the primary differentiating features. Unfortunately, these very basic differences prevent direct comparison of fields generated by the two instruments.

Patient Reliability Factors

Patient reliability factors include positive catch trials (false positives), negative catch trials (false negatives), short-term fluctuation (in phase two only), and a measured reliability factor (RF) presented as a percentage.

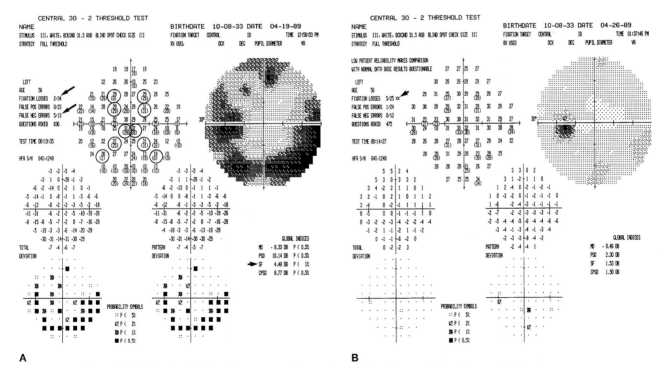

A   **B**

Figure 2–78. Left visual fields of the same patient performed 1 week apart. In one instance **(A)**, there were 2 of 34 fixation losses, 5 of 19 false-negative errors, and a short-term fluctuation of 4.48. The circles illustrate the points of test/retest for the determination of short-term fluctuation. In the other case **(B)**, there were 5 of 25 fixation losses. The fields are remarkably different and neither is valid because of poor patient reliability.

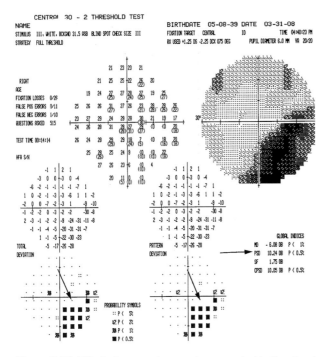

Figure 2–79. Effect of a very deep scotoma created in the visual field. The scotoma that is deep will be similar in appearance in both the total deviation and pattern deviation probability plots.

Positive Catch Trials. Positive catch trials indicate when the patient reports seeing the target even when it is not presented. The Humphrey/Zeiss equivalent is the false positive.

Negative Catch Trials. Negative catch trials indicate when the patient reports seeing no target at maximum intensity even though the patient has seen the target previously at that location. The Humphrey/Zeiss equivalent is the false negative.

Short-term Fluctuation. Short-term fluctuation represents the drift or scatter of threshold values when measured more than once. This not automatically performed on all threshold fields.

Reliability Factor. The reliability factor (RF) is an indication of the percentage of positive and negative catch trials missed by the patient. If the RF exceeds 15 percent, it is recommended that the field test be repeated.

Visual Field Printouts

Upper Left—Raw Data. If patient reliability factors are acceptable, you may then proceed to the analysis of the printouts. The Interzeag/Octopus device gives three separate field displays on its composition printout. The upper left field displays the true threshold decibel levels at the specific tested points. This is raw data and as such is difficult to interpret.

Upper Right—Comparison Field. This display has significance from the standpoint that it is a display of deviation from "normal" expecteds. The difference from the expecteds is displayed at each point. Any deviation over 5 decibels will be displayed.

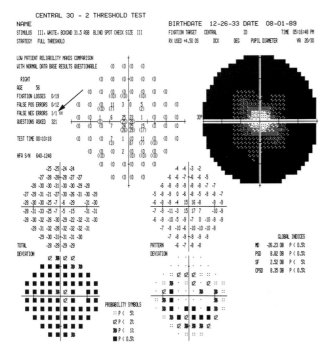

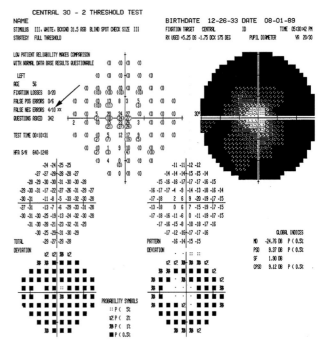

Figure 2–80. A patient with end-stage glaucoma and severe visual field defects. The patient reliability is flagged because of a high proportion of false-negative errors. These exist because the test/retest points to generate this index are within an area of nerve fibers desensitized by prior testing. This field is, in fact, a perfectly reliable visual field.

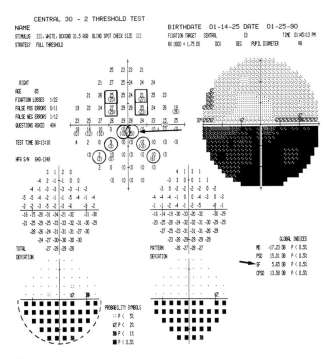

TABLE 2–14. PRINTOUT SUMMARY FOR THE INTERZEAG/OCTOPUS DEVICE

Top left: Display of true decibel values (inverse of apostilbs)

Top right: Comparison field, which is a display of decibel deviation from expected normals

Lower left: Gray scale

Lower right: Display of indices and reliability factors

Bottom: Patient reliability factors and demographic data

Lower Left—Gray Scale. The gray scale is a substitute for the isopter display of the Goldmann-type perimetry. The gray scale is a representation of threshold values. The darker the printout, the poorer the retinal sensitivity. Gray-scale printouts are potentially dangerous as they do not take age-matched comparisons into account!

Lower Right—Indices. This portion of the printout indicates patient reliability as well as indices. The short-term fluctuation and reliability factors are only generated when the perimetrist advances into phase 2. All other patient reliability factors including catch trials are indicated at the bottom of the printout. Table 2–14 represents a summary of the printout.

Figure 2–81. A patient with a severe altitudinal defect can demonstrate a high short-term fluctuation level that can falsely lead the clinician to discount the value of the test. The high error is secondary to test/retest in an area of desensitized nerve fibers. This visual field is perfectly reliable and represents anterior ischemic optic neuropathy.

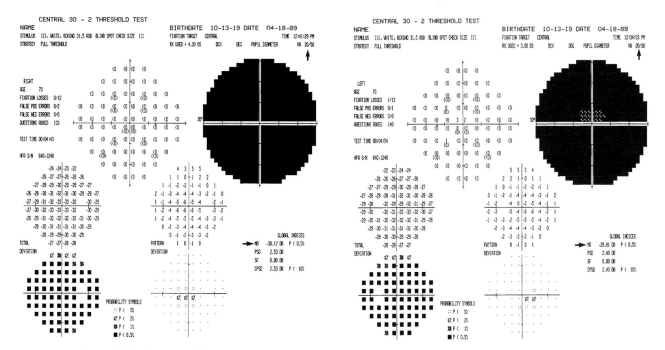

Figure 2–82. A patient with end-stage glaucomatous optic atrophy and severe visual field defects. These fields also demonstrate the potential danger encountered with artificial intelligence. If the clinician were to read the pattern deviation probability plot, which assumes that the field defect is secondary to an overall depression of the field secondary to media opacities, the field would be interpreted as being totally normal. The MD in both fields is very high while the PSD is within normal limits. The pattern deviation probability plot should be reserved for patients with media opacities.

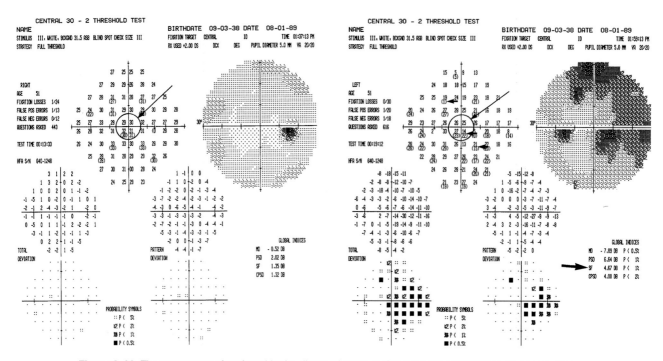

Figure 2–83. The asymmetry often found in the diseased state. In this case the condition is glaucoma. The arrows point to the perifoveal test areas demonstrating the depression in these zones that will often occur with glaucoma. Note as well the difference in the short-term fluctuation between the two eyes that often occurs in asymmetrical diseased states.

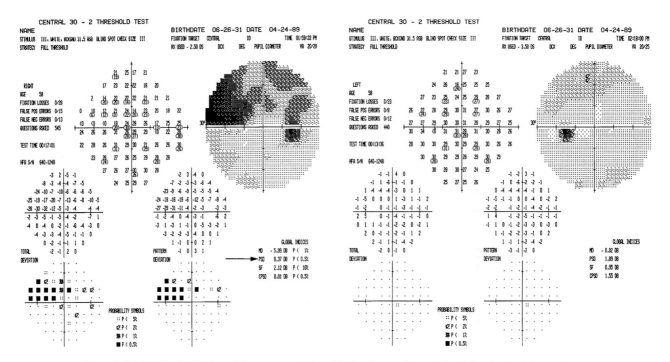

Figure 2–84. Another illustration of the asymmetry found in the diseased state. The defect in the right eye is secondary to ischemic optic neuropathy and is very deep as evidenced by the presence in both the total deviation probability plot and the pattern deviation probability plot.

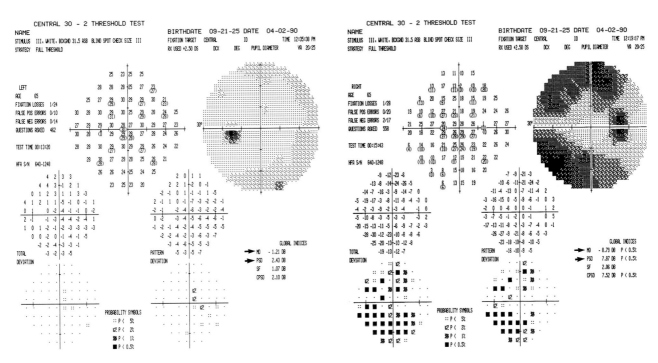

Figure 2–85. Effect of defects on the generation of the global indices of MD and PSD. The arrows point to the increase in the index in both instances with increases in the number of defects.

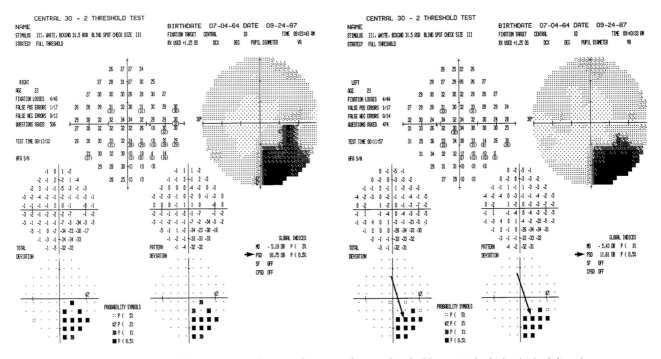

Figure 2–86. Right inferior congruous deep quadrantanopsia associated with a posterior lesion in the left parietal area. Note the similarity in the global indices in both fields associated with the congruity.

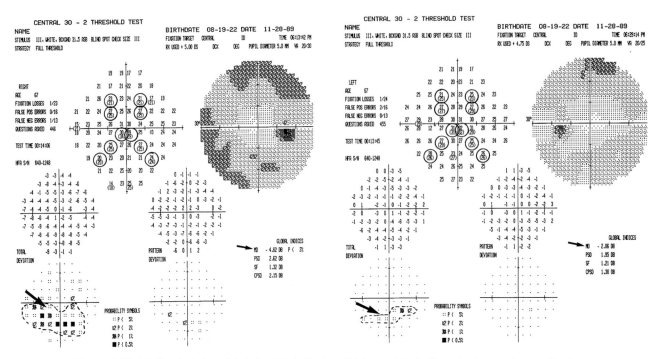

Figure 2–87. Inferior clustering of defect points in the hemifield associated with early glaucomatous optic atrophy. The patient does not have media opacities.

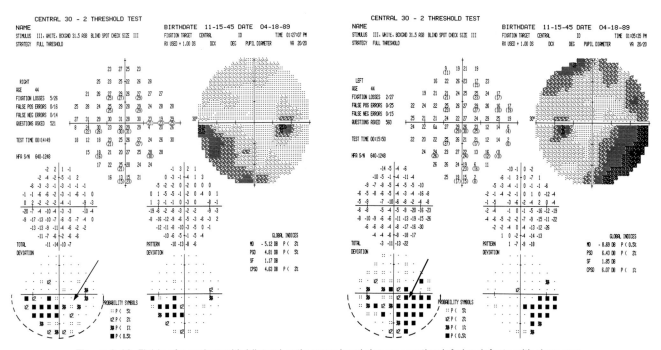

Figure 2–88. Fields of a patient with bilateral optic nerve head drusen creating inferior defects with deep scotomas in the binasal zones of each eye, as evidenced in the pattern deviation probability plots.

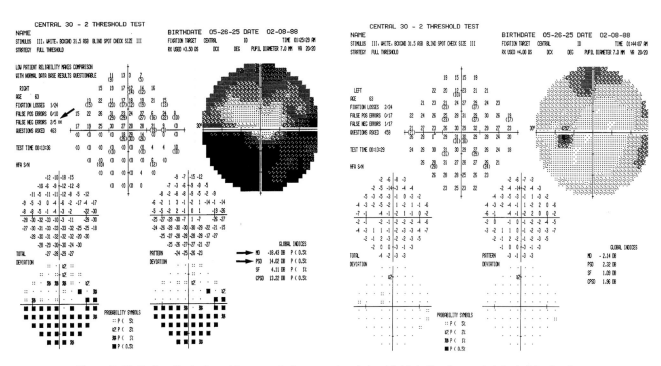

Figure 2–89. Further illustration of the expected asymmetry of visual fields in the diseased state. In this situation, the patient has ischemic optic neuropathy in the right eye. Note the high false negatives that would prompt one to discount the value of the field, when the field is actually very reliable.

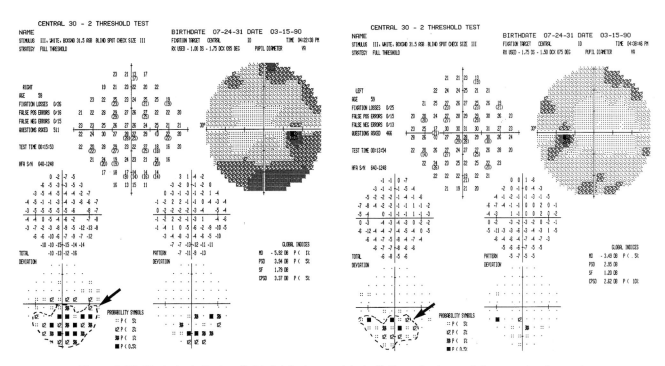

Figure 2–90. Clustering in the hemifield of defects associated with the early stages of glaucoma development.

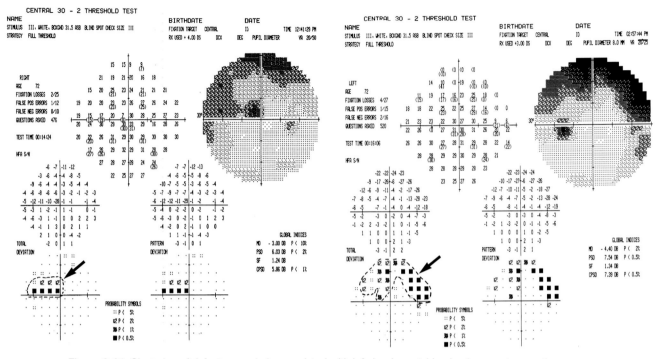

Figure 2–91. Clustering of defects superiorly associated with inferior rim notching in glaucomatous optic neuropathy. Again, there is the characteristic asymmetry associated with optic nerve and retinal disease.

Global Indices

The Interzeag/Octopus system has a set of global indices that serve as guidelines for the interpretation of the visual fields. These include mean sensitivity, mean deviation, loss variance, and corrected loss variance. Not all global indices are calculated against age-matched "normals." Ranges for "normals" are indicated on the printout.

Mean Sensitivity. Mean sensitivity is the average overall mean sensitivity level in decibels. It would be expected that the mean sensitivity level would decrease with age.

Mean Deviation. The mean deviation is the difference between the measured mean sensitivity level for the patient and that for age-matched normal levels. The mean deviation index is increased greatly by overall hill of vision depressions, but only slightly by isolated small scotomas. The Humphrey/Zeiss equivalent is the mean deviation.

Loss Variance. Loss variance is a measure of the departure from the age-corrected standard normal-shaped hill of vision. Loss variance is large with isolated scotomas and small with overall depressions. If the loss variance is increased outside of the normal ranges indicated, you must determine if patient reliability (short-term fluctuation) is the problem. This is achieved by going into phase 2 in the global analysis program. The Humphrey/Zeiss equivalent is the pattern standard deviation (PSD). High levels are indicated in parentheses ( ).

Corrected Loss Variance. Corrected loss variance is a measure of the departure from the age-corrected standard normal-shaped hill of vision corrected for patient intratest reliability (SF). This index can only be generated through phase 2 in the global analysis program. The Humphrey/Zeiss equivalent is the corrected pattern standard deviation (CSPD).

Several new sophisticated features are available for data analysis for the Humphrey/Zeiss and Interzeag/Octopus units. The systems go by different generic names but all function to provide the practitioner with numerous methods for manipulating and analyzing the basic data obtained through threshold visual field testing.

PHYSICAL DIAGNOSTIC TESTING

Because most ocular disease is a manifestation of systemic disease, it is important for the primary care practitioner to have some understanding of simple physical diagnostic tests to assist in proper diagnosis and management. The topic cannot be fully addressed here; however, the basics will be discussed. Other sources listed in the references provide a more indepth discussion of the topics.

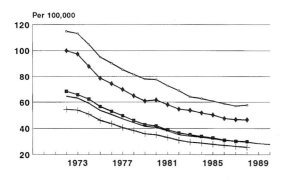

−Total −◦− Black Men −♦− Black Women −■− White Men −+− White Women

Figure 2–92. Age-adjusted mortality rates for stroke by race and sex, 1972–1990.

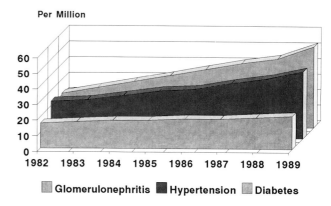

▨ Glomerulonephritis   ■ Hypertension   ▥ Diabetes

Figure 2–94. Incidence rates per million population of reported end-stage renal disease therapy by primary diagnosis, 1982–1989.

Blood Pressure and Pulse Evaluation

There are currently over 50 million persons in the United States with systemic hypertension. Approximately 45 percent of patients over the age of 65 years have systolic blood pressure (BP) of 160 mm Hg or greater or diastolic BP of 95 mm Hg or greater. The systolic hypertension in the elderly study (SHEP) has shown that controlling systolic hypertension above 160 mm Hg in older patients definitely reduces morbidity and mortality. It is recommended that patients over the age of 65 with diastolic BP of 90 or greater will benefit from treatment. Having three separate clinical BP readings over 140/90 is associated with a 37 percent increase in mortality in men and a 53 percent increase in mortality in women. Prevalence of hypertension is 33 percent higher in blacks, is more severe in blacks, and causes a higher death rate in young blacks. To complicate the picture, blacks also have 2.5 times the incidence of asthma as whites.

Systolic hypertension is the major risk factor for stroke, and patients with the combination of hyper-

tension and diabetes are at increased risk for both systemic vascular disease and retinopathy. Figures 2–92 and 2–93 illustrate the positive effect of controlling hypertension in this country over the past few years. Figure 2–94 illustrates the increase in the incidence of end-stage renal disease secondary to hypertension, diabetes, and glomerulonephritis. Hypertension is a major morbidity factor in ocular disease and all patients should be screened in office for hypertension. Table 2–15 lists some of the ocular complications of hypertension, and Table 2–16 outlines the proper procedure for taking routine blood pressure measurements. Table 2–17 gives recommendations regarding management of specific blood pressure levels for patients over the age of 18 years.

Figures 2–95 to 2–97 illustrate the results of the Trials of Hypertension Prevention, Phase I (TOHP-I) study on the effects of life-style modification in hypertension and hypertensive events.

Palpation for the radial pulse is of value in that it gives the clinician some sense of the possibility of

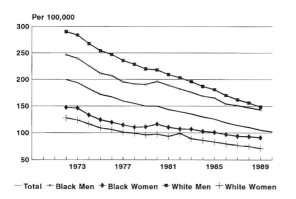

−Total −◦− Black Men −♦− Black Women −■− White Men −+− White Women

Figure 2–93. Age-adjusted mortality rates for coronary heart disease by race and sex, 1972–1990.

TABLE 2–15. SYSTEMIC HYPERTENSION: SOME OCULAR SIGNS AND SYMPTOMS

Anomalous A/V crossings
Arterial sheath changes
Branch retinal artery occlusion
Branch retinal vein occlusion
Central retinal artery occlusion
Central retinal vein occlusion
Hemicentral retinal vein occlusion
Headaches
Ischemic optic neuropathy
Isolated preretinal hemorrhages
Isolated cotton-wool spots
Malignant hypertensive retinopathy
Postural vision changes
Retinal macroaneurysms
Subconjunctival hemorrhages
Transient vision loss
Enhancement of the development of diabetic retinopathy

TABLE 2–16. GUIDELINES FOR TAKING BLOOD PRESSURE

- Patients should be seated with their legs uncrossed, arm bare, free of constrictive clothing, and supported at approximately heart level
- Patients should not have smoked or ingested caffeine within 30 minutes prior to the test
- Patients should rest for 5 minutes prior to the test
- Use a mercury sphygmomanometer or other routinely calibrated device
- Use the proper-sized cuff—the rubber bladder should encircle at least 80 percent of the arm circumference
- Technique
  Take the pulse rate
  Place the cuff on the upper arm 1 inch above the crease of the elbow
  Palpate the brachial artery at the crease of the elbow, then place the bell head of the stethoscope over this site—you should hear the pulse
  Determine the level for maximal inflation by observing the pressure at which the palpated radial pulse disappears as the cuff is rapidly inflated and then add 30 mm Hg. Quickly deflate the cuff and wait 15 to 30 secs before reinflating
  Slowly release the air allowing the pressure to fall smoothly at the rate of about 2 mm Hg per second
  Both systolic (appearance of sound) and diastolic (disappearance of sound) should be recorded—then the cuff rapidly deflated
  Wait at least 1 minute
  Then repeat
  Average two or more readings
  If the readings differ by more than 5 mm Hg, additional readings should be obtained

TABLE 2–17. CLASSIFICATION AND FOLLOW-UP OF BLOOD PRESSURE MEASUREMENTS IN ADULTS OVER AGE 18 YEARS

Blood Pressure Range (mm Hg)	Recommended Follow-up
Diastolic	
<85	Recheck in 2 years
85–89	Recheck in 1 year
90–99	Confirm in 2 months and refer for care if repeatable
100–109	Refer within 4 weeks for care
110–119	Refer within 1 week for care
>120	Refer immediately for care
Systolic When Diastolic >90	
<130	Recheck in 2 years
130–139	Recheck in 1 year
140–159	Confirm in 2 months
160–179	Refer within 1 month for care
180–209	Refer within 1 week for care
>210	Refer immediately for care

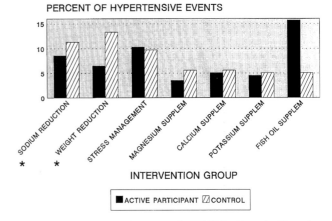

Figure 2–95. Hypertensive events in TOHP-I with and without intervention. Asterisks indicate effective modalities of treatment. Supplem, supplement.

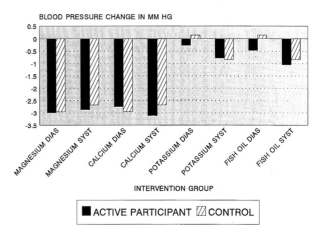

Figure 2–96. Mean changes from baseline blood pressure in TOHP-I associated with nutritional supplements. Dias, diastolic; Syst, systolic.

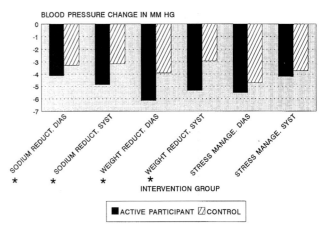

Figure 2–97. Mean changes from baseline blood pressure in TOHP-I associated with life-style alterations. Asterisks indicate effective modalities of treatment. Dias, diastolic; Syst, systolic.

heartbeat abnormalities and is also grossly elevated in systemic conditions such as thyroid disease and malignant hypertension. The pulse rate is also important in all glaucoma patients placed on beta-blocking drugs, as these drugs have the potential to significantly alter pulse rates. The rate can be taken over a 15 second time frame, multiplied by four, and recorded as beats per minute (BPM).

Palpation and Auscultation of the Carotid System

The carotid system has a very direct relationship to the eye, and as such alterations in the system often create significant ocular signs and symptoms. Evaluation of the system can be accomplished in a screening fashion by palpation and auscultation of the carotid pulse. The common carotids branch off of the aortic arch and course up the neck between the trachea and the sternocleidomastoid muscles to bifurcate at the angle of the jaw into the external and internal carotid arteries. The external system supplies the scalp and face and represents a collateral system for the internal carotid supply. The internal carotid system supplies both the brain and the eye via the ophthalmic division. As such, the formation of plaques within the system can impact directly on vision function. Although imprecise, palpation of the carotids can give some idea of the flow characteristics within the system, especially if the right system is compared to the left. Care must be exercised when comparing one side to the other, as excessive pressure in a stenotic system can create an artificial transient reduction in blood supply to the brain and manipulation may even dislodge emboli. Asymmetry of the pulse coupled with ocular signs and symptoms can be an indication of the need to further investigate the carotid system. When palpating, it is important to position the fingers at approximately the same location on both sides ascending from near the clavical area to the angle of the jaw, which represents the carotid sinus (Fig. 2–98). Assure that the patient's head is not torted or tilted as the physical alteration of the carotid system can elicit pulsation variation.

Auscultation for bruits, which are swishing or rumbling sounds within the major vessels, may also be an indication of obstructed flow. When plaque forms at vessel bifurcations, flow is altered, allowing for the change in the normal sound of blood flow. Again, auscultation is an inexact science, as bruits often do not occur until there is approximately 50 percent occlusion and may actually disappear when occlusion reaches 75 percent. To auscultate for bruits, initially use the open bell portion of the stethoscope to attempt to pick up the low-frequency bruit. Palpate

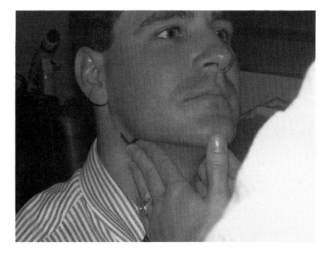

Figure 2–98. Technique for palpation for asymmetry of the carotid arteries.

for the pulse to locate the position of the carotids. Start low in the neck near the clavicle, gently placing the bell over the carotid while asking the patient to hold his or her breath. Listen for 10 to 15 seconds, ask the patient to breathe, and then move up the sternocleidomastoid toward the angle of the jaw and the carotid sinus. Listen for the swooshing sound of the bruit and for changes in pulse characteristics throughout the system. Take care not to tort or tilt the patient's head as this maneuver can create an anatomical bruit. The presence of a bruit is indicative of stenosis but the absence does not indicate a system free from stenosis. Refer to Figure 2–99.

The orbit may also be auscultated to investigate for orbital vascular abnormalities or congestion. The technique is performed through the closed eyelid

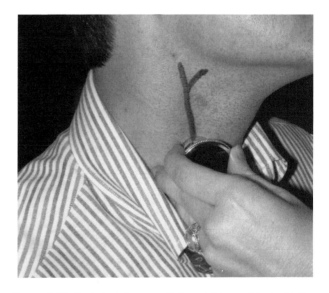

Figure 2–99. Technique for auscultation of the carotid arteries for bruits. The distribution of the carotid system is drawn on the neck.

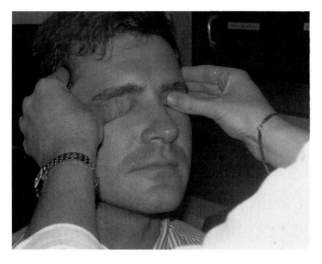

Figure 2–100. Technique for performing retropulsion of the ocular contents to assess orbital contents and resistance.

Certainly, real-time ultrasound evaluation of the carotid system is indicated in cases of both symptomatic and asymptomatic Hollenhorst plaque, transient ischemic attacks, transient monocular blindness, and unilateral or asymmetrical retinal vascular disease; and possibly in ischemic optic neuropathy and in situations when bruits have been auscultated. It has been shown that real-time ultrasonography demonstrates a 95 percent agreement with angiography in identifying carotid stenosis of greater than 50 percent. Although angiography is more specific in diagnosis, it carries a higher morbidity and mortality rate than ultrasonography. Refer to Figure 2–101 for an example of diagnostic ultrasonography demonstrating carotid stenosis.

while the patient holds his or her breath. A detection of an orbital bruit suggests a vascular anomaly and indicates the necessity to rule out this possibility. Globe repositioning (retropulsion) may also be of value in conditions that create orbital bruits (Fig. 2–100). This test is simply an evaluation of resistance to external pressure to push the eye gently back into the orbit. Simultaneous gentle repositioning is accomplished with the thumbs while the clinician notes differences in resistance and the patient response of pain or discomfort. This test is of value in conditions that may create proptosis and in conditions of inflammation that may create pain. Obviously, this test is contraindicated in cases of recent trauma that may have created a penetrating wound.

Diagnostic Doppler Ultrasonography

A more precise method of assessing the carotid system is through Doppler ultrasonography. This test is a noninvasive evaluation that is of no discomfort to the patient and can be quite valuable when assessing for stenosis of the system. The test goes by many names, often called "duplex" because the test is a combination of high-resolution, real-time B-mode echography and pulsed Doppler sonography. The B-mode is used to image the arterial structure and to assess the degree of stenosis while the Doppler mode measures blood flow velocity. During Doppler ultrasonography the sound signal is scattered by red blood cells, causing a shift in frequency. If stenosis is present, the red blood cell velocity increases. If stenosis exceeds 50 to 70 percent, the increased velocity is no longer sustained. Color imaging may also be used for the Doppler measurements to allow a more accurate evaluation.

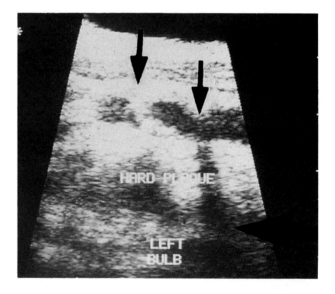

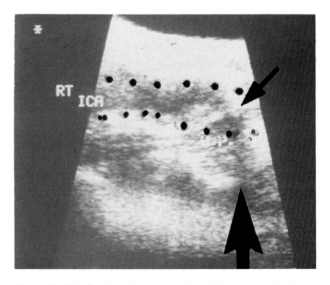

Figure 2–101. Duplex ultrasonography with arrows pointing to plaque formation and the shadow created by the plaque.

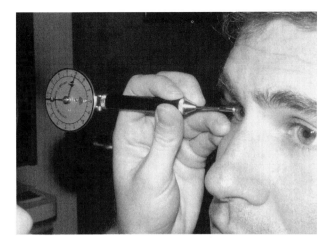

Figure 2–102. A technique for one-person performance of ophthalmodynamometry. The shaft of the ODM must be perpendicular to the globe to exert exact pressures.

Ophthalmodynamometry (ODM)

Ophthalmodynamometry (ODM) is a testing technique for the indirect measurement of ophthalmic artery pressure. It is a test that may be of value in the same clinical situations as duplex ultrasonography, but the test has severe limitations. Proper technique is so crucial because something as simple as not applying perpendicular pressure to the globe can result in artificially elevated readings. The test is based on the fact that artificially elevating the intraocular pressure to the level of the diastolic pressure in the retinal arteries will result in a collapse (blanching) or pulsation of that artery. Venous pulsation occurs at a much lower intraocular pressure; in fact, in a high percentage of patients it is spontaneous, because the walls of the veins are very thin.

The test is performed on a dilated anesthetized eye by placing the footplate of the ODM instrument on the lateral aspect of the globe, taking care not to exert too much pressure (Fig. 2–102). Then while observing an artery at the point where it crosses the edge of the disc with a direct ophthalmoscope, the clinician increases the pressure on the footplate perpendicular to the globe until first observing the arterial collapse. Pressure may then be further increased to the point of total loss of the pulse. Pressure is then released and the instrument removed to observe and record the reading on the self-recording dial or linear slide. The first arterial pulse indicates the diastolic pressure and the loss of the pulse indicates the systolic pressure. Another method may be used employing a binocular indirect view with an assistant increasing the pressure on the footplate. Three readings should be taken and averaged. A conversion nomogram is then plotted against the intraocular pressure to give the BP in mm

Hg. The diastolic value should lie in the range of 45 to 60 percent of the brachial blood pressure (values between 30 and 50 mm Hg), whereas the systolic value should be between 54 and 70 percent of the brachial pressure (values between 60 and 85 mm Hg). If the measured value is 20 percent under that expected, the test is considered positive. The true value of ODM lies in comparison between the two eyes. In healthy individuals the difference between the two eyes should not be more than 10 to 15 percent. Both diastolic and systolic readings are necessary for definitive diagnosis, but in reality this is not a definitive test for carotid stenosis but rather a screening test. If symptoms are there, ODM should not be the sole basis of differential diagnosis.

More sophisticated instruments use suction to artificially elevate the intraocular pressure and have built-in recording systems to eliminate the necessity to observe the retinal vascular system while increasing the pressure. Some of the suction systems (oculopneumoplethsmography) may also be used to more closely evaluate the status of the ophthalmic artery system after it branches from the internal carotid.

Neurologic and Ocular Imaging

The sophistication and technology of neurologic and ocular imaging is changing on a daily basis. Computed tomography (CT) or computed axial tomography (CAT) is a relatively new procedure but has already been supplanted by magnetic resonance imaging (MRI). In fact the changes are occurring so rapidly that, as a primary care clinician, I would recommend deferring to the neurologist, neuroradiologist, or neurosurgeon to determine the test of choice. CT does have its place, especially when calcified structures need further study or repeated studies are expected and the clinician wants to minimize the amount of x-ray radiation delivered to the patient. Figures 2–103 to 2–113 illustrate CT scans and MRI scans, demonstrating their diagnostic efficacy.

With CT, a collimated x-ray is sent through the tissue and received by a detector minus the absorbed radiation. Slices are made through the area studied and the difference between emitted and received radiation are calculated for each segment. These calculations are then displayed in a gray scale equivalent and are recorded on films as desired. Coronal scans show orbital detail and allow for ready comparison between the two orbits. The coronal scan is especially useful in the evaluation of extraocular muscles in thyroid eye disease. This scan is also valuable in evaluation of the pituitary area. The neuro-ocular plane, which is the visual pathway from the cornea to the calcarine fissure oriented at −7 degrees to the orbito-

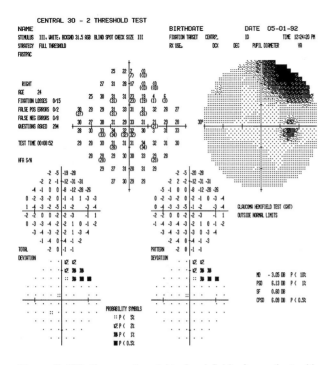

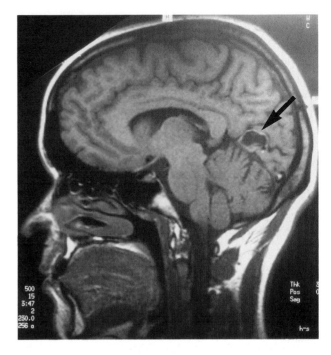

Figure 2–103. Preoperative right visual field of a patient with a left occipital lobe lesion as shown in Figures 2–105 through 2–107).

Figure 2–105. Preoperative MRI without contrast of the patient whose visual fields are shown in Figures 2–103 and 2–104. The arrow points to a calcified lesion shown in the T1 phase of the MRI.

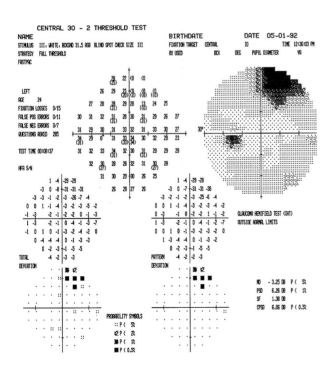

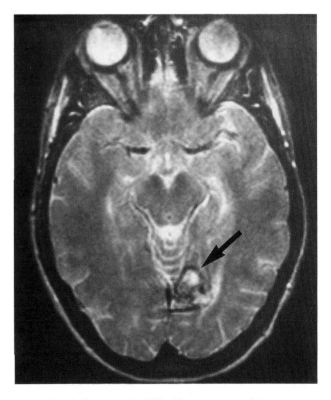

Figure 2–104. Preoperative left visual field of the patient shown in Figure 2–103. Together the figures form a right superior quadrantanopsia with fair congruity implying a lesion posterior in the cortex.

Figure 2–106. Preoperative MRI without contrast of the same patient shown in Figure 2–105 with the arrow again pointing to the lesion. The dark ring surrounding the lesion was thought to be old blood.

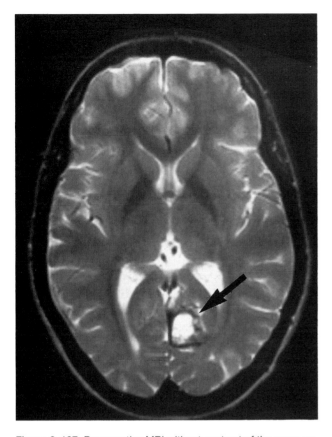

Figure 2–107. Preoperative MRI without contrast of the same patient shown in Figure 2–106, but at a different level, with the arrow again pointing to the lesion in the T2 (2nd echo) phase of the MRI.

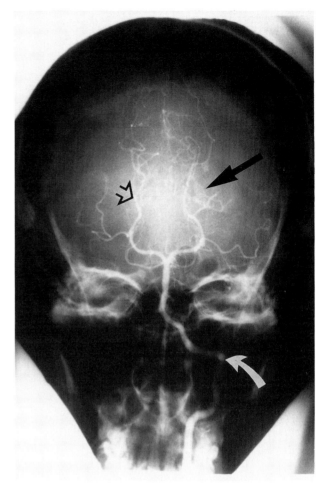

Figure 2–108. Preoperative cerebral arteriogram of the patient shown in Figures 2–105 through 2–107; view is of a selective left vertebral injection (*white arrow*). The large dark arrow points to the zone of the lesion and, according to the report, demonstrates slight decreased vascularity as compared to the open arrow. This could, however, be nothing more than an anatomic variation.

meatal line, will give a view of the orbit and pathway simultaneously with minimal x-ray dosage. CT is useful in assessment of the possibility of invasive foreign bodies, craniopharyngiomas, and buried drusen of the optic nerve head that are difficult to view clinically. Contrast media injected intravenously is useful in the differential diagnosis of vascular lesions, but MRI is the preferred modality in soft-tissue disorders.

MRI uses analysis of radiowaves emitted by protons within a strongly magnetic field for generation of a study. There is no radiation involved. The receiving portion of the scanner is tuned to receive the deflections of specific atoms of the tissues that are being scanned. MRI may achieve direct multiplane image formation, which is an advantage over CT scanning and also gives an accurate image of the contrast of white and gray matter in the central nervous system while imaging the cerebral spinal fluid (CFS) as black. This black background of the CSF also provides a good contrast for viewing blood vessel detail, and alteration of this detail (localized infarcts), without the necessity for contrast injection, whereas CT is preferable for fresh hemorrhages. Plaques of demyelinizing

diseases are also more easily viewed with MRI—in fact the technique has become an important diagnostic feature in the workup of suspected multiple sclerosis patients.

The magnetic resonance angiogram (MRA) is also a valuable tool for the evaluation of the carotid system and the intracranial vasculature but selective cerebral angiography, which carries significant risk, is still the definitive diagnostic test for suspected vascular alterations. Digital subtraction angiography is often used as an adjunct to angiography, employing computer enhancement of the data while requiring less contrast medium. Gadolinium is a contrast agent used in MRI specific for the blood–brain barrier to distinguish differing types of lesions. MRI is superior to CT for imaging all parenchymal abnormalities, espe-

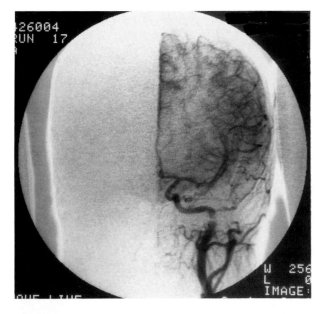

Figure 2–109. Preoperative AP digital subtration imagery of the patient shown in Figure 2–108 showing no evidence of abnormal intracranial vasculature in the distribution of the left internal carotid system.

cially in the posterior fossa and brainstem because of the interference set up there by the bony structures. CT is excellent for calcified alterations whereas MRI is the choice for soft-tissue problems. Often a combination of the two is necessary to discern the cause for alarm, and even at that the cause is still obscure.

Exophthalmometry

Exophthalmometry is a testing technique used when there is suspicion that proptosis is a feature of a disease process or when ruling out anatomical variations as a cause of pseudoptosis. The most obvious indication is when thyroid eye disease is suspected, but the test is also of value in any space-occupying orbital lesion. The measurement may be accomplished in many ways from a screening technique using a device called the Luedde exophthalmometer to a more precise technique using the Hertel exophthalmometer. Both instruments measure the forward protrusion of the corneal surface using the lateral orbital rim as a point of reference. The Luedde exophthalmometer comes with instructions, but the basic technique is to place the notched end of the lucite at the lateral orbital rim and to view with parallax the corneal apex from the side and use the scale to determine the degree of protrusion. Each eye measurement is determined independently. The Hertel exophthalmometer uses a mirror

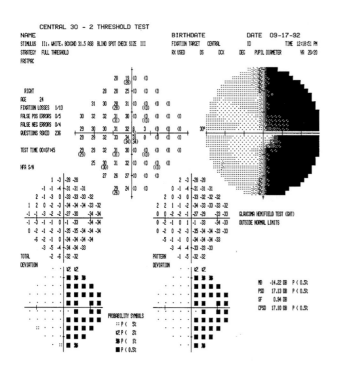

Figure 2–110. Postoperative right visual field of the patient shown in Figures 2–103 through 2–109.

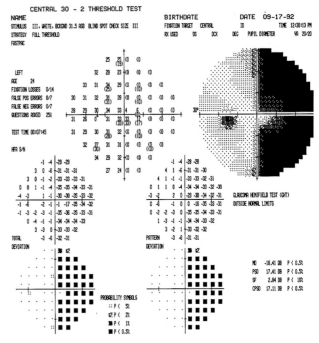

Figure 2–111. Postoperative left visual field of the patient shown in Figures 2–103 through 2–109. Note that Figure 2–110 and this figure form a total right homonymous hemianopsia with macular sparing. Vision has been maintained at 20/20 OU.

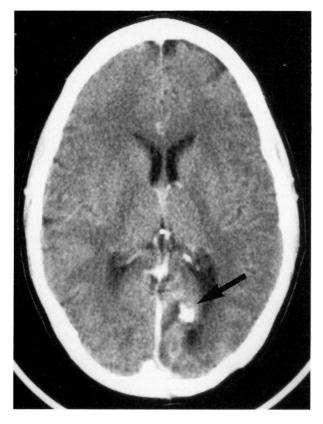

Figure 2–112. Postoperative and postradiation CT scan with contrast of the patient shown in Figures 2–103 through 2–111. The scan was performed approximately 3 months after surgery. The arrow points to the remnants of the calcified lesion.

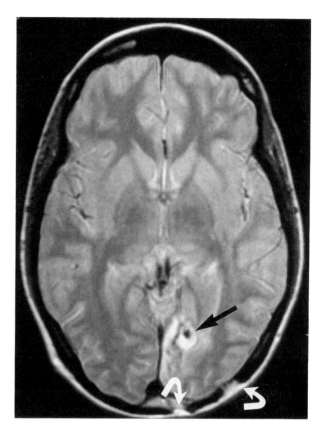

Figure 2–113. 6-Month postoperative MRI without contrast at spin density of the patient shown in Figures 2–103 through 2–112. The arrow points to the lesion and can be reasonably compared to the preoperative Figure 2–107. The white arrows point to the craniotomy sites.

system to enable the clinician to observe both eyes with parallax without moving the instrument. The Hertel device also employs a scale to determine baseline for future settings regarding the distance between the lateral orbital rims. Normal exophthalmometry readings range from 12 to 20 mm for whites and 12 to 24 mm for blacks, as blacks often have anatomically shallower orbits. Multiple averaged readings improve the diagnostic ability of this as well as many other procedures.

Forced Ductions

Forced ductions are an important test to differentiate between neurogenic and mechanical extraocular muscle restrictions. Forced ductions are necessary in cases of sudden-onset diplopia, the possibility of trauma-induced diplopia, and in noncomitant diplopia. The test is performed after anesthesia is attained with 10% topical cocaine solution at the site on the conjunctiva near the insertion of the recti muscle to be tested. A toothed forceps is used to grasp the conjunctiva and fascia of Tenon opposite to the direction of the desired rotation of the globe at the insertion of the muscle. This is usually approximately 5 mm posterior to the lim-

bus. The patient is then asked to look in the direction of the intended rotation while applying gentle force to rotate the eye in the same direction. Restriction in movement of the globe indicates a mechanical problem versus a neurogenic cause.

Pain on Gross Excursion

Pain on motion of the eyes is often associated with optic neuritis. About 20 percent of patients with optic neuropathy have pain on motion of the globe, and some sources cite the percentage as being closer to 50 percent. Two important points concerning this symptom are (1) this is not an absolute sign of optic neuropathy, and (2) the clinician must elicit gross movements of the eyes to put enough stretch on the nerve to stimulate the pain receptors attached to the orbital wall. This symptom in the absence of other signs or symptoms is nebulous at best.

Uhthoff's Symptom

Uhthoff's symptom is a loss or dimming of vision or an increase in the size of a scotoma when the body temperature is increased. This can occur while lying in the sun, while in a steam bath, or while exercising strenuously. This symptom is most often associated with loss of the myelin insulation of nerve fibers commonly occurring in demyelinizing disease. The symptom can, however, present in many conditions; therefore, its presence should not trigger the diagnosis of demyelinizing disease (multiple sclerosis).

Lhermitte's Symptom

Lhermitte's symptom is the sensation of electric-like shocks in the limbs and trunk when the head is flexed forward, placing the chin on the chest. This symptom is strongly suggestive of demyelinizing disease because of loss of the myelin insulation around the nerve fibers. This can also be a sign of cervical injury, and as such the test should be performed with great care. Again, this test on its own is not specifically diagnostic of any disease process.

Screening Tests for Motor Function

Several tests of motor function are available, including walking heel–to–toe down a straight line (tandem walking), finger-to-nose and finger-to-finger testing, and standing with heels and toes together with eyes closed and arms outstretched (Romberg's sign). These tests usually relate to demyelinizing disease or vascular compromise or insufficiency, in that coordination and balance are often compromised. These tests are of value in assessing any potential neurologic/optic nerve lesion.

Tandem Walking. A gait that lacks coordination is called ataxic. Ataxia can be the result of cerebellar disease, loss of sense of position, or intoxication. Tandem walking is performed by asking the patient to walk heel-to-toe on a straight line (Fig. 2–114). Observe the patient's ability to perform this without too much imbalance. A variation is to ask the patient to hop in place on each foot, which is a test of not only cerebellar function but also muscle strength.

Gait Evaluation. Observation of the patient's gait on entering the office or examination room can give the clinician some clues as to possible problems. The more common gaits are described below.

The gait associated with spastic hemiparesis (often a unilateral upper motor neuron problem) is described as the patient dragging the foot or performing circumduction (moving the foot outward in a circle). One arm is also usually immobile, held close to the side, and the joints are flexed. This gait is often associated with stroke.

The parkinsonian gait is characterized by a stooped posture with the head and neck forward and

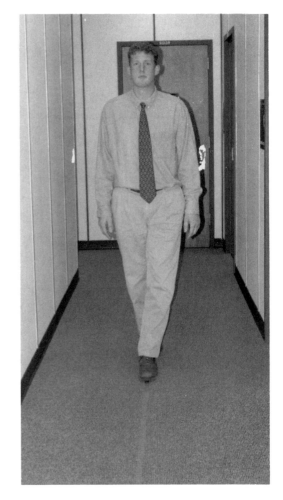

Figure 2–114. Performance of the tandem walk. The patient is walking heel-to-toe on a masking tape line.

the arms flexed at the elbows and wrists. The patient stutters at the start of ambulation followed by short shuffling steps. The movement is very stiff.

The gait of cerebellar ataxia has been described in tandem walking as staggering, unsteady, and wide-based, with difficulty in position sense.

The gait of sensory ataxia is characteristic of peripheral neuropathy or posterior column disease. This gait is unsteady and wide-based as with cerebellar ataxia. The patient kicks the feet forward and outward, and then brings them down on first the heel and then the toes, making a double tap sound. The patient relies strongly on the sense of sight for ambulation.

The steppage or foot-drop gait is associated with lower motor neuron disease such as syphilis. The patient either drags the feet or lifts them high to compensate, and the heels are not involved in the ambulatory process. After lifting high with the knees flexed, the patient slaps the feet to the floor as if climbing stairs.

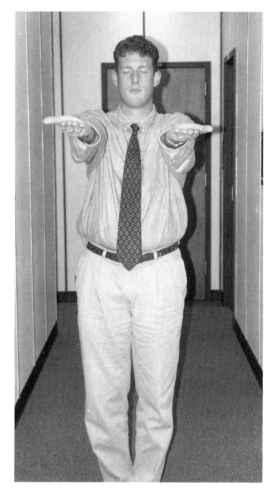

Figure 2–115. One method of eliciting Romberg's sign with the arms extended and the palms up while the eyes are closed.

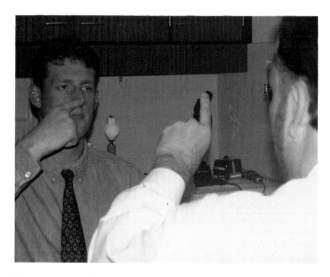

Figure 2–116. One technique for performance of finger-to-finger/finger-to-nose testing.

Romberg's Sign. Romberg's test is performed by asking the patient to stand with heels and toes together without support. This is performed with the eyes open and then closed. The test can be modified by asking the patient to extend the arms forward with palms up and eyes closed for about 30 seconds (Fig. 2–115). Be sure to stay close to the patient, as this test can be very dramatic in affected patients, causing them to reel considerably. The patient with cerebellar ataxia from a loss of position sense can perform this test well with the eyes open but fails when the eyes are closed. Also observe the action of the arms during this period, as the tendency of one forearm to pronate suggests a mild hemiparesis. The arm may also drift downward (pronator drift) with flexing of the fingers.

Point-to-Point Testing. Many variations of point-to-point testing can be performed. The clinician can ask the patient to touch his or her index finger and nose alternately several times (Fig. 2–116). The clinician may then move the index finger around to challenge the patient in altering directions. In cerebellar disease, movements are unsteady and vary in speed and direction, creating overshooting, which is known as dysmetria. Observe for any altered movements or tremor. Remember to modify expectations according to patient age and health status. You may also ask the patient to alternately touch your index finger and the patient's nose with the eyes closed. Testing with the eyes closed gives some assessment of position sense controlled by the cerebellar system. Repeatable deviation with the eyes closed is called past pointing.

A variation of point-to-point testing can be performed by asking the patient to remove both shoes, stand, place one heel on the opposite knee, and run it down to the foot. In cerebellar disease, the heel first misses the knee and then poorly follows the shin down to the foot. The loss of position sense is enhanced by closing the eyes.

Screening Tests for Sensory Function

Numerous tests for sensory function are available, but for screening purposes the clinician may assess pain and vibration sense in the hands and feet, light touch, and stereognosis. Regardless of the tests chosen, results must be compared symmetrically on the two sides of the body. Also, some assessment should be made comparing distal to proximal sensory function.

Pain and Light Touch. Using two sharp tips of disposable cotton applicators, stimulate the areas of interest supplied by the specific nerves, asking if the stimulus is sharp or dull and if the two sides feel the same. Analgesia is an absence of the pain sensation, hypoalgesia is decreased sensitivity to pain, and hy-

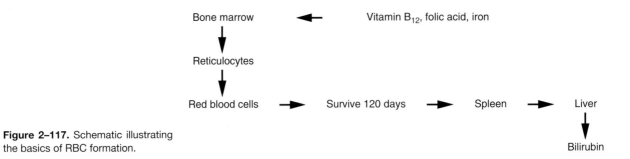

Figure 2–117. Schematic illustrating the basics of RBC formation.

peralgesia is an increased sense of pain. Likewise the sense of light touch may be performed in the same way by using the cotton-tipped applicator end pulled into a wisp. Anesthesia is the absence of light touch sensation, hypoesthesia is decreased sensitivity, and hyperesthesia is increased sensitivity.

Vibration Sense. To test for vibration sense, tap a low-pitched tuning fork on your hand and place it over the distal interphalangeal joint of the patient's finger and ask what the patient feels and when the sensation ceases. Perform the same test over the interphalangeal joint of the big toe. If equivocal, repeat over a bony prominence more proximal until the vibration is sensed. Loss of vibratory sense occurs first in peripheral neuropathies such as those in diabetes.

Stereognostic Testing. Stereognosis is the patient's ability to identify an object placed in the hand with the eyes closed. Astereognosis is the inability to identify the object and indicates a lesion in the sensory cortex. Graphesthesia, or number recognition, may also be used to test for astereognosis by drawing a number or letter on the patient's palm with the eyes closed and asking the patient to identify it.

CLINICAL LABORATORY DIAGNOSTIC TESTING

Laboratory diagnostic testing is the language, backbone, and support system for physical diagnosis. Although the primary eyecare practitioner cannot

---

TABLE 2–18. RED BLOOD CELL (RBC) COMPONENTS OF THE COMPLETE BLOOD COUNT (CBC)

Red Blood Cell Count (RBC)

Numbers of erythrocytes/μL
Used to detect anemias/polycythemias
Used as part of the erythrocyte indices

Hematocrit (HCT)

The volume of packed RBCs in 100 μL of blood
Used to establish presence and severity of anemia along with erythrocyte indices
Elevated in polycythemias, depressed in anemias

Hemoglobin (Hgb)

Measure of amount of oxygen-carrying pigment in blood
Depression indicates possibility of decreased oxygen to peripheral tissues
Consider glycated Hgb

Mean Corpuscular Volume (MCV)

Measure of relative cell size—normocytic, macrocytic, microcytic
Used to evaluate type of anemia

$$MCV = \frac{HCT \times 10}{RBC \times (10^6)}$$

$$= \frac{45\% \times 10}{5}$$

$$= 90 \ \mu m^3$$

Mean Corpuscular Hemoglobin (MCH)

Measures amount of hemoglobin in the average RBC—normochromic, hyperchromic, and hypochromic
Used to evaluate hemoglobin content

$$MCH = \frac{Hgb \times 10}{RBC \times (10^6)}$$

$$= \frac{15 \times 10}{5} = 30 \ pg$$

Mean Corpuscular Hemoglobin Concentration (MCHC)

Measure of chromicity or a percentage of the average RBC which is Hgb

$$MCHC = \frac{Hgb \times 100}{HCT}$$

$$= \frac{15 \times 100}{45}$$

$$= 33 \ \%$$

Reticulocyte Count

Immature RBCs
Indication of RBC production and are a proportion of 1000 RBCs
Normal range is 0.2 to 1.5%

be expected to know the nuances of clinical laboratory diagnosis, it is crucial to have a basic understanding to assure that the patient with an ocular sign of systemic disease receives the proper workup. The following presents a synopsis of clinical laboratory testing that is essential for the practice of primary eyecare.

Complete Blood Count (CBC)

The complete blood count (CBC) is the anchor of clinical laboratory diagnosis. Components include red blood cell, white blood cell, and platelet evaluation. The CBC provides the initial point of entry into the differential diagnosis of a number of disorders. It is important to understand the component features of the CBC to fully appreciate the extent of the capabilities. Understanding the components of the CBC that provide the analysis of red blood cells (RBCs) depends on an appreciation of the formation of the RBCs (Fig. 2–117).

The individual components of the RBC analysis of the CBC are summarized in Table 2–18. These are usually reported by the reference laboratory on a form including the normal values for the testing site. Not all values, such as the mean corpuscular hemoglobin (MCH), are routinely used in everyday practice.

RBC distribution width is a feature sometimes included in the analysis of RBCs. This test is a measure of the width of the RBCs to establish size variation among them. If this value is elevated it may indicate a component deficiency.

Erythrocyte Sedimentation Rate (ESR)

Another absolutely crucial laboratory test in primary eyecare is the erythrocyte sedimentation rate (ESR). Although there are different varieties, the Westergren method is a measure of the speed of RBCs settling in mixed uncoagulated venous blood. This test can now be performed in office. This test is a reflection of increases in plasma protein, especially fibrinogen and the immunoglobulins. It is a nonspecific test in infections, cancer, giant cell arteritis, and rheumatic diseases, and is used as a gauge of the efficacy of steroid treatment in ocular diseases such as temporal arteritic optic neuropathy. The average normal values for the

Westergren method can be approximated by the following formulas:

$$\text{Average for Males} = \text{Age}/2$$

$$\text{Average for Females} = (\text{Age} + 10)/2$$

Sickledex Test

The flocculation test that is used as a screener for the sickling of RBCs is the Sickledex test. Should this test be positive or equivocal, the definitive diagnosis is achieved through serum electrophoresis.

Studies of White Blood Cells

The status of the white blood cells (WBCs) is also evaluated with the CBC. Although in no way a detailed analysis, the CBC does give a general impression of the white blood cell status. Figure 2–118 illustrates the basics of WBC formation. The individual components of the WBC analysis are outlined in Table 2–19. The normal ranges for the white blood cell evaluation in the CBC are listed in Table 2–20.

THE ANEMIAS AND LEUKEMIAS

The anemias result in a decreased RBC mass, creating a decreased oxygen-carrying capacity. The general clinical changes experienced are the consequence of the resulting hypoxia. Retinal changes typically occur when the hemoglobin level is decreased below half of normal. Anemia can occur as the result of (1) a reduced metabolite necessary for the production of RBCs, (2) a failure of proper blood formation, or (3) RBC loss. The leukemias are the result of the proliferation and/or accumulation of WBCs that may then alter tissue and bone marrow function. The results of the altered tissue, vascular integrity, and altered platelet function are retinal hemorrhages and cotton-wool spots. Figures 2–119 to 2–122 illustrate examples of some of the anemias, with common ocular and systemic manifestations as well as expected laboratory results. Table 2–21 gives representative examples of some of the results found in anemia analysis, and Table 2–22 gives recommendations for specific differential diagnostic tests to assist in pinpointing the anemia type.

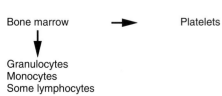

Figure 2–118. Schematic illustrating the basics of WBC formation.

TABLE 2–19. FEATURES OF WHITE BLOOD CELL(WBC) ANALYSIS

Total White Blood Count

1. Measures the number of leukocytes per μL of whole blood
2. Leukocytosis is an elevation of WBCs
   Leukemoid reaction is leukocytosis in cases of nonmalignancies
   Leukemia is leukocytosis in cases of malignancy
3. Leukopenia is a nonspecific reduction of WBCs

Differential White Blood Count

1. Inspection of the peripheral blood smear reported as the percentage of the total WBCs—represents a look at the first 100 WBCs across the screen
2. Neutrophils increase with bacterial infection, tumors, and drugs
   Segs are mature neutrophils
   Bands are immature neutrophils
   A high percentage of bands (left shift) indicates an active infection
3. Basophils increase in hypersensitivity reactions and secondarily in leukemias, hyperthyroidism, and pregnancy
4. Eosinophils increase in allergies but also in many other disorders

5. Lymphocytes must be evaluated in relation to an overall increase in WBCs
   Lymphocytosis if severe is leukemia, a viral infection, or a drug reaction
   Lymphocytosis if moderate is an infectious disease such as hepatitis or mononucleosis
   Lymphocytopenia in systemic lupus erythematosus, Hodgkin's disease, or steroid therapy
6. Monocytes serve as phagocytes to remove debris
   May be elevated in monocytic leukemia, lymphomas, sarcoidosis, and collagen diseases

Platelet Evaluation (Thrombocytes)

1. Platelet count and platelet survival time is an evaluation of the ability of blood to clot
2. Reduced in thrombocytopenia and elevated in polycythemia
3. Clottability is related to extravascular tissue integrity, vascular integrity, and platelets and other blood coagulation factors
4. Other clotting factors are synthesized in the liver with the help of vitamin K
   Prothrombin time is a measure of extrinsic clotting ability or that which is activated in injury to the tissue
   Partial thromboplastin time is a measure of intrinsic clotting ability

HYPERVISCOSITY SYNDROMES

Increased blood viscosity (hyperviscosity) results from an abnormally high accumulation of varieties of blood components. This results in decreased oxygen-carrying capacity of the blood, creating dilated tortuous veins and the increased likelihood for vascular occlusion. Figure 2–123 illustrates one example of a hyperviscosity syndrome, polycythemia vera, in which there is an increase in abnormal RBCs and a deletion of clotting factors.

Blood Chemistry Analyses

Blood chemistry analyses involve a number of tests, often complex and difficult to interpret. A few of the basic tests that are particularly applicable to primary eyecare practice will be discussed. A number of these tests are routinely "packaged" in panels that represent an overall cost savings to the patient. Individual reference laboratories will provide manuals on their particular combinations for the panels. As with all diagnostic tests, the primary eyecare practitioner should be looking for results to support a diagnostic hypothesis rather than for a diagnosis buried within a group of test results.

TABLE 2–20. NORMAL RANGES FOR CBC AND DIFFERENTIAL VALUES

Test	Males	Females
Red blood cell count	4.6–6.2 million/μL	4.2–5.4 million/μL
Hemoglobin	14–18 g/dL	12–16 g/dL
Hematocrit	42–52%	37–47%
Mean corpuscular volume (MCV)	80–94 μm³	87–99 μm³
Mean corpuscular hemoglobin (MCH)	27–31 pg	27–31 pg
Mean corpuscular hemoglobin concentration (MCHC)	32–36%	32–36%
Reticulocyte count	0.5–1.5%	0.5–1.5%
Platelet count	140,000–440,000/μL	140,000–440,000/μL
Total WBC		
Children	4500–13,500/μL	4500–13,500/μL
Adults	4500–11,000/μL	4500–11,000/μL
Differential Values		
Seg neutrophils	56% of total WBCs	
Band neutrophils	3% of total WBCs	
Lymphocytes	21–35% of total WBCs	
Monocytes	4% of total WBCs	
Eosinophils	2.7% of total WBCs	
Basophils	0.3% of total WBCs	

Ocular manifestations
Flame hemorrhages, cotton wools spots, distended tortuous veins

Systemic manifestations
Ease of fatigablility, dyspnea, palpitations, tachycardia

Lab results
Decreased HgB, decreased RBCs, decreased serum iron, and increased total iron binding capacity (TIBC)

Figure 2–119. Ocular and systemic manifestations of iron deficiency anemias.

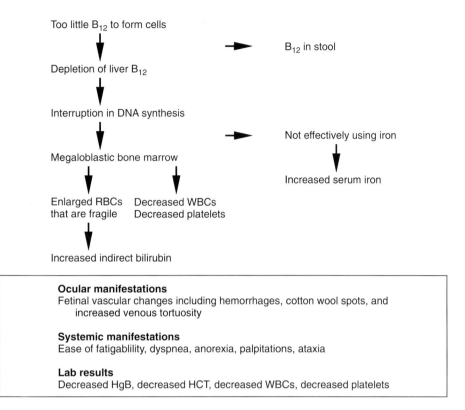

Too little B$_{12}$ to form cells

→ B$_{12}$ in stool

Depletion of liver B$_{12}$

Interruption in DNA synthesis

→ Not effectively using iron

Increased serum iron

Megaloblastic bone marrow

Enlarged RBCs that are fragile   Decreased WBCs Decreased platelets

Increased indirect bilirubin

Ocular manifestations
Fetinal vascular changes including hemorrhages, cotton wool spots, and
   increased venous tortuosity

Systemic manifestations
Ease of fatigablility, dyspnea, anorexia, palpitations, ataxia

Lab results
Decreased HgB, decreased HCT, decreased WBCs, decreased platelets

Figure 2–120. Ocular and systemic manifestations of pernicious anemia as well as its scheme of etiology.

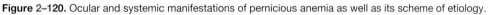

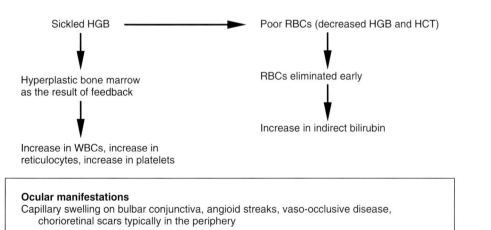

Sickled HGB → Poor RBCs (decreased HGB and HCT)

Hyperplastic bone marrow
as the result of feedback

RBCs eliminated early

Increase in indirect bilirubin

Increase in WBCs, increase in
reticulocytes, increase in platelets

Ocular manifestations
Capillary swelling on bulbar conjunctiva, angioid streaks, vaso-occlusive disease,
   chorioretinal scars typically in the periphery

Systemic manifestations
Pain in arms, legs, and abdomen with acute attacks

Lab results
Decreased HgB and HCT during crisis, increased WBCs and platelets, and increased
   indirect bilirubin

Figure 2–121. Ocular and systemic
manifestations of sickle-cell disease
as well as its scheme of etiology.

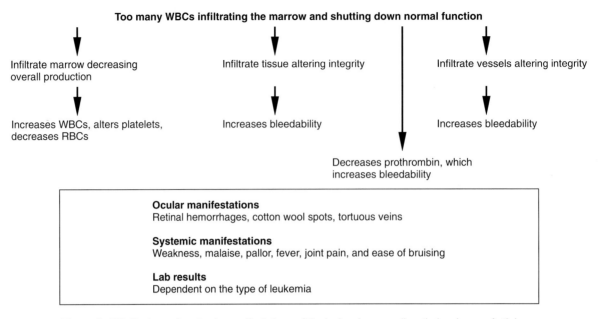

Too many WBCs infiltrating the marrow and shutting down normal function

Infiltrate marrow decreasing overall production

Infiltrate tissue altering integrity

Infiltrate vessels altering integrity

Increases WBCs, alters platelets, decreases RBCs

Increases bleedability

Increases bleedability

Decreases prothrombin, which increases bleedability

Ocular manifestations
Retinal hemorrhages, cotton wool spots, tortuous veins

Systemic manifestations
Weakness, malaise, pallor, fever, joint pain, and ease of bruising

Lab results
Dependent on the type of leukemia

Figure 2–122. Ocular and systemic manifestations of the leukemias as well as their scheme of etiology.

Blood Glucose Testing. Blood glucose testing is the cornerstone for the diagnosis of diabetes as well as the assessment of the degree of control of patients with diabetes. Unfortunately, controversy surrounds the issue of blood glucose testing, with considerable change occurring in the field. However, in primary care it is essential to have a grasp of the rudimentary aspects of the testing procedures as well as an understanding of the best method to assess control. Several tests exist, but this discussion will be limited to the basics.

The **fasting blood glucose (fasting blood serum, or FBS) test** is currently the standard for the diagnosis of both type 1 (insulin-dependent) and type 2 (non-insulin-dependent) diabetes mellitus. It is not that ef-

fective for assessment of the efficacy of control. The test is based on a venous blood draw after a 12-hour overnight fast. Laboratory standards vary somewhat, but a reading over 140 mg/dL on two separate occasions is considered diagnostic of diabetes. Often hand-held instruments using a finger prick and capillary draw are used for this test, but recent work indicates that unless these instruments are routinely calibrated, they should not be used for diagnosis and may even be erroneous in self-monitoring of glucose levels.

The **2-hour postprandial test** is a much misused and misunderstood test. It was originally designed to assess the level of blood glucose 2 hours after eating. It is best to view this test as a random sample of glu-

TABLE 2–21. EXAMPLES OF RESULTS IN ANEMIA ANALYSIS

Test Results	Indications
Decreased Hgb Decreased HCT	Presence and severity of anemia
Peripheral smear	Morphologic type of anemia (macro, micro, normocytic)
Increased reticulocytes Increased indirect bilirubin	Anemia of RBC destruction
Decreased WBCs Decreased platelets	Anemia of decreased RBC production

Levels of
  Iron
  Gastric B$_{12}$
  Urine tagged B$_{12}$
	Anemia related to nutritional deficiencies

Stool for occult blood	Establishes anemias related to blood loss

TABLE 2–22. CHARACTERISTICS OF SOME ANEMIAS WITH RECOMMENDED SPECIALIZED TESTS

Type of Anemia	Characteristics	Recommended Differential Tests
Pernicious	Macrocytic, normochromic, or hyperchromic	Bone marrow, Schilling test, serum iron
Iron deficiency	Microcytic, hypochromic	Serum iron, total iron-binding capacity
Thalassemia	Microcytic, hypochromic	Fetal Hgb, electrophoresis
Sickle cell	Normocytic, normochromic	Sickledex, electrophoresis

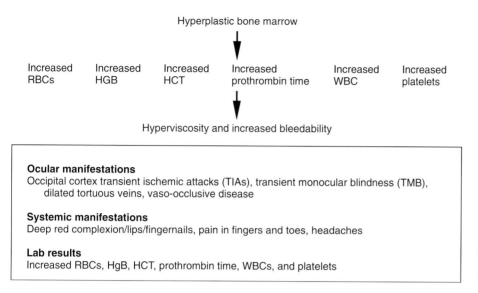

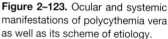

Figure 2–123. Ocular and systemic manifestations of polycythemia vera as well as its scheme of etiology.

cose levels, which should never exceed 200 mg/dL even in the "well-controlled" patient with diabetes.

The **oral glucose tolerance test (OGTT)** may be run over varying lengths of time but is usually a 3-hour test. The patients are placed on an unrestricted diet and physical activity for 3 days prior to testing. The patient is then asked to fast for 10 hours the night before, and then enters in the morning to be given a 75-gram glucose load. Blood is then drawn on a regular basis and the levels are assessed. The fasting level should be less than 115 mg/dL and the 2-hour level should be less than 140 mg/dL, with glucose levels never exceeding 200 mg/dL during the test. The test is a reasonable diagnostic test, even crucial for the diagnosis of hypoglycemia, but should not be ordered in a cavalier fashion because of the relative discomfort to the patient.

The **gestational oral glucose tolerance test** is now recommended for all pregnant women between the 24th and 28th weeks regardless of the results of previous screening tests. The test varies slightly from the basic OGTT in that a 100-mg glucose load is given after a fast of 10 hours. At least two of the following criteria must be met for diagnosis of gestational diabetes: (1) fasting glucose levels of 105 mg/dL, (2) 1-hour glucose levels greater than 190 mg/dL, (3) 2-hour glucose levels above 165 mg/dL, and (4) 3-hour glucose levels above 145 mg/dL.

The **glycated (glycosylated) hemoglobin level test** has become the standard to assess the level of blood glucose control over a time frame. This test goes by different terminology (glycosylated Hgb, hemoglobin A₁C) and unfortunately does not have a universal standardization. The test is a measure of the degree of glycemic control over the past 60 days and is expressed in a percentage. It is a test that does not rely

on the results of the patient's home monitoring and will not allow the patient the opportunity of cheating a couple of days before the visit for an improved fasting glucose level. The glycosylation of the hemoglobin decreases the oxygen-carrying capacity and represents a situation of hypoxia. There is therefore a correlation of increased levels of glycosylated HgB and increased incidence of preproliferative and proliferative diabetic retinopathy. Although laboratory values differ, excesses over 11 percent are related to increases in retinopathy. As the value is a representation of hypoxia, it is logical that elevated levels are also strongly related to cardiovascular disease. Along the same lines is the test for **fructosamine levels.** This is an evaluation of blood glucose levels over the past week. This test is more standardized, resulting in less confusion between labs. Table 2–23 gives some examples of some other blood chemistry tests as well as some of their uses in primary care.

Blood Lipid Testing

Lipids are necessary to the body because they serve as a source of energy for metabolism, building blocks in the construction of cell membranes, precursors of steroid hormones and bile acids, and a transport medium for essential vitamins (vitamin A). Many factors affect blood lipid levels, including insulin, which increases the synthesis of fatty acids in the liver; and cortisol, which contributes to the breakdown of fatty acids and increases mobilization of the fats. Altered lipids increase the risk of coronary heart disease, which is the leading cause of death in the United States, and also increase the complications of several other systemic diseases. The Lipid Research Clinics Coronary Primary Prevention Trial found that a 1 per-

TABLE 2–23. SELECTED BLOOD CHEMISTRY TESTS

Test	Value
Cardiac Enzymes	
Asparate amino-transferase (AST)	In heart, liver, skeletal muscle, and kidney; is released after insult
Creatine kinase (CK)	First to be elevated after acute cardiac insult (within 4–8 hr)
Lactate dehydro-genase (LD)	Peaks 1 day after acute cardiac insult
Liver Enzymes	
Alanine amino-transferase (ALT)	Elevated in liver, obstructive biliary disease, and neoplasia
Alkaline phos-phatase (ALP)	Elevated in hepatic disease, Paget's disease, neoplasia, bone fracture, melanoma
Others	
Blood urea nitrogen (BUN)	End product of protein metabolism produced in the liver traveling to kidneys; increased in renal disease
Uric acid	End product of nucleoprotein metabo-lism; elevated in gout, toxemia, leukemia, Down syndrome, polycythemia
Bilirubin	End product of RBC destruction; indirect or unconjugated is elevated by liver disease and direct or conjugated by obstructive disease
Calcium	Associated with parathyroid disease, Paget's disease, malabsorption, cataracts
Phosphorus	Inverse relationship to calcium changes; elevated in Paget's disease, reduced in hyperparathyroidism, and rapid change in diabetic ketoacidosis
Potassium (electrolyte)	Hypokalemia may alter cardiac, neuro-logic function; carbonic anhydrase inhibitors and diuretics may alter potassium levels
Sodium (electrolyte)	Necessary for proper bodily function; may be altered by many medications and in hypo- and hypernatremia
Angiotensin-convert-ing enzyme (ACE)	Elevated in patients with sarcoidosis

cent reduction in serum cholesterol in hyperlipidemic men was correlated to a 2 percent reduction in coronary heart disease death rates. The four major lipo-proteins include (1) very-low-density lipoproteins (VLDL), (2) low-density lipoproteins (LDL), (3) high-density lipoproteins (HDL), and (4) chylomicrons. Al-though very complex, the HDLs act to offset the neg-ative effects of the other lipid constituents. A cardiovascular risk ratio may be generated using the HDL levels compared to the LDL levels, which is sup-posed to be below 3 to 1.

It should be noted that virtually all diabetic pa-tients have the potential for elevated lipid levels, be-cause when the body cannot effectively utilize glucose for the generation of energy, it must go to the lipid stores. Upon metabolism of these stores, the free lipids are liberated into the system, creating elevated lipid factors.

A **fasting serum lipid level test** is the definitive lipid test to run when concerned about increased risk, as random catches or screens are thought to be of minimal value. Triglycerides are only to be deter-mined under fasting situations. Reference laborato-ries differ in their normal ranges and will indicate their parameters on the report. Further differenti-ation of the type of lipid problem is determined by electrophoresis. Familial hyperlipoproteinemias are not only complex to diagnose but are extremely complex regarding treatment. Table 2–24 lists some of the more common ocular manifestations of lipid disorders.

Serologic Testing

Serologic testing consists of several fairly sophisti-cated procedures with diagnostic abilities particularly

TABLE 2–24. LIPID DISORDERS: OCULAR MANIFESTATIONS

Disorder	Characteristics
Arcus senilis	May occur associated with elevated lipid levels
Palpebral xanthoma	May occur associated with elevated lipid levels especially if elsewhere on body
Branch retinal vein occlusion	More strongly associated with hypertension but may also occur in thick blood syn-dromes; visual loss with macular edema or neovascularization
Central retinal vein occlusion	Strong association with hyperlipidemia and ipsilateral ICA stenosis; visual loss with macular edema; develops neovascular glaucoma
Hemicentral retinal vein occlusion	Strong association with hyperlipidemia and ipsilateral ICA stenosis; visual loss with macular edema; strong tendency for disc/retinal neovascularization
Transient mon-ocular blindness	Strong association with atheroma buildup at the ipsilateral carotid sinus
Asymmetrical retinal vasculopathy	
Central/branch retinal artery occlusion	Strong association with eroding emboli from cardiac or internal carotid system
Hollenhorst plaque	
Lipemia retinalis	Association is with familial hyperlipopro-teinemia necessitating electrophoresis for specific diagnosis
Diabetic exudative macular disease	Hard exudate formation may worsen with the increase in serum lipid levels

HTN = hypertension; ICA = internal carotid artery.

applicable to a number of ocular conditions. The direct **fluorescent antibody test** detects the presence of an antigen in a patient's blood sample, whereas the indirect fluorescent antibody test detects the presence of antibodies occurring as the result of an antigen. In either case the method of detection depends on fluorescence. The direct test is often used for chlamydia and herpes, whereas the indirect is useful for toxoplasmosis, toxocara, cytomegalovirus, and most often for treponema—the **fluorescent treponemal antibody absorption test (FTA-ABS).** The FTA-ABS is especially useful in all stages of syphilis.

The **enzyme immunoassay (EIA)** or **enzyme-linked immunoassay (ELISA)** is like the fluorescent antibody tests with the exception the color change rather than fluorescence is used in the detection. EIA may be used to assist in the differential diagnosis of many of the same conditions as the fluorescent antibody test—toxoplasmosis, toxocara, Lyme disease, and so forth.

The **Western blot test** enhances the differential diagnostic ability of the immunoassay tests by fractionating the antigen by gel electrophoresis before testing. The Western blot test is used to specify the FANA (fluorescent antinuclear antibody test), to detect the HIV, to monitor AIDS patients' immune systems, and to detect the antibodies to the spirochete in Lyme disease.

Human leukocyte antigen (HLA) typing is used to detect the specific histocompatability antigenic markers on lymphocytes that often have characteristics for specific diseases and are often used to predict the likelihood of these diseases. HLA typing is used extensively to assist in diagnosis in diabetes and ankylosing spondylitis (HLA-B27).

Venereal disease research laboratory (VDRL) and **rapid plasma reagin (RPR) tests** detect a nonspecific rise in reagin levels in patients with an acute inflammation, but are often used as screening tests for syphilis. When the FTA-ABS or MHA tests are negative and syphilis is suspected, the VDRL or RPR tests may be used to cover the possibility of activation. These tests are often necessary in the differential diagnostic clarification in Lyme disease.

Microhemagglutination (MHA) tests are used to detect the antibody–antigen reaction by the clumping of sheep erythrocytes. This test is used in the determination of the patient's immunoglobulin G (IgG) antitreponemal antibody, and therefore is of use in the diagnosis of syphilis.

The **purified protein derivative (PPD)** of tubercle bacilli is used as a skin test for screening for tuberculosis. This test is often combined with the chest x-ray in the differential diagnosis of granulomatous anterior uveitis. As the incidence of tuberculosis is again on the rise in the world, this should always be a consideration in the presence of granulomatous anterior uveitis.

Specific Rheumatologic Screening Techniques

The majority of rheumatologic testing techniques related to eyecare will be ordered relative to external disease processes such as dry eye. It is important to recognize these tests relative to the posterior segment, however, because of some of the retinal manifestations of the rheumatologic diseases. It is also important for the primary care practitioner to be familiar with these findings, because a number of therapeutic modalities in rheumatologic diseases have an impact on retinal and optic nerve function.

The **latex agglutination (LA)** test is used to detect the presence of the rheumatoid factor (RF) in the blood. This is a commonly used screening test when a rheumatologic process is thought to create a specific reaction in the eye.

The **antinuclear antibody (ANA)** test detects antibodies to cell nuclei caused by collagen vascular disease but is not specific enough to be totally diagnostic. Interpretation is difficult and can be positive in numerous conditions. It has 90 percent sensitivity but a very low specificity.

The complexity of differential diagnosis in rheumatologic diseases is represented by the recommendations for the differential diagnosis of Sjögren's syndrome (Table 2–25). Table 2–26 lists the gamut of systemic diseases known to be associated with Sjögren's syndrome and Table 2–27 illustrates the neurologic complications. Clearly, rheumatologic diagnosis is the realm of the rheumatologist.

TABLE 2–25. SJÖGREN'S SYNDROME: RECOMMENDED DIFFERENTIAL DIAGNOSTIC TESTS

Lupus erythematosus prep (LE prep)
Erythrocyte sedimentation rate (ESR)
Gammaglobulin concentration
Alkaline phosphatase
SGOT
Chest x-ray
Electrocardiogram
Serum creatinine level
Thyroid studies
Complete blood count (CBC)
Rheumatoid factor
Antinuclear antibodies
Bilirubin
Anti SS-A, SS-B antibodies
Urinalysis
BUN
VDRL
C3 and C4 complement

Reprinted with permission from Alexander LJ. Keratoconjunctivitis sicca. In: Onofrey B, ed. *Clinical Optometric Pharmacology and Therapeutics.* Philadelphia: Lippincott; 1992.

TABLE 2–26. SJÖGREN'S SYNDROME: SYSTEMIC CONDITIONS

Rheumatoid arthritis	Hemochromatosis
Scleroderma	Systemic lupus erythematosus
Polymyositis	Polyarteritis nodosa
Panarteritis	Thyroid eye disease
Wegener's granulomatosis	Interstitial pulmonary fibrosis
	Lymphoproliferative disorders
Paraproteinemias	Raynaud's disease
Primary biliary cirrhosis	Graft versus host disease
	Sarcoidosis
AIDS	Pemphigoid syndrome
Amyloidosis	Stevens–Johnson syndrome
Leprosy	Thermal and chemical burns
Riley–Day syndrome	Kidney transplant
Cystic fibrosis	Epstein–Barr virus
Lyell's syndrome	Fabry's disease

Reprinted with permission from Alexander LJ. Keratoconjunctivitis sicca. In: Onofrey B, ed. *Clinical Optometric Pharmacology and Therapeutics.* Philadelphia: Lippincott; 1992.

TABLE 2–28. GRANULOMATOUS ANTERIOR UVEITIS: SYSTEMIC CONDITIONS AND RECOMMENDED LABORATORY TESTS

Condition	Appropriate Laboratory Tests
Multiple sclerosis	MRI, myelin basic protein in cerebrospinal fluid by electrophoresis
Sarcoidosis	Angiotensin-converting enzyme (ACE), CBC, ESR, x-ray, biopsy of nodules, gallium scan
Syphilis	FTA-ABS (most sensitive at all stages), MHA-TP, and VDRL or RPR to rule out activity with a negative FTA-ABS or MHA-TP
Toxocariasis	Enzyme-linked immunoassay (EIA) IgG/IgM specific
Toxoplasmosis	Fluorescent antibody, Enzyme-linked immunoassay (EIA) IgG/IgM specific
Tuberculosis	PPD with anergy panel, chest x-ray

Laboratory Workup of Anterior Uveitis

Granulomatous and certainly some nontraumatic nongranulomatous anterior uveitis is often a manifestation of a systemic disease, and is often associated with optic nerve and retinal anomalies. The clinician is therefore often faced with the task of a differential diagnosis of ocular and systemic disease as well as managing the acute inflammatory reaction. The following is a summary of the workup necessary for some of these conditions. Table 2–28 lists the more common systemic conditions associated with granulomatous anterior uveitis, and Table 2–29 reflects the conditions associated with nongranulomatous anterior uveitis. The general workup is indicated when the uveitis is recurrent, when you cannot readily identify the associated ocular or systemic condition, or when you are looking for a confirmation of reactivation in conditions such as toxoplasmosis. Mandatory tests in previously undiagnosed conditions include a treponemal test (FTA-ABS or MHA) and a chest x-ray for the granulomatous variety of anterior uveitis.

Urinalysis

Urinalysis has been the cornerstone of laboratory diagnosis for decades. Initially, diabetes was diagnosed solely by urinalysis, and urinalysis still provides considerable insight into the diagnosis and management of many disease processes. Protein in the urine or proteinuria is important in the assessment of kidney function and is an indicator of poor control or breakdown of the glomerular system in diabetes and hypertension. New testing systems to assess small amounts of protein in the urine—**microalbuminuria**—are currently being extensively used, and positive results are often associated with the development of diabetic retinopathy.

TABLE 2–27. SJÖGREN'S SYNDROME: NEUROLOGIC DISORDERS

Focal neurologic defects	Seizures
Movement disorders	Recurrent aseptic meningitis
Encephalopathy	Cognitive dysfunction
Dementia	Mimicker of multiple sclerosis
Chronic progressive myelopathy	Transverse myelopathy
Polysensory neuropathy	Peripheral neuropathy

Reprinted with permission from Alexander LJ. Keratoconjunctivitis sicca. In: Onofrey B, ed. *Clinical Optometric Pharmacology and Therapeutics.* Philadelphia: Lippincott; 1992.

TABLE 2–29. NONGRANULOMATOUS ANTERIOR UVEITIS: SYSTEMIC CONDITIONS AND RECOMMENDED LABORATORY TESTS

Condition	Appropriate Laboratory Tests
Ankylosing spondylitis	ESR, HLA (HLA-B27), Sacroiliac x-rays
Behçet's disease	HLA testing (HLA-B5), Behçet's skin puncture test
Juvenile rheumatoid arthritis	HLA testing (HLA-B27), x-rays of affected joints, antinuclear antibody testing (ANA), rheumatoid factor (RF)
Inflammatory bowel disease	HLA testing (HLA-B27), x-rays of affected joints
Lyme disease	Western blot, ESR, aspartate transamine level, EIA, x-rays of affected joints
Psoriatic arthritis	HLA testing (HLA-B27)
Reiter's syndrome	HLA testing (HLA-B27), ESR, x-rays of sacroiliac spine

TABLE 2–30. PITUITARY GLAND DISORDERS

Type of Tumor Cell	Normal Secretions	Ocular Signs	Systemic Signs	Neurologic and Lab Tests
Chromophobe	None	Bitemporal hemianopsia optic atrophy	Amenorrhea, sexual impotence	Expanded sella turcica
Eosinophilic	Growth hormone, luteinizing prolactin	Possible bitemporal hemianopsia	Gigantism, acromegaly, headache, hyperthyroidism, diabetes	Expanded sella turcica, FBS, serum growth hormones
Basophilic	ACTH, TSH, FSH	Usually none	Cushing's syndrome, truncal obesity, amenorrhea, hirsutism, diabetes, hypertension	No neurologic tests; FBS, incr. serum cortisol, elevated plasma 17-hydro-corticoid levels

Urinalysis may also involve assessment for **galactose** elevation in the urine associated with galactosemia. This elevation may reflect cataract development in children and at an early age in adults. This test is highly specialized, and is not readily available from all laboratories.

Hypocalcemia, or decreases in calcium in the urine, may also be associated with early-onset cataract development, whereas other alterations of calcium in the urine occur in diseases such as sarcoidosis.

Although urinalysis was instrumental in the history of the diagnosis of diabetes, it is now recognized as an insensitive screen for diabetes, because spillage often does not occur until serum levels reach 180/dL. The value of urinalysis in the diabetic is associated with the previously mentioned microalbuminuria assessment and in the detection of **ketones** in the urine. The ketones represent the end products from the metabolism of fat and fatty acids that occurs when the diabetic needs energy and has to go to stored fats to release that energy. Ketonuria may also reflect overall fever, anorexia, diarrhea, starvation, vomiting, and reactions to certain drugs, but is especially apparent in poorly controlled diabetes.

The **nitroprusside** test is a urinalysis test of value in the screening for homocystinuria. Homocystinuria presents in the eye as dislocation of the crystalline lens, and the basic disease puts the patient at risk for death during general anesthesia. The other major cause for lens dislocation is Marfan syndrome. Both conditions put the patient at risk for systemic complications.

Disorders of the Pituitary System

The most obvious consequence of a disorder of the pituitary system that would present in the eyecare office is the visual field defect. Approximately 10 percent of intracranial tumors affect the pituitary system. The active secretory varieties usually secrete only one hormone in excess, typically creating endocrine problems. The basophilic adenomas may also alter the CBC because of the action of the glucocorticoids on blood formation, and may also increase the blood glucose levels. Table 2–30 describes some of the more common characteristics of pituitary disorders, with indications of what types of alterations of specific hormone levels may occur.

Disorders of the Thyroid System

Disorders of the thyroid system can produce fairly significant ocular side effects and signs (Tables 2–31 and 2–32). Thyroxine, which increases the rate of metabolism, is produced by the thyroid gland, and its production is stimulated by the thyroid-stimulating hormone (TSH) produced by the pituitary gland. The pituitary gland is stimulated by the thyrotropin-releasing hormone (TRH) secreted by the hypothalmus. An alteration anywhere within this system has

TABLE 2–31. HYPOTHYROIDISM: OCULAR AND SYSTEMIC CHARACTERISTICS

- Nonpitting edema of the eyelids, face, and extremities
- Loss of outer one third of eyebrows
- Fatigue, lethargy
- Cold, dry skin
- Loss of hair

TABLE 2–32. HYPERTHYROIDISM: OCULAR AND SYSTEMIC CHARACTERISTICS

- Lid retraction
- Lid lag
- Proptosis
- Diplopia and restricted gaze
- Variable intraocular pressure
- Compressive optic neuropathy
- Tachycardia
- Hypertension
- Tremor
- Hot skin

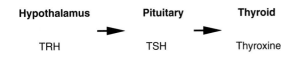

Hypothalamus	Pituitary	Thyroid
TRH	TSH	Thyroxine

Figure 2–124. Flow of stimulation through the thyroid system.

the potential to produce the signs and symptoms of hypothyroidism or hyperthyroidism. Figure 2–124 illustrates the flow of stimulation through the system.

Tests for thyroid status are complex and should be in the hands of a qualified endocrinologist. The tests include thyroxine (T4) levels, thyroid stimulating hormone (TSH) levels, and T7, which is an indirect measure of free T4, T3, and T3 uptake.

REFERENCES

Fluorescein Angiography

Alexander LJ. How to perform and interpret fluorescein angiography. *Rev Optom.* 1988;125:72–82.

Alexander LJ. Diseases of the retina. In: Bartlett JD, Jaanus SD, eds. *Clinical Ocular Pharmacology.* Boston: Butterworths; 1984.

Balogh VJ. The use of oral fluorescein angiography in idiopathic central serous chorioretinopathy. *J Am Optom Assoc.* 1986;57:909–913.

Brown RE, Sabates R, Drew SJ. Metochlopramide as prophylaxis for nausea and vomiting induced by fluorescein. *Arch Ophthalmol.* 1987;105:658–659.

Butner RW, McPherson AR. Adverse reactions in intravenous fluorescein angiography. *Ann Ophthalmol.* 1983;15:1084–1086.

Ellis PP, et al. Antihistamines as prophylaxis against side reactions to intravenous fluorescein. *Trans Am Ophthalmol Soc.* 1980;78:190–205.

Hedges TR Jr, et al. Intravenous digital subtraction angiography and its role in ocular vascular disease. *Arch Ophthalmol.* 1985;103:666–669.

Hunter JE. Oral fluorography in papilledema. *Am J Optom Physiol Opt.* 1983;60:908–910.

Hunter JE. Oral fluorography in retinal pigment epithelial detachment. *Am J Optom Physiol Opt.* 1982;59:926–928.

Noble MH, et al. Oral fluorescein and cystoid macular edema: Detection in aphakic and pseudophakic eyes. *Br J Ophthalmol.* 1984;68:221–224.

Novotny HR, Alvis DL. A method of photographing fluorescein in circulating blood in the human retina. *Circulation.* 1961;24:82–86.

Oral Fluorescein Study Group. Oral fluorography. *J Am Optom Assoc.* 1985;10:784–792.

Pacurariu RI. Low incidence of side effects following fluorescein angiography. *Ann Ophthalmol.* 1982;14:32–36.

Patz A, Fine SL. *Interpretation of the Fluorescein Angiogram.* Boston: Little, Brown; 1977.

Schatz H. *Interpretation of Fundus Fluorescein Angiography.* St. Louis: Mosby; 1978.

Starup K, et al. Fluorescein angiography in diabetic children. *Acta Ophthalmol.* 1980;58:347–354.

Yamana Y, et al. Early signs of diabetic retinopathy by fluorescein angiography. *Jpn J Ophthalmol.* 1983;27:218–227.

Diagnostic Ultrasonography

Rinehart CA, Talley DK. Ocular ultrasonography and biometry: Examination and indications. *S J Optom.* 1990;8:23–30.

Rinehart CA, Talley DK. Ocular ultrasonography and biometry: Introduction and instrumentation. *S J Optom.* 1989;7:19–27.

Visual Fields Testing

Alexander LJ. Primary open-angle glaucoma. *Optom Clin.* 1991;1:19–102.

Comer G, et al. Clinical comparison of the threshold-related and single-intensity strategies of the Humphrey field analyzer. *J Am Optom Assoc.* 1988;59:605–609.

Enger C, Sommer A. Recognizing glaucomatous field loss with the Humphrey Stat-Pac. *Arch Ophthalmol.* 1987;105:1355–1357.

Katz J, Sommer A. Reliability indexes of automated perimetric tests. *Arch Ophthalmol.* 1988;106:1252–1254.

Lalle PA. Visual fields. In: Lewis TL, Fingeret M, eds. *Primary Care of the Glaucomas.* Norwalk, CT: Appleton & Lange; 1992.

Lalle PA, et al. Automated perimetry in the management of glaucoma. *J Am Optom Assoc.* 1989;60:901–911.

Miller KN, et al. Automated kinetic perimetry with two peripheral isopters in glaucoma. *Arch Ophthalmol.* 1989;107:1316–1320.

Odberg T. Visual field prognosis in advanced glaucoma. *Acta Ophthalmol.* 1987;182:27–29.

Wirtschafter JD. Examination of the peripheral visual field: Obligatory, helpful, or a waste of resources? *Arch Ophthalmol.* 1987;105:761–762.

Blood Pressure Evaluation

Alexander LJ. National health care issues: Hypertension update. *J Am Optom Assoc.* (in press)

Alexander LJ. National health care issues: Stroke. *J Am Optom Assoc.* 1992;63:361–364.

Alexander LJ. Variations in physician response to consultation requests for Hollenhorst plaques: A pilot study. *J Am Optom Assoc.* 1992;63:326–332.

Classe JG. Hypertension and diabetes: A clinicolegal review. *Optom Clin.* 1992;2:15–30.

Hypertension Prevention Trial Research Group. The Hypertension Prevention Trial: Three year effects of dietary changes on blood pressure. *Arch Intern Med.* 1990;150:153–162.

Joint National Committee on Detection, Evaluation, and Treatment of High Blood and Treatment of High Blood Pressure. Bethesda, MD: NIH Publication No. 93-1088; January, 1993.

Joint National Committee on Detection, Evaluation, and Treatment of High Blood and Treatment of High Blood Pressure. *Arch Intern Med.* 1988;148:1023–1038.

Newcomb RD. Epidemiology of essential hypertension and diabetes mellitus. *Optom Clin.* 1992;2:1–14.

Schwartz GL. Diagnosis, pathogenesis, and management of essential hypertension. *Optom Clin.* 1992;2:31–46.

SHEP Cooperative Research Group. Prevention of stroke by antihypertensive drug treatment in older persons with isolated systolic hypertension. *JAMA.* 1991;265: 3255–3264.

Stamler, R. Implications of the INTERSALT Study. *Hypertension.* 1991;17(suppl I):16–20.

Stamler R, et al. Primary prevention of hypertension by nutritional–hygienic means. Final report of a randomized, controlled trial. *JAMA.* 1989;262:1801–1807.

Trials of Hypertension Prevention Collaborative Research Group. The effects of nonpharmacologic interventions on blood pressure of persons with high normal levels. Results of the trials of hypertension prevention, phase I. *JAMA.* 1992;267:1213–1220.

Clinical Laboratory Testing

Alexander LJ. Keratoconjunctivitis sicca. In: Onofrey B, ed. Clinical Optometric Pharmacology and Therapeutics. Philadelphia: Lippincott; 1992.

Bates B. *A Guide to Physical Examination and History Taking.* Philadelphia: Lippincott; 1991.

Classe JG. Legal aspects of clinical laboratory testing. *Optom Clin.* 1992;2:15–26.

Dayhaw-Barker P. Hematological testing. *Optom Clin.* 1992;2:41–51.

Fingeret M, Casser L, Woodcome HT. *Atlas of Primary Eyecare Procedures.* Norwalk, CT: Appleton & Lange; 1990.

Mathews DE, et al. Blood chemistries, serology, and immunology. *Optom Clin.* 1992;2:53–69.

Nowakowski R. A review of theoretical and practical aspects of clinical laboratory testing. *Optom Clin.* 1992;2:1–14.

Nowakowski R. Urinalysis. *Optom Clin.* 1992;2:71–86.

Talley DK. Clinical laboratory testing for the diagnosis of systemic disease associated with anterior uveitis. *Optom Clin.* 1992;2:105–123.

Chapter Three ■ ■ ■ ■ ■ ■

Congenital and Acquired Anomalies of the Optic Nerve Head

To the health care practitioner looking inside the eye, the optic nerve head usually is the easiest landmark to view, and is one of the most important of all structures within the eye because of its intimate relationship to the neurologic system and the importance of accurate analysis related to the development of glaucomatous optic atrophy. Diseases and disorders of the optic nerve, however, can be the most difficult to differentially diagnose because of the subtleties associated with alteration of structure

as well as the myriad of congenital variations present in the healthy population. Fortunately, observation techniques have improved considerably over the past few years, allowing for the development of more precise diagnosis.

This discussion provides the clinician a good basis for recognition and implications of congenital variations of the optic nerve head as well as a sound background for effective differential diagnosis of acquired variations.

RELEVANT CLINICAL ANATOMY OF THE OPTIC NERVE HEAD

Gross Anatomy

The optic nerve actually is a white-matter tract of the brain that is grossly divided into four portions: (1) intraocular, which is 1 mm in length and 1.60 mm in diameter and is about 4 mm superior and nasal to the fovea; (2) intraorbital, which is 25 to 30 mm in length traversing a tortuous course and about 3 to 4 mm in diameter (the diameter increases in back of the lamina because of the myelin sheathing of the nerve fibers); (3) intraosseus, which is 4 to 10 mm in length; and (4) intracranial, which is 14 to 20 mm in length. The retrobulbar optic nerve is surrounded by the same layers as the brain—the pia, arachnoid, and dura—and as such is subject to alterations from pressure and diseases in these areas.

The physiologic cup is apparent on most optic discs and varies considerably from person to person, but is most often a mirror image of the fellow eye. Comparison of the structure of the optic nerve and comparison of the physiologic cups often will give a clue to the anomaly of the disc. There seems to be a larger physiologic cup in some races than in others. The status of the physiologic cup is not as important as the status of the neuroretinal rim in most acquired diseases of the optic nerve head. The key to differential diagnosis of most anomalies of the optic nerve head is the side-by-side comparison of one nerve head to the other.

The Neuroretinal Rim

The neuroretinal rim (Fig. 3–1) is classically described as the pink ring of capillary-rich tissue present on healthy optic nerve heads. In most cases, the rim is pinker or denser nasally than temporally. Just envision the neuroretinal rim as a donut and the physiologic cup as the hole in the donut. The appearance of this donut will vary from person to person, but the donut of the right eye should be a mirror image of the donut of the left eye. Optic nerve diseases, such as glaucoma or anterior ischemic optic neuropathy, cause bites to be taken out of the donut from the inside out (Figs. 3–2 to 3–4). This bite reflects compromised nerve fibers, resulting in visual field defects. Often this bite is not pasty white in color but rather a desaturation of the normally pink neuroretinal rim. Observation of bites out of the neuroretinal rim can be enhanced by using the red-free filter in the direct or binocular indirect ophthalmoscope. Again, variations in the neuroretinal rim are best seen by side-by-side comparisons of the two nerve heads.

Vascular Supply

Alteration of the larger vessels of the disc can also provide a clue to the cause of a funny-looking disc. The

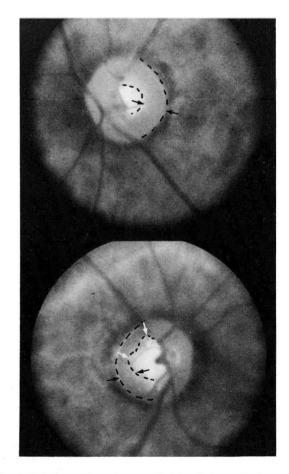

Figure 3–2. Comparison of neuroretinal rims between the two eyes is the key to diagnosis. The rim of the left disc (*top*) is intact, but the rim of the right disc (*bottom*) shows areas of notching (*white arrows*) secondary to glaucoma.

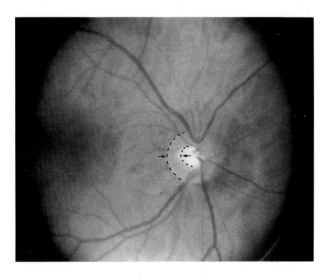

Figure 3–1. The dotted lines demarcated by the small arrows illustrate the neuroretinal rim.

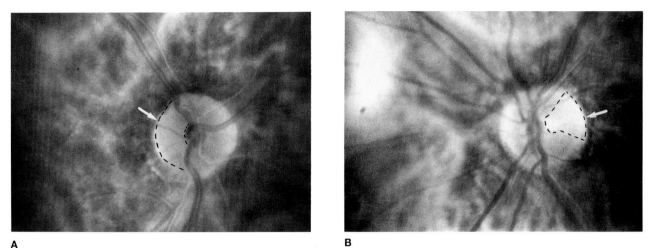

Figure 3–3. A. The neuroretinal rim of the right disc is intact in the temporal area. **B.** The neuroretinal rim of the left disc shows a bite taken at the edge of the disc. This pattern is characteristic of optic neuropathies.

vascular supply to the optic nerve originates from the ophthalmic artery, which is a branch of the internal carotid system. This explains the direct relationship of internal carotid disease to retinal and nerve head emboli and infarcts. The central retinal artery enters the nerve posterior to the globe and runs forward, constricting at the lamina and entering the globe through the optic nerve head, commonly nasal to the ingress of the central retinal vein. The artery bifurcates to the superior and inferior papillary arteries to run out into the retina to supply the inner retinal layers. The central retinal vein usually forms on the disc, coursing back through the lamina, but there are occasions when this vein does not form until after passing through the lamina. The clinical example of this anomalous for-

mation of the central retinal vein is a hemicentral retinal vein occlusion. The vein is thin-walled and very susceptible to external pressures. Most of the blood supply to the nerve head emanates from the short posterior ciliary arteries, the posterior ciliary arteries, and the pial artery. Small branches from the central retinal artery supply the most superficial layers of the optic nerve head. The blood supply to the optic nerve head is somewhat compartmentalized in nature, explaining sectoral-like nerve head infarcts associated with such entities as anterior ischemic optic neuropathy.

Microscopic Anatomy

Nerve Fiber Layer.
The optic nerve head can be separated into several regions microscopically. The sur-

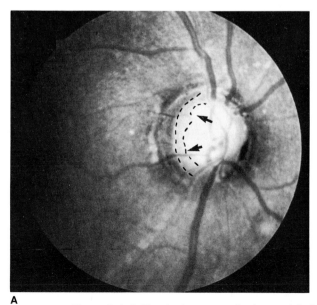
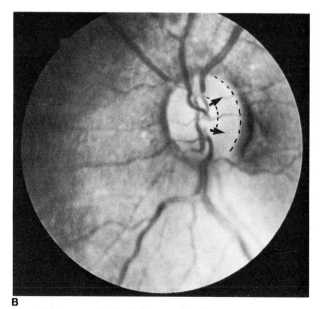

Figure 3–4. A. The rim is compromised, especially in the area of the arrows. **B.** The fellow eye is not compromised. This asymmetrical compromise of the neuroretinal rim is characteristic of glaucomatous optic atrophy. Asymmetrical visual fields usually occur as well.

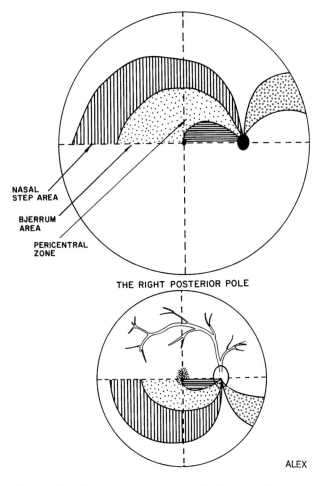

FIELD PROJECTION OF THE RIGHT POSTERIOR POLE

NASAL
STEP AREA

BJERRUM
AREA

PERICENTRAL
ZONE

THE RIGHT POSTERIOR POLE

ALEX

Figure 3–5. Bottom. The pattern followed by the nerve fibers emanating from the right optic nerve head. **Top.** Corresponding field projection of the emanating nerve fibers.

face nerve fiber layer is the most superficial of the regions. This layer consists of nonmyelinated nerve fibers entering the optic nerve from the various areas of the retina. The different areas of the retina have a specific locus on the nerve head (Fig. 3–5). The nerve fibers are separated from the overlying vitreous by a thin membrane derived from astrocytes. The nerve fibers can be envisioned as garden hoses running from a synapse at the ganglion cell to a synapse at the lateral geniculate body. The nerve impulse travels along the wall of the hose, and the center of the hose is filled with an ever-flowing protoplasm (axoplasm) that supplies nutrients to the fiber. Pressure on the hose, such as from increased intracranial pressure, can cause axoplasmic stasis and swelling of the nerve fibers (papilledema). Actual insult to the wall, such as that occurring with retrobulbar neuritis, can alter nerve transmission, resulting in loss or reduction in vision.

Prelaminar or Glial Region. The prelaminar or glial region is the supportive and nutritive area for the nerve fibers. This area occupies over half of the optic nerve head volume. Encircling this region is the border tissue of Elschnig, which is collagenous and acts to separate the choroid from the optic nerve.

Lamina Cribrosa Region. The lamina cribrosa region is collagenous connective and glial tissue that is continuous with and bridges the scleral canal. This sievelike tissue provides support for the exit of the nerve fibers. This can be visualized in about 35 percent of normal eyes as laminar dots at the base of the cup.

Retrolaminar Optic Nerve. The retrolaminar optic nerve is about twice the diameter of the intraocular portion because of the presence of the myeline or insulating sheath around the nerve fibers. Compromise of this myelin occurs in diseases such as multiple sclerosis. This portion of the nerve is enclosed by the sheath of dura, arachnoid, and pia—a direct extension of the brain.

CONGENITAL VARIATIONS OF THE OPTIC NERVE

Because of their significance in differential diagnosis, the important congenital abnormalities of the optic nerve are discussed here. Most of these anomalies are stationary rather than progressive, and many are completely benign. The majority of them are managed simply by observation alone, although a few may require surgical intervention.

Persistence of the Hyaloid System

Introduction and Description. The hyaloid artery is derived from a branch of the internal carotid artery entering the optic stalk at the 3- to 4-week embryonic

Pearls

Persistence of the Hyaloid System

Characteristics
△ Regression of the hyaloid system usually complete by the eighth month
△ Incomplete regression leaves varying amounts of glial tissue, usually nasally on the disc
△ Usually there are no symptoms, only a rare associated vitreous hemorrhage

Management
△ Rule out persistent hyperplastic primary vitreous (PHPV), retinopathy of prematurity (ROP), and retinoblastoma
△ Routine eye examinations are indicated

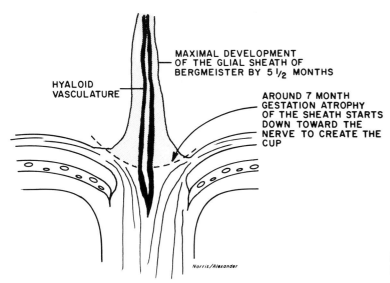

Figure 3–6. An illustration of the development of Bergmeister's papilla.

stage. It typically courses forward to the lens near the end of the 4-week stage to form the tunica vasculosa lentis, the vascular supply to the developing eye. Regression of this artery usually begins at the third month and is totally regressed by the eighth month.

At the same time, the primitive epithelial papilla develops. By 7 weeks, the nerve fibers have reached the optic stalk. Bergmeister's papilla is the result of isolation of a group of primitive epithelial cells allowed to multiply to form a glial sheath around the hyaloid artery at around 4 months (Figs. 3–6 to 3–8). By the sixth month, this structure may occupy a full one third of the artery from the disc forward. During the seventh month, this structure begins to atrophy. The degree to which it atrophies and regresses determines, in part, the amount of physiologic cupping.

Incomplete regression can leave varying amounts of glial tissue on the disc or above the disc in the form of epipapillary membranes. The epipapillary membranes are usually white and almost always on the nasal side of the disc (Fig. 3–9).

A persistent hyaloid vessel (Fig. 3–10) may remain beyond full gestation. As such, it can present many pictures, from a shriveled thread trailing away from the lens (at Mittendorf's dot) to a ghost sheath coursing forward from the optic nerve head. Hyaloid artery remnants are present in 95 percent of premature infants and about 3 percent of full term infants.

Signs and symptoms of persistence of the hyaloid system are usually limited to the complaint of vitreous floaters.

Management. Persistence of the hyaloid system is usually a benign condition except for the occasional vitreous hemorrhage that may occur should there be a patent vessel remaining in the hyaloid system.

Effective clinical management for this condition consists of patient education and routine eye exami-

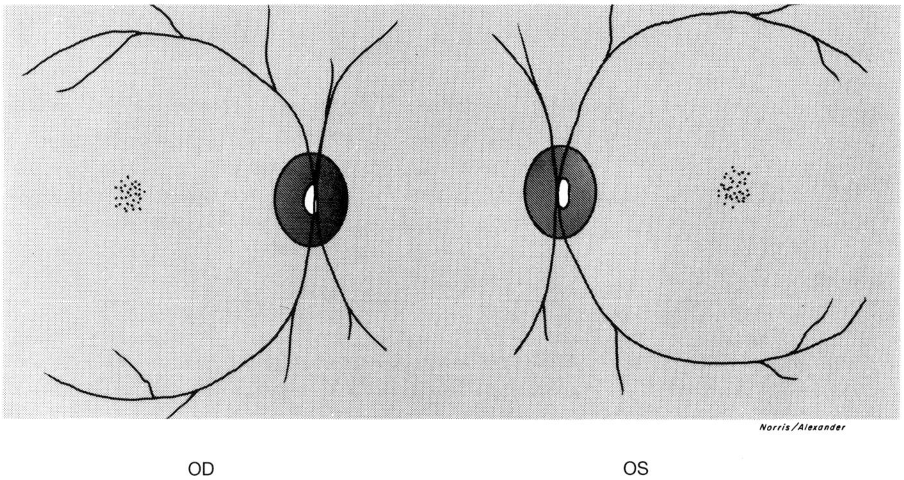

Figure 3–7. A schematic of normal optic nerve head appearances. This serves to illustrate the basic concept of simultaneous comparison of optic nerve heads crucial in differential diagnosis of optic nerve head disorders.

OD

OS

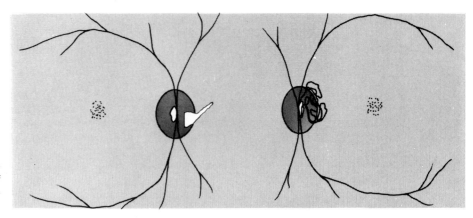

Figure 3–8. Illustration of the typical opthalmoscopic presentation of Bergmeister's papilla and prepapillary vascular loops.

Norris/Alexander

nations. Should a vitreous hemorrhage occur, management would consist of a retinal consultation for possible employment of photocoagulation and/or vitrectomy.

Prepapillary Vascular Loops

Introduction and Description. Prepapillary vascular loops (Fig. 3–11) may occur on either the arterial or the venous side of the vascular system, although about 95 percent are considered arterial. These vessels appear as loops or twists extending from the optic nerve into the vitreous cavity. In 30 percent of the cases, a cloudy sheath encases the loop, indicating glial tissue and the embryonic nature of the vessel.

Arterial loops project varying distances into the vitreous and may move with eye movements. They usually ascend from the disc and descend back into

the disc. Cilioretinal arteries also are present in about 75 percent of eyes with arterial loops emanating from the disc. There is a low incidence of bilaterality with arterial loops and no apparent association with any other ocular or systemic abnormality. These vessels most often supply the inferior retina.

Prepapillary arterial loops originate and terminate as a true branch of the central retinal artery that typically develops with but is independent of Bergmeister's papilla. Following atrophy and regression of Bergmeister's papilla, the loop remains free in the vitreous. A sheath around the loop represents incomplete regression of Bergmeister's papilla.

Prepapillary venous loops occur at about a 5-percent rate. Venous loops appear very similar to arterial loops, with the exception that the walls glisten more than arterial wells. Again, there is no apparent

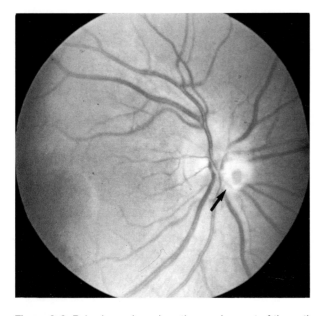

Figure 3–9. Raised area (*arrow*) on the nasal aspect of the optic nerve head, the typical location of Bergmeister's papilla.

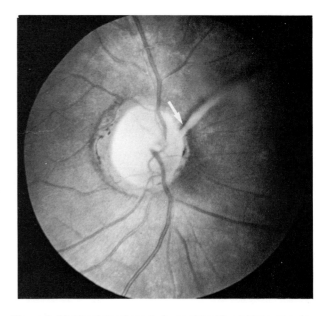

Figure 3–10. Nasal attachment of a persistent hyaloid structure (*arrow*).

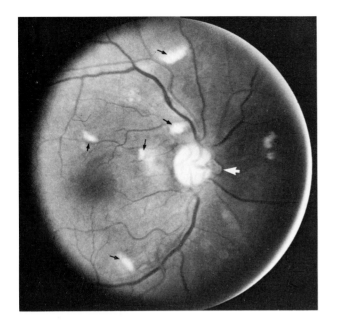

Figure 3–11. The large white arrow points to a prepapillary vascular loop, and the small black arrows point to cotton-wool spots.

Pearls

Prepapillary Vascular Loops

Characteristics

△ Usually unilateral, arterial, and of embryonic origin, developing independent of Bergmeister's system

△ Cilioretinal arteries present in 75 percent of cases, which hook out of the temporal edge of the optic nerve head

△ Usually benign but may be associated with transient monocular blindness, retinal artery occlusion, and vitreous hemorrhage when there is the potential for altered pressure–perfusion ratios

Management

△ Rule out acquired loops including chronic glaucoma, tumors causing retrobulbar compression, vaso-occlusive disease

△ Educate the patient

△ Perform routine eye examinations

association of prepapillary venous loops with any systemic or ocular abnormality. Embryologic development is similar to prepapillary arterial loops.

Acquired prepapillary vascular loops are usually associated with venous obstruction or a compressing optic nerve tumor. These loops or collaterals may also present in chronic open-angle glaucoma. Multiple loops are usually present in the acquired variety, and the loops usually do not extend very far into the vitreous cavity. The acquired loops are usually referred to as "optociliary shunts." Shunt vessels may also occur in chronic primary open-angle glaucoma.

Prepapillary vascular loops usually do not create symptoms but may on occasion be associated with transient monocular blindness, retinal artery obstruc-

tion, and vitreous hemorrhage, especially in conditions with altered pressure–perfusion ratios such as increased intraocular pressure or internal carotid stenosis. This occurs because the vessels are "anatomically exposed" to external pressures.

Management. The incidence of associated retinal vascular disease with prepapillary vascular loops is thought to be very low. In general, it can be said that prepapillary vascular loops are of no immediate threat to vision.

Management of the vascular loops consists of ruling out acquired loops, routine eye examinations, and management of any potential complications (Table 3–1).

TABLE 3–1. COMPARISON OF PERSISTENT HYALOID ARTERIES, CONGENITAL PREPAPILLARY VASCULAR LOOPS, AND ACQUIRED PREPAPILLARY VASCULAR LOOPS

	Persistent Hyaloid Arteries	Congenital Prepapillary Vascular Loops	Acquired Prepapillary Vascular Loops
Ophthalmoscopic appearance	Single vessel, no return to disc	Vessel arising from disc and returning to disc	Often multiple loops
Extension into vitreous cavity	May run forward to lens	Usually up to one third of posterior vitreous cavity	Less than 0.5 mm
Presence of blood in vessel	Sometimes	Yes	Yes
Association with retinal vascular disease	No	No	Yes, especially venous occlusive
Complications	Vitreous hemorrhage rare	Branch arterial obstruction rare	Usually indicative of other disease processes

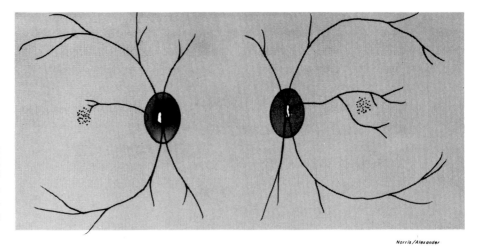

Figure 3–12. Schematic illustrating the typical appearance of a cilioretinal artery (note the hook at the edge of the disc) and a congenital macrovessel (note the crossing over the horizontal raphe and invasion into the macula).

Norris/Alexander

MISCELLANEOUS CONGENITAL VASCULAR ANOMALIES ASSOCIATED WITH THE OPTIC NERVE HEAD

Congenital Macrovessels

Introduction and Description. An enlarged single retinal vessel can at times be seen to enter or exit the nerve head and course across the macula with branches both inferior and superior to the horizontal raphe. These vessels have been given the name congenital macrovessels. These are most often veins, frequently with arteriovenous anastomoses. There appears to be no association with systemic or ocular abnormalities. There are usually no signs or symptoms of enlarged single retinal vessels unless the vessel actually passes through the fovea, contributes to the formation of a macular cyst or hemorrhages. Refer to Figures 3–12 and 3–13.

Management. Management of congenital macrovessels consists of routine eye examinations. When the vessel demonstrates leakage, a fluorescein angiogram may be performed to ascertain if photocoagulation

would assist in sealing the leakage. There is also the suggestion that if the macrovessel assumes the appearance of gross convolutions (racemose angioma), a neurologic investigation is in order.

Racemose Angioma

Introduction and Description. Racemose angioma is an arteriovenous malformation leaving the optic nerve as an enlarged vessel, coursing through the retina, and returning to the optic nerve. This may affect vision and is usually unilateral. In more severe forms, the vessels may be so predominant as to actually obliterate vision. There is a high association with arteriovenous malformation in the central nervous system and in the skin of the face and head. These angiomas typically form at the 16th week of gestation, with the stimulus for formation being obscure.

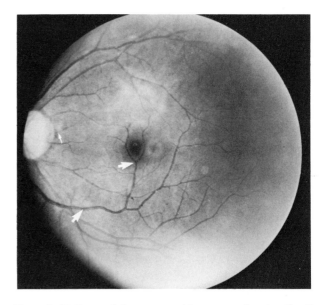

Figure 3–13. Congenital macrovessel (*large arrows*) and a cilioretinal artery (*small arrow*).

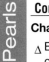

Congenital Macrovessels

Characteristics

Δ Enlarged single vessel leaving the disc and crossing over the horizontal raphe

Δ Usually veins with possible arteriovenous anastomoses

Management

Δ Recognition and routine examinations with consideration of fluorescein angiography if leakage is present

Δ Consider neurologic consultation if gross appearance, which may suggest racemose angioma

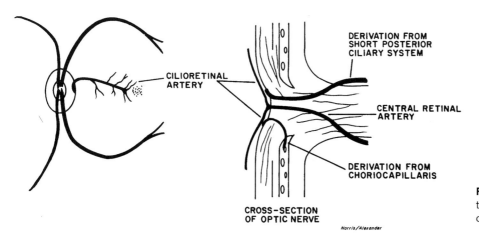

Figure 3–14. Schematic illustrating the clinical appearance and proposed origin of the cilioretinal artery.

Accompanying systemic signs may include seizures, hemiparesis, and psychological changes. Hemangiomas may also occur in the midbrain associated with the retinal AV malformation (Wyburn–Mason syndrome), as may hemangiomas in the ipsilateral pterygoid fossa, mandibular, and maxillary regions.

Management. Management of racemose angiomas includes careful observation, as the condition is congenital and typically does not progress. In addition, investigation for angiomas elsewhere in the system by MRI and electroencephalogram are indicated. The patient should also be warned that other hemangiomas in the mandibular and maxillary region could hemorrhage with dental procedures on the same side as the ocular lesion. Refer to a further discussion in Chapter 4.

Cilioretinal Vessels

Introduction and Description. The cilioretinal artery (Figs. 3–14 and 3–15) is not derived from the central retinal artery. It may be derived from the short posterior ciliary system or the choroidal system. Cilioretinal arteries are relatively common, occurring in at least 20 percent of eyes. Nearly 90 percent are positioned temporally and supply the inner retina in the papillomacular bundle. Cilioretinal veins occur with less frequency than do cilioretinal arteries. From an ophthalmoscopic standpoint, the cilioretinal artery appears to hook out of the temporal edge of the disc and course toward the macula. The cilioretinal artery is most easily seen in a central retinal artery occlusion, because flow is maintained in the distribution area whereas the rest of the retina becomes opaque because of oxygen starvation.

The cilioretinal vascular system is of no concern

Pearls

Racemose Angioma

Characteristics

△ Arteriovenous malformation leaving the optic nerve as an enlarged vessel and returning to the nerve

△ Usually unilateral; if large enough, may affect vision

△ Often associated hemangiomas in the midbrain (Wyburn–Mason Syndrome), ipsilateral pterygoid fossa, ipsilateral mandibular, and maxillary regions

△ May have associated systemic neurologic signs and symptoms

Management

△ Recognition and careful routine observation
△ A neurologic consultation to rule out angiomas in the central nervous system including MRI/MRA and EEG
△ Warn of dental procedures on the ipsilateral side

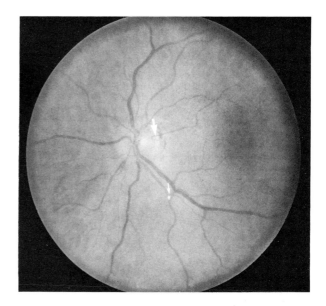

Figure 3–15. The large arrow points to the hook of a cilioretinal vessel. The small arrow points to a Hollenhorst plaque.

Cilioretinal Vessels

Characteristics

△ Usually derived from the short posterior ciliary artery system or choroidal vascular system
△ Occur in 20 to 25 percent of the population
△ 90 percent positioned temporally, hooking out of the edge of the disc and running in the papillo-macular bundle
△ May remain patent in a central retinal artery occlusion, as the vessel is derived from a different vascular network
△ May become occluded, creating a central scotoma

Management

△ Proper recognition
△ Similar workup to central and branch arterial occlusions if an occlusion or arterial plaque is noted
△ Routine eye examinations

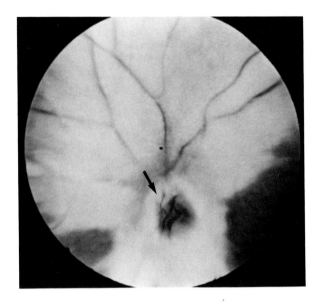

Figure 3–17. A dramatic case of myelinated nerve fibers. The arrow points to the optic disc.

in the long-term management of the patient. It is of some benefit to patients with a central retinal artery occlusion, because a degree of vision is maintained in the distribution pattern of the patent cilioretinal artery. There also are instances when the cilioretinal artery may be obstructed, creating a central scotoma.

Myelinated Nerve Fibers

Introduction and Description. Myelinated nerve fibers (also called medulated nerve fibers) appear in many patterns and may be distributed throughout the eye. The myelination occurs in approximately 1 percent of the population, representing extended proliferation of normal tissue. The structural changes are confined solely to the nerve fiber layer. In embryonic development, myelination of the nerve fibers usually ceases at the level of the lamina cribrosa. If, however, the myelination persists into the eye, the characteristic appearance is that of superficial opacification with

Myelinated Nerve Fibers

Characteristics

△ Represent the continuation of totally normal myelinated tissue anterior to the lamina cribrosa
△ Superficial retinal opacification with feathered edges
△ May totally surround the optic nerve
△ May exist separated from the optic nerve head within the posterior pole
△ May create visual field loss at threshold

Management

△ Rule out cotton-wool spots and any other potential associated conditions
△ Differentiate from cotton-wool spots
△ Perform routine examinations

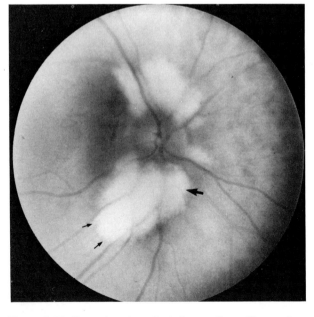

Figure 3–16. Illustration of myelinated nerve fibers. The small arrows point to the feathered or flayed edges.

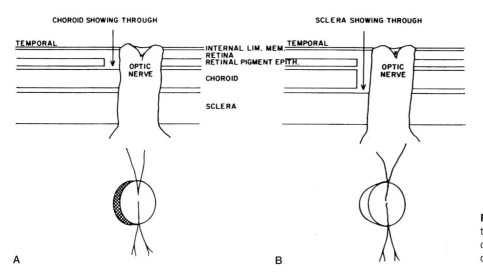

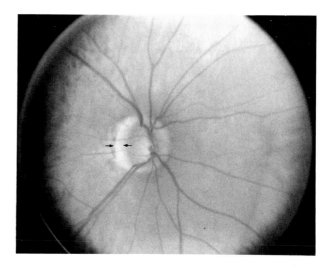

Figure 3–18. Schematic illustrating the reason for development of a choroidal crescent (**A**) and a scleral crescent (**B**).

flayed edges (Fig. 3–16). This feathery pattern is very superficial and will thus block visualization of all underlying structures, such as retinal blood vessels. Often the presentation is so dramatic that the affected area is totally opaque, creating a scotoma at threshold. It may totally surround the optic nerve (Fig. 3–17). Myelination may also exist separated from the area of the optic nerve head, but is usually within the posterior pole.

Usually, myelination of nerve fibers is of no consequence, although it has the potential to cause visual field compromise at threshold levels. There have been some reports of the association of myelinated nerve fibers with myopia, amblyopia, and strabismus. Some authors have cited examples of spontaneous appearance of myelination and of disappearance with demyelinating disease.

Management. Myelinated nerve fibers are typically benign and stable, creating no long-term problems. Management consists of definitive diagnosis and routine eye examinations. Variations have been reported with numerous conditions including demyelinating optic neuropathy, but most instances represent total normalcy.

Choroidal and Scleral Crescents: Circumpapillary Changes

Introduction and Description. Crescents are usually isolated anatomic alterations but may be associated with other congenital and acquired optic nerve head anomalies. A choroidal crescent is a different color (usually darker) than the adjacent optic nerve head and retina. The choroidal crescent occurs because the retinal pigment epithelium is not abutted to the disc tissue, allowing the underlying choroid or retinal pigment epithelium to show through (Fig. 3–18). The scleral crescent is a variation of white coloration be-

cause neither the retinal pigment epithelium nor the choroid abuts the nerve head, revealing the underlying white sclera (Fig. 3–19). The scleral crescent is often associated with high myopia because of the elongation of the eyeball. As the eye stretches, the retinal pigment epithelium and choroid are pulled away from the disc tissue. The crescents usually occur at the temporal aspect of the disc. The scleral crescent may also be a feature of other acquired conditions that may pull the retina toward the periphery, such as retinopathy of prematurity and proliferative sickle-cell retinopathy.

There are no particular signs or symptoms associated with crescents other than those occurring with diseases such as progressive myopia, retinopathy of prematurity, and proliferative sickle cell retinopathy. The physiologic blind spots may be enlarged on threshold perimetry.

Figure 3–19. Scleral crescent (*arrows*).

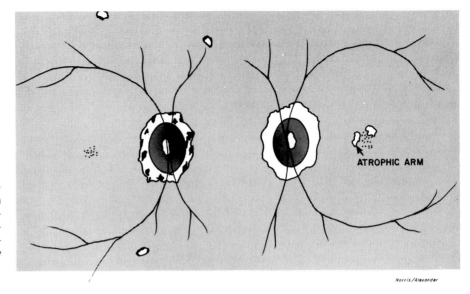

Figure 3–20. This schematic illustrates the expected patterns in circumpapillary choroiditis often associated with presumed ocular histoplasmosis, and in circumpapillary atrophy often associated with dry age-related maculopathy.

Norris/Alexander

Management. Choroidal and scleral crescents are benign, and management consists of proper differential diagnosis of any associated conditions. The differential diagnosis must include circumpapillary atrophy, which may occur in elderly patients. Circumpapillary atrophy is the histopathologic equivalent of dry age-related maculopathy. Circumpapillary atrophy can be differentiated from the circumpapillary choroiditis associated with presumed ocular histoplasmosis by the presence of pigment clumping in the choroiditis (Figs. 3–20 to 3–25). A summary of differential diagnostic features of circumpapillary changes is outlined in Table 3–2. It should be noted that it is the responsibility of the primary care practitioner to recognize the implications of associated conditions that might precipitate the development of any crescent. If the crescent is associated with progressive myopia, one must consider the association of peripheral retinal disease. If the crescent is associated with a posterior staphyloma, one must consider the concomitant association of non-rhegmatogenous retinal detachment.

Pearls

Choroidal and Scleral Crescents

Characteristics

△ Choroidal crescent is usually darker than the retina, occurring because the retinal pigment epithelium is not abutted to the optic nerve

△ Scleral crescent is white, occurring because the retinal pigment epithelium and choroid are not abutted to the optic nerve

△ Scleral crescents may be associated with ectasia of the posterior pole, proliferative retinal vascular conditions of the peripheral temporal retina such as ROP, or sickle-cell proliferation

Management

△ Recognize the cause for the crescent if not just an anatomical variant

△ Follow the patient at routine eye examinations

△ Ask for a consultation if there is an active retinal condition or if there is the threat of non-rhegmatogenous retinal detachment

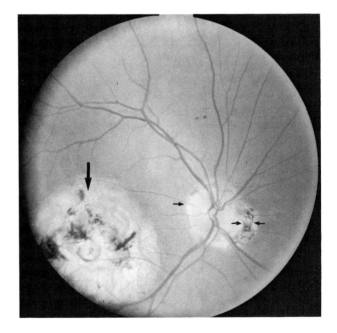

Figure 3–21. The large arrow points to a disciform macular scar, and the small arrows point to the circumpapillary choroiditis associated with this case of presumed ocular histoplasmosis syndrome.

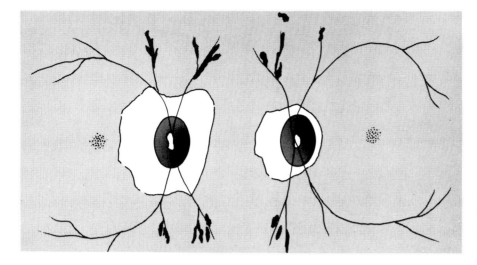

Figure 3–22. This schematic illustrates both the circumpapillary changes and the pigmented paravenous changes in pigmented paravenous retinochoroidopathy.

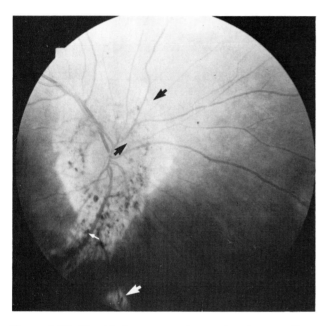

Figure 3–23. The black arrows point to the circumpapillary changes, and the white arrows point to the paravenous changes, in this case of pigmented paravenous retinochoroidopathy.

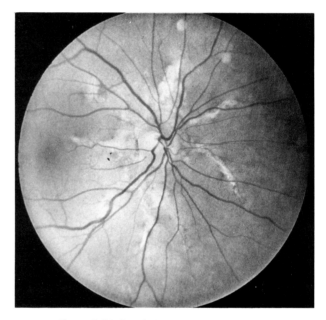

Figure 3–24. A typical case of angioid streaks.

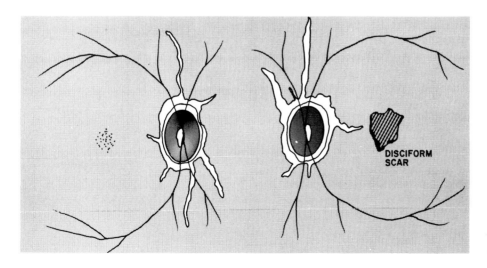

DISCIFORM SCAR

Figure 3–25. A schematic representation of angioid streaks with the circumpapillary hub from which spokes emanate. Often, a disciform scar is the result of choroidal neovascular nets.

TABLE 3–2. COMPARISON OF CIRCUMPAPILLARY CHANGES

Characteristics	Choroidal Crescent	Temporal Scleral Crescent	Circumpapillary Atrophy	Temporal Isolated Zones of Peripapillary Atrophy	Circumpapillary Choroiditis	Nasal Scleral Crescent	Angioid Streaks	Pigmented Paravenous Retinochoroidopathy
Refractive status	Not applicable	High myopia	Not applicable, possible reduced visual acuity or amblyopia	Not applicable	Not applicable	Oblique myopic astigmatism	Not applicable	Not applicable
Associated ophthalmoscopic signs	Not applicable	Thinned retina, dragged disc vessels, isolated choroidal atrophy	Possible Dry ARM, peripheral drusen, CONH	Atrophy of the neuroretinal rim	Possible peripheral chorioretinitis, disciform maculopathy	Situs inversus, nasal staphyloma	Streaks emanating from disc, possible disciform maculopathy	Pigment hyperplasia attached to veins
Associated systemic signs	Not applicable	Not applicable	Age or in CONH, neurologic and endocrine signs possible	Not applicable	Possible systemic histoplasmosis	Not applicable	Pseudoxanthoma elasticum, Paget's disease, sickle-cell disease	Not applicable
Associated visual field signs	Not applicable	Possible scotomas in late stages	Enlarged blind spot	Pericentral scotomas, nasal steps	Possible central scotoma, enlarged blind spot	Bitemporal field defects crossing verticals	Possible central scotoma, field defects with streaks	Field defects in areas of pigment change
Associated diagnosis	Normal anatomical variant	Degenerative myopia	Age-related choroidopathy	Glaucoma	POHS	Tilted disc syndrome	Angioid streaks	Pigmented paravenous retinochoroidopathy

ARM, age-related maculopathy; CONH, congenital optic nerve hypoplasia; POHS, presumed ocular histoplasmosis syndrome.

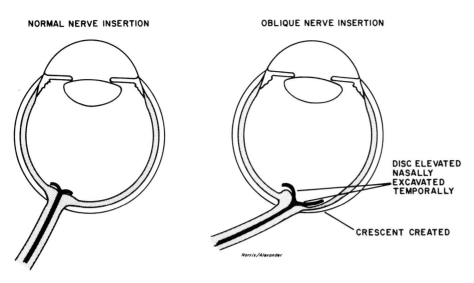

NORMAL NERVE INSERTION

OBLIQUE NERVE INSERTION

DISC ELEVATED
NASALLY
EXCAVATED
TEMPORALLY

CRESCENT CREATED

Norris/Alexander

Figure 3–26. Schematic illustrating the results of oblique entry of the optic nerve into the eye.

Tilted and Malinserted Discs

Introduction and Description. Anomalies of disc insertion can create a very interesting and confounding picture for the clinician. Usually the alteration is seen in myopic eyes, but it may occur in emmetropic or hyperopic eyes. The optic nerve head can be tilted in any direction and usually has a crescent at the border in the direction of the downward tilt. In fact, the presence of a crescent becomes an important differential diagnostic sign in discs that are confusing to the clinician. The presence of the crescent actually indicates a tugging of retinal tissue away from the edge of the disc in the involved area. The tilt may be so dramatic that a staphyloma is associated with the downward tilting. The tilt is usually inferior nasal in the true tilted disc syndrome, whereas it usually is tilted temporally (the nasal aspect of the disc is raised) in the malinsertion syndrome. The malinsertion syndrome is very common, creating a raised nasal aspect of the disc and a depressed temporal aspect. Variations can occur, allowing for superior elevation and inferior depression or any other presentation. This picture gives a papilledema-like appearance to the disc by direct ophthalmoscopy because the raised portion creates blurred disc margins. Often, however, the right and left disc become mirror images in tilted disc variants because of the congenital nature of the condition. The comparison of the two discs therefore becomes an important differential diagnostic tool. The malinsertion is actually an oblique insertion of the optic nerve through the scleral canal (Fig. 3–26) and is of no consequence except for confounding the differential diagnosis. Figures 3–27 through 3–31 illustrate various types of tilted discs.

The tilted disc syndrome is a variation composed of tilting of the vertical axis of the nerve head off 90 degrees, accompanied by a horizontal tilting that is sometimes attributed to incomplete closure of the fetal fissure, similar to the more familiar optic disc coloboma. The tilt is usually toward the inferonasal

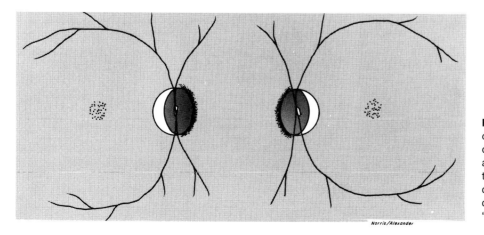

Norris/Alexander

Figure 3–27. Schematic illustrating a case of bilateral malinsertion of the discs. The nasal borders of the discs are tilted up and are blurred, and the temporal aspects of the discs are excavated, with a resultant scleral crescent. This is at times referred to as "tilted discs."

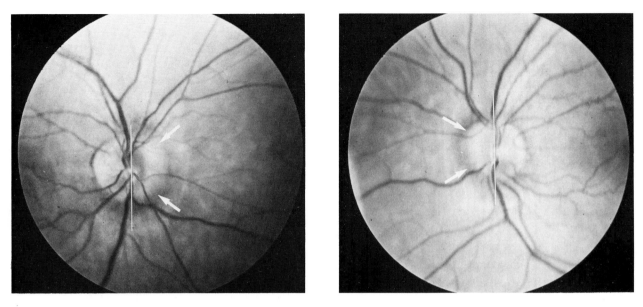

Figure 3–28. Photographs of bilaterally tilted discs (malinsertion) with the arrows pointing to elevated nasal disc margins. The tilting occurs along the vertical axis of the discs.

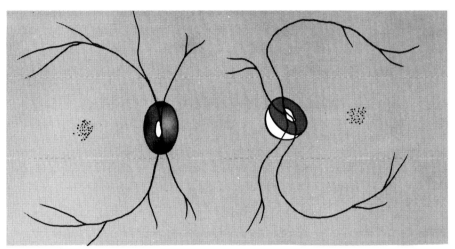

Norris/Alexander

Figure 3–29. Schematic illustrating tilting of the vertical axis of the disc.

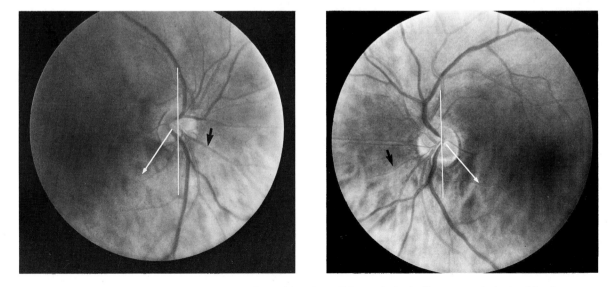

Figure 3–30. These photographs illustrate tilting of the discs off the vertical axis. The true vertical axis of the disc is illustrated by the white arrow. Often, there is a staphylomatous area of the retina in the inferior nasal zone (*black arrows*).

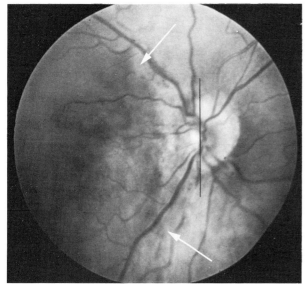

A

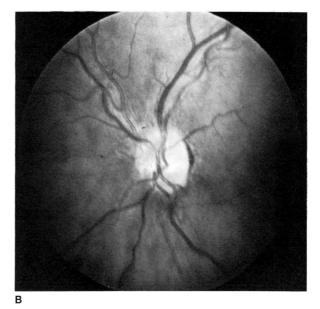

B

Figure 3–31. A. The disc appears tilted in this right eye. Actually, there is a staphyloma in the macular area (*arrows*) that creates a depression temporal to the black line. **B.** The disc in the fellow eye is normal by comparison.

direction, resulting in a nasal area of fundus ectasia (staphyloma) and an accompanying crescent. If bilateral (75 percent), there also is an associated pseudo-bitemporal field defect that corresponds to the area of ectatic fundus. The field defect is differentiated from a neurologic defect by virtue of the fact that the defect crosses the vertical and can be made to improve by increasing the myopic correction when retesting the field. With the retest, the field defect becomes less apparent. There may, however, be enough of an ectasia to physically misalign the photoreceptors, rendering them subject to the Stiles–Crawford effect. If torted enough, the receptors are desensitized, which reduces visual acuity. Oblique myopic astigmatism with slight reduction in visual acuity is often associated with the

condition. Ocular situs inversus, the vessel pattern on the nerve head, is a feature of the tilted disc syndrome. In normal optic discs, the vessels leave the disc in a direct path toward the quadrants that they supply. In situs inversus, the temporal vessels first course toward the nasal retina before making their sharp temporal turn. Situs inversus is of no significance except for the strange appearance of the nerve head. With situs inversus the nasal retina appears similar to a normal temporal retina because of the strange vascular pattern. **See color plates 2 and 3.**

There are no particular signs and symptoms of the tilted disc syndrome other than the bitemporal visual field defects when the condition is bilateral. The clinician must rule out chiasmal compromise in the case of bitemporal visual field defects. With tilted discs, the field defects cross over the vertical. Chiasmal compromise respects the vertical meridians of the visual field until the latter stages of chiasmal invasion.

Pearls

Tilted Disc Syndrome

Characteristics

Δ Thought to be a variation of incomplete closure of the fetal fissure

Δ Tilting of the vertical axis of the disc with situs inversus

Δ Usually there is an area of nasal retinal–choroidal ectasia (staphyloma)

Δ Visual field defect corresponding to ectasia, often a pseudo-bitemporal defect that crosses over the verticals

Management

Δ Rule out other causes of bitemporal field defects

Δ Encourage routine examinations

Pearls

Malinserted Discs

Characteristics

Δ Elevation of the nasal aspect of the disc with temporal depression

Δ Usually an associated scleral and/or choroidal crescent

Δ Possible visual field alteration

Management

Δ Rule out causes of optic disc edema

Δ Encourage routine examinations

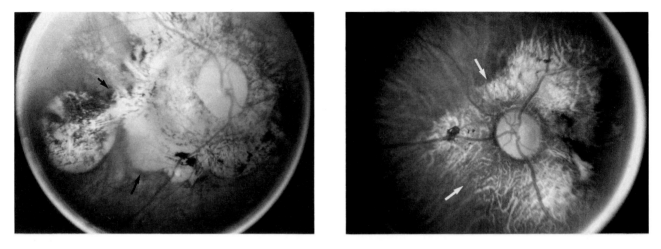

Figure 3–32. Examples of circumpapillary staphylomas (*arrows*).

There may also be systemic endocrine problems associated with chiasmal compromise.

Management. Tilted discs are benign, stable anatomic variations. Although they are considered by some to be variations of colobomas, there does not seem to be an increased risk for retinal detachment as there is with other optic nerve head coloboma variations. Differential diagnosis is crucial, coupled with routine eye examination followup especially when considering the possibility of neurologic compromise. A good rule to follow in all optic nerve anomalies where the diagnosis is not definitive is a routine follow-up of visual field in 1 to 3 months.

Circumpapillary Staphyloma

Introduction and Description. Although rare, the circumpapillary staphyloma can cause confusion from a diagnostic standpoint. This condition is characterized by an optic nerve head, usually fairly normal in appearance, lying elevated at the base of a staphyloma. Because of the stretching in the area, the surrounding retina and choroid usually show retinal pigmentary changes in the form of thinning and increased ability to view the underlying choroid and RPE migration (Fig. 3–32). The diagnosis is enhanced by stereoscopic viewing techniques and B-scan ultrasonography, which will actually picture the elevated nerve head within the elongation of the globe (Fig.

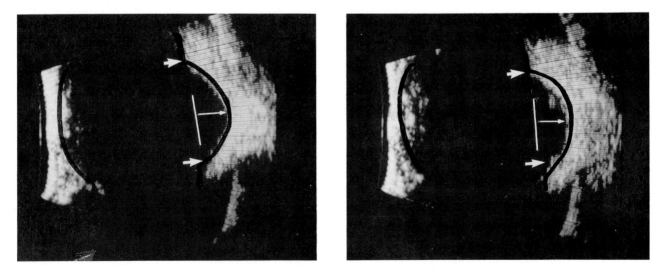

Figure 3–33. B-scan ultrasonography of posterior staphylomas. The large white arrows point to the normal retinal surface, the white lines show the expected area for the retinal surface, and the small arrows indicate the depth of the depression.

Circumpapillary Staphyloma

Characteristics

△ Usually unilateral
△ Optic nerve lying elevated at the base of an area of staphyloma
△ The area around disc is depigmented and may have pigmentary migration
△ Variably reduced vision or constricted fields
△ The differential diagnosis is assisted by ultrasonography (A and/or B-scan)

Management

△ Patient education and provision of safety eyewear
△ Routine eye examinations are indicated

Pearls

3–33). The B-scan and A-scan can also be useful in comparison of the actual length of the globes, as the condition is usually unilateral and is often misdiagnosed as refractive amblyopia. The acuity usually is reduced but is variable depending on the involvement of the macula. Threshold visual fields are affected to varying degrees and may present constriction in the periphery.

The condition is most often unilateral and is considered to be the result of failure of development of the sclera. Tissue is not missing as it is in a coloboma, but rather the sclera is bulging or ectatic.

If the circumpapillary staphyloma is unilateral, the patient has reduced vision in the affected eye, with a possible strabismus. There is no strong predilection toward retinal detachment as with colobomatous defects.

Management. Circumpapillary staphylomas must first be properly diagnosed. The condition is benign and self-limited. The patient should wear safety glasses to protect the unaffected eye, and should be educated regarding the condition and the importance of protecting the unaffected eye. The patient should have routine eye examinations. **See color plate 1.**

Congenital Coloboma of the Optic Nerve Head

Introduction and Description. A coloboma is a depression of the retina, choroid, optic nerve, or a combination of these, that is the result of absence of tissue (Fig. 3–34). The varieties of colobomas of the optic nerve include the tilted disc syndrome as well as many others, and are discussed separately. There is a fairly common thread that runs through all of these defects. In all varieties of coloboma, the affected nerve head is larger than its fellow, and invariably has vessels with an unusual appearance emanating from the disc. There are often an increased number of vessels leaving the disc. With stereoscopic viewing, the clinician can also expect variable excavation at some location within the nerve head.

The true congenital coloboma of the optic nerve head (Fig. 3–35) is secondary to incomplete closure of the embryonic fissure. The coloboma can be confined to the nerve head or can be present in combination with a retinochoroidal coloboma (Fig. 3–36). In either case, the site of presentation is usually the inferior portion of the disc or retina, which coincides with the expected final aspect of closure of the fetal fissure. As stated previously, some form of unusual vessel arrangement present in most ocular congenital variants is also present, as is enlargement of the affected nerve head. There are usually pigmentary anomalies surrounding the coloboma due to stretching of the retinal tissue with subsequent reactive retinal pigment epithelial hyperplasia. Visual acuity is variable with colobomas, but can be reduced to light perception. Visual field changes are likewise related to the position and extent of the colobomatous defect, but are often very dramatic and can occupy a considerable aspect of the visual field.

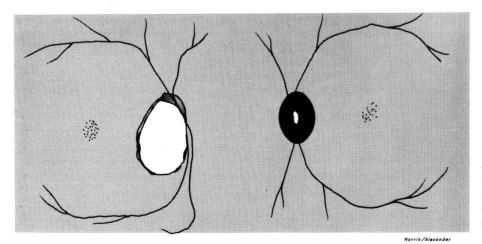

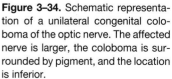

Figure 3–34. Schematic representation of a unilateral congenital coloboma of the optic nerve. The affected nerve is larger, the coloboma is surrounded by pigment, and the location is inferior.

Norris/Alexander

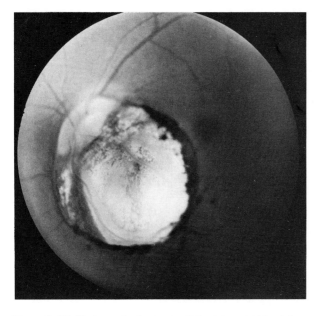

Figure 3–35. Photograph of a congenital coloboma of the left optic nerve. Note the retinal pigment epithelial hyperplasia surrounding the defect.

Congenital Coloboma of the Optic Nerve Head

Characteristics

△ Affected nerve head always is larger than its fellow, with unusual vascular pattern

△ Usually inferior portion of optic nerve head affected with significant excavation and surround of pigment hyperplasia

△ Reduced visual acuity and visual field defects variable but are present

△ Often associated with systemic abnormalities

△ Strong association with non-rhegmatogenous retinal detachment in optic nerve variety and rhegmatogenous retinal detachment in retinochoriodal variety

Management

△ Rule out systemic abnormalities

△ Protective eyewear

△ Patient education about signs and symptoms of retinal detachment as well as the importance of safety eyewear and being safety conscious

△ Routine yearly examinations

At times, glial tissue will fill the depths of the coloboma, giving an unusual appearance approaching that of the morning glory disc. The morning glory disc and the full-blown optic nerve coloboma may represent opposite limits of a continuous spectrum. There should be little difficulty in making a differential diagnosis if stereoscopic observation techniques are used. Comparison of disc size will also reveal a difference in the size of the discs even if the condition is bilateral. B-scan ultrasonography (Fig. 3–37) is also of value in differential diagnosis. Colobomas may occur elsewhere in the ocular system, as with a coincidental iris coloboma, but their presence elsewhere is not necessarily the rule (Figs. 3–38 and 3–39).

Because the condition is congenital, the problem may appear on a routine screening for visual acuity. The patient with a coloboma of the nerve head often will report some reduction in visual acuity. If the con-

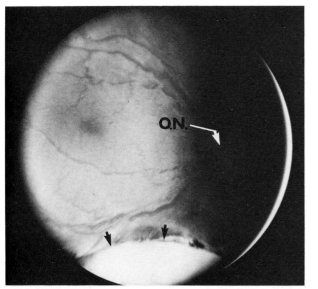

A

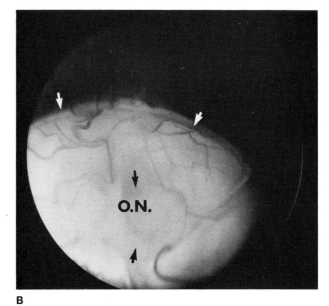

B

Figure 3–36. A. A retinal-choroidal coloboma (*black arrows*). **B.** A combined retinal-choroidal-optic nerve coloboma in the fellow eye.

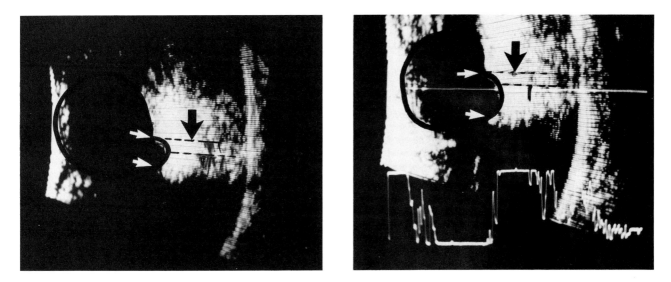

Figure 3–37. B-scan ultrasonography of the eye in bottom of Figure 3–36, taken at slightly different angles. The dotted lines demarcate the optic nerve. The white arrows point to the extent of the coloboma.

dition is bilateral, the clinician should expect nystagmus due to congenital reduction in visual acuity. There are other ocular associations with optic nerve coloboma, including myopia, hyaloid system remnants, and posterior lenticonus. Systemic associations include transphenoidal encephalocele, cardiac defects, and drug-related congenital anomalies.

Retinochoroidal colobomas (Figs. 3–38 and 3–39) have numerous associated systemic conditions involving the cardiovascular, central nervous, musculoskeletal, gastrointestinal, genitourinary, and na-sopharyngeal systems. Chromosomal anomalies have also been linked to retinochoroidal colobomas. **See color plate 4.**

Management. There is a strong association between optic nerve head coloboma and non-rhegmatogenous retinal detachment usually occurring early in life. The association is even more common in the retinochoroidal coloboma. The retina is severely stretched as it dives down into the coloboma. The physical evidence for this retinal compromise is the pigment hy-

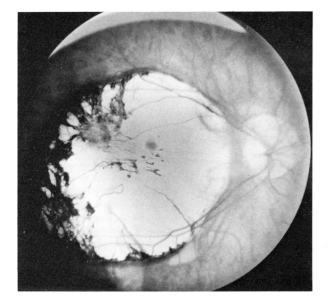

Figure 3–38. Example of a retinal–choroidal coloboma in the macular area. Note the retinal pigment epithelial hyperplasia surrounding the coloboma.

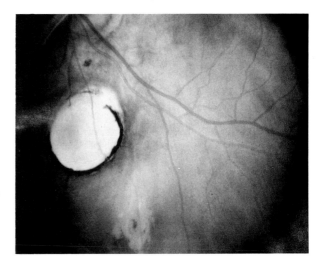

Figure 3–39. Example of a small retinal–choroidal coloboma inferior to the optic nerve.

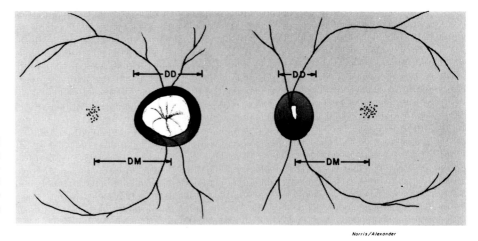

Figure 3–40. Schematic of a unilateral morning glory disc anomaly. As with all congenital optic nerve head defects, the affected disc is larger than the normal disc. Note also the reduced DM/DD ratio associated with morning glory disc anomalies.

Norris/Alexander

perplasia that is usually present at the borders of the coloboma. The detachment often occurs in the second to third decade, involving subretinal fluid in the papillomacular area. Perhaps liquefied vitreous may leak through the areas of retinal structure compromise at the borders of the coloboma, allowing the retina to lift away. One fourth of patients with colobomas and retinal detachment lose vision permanently. The detachments associated with optic nerve colobomas are usually non-rhegmatogenous, whereas those in retinochoroidal colobomas are usually rhegmatogenous. There are reports of circumpapillary retinal traction associated with optic nerve colobomas.

Although the coloboma is benign and self-limited, there is concern for the development of an associated retinal detachment. The clinician must protect the affected eye by dissuading the patient from participation in contact sports and by the provision of maximal protective eyewear. A crucial aspect of management is the assurance that the patient understands the potential severity of the situation. The primary care practitioner must also assure that the patient has no related neurologic anomalies such as midline defects. If these are apparent, it is important to assure that the other manifestations of these conditions, such as endocrine imbalance, are properly managed. Routine yearly eye examinations are indicated.

In patients with retinochoroidal coloboma, it is important that the clinician rule out the many possible associations with systemic abnormalities and chromosomal disorders, as well as carefully manage for the potential of rhegmatogenous retinal detachment. Again, patient education and provision of protective eyewear become crucial.

Morning Glory Disc

Introduction and Description. The morning glory disc (Figs. 3–40, to 3–42) is a unilaterally enlarged, funnel-shaped or scalloped area of the optic nerve head that is surrounded by an elevated ring of chorioretinal pigmentary disturbance. The condition gets its name from its resemblance to the flower. As in the optic nerve head coloboma, there is an associated enlargement of the affected disc, an abnormal vascular pattern (the vessels appear to enter and exit the disc at the margins), and an excavation when viewed using stereoscopic techniques. The vessels of the nerve head are often hidden by white central glial tissue and appear to exit the nerve head in a radial fashion. There may also be narrowing and sheathing of the arteries. Although the number of disc vessels is normal, it appears that there are too many on the nerve head because of multiple bifurcations prior to leaving it. The right eye is involved most often, and morning glory disc is seen in females twice as frequently as in males.

The embryologic origin of the morning glory disc anomaly is somewhat controversial. It is thought by

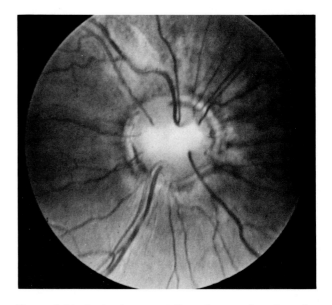

Figure 3–41. A classic presentation of a morning glory disc anomaly.

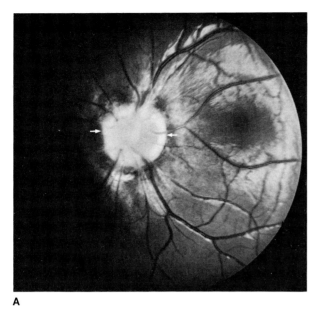

A

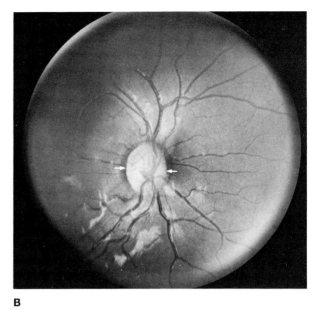

B

Figure 3–42. A. The left eye with a morning glory disc. The extent of the disc is demarcated by arrows. **B.** The fellow right eye has a normal-sized disc. The key to the diagnosis of congenital variations of the optic nerve is a comparison of disc sizes.

some to be a variant of an optic nerve coloboma (central coloboma), and others believe it to be a variety of optic nerve dysplasia originating from a large scleral canal with backwards displacement of the lamina cribrosa.

Visual acuity varies from just barely reduced to hand motion in the morning glory disc anomaly. Be-

cause morning glory disc is most often unilateral, it is usually asymptomatic and may be discovered on routine vision screening. At the point of discovery, the misdiagnosis of refractive amblyopia is often given. The unilateral version usually presents poor vision and a centrocecal scotoma, while the bilateral version is characterized by only moderate reduction of vision. There may be an associated strabismus (50 percent), and there is often an association with myopia. Many ocular abnormalities have been associated with the morning glory disc anomaly, including cataracts, persistent hyaloid system and Bergmeister's papilla, persistent pupillary membrane, ciliary body cysts, microcornea and micro-ophthalmos in the contralateral eye, and Duane's retraction syndrome.

There are also related systemic abnormalities, including basal encephalocele and hypertelorism. For this reason, radiologic studies may be indicated in patients with morning glory disc anomaly should questionable neurologic signs be present. **See color plate 5.**

Management. The morning glory disc anomaly is a relatively benign condition, although there is a strong association with the development of non-rhegmatogenous retinal detachment confined to the posterior pole as in other forms of optic nerve head colobomas. The detachments appear to be somewhat resistant to repair. In addition, the glial tissue in the cup may actually proliferate and create additional traction similar to persistent hyperplastic primary vitreous (PHPV).

The most important aspect of management of the morning glory disc anomaly is proper diagnosis. Be-

Pearls

Morning Glory Disc

Characteristics

Δ Affected nerve head is larger than its fellow when unilateral

Δ Unusual vascular pattern actually radiating from the disc

Δ Funnel-shaped nerve head surrounded by elevated chorioretinal pigmentary disturbance

Δ Variable visual acuity and visual field disturbance
 If unilateral, usually severe vision loss
 If bilateral, usually only mild to moderate vision loss

Δ Related systemic abnormalities may occur

Δ Strong association with non-rhegmatogenous retinal detachment

Management

Δ Rule out systemic abnormalities

Δ Protective eyewear and caution about trauma and safety

Δ Patient education about signs and symptoms of retinal detachment as well as morbidity of condition

Δ Routine yearly examinations

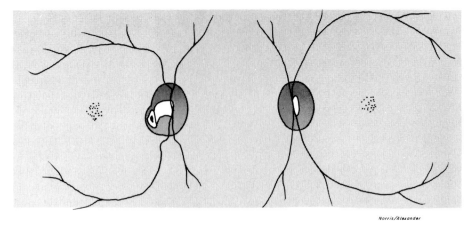

Figure 3–43. Schematic presentation of a unilateral congenital pit of the optic nerve. As with other congenital variations, the affected optic nerve is larger. The pit is usually inferior temporal.

Norris/Alexander

cause of the association with retinal detachment, contact sports should be avoided, and protective eyewear should be prescribed. Patient education regarding the signs and symptoms of retinal detachment and the relative morbidity of the condition is also very important. It is also important to assure yourself that there are no associated systemic problems that may present with optic nerve coloboma variations. Routine yearly examinations are indicated.

Congenital Pits of the Optic Nerve Head

Introduction and Description. Congenital pits of the optic nerve head may vary considerably in their presentation (Figs. 3–43 to 3–45). Pits appear as a discolored area of the nerve head, varying from yellowish white to olive-gray (60 percent are gray). This color

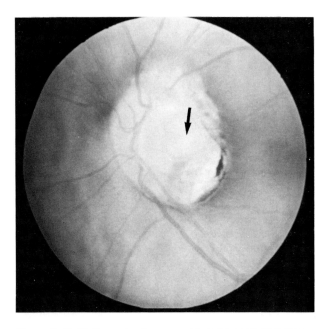

Figure 3–44. Photograph of an unusually large optic pit that borders on being classified as a coloboma. The arrow points to two very deep depressions located within the defect.

variation is thought to be related to the remnants of glial retinal elements at the base of the pit. Membranous coverings over the pit may also alter the color. Pigmentation may occur in the area of the pit. However, color and shape are not reliable for differential diagnosis. Retinal pigment epithelial migration and hyperplasia may also be present adjacent to the pit in the retinal area, and represent areas of retinal traction. In addition, it has been noted that with careful observation the base of the pit may be seen to pulsate. The shape may vary from a slit-like pit, known as the "6:45 syndrome," to round or oval. The 6:45 syndrome refers to the o'clock position of the pit on the right optic nerve head.

Size can be variable from 0.1 to 0.7 disc diameters, with depths from 0.5 diopters and deeper. The most common size is approximately 0.3 disc diameters. The size of the affected optic nerve head is larger than that of the unaffected eye and has an accompanying abnormal vascular pattern that is consistent with other congenital anomalies. Circumpapillary chorioretinal atrophy in the area of the pit is another characteristic finding, as is a cilioretinal artery (60 percent).

Pits may be located at any position on the disc, but the inferior and temporal areas are the most common. About 20 to 33 percent of pits are located centrally and resemble glaucomatous optic atrophy. The differentiation from glaucomatous optic atrophy is best achieved by simultaneous comparison of the discs, and as with all other congenital variations the affected disc is larger. Even if bilateral, there is an appreciable size difference between the two affected optic nerve heads. It is rare to find more than one pit per nerve head, and about 85 percent of patients have only a unilateral pit.

There is a loss of retinal ganglion cells and nerve fibers in the area of the pit that accounts for the associated visual field defect. This loss may be secondary to atrophy associated with the extreme attenuation of the nerve fibers in the area of the pit. Paradoxically, in

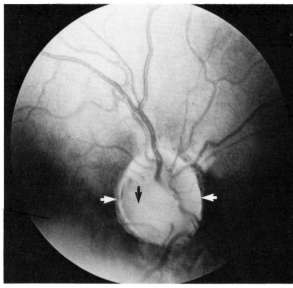

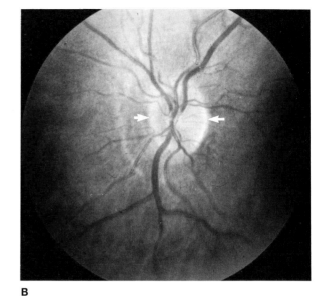

Figure 3–45. A. Right optic nerve head with an optic pit (*black arrow*). Compare the size of the affected disc with the fellow left eye (**B**).

Congenital Pits of the Optic Nerve Head

Characteristics

△ Affected disc is larger than its fellow with un-usual vascular pattern

△ 60 percent of discs with pits have cilioretinal ar-teries

△ Most often an inferior temporal discoloration (olive-gray) that is excavated—about one-quar-ter to one-third are central

△ Often associated adjacent retinal pigment ep-ithelial alterations representing reactive hyper-plasia secondary to tugging of the retinal tissue

△ Usually 0.3 disc diameters in size, but size varies from 0.1 to 0.7 disc diameters

△ Visual field defect corresponds to the pit loca-tion

△ Strong association with non-rhegmatogenous retinal detachment (40 to 60 percent), mean age 30 years

Management

△ Patient education about signs and symptoms of retinal detachment

△ Home monitoring by Amsler grid

△ Patient education regarding the relative morbid-ity of the condition

△ Patient education regarding the potential effects of trauma

△ Routine yearly examinations

spite of the loss of nerve fibers, there is usually no as-sociated nerve fiber conduction defect.

The origin of the pit is controversial. Pits have been associated with incomplete closure of the fetal fissure, a coloboma-like origin. Other investigators propose that the pits result from an abnormal dif-ferentiation of the primitive epithelial papilla. Some clinicians believe that there is an associated malcom-munication between the subarachnoid space sur-rounding the optic nerve and the optic pit. Regardless of the origin, the signs, symptoms, and prognosis are clinically well founded.

The patient is often unaware of the presence of an optic pit because vision is usually unaffected until the associated complication of a non-rhegmatogenous retinal detachment. The pit is often discovered on a routine eye examination, especially if routine auto-mated perimetry is performed. Approximately 60 to 70 percent of patients with pits of the nerve head have arcuate scotomas corresponding to the location of the pit. The 6:45 syndrome classically presents a pistol-grip visual field defect, which is a variation of an ar-cuate scotoma.

Unfortunately, a high percentage (40 to 60 per-cent) of patients with optic pits of the nerve head de-velop non-rhegmatogenous retinal detachments in the macular area extending toward the disc. The ma-jority of these patients have temporal pits. Those pa-tients with central pits rarely have detachments. The detachments associated with pits often are difficult to view because they are flat (non-rhegmatogenous) and usually do not undulate because of the high viscosity of the subretinal fluid. Cystic changes are seen in the elevated retina in about two thirds of the patients. These cystic changes in the inner nuclear layer may develop into lamellar macular holes. In approximately one third of the detachments, small subretinal yellow precipitates occur on the retinal surface. There appears to be a high incidence of posterior vitreous detachment associated with the serous maculopathy. The mean age of incidence of the serous maculopathy associated with a congenital pit of the optic nerve head is about 30 years. Symptoms of the detachment include metamorphopsia and vision reduction.

The etiology of the subretinal fluid is very controversial. Fluorescein angiography demonstrates that the serous detachment associated with a pit is distinctly different from that associated with idiopathic central serous choroidopathy and choroidal neovascularization. Virtually all pits hyperfluoresce during fluorescein angiography. With detachment, there may be a mottled macular hyperfluorescence during the venous phase. There are proponents of the theory that liquefied vitreous is responsible for the subretinal fluid. Others argue that the fluid emanates from leaking vessels within the pit. An unsubstantiated theory is the leakage of cerebrospinal fluid from the subarachnoid sheath surrounding the optic nerve. The majority of work supports the theory of a vitreous communication via the pit. **See color plate 6.**

Management. There is a very high incidence of serous maculopathy (non-rhegmatogenous retinal detachment) associated with congenital pits in the temporal aspect of the optic nerve head. Some reports state that the condition waxes and wanes, with a high percentage of spontaneous reattachment; whereas others cite the presence of subretinal fluid in up to 75 percent of cases over a 5-year follow-up. The primary prognostic indicators are size and location of the pit. There is no particular association of optic pits to any

other ocular or systemic abnormality. There also appears to be some propensity toward the development of low-tension glaucoma in patients with congenital pits of the optic nerve head.

The controversy surrounding congenital pits of the optic nerve head continues with management. Prophylactic photocoagulation near the pits has been advocated, but results were not beneficial. In addition to photocoagulation, oral corticosteroids, optic nerve decompression, scleral buckling, and vitrectomy have been tried in the treatment of the serous maculopathy secondary to optic pits. The only mode of therapy that may be of value is photocoagulation. Photocoagulation applied in cases of serous maculopathy results in flattening of the retina and elimination of subretinal fluid, but visual acuity does not improve significantly.

The clinician should routinely monitor the patient with a congenital pit of the optic nerve head. The follow-up examination should be on a yearly basis. Patient education regarding the relative morbidity of the condition is important as well as advice regarding avoidance or minimizing of trauma to the head. When faced with eye hazard situations, the patient with the congenital pit of the optic nerve head should wear protective eyewear. The patient should be given some method of monitoring the vision monocularly and should report metamorphopsia or vision loss as soon as it occurs. The longer the macula is detached, the poorer the long-term prognosis.

Congenital Optic Nerve Hypoplasia

Introduction and Description. Congenital optic nerve hypoplasia (CONH) may occur unilaterally or bilaterally (Figs. 3–46 to 3–48). CONH is thought to occur in 2 of 100,000 births with no sexual predilection. The nerve head is typically one-third to one-half the size of a normally developed optic nerve. The normal disc size range is between 3.44 and 4.70 mm, whereas

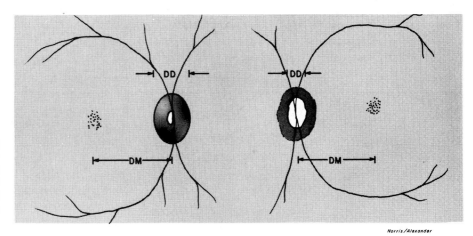

Figure 3–46. Schematic illustrating unilateral congenital optic nerve hypoplasia. The affected disc is reduced in size, which increases the DM/DD ratio. The affected disc is surrounded by a discolored area that corresponds to the size of the unaffected disc.

Norris/Alexander

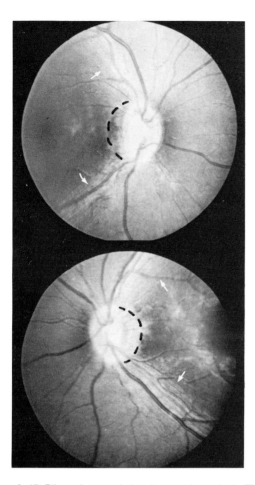

Figure 3–47. Bilateral congenital optic nerve hypoplasia. The dotted lines represent the expected disc size. The arrows point to the edges of the intact nerve fiber layer. The macular zones have a severe reduction in nerve fiber layer reflex. This patient had nystagmus.

hypoplastic discs range from 1.80 to 3.27 mm on a 35-mm slide taken at 30 degrees and viewed at 2.5 × magnification. The nerve head is usually pale in comparison to the normal nerve head, and is usually surrounded by a yellow zone that may be variably pigmented. This surrounding zone approximates the size of the optic nerve head if it were normal in its development. This is referred to in some reports as a "double-ring sign." The reduction in size is the result of an absent or severely reduced nerve fiber layer with a corresponding absence of ganglion cells. This is all thought to be related to a failure of development of the ganglion cell layer of the retina secondary to interruption in fetal development. The alteration results in a reduction of nerve fibers from the ganglion cell layer to the lateral geniculate body. There is also referral to a condition known as segmental optic nerve hypoplasia, where only a portion of the disc is hypoplastic, resulting in visual field defects more than in reduction of visual acuity.

The majority of patients with congenital optic nerve hypoplasia have relatively normal optic nerve head vasculature that exits and enters the disc centrally. The disc-macula/disc-disc (DM/DD) ratio is altered in cases of congenital optic nerve hypoplasia and may serve as a means of quantification of the condition. The normal DM/DD ratio is 2:1 to 3:2, and values greater than 3:2 are strongly suggestive of congenital optic nerve hypoplasia.

Because there is a maldevelopment of the nerve fiber layer, there is a resultant variable visual acuity from normal to no light perception. Interestingly, there is a higher prevalence of astigmatism in eyes with CONH. The patient may often have amblyopia or strabismus (50 percent), and the majority manifest

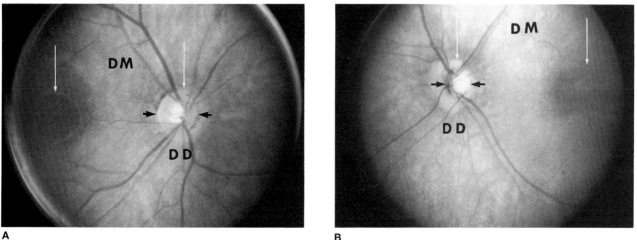

A   B

Figure 3–48. A. The unaffected right eye with DM and DD distances indicated. **B.** The fellow left eye with congenital optic nerve hypoplasia and the expected increased DM/DD. Acuity was reduced to 20/200.

Congenital Optic Nerve Hypoplasia

Characteristics

△ Nerve head is usually one-half to one-third the size of the fellow eye and pale by comparison

△ May be a variation called segmental hypoplasia

△ Surrounded by a discolored zone the size of the normal optic nerve head

△ Altered DM/DD ratio

△ Reduced vision because of maldevelopment of the nerve fiber layer

△ Higher prevalence of astigmatism in affected eyes

△ Variable visual fields usually nasal or altitudinal defects

△ Association with multiple systemic abnormalities especially if bilateral

△ Present in approximately 50 percent of fetal alcohol syndromes

Management

△ Proper differential diagnosis to prevent unnecessary treatment, such as amblyopia therapy

△ Rule out systemic abnormalities

△ Patient education

△ Provision of protective eyewear if unilateral

△ Communication with other providers of health care managing the patient

△ Routine eye examinations

esotropia. The pupillary response in the affected eye is usually absent or very slowly reactive to direct light. A Marcus Gunn pupil may then be present in cases of unilateral congenital optic nerve hypoplasia. As one would expect, nystagmus is present in a majority of bilateral cases because of poor acuity from birth. Visual fields vary considerably depending on the areas of the nerve head affected and the extent of the hypoplasia. The more common field defects are nasal and inferior altitudinal defects. The author has seen a teenage patient with total inferior altitudinal hemianopsias secondary to bilateral congenital optic nerve hypoplasia with a totally unremarkable neurologic work-up. It is important to remember that there is a gradient regarding the degree of hypoplasia from just clinically observable to almost total absence of the nerve head.

Congenital optic nerve hypoplasia has been related to many ocular and systemic anomalies, including strabismus, nystagmus, persistent hyperplastic primary vitreous, anencephaly, hydranencephaly, septo-optic dysplasia (De Morsier's syndrome), pituitary dysfunction (13 percent), cerebral palsy, epilepsy, porencephaly, absence of the septum pellucidum (27 percent), intracranial tumors, and facial and head abnormalities. There also has been an association with maternal ingestion of quinine to induce abortion, and use of dilantin, lysergic acid diethylamide (LSD), phencyclidine (PCP), and ethanol (CONH is thought to occur in approximately 50 percent of fetal alcohol syndromes) as well as other pharmacologic implications. There is thought to be some association with maternal cytomegalovirus, syphilis, rubella, and diabetes. It should be noted, however, that the majority of patients with congenital optic nerve hypoplasia have no associated systemic abnormalities. **See color plates 7 and 8.**

Management. Congenital optic nerve hypoplasia is a benign, self-limited condition that will not respond to intervention from an ocular standpoint. The only possible concern surrounds the associated systemic anomalies.

Management of congenital optic nerve hypoplasia involves, most importantly, proper differential diagnosis to prevent unnecessary amblyopic or strabismic therapy or unnecessary extensive neurologic investigations because of a small pale optic disc and reduced vision.

Additional studies may be indicated when there is the suspicion of associated systemic anomalies. It should be noted that systemic anomalies are more likely if the condition is bilateral. Axial tomograms, skull x-rays, CT scans, and magnetic resonance imaging may be employed to assist in the discovery of neurologic malformations and dysfunction. An extensive endocrinology work-up is indicated if there is evidence of hormonal alterations, sexual precocity, sexual infantilism, diabetes insipidus, hypoglycemia, and/or hypoadrenalism.

Should the condition be unilateral, protective eyewear is indicated. Extensive patient education is warranted as well as routine visual assessments to assure that a neurologic problem is not lurking behind the diagnosis of CONH.

■ ■ ■ ■ ■ ■

Clinical Note: Differential Diagnosis for Optic Nerve Aplasia

Optic nerve aplasia is a rare condition in which there is total absence of the optic nerve, ganglion cells, and retinal vessels. Aplasia is considered to occur as the result of interference in the development of the optic nerve at an earlier point in gestation than that which would result in optic nerve hypoplasia.

The eye affected with aplasia is often microophthalmic with cataracts and retinal–choroidal colobomas. There is no vision at all and no pupillary response. This condition is usually unilateral. Optic nerve aplasia may or may not have related systemic abnormalities.

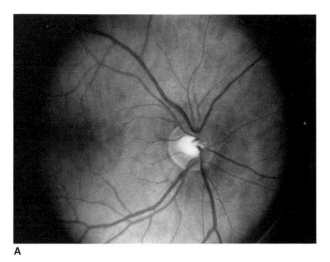 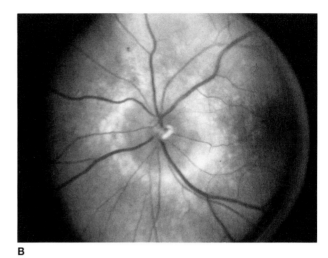

A   B

Figure 3–49. The normal-sized optic nerve head (**A**) compared to the megalopapillic left nerve head (**B**). Acuity was not reduced.

Megalopapilla

Introduction and Description. Clinically, megalopapilla (Figs. 3–49 and 3–50) is a term used to describe any nerve head that is larger by observation than its fellow nerve head. As discussed previously, many congenital nerve head anomalies can appear as an associated enlargement of the affected nerve. Among these variations are congenital optic nerve coloboma, congenital optic pits, the morning glory disc anomaly, and buried drusen of the nerve head. When the clinician is faced with the unilaterally enlarged optic nerve, it is important to rule out any acquired condition creating enlargement of the nerve head secondary to optic disc edema or associated with the other developmental anomalies previously mentioned. Once congenital and acquired anomalies have been ruled out, the clinician is left with megalopapilla as a diagnosis.

The megalopapillic nerve head can have any number of appearances but usually has an unusual vascular pattern similar to other congenital disc anomalies. The DM/DD ratio will be reduced below 2:1. The condition is usually unilateral, but bilateral megalopapilla is seen occasionally. Acuity is usually unaffected, and nerve conduction defects are absent. Circumpapillary retinal pigment epithelium defects are often present.

Simultaneous comparison of the view of the nerve heads is often necessary for a differential diagnosis. This is difficult with direct ophthalmoscopy, and fundus lens evaluation is enhanced with binocular indirect ophthalmoscopy and is maximized with fundus photography.

The condition is thought to evolve as the result of abnormal development of the primitive epithelial papilla. Visual acuity is usually normal, and visual

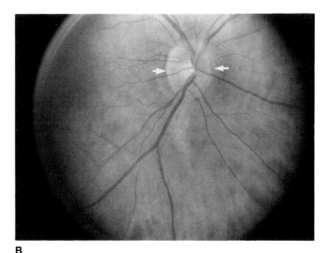

A   B

Figure 3–50. A. The left nerve head is enlarged but flat, and acuity is normal. The long white arrow points to a retinal–choroidal coloboma. The right nerve head (**B**) is of normal size.

Megalopapilla

Characteristics

△ Unilaterally enlarged optic nerve of congenital origin, possibly secondary to abnormal development of the primitive epithelial papilla

△ Reduced disc macula/disc disc (DM/DD) ratio

△ May simulate asymmetrical CD ratios of glaucomatous optic atrophy

Management

△ Benign nonprogressive anomaly requiring routine eye examinations

fields are unaffected except for enlarged physiologic blind spots. There are no associated severe systemic anomalies. Other congenital anomalies, such as cleft palate, may coexist. The importance of the recognition of an enlarged disc lies in the fact that with the large disc there is often a corresponding increase in the cup. The scleral canal is larger, allowing for more of a spread of the nerve fibers, creating a correspondingly enlarged cup. This enlarged cup, which is usually asymmetrical with the fellow eye, can easily be misinterpreted as glaucomatous optic atrophy. Simultaneous comparison of the nerve heads and threshold visual fields will put the diagnosis in the proper category.

Management. Megalopapilla is a benign, nonprogressive congenital anomaly that requires no management beyond proper differential diagnosis. **See color plate 9.**

Buried Drusen of the Optic Nerve Head

Introduction and Description. Buried drusen of the nerve head (Figs. 3–51 to 3–56) can create a diagnostic dilemma that certainly does not represent a benign, nonprogressive condition. Unfortunately the term pseudopapilledema is applied to this condition as well as other congenital variations of the disc presenting small hyperemic discs. Buried drusen of the nerve head occur congenitally with variable clinical presentation. The drusen of the nerve head have no histopathologic correlation to retinal drusen and as such are not age-related aside from the fact that they have a tendency to become more visible ophthalmoscopically with age. Optic nerve head drusen are inherited in an autosomal irregular dominant pattern with incomplete penetrance, are bilateral in over 70 percent of the patients, and occur primarily in whites. Drusen appear in approximately 1 percent of the population.

Drusen evolve slowly, often requiring decades to fully develop. In childhood, the discs appear papilledema-like, with no physiologic cupping. Later, the discs become yellowish, with spherical refractile structures surfacing. These refractile bodies transilluminate (glow) and appear more often near the nasal

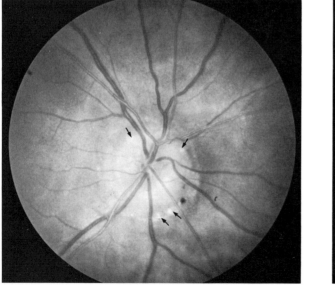 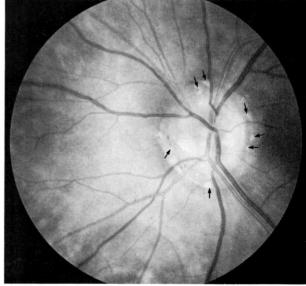

Figure 3–51. An example of bilateral optic nerve head drusen in an older patient. Both nerve heads were elevated. The arrows point to glowing buried drusen.

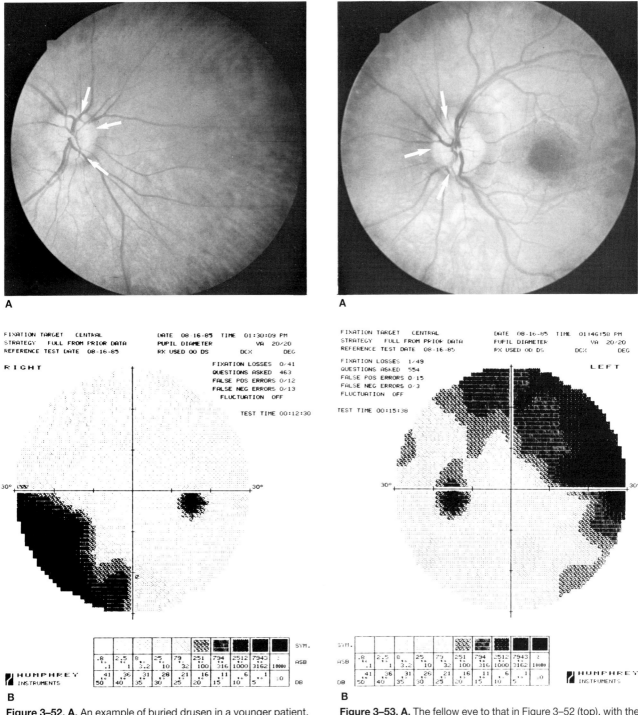

Figure 3–52. A. An example of buried drusen in a younger patient. The arrows point to areas of gross optic nerve head elevation where no drusen were readily visible. **B.** The field corresponding to that in top figure, demonstrating a dense defect.

Figure 3–53. A. The fellow eye to that in Figure 3–52 (top), with the arrows again pointing to gross elevation. **B.** The corresponding field defect.

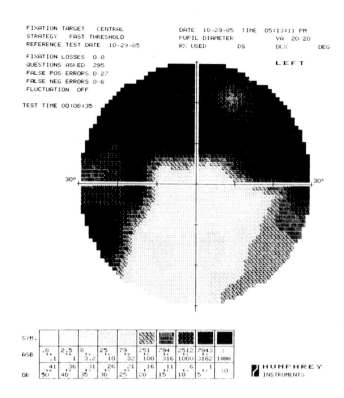

Figure 3–54. Within 3 months, the field defect in Figure 3–53B had progressed to this stage. This illustrates the potential for vision loss with buried drusen of the optic nerve head.

disc margin, although they can be seen at any location. There is often an anomalous vascular pattern on the nerve head (about 10 percent of cases), again similar to the presentation of vascular anomalies in other congenital optic nerve head conditions.

The drusen of the optic nerve are confined anterior to the lamina cribrosa. The calcium-like globular deposits (thought to be calcified mitochondrial mate-

rial) may be associated with alterations of axoplasmic flow and subsequent damage to the axons. It has been postulated that alteration of the axons occurs before the calcific deposition. The calcific deposits can then compromise (are actually thought to shear) the nerve fibers and vascular supply, leading to visual field defects and circumpapillary hemorrhages.

Buried drusen of the nerve head give a pa-

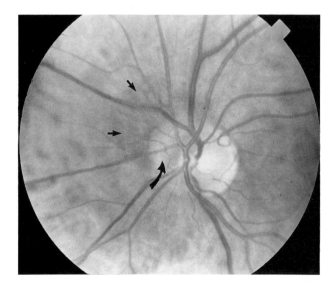

Figure 3–55. The curved arrow points to an area of disc elevation. The small arrow points to an area of sub retinal hemorrhage secondary to the buried drusen.

pilledema-like appearance to the discs in younger patients and ascend within the disc to assume their refractile properties as the patient ages. The buried drusen often become more visible even at the second decade of life. The increased visibility with age is not always an absolute characteristic of the aging drusen but is the rule. Visual field defects are often present and are known to progress. The defects may be scotomas, concentric constriction, or generalized depressions. Most often the defects are arcuate, sector, or altitudinal in presentation. The visual field defects, although usually slow in progression, can compromise mobility and can become a danger when operating motor vehicles. Most often the patients do not even notice the field defect because of its slow progression. The sharpness of the drusen can shear the blood vessels, leading to hemorrhages in, around, and over the optic nerve head.

The drusen are known to autofluoresce, which aids in differential diagnosis. This autofluorescence is achievable by using the exciting and barrier filter available in cameras equipped to perform fluorescein angiography. During fluorescein angiography, the drusen typically hyperfluoresce but do not leak. Ultrasonography (see Fig. 3–56) is of tremendous assistance in the differential diagnosis from optic disc edema. The buried drusen are highly reflective with ultrasound. Unfortunately, the reflectivity is not as dramatic in the younger patient with buried drusen and often is not effective in assisting in differential diagnosis. Even when the frequency of the ultrasound wave is reduced so that soft tissue is no longer reflective, the drusen will continue to reflect because of their calcific composition. In extremely large buried drusen, the CT scan will also demonstrate the abnormality. **See color plates 11 and 12.**

Although usually not associated with systemic abnormalities, there are reports of migraine headaches, seizures, motor clumsiness, retardation, cerebellar astrocytoma, and learning disorders in patients with buried drusen of the nerve head. The diagnosis must always consider the possibility of associated neurologic disorders and as such should always be carefully followed until establishing that the disorder is not progressing and does not have other soft signs.

Management. Buried drusen of the optic nerve head can be visually devastating. Hemorrhages secondary to the drusen can compromise vision. Juxtapapillary choroidal neovascular membranes with their potential sequelae are also a potential complication of buried drusen of the optic nerve head. The most severe complication is, however, progressive compromise of the nerve fibers and slowly progressive optic atrophy. The changes can cause a progressive visual field defect that can ultimately result in total loss of visual function.

Unfortunately, buried drusen of the optic nerve head progress unchecked. Interventive therapy is currently not available to prevent either the associated nerve fiber loss or the hemorrhages.

It is important to make the proper differential diagnosis to avoid costly and unnecessary neurologic evaluations. Buried drusen of the optic nerve can occur in retinitis pigmentosa and angioid streaks and are also simulated by an astrocytic hamartoma of the optic nerve head and meningiomas of the optic nerve.

Pearls

Buried Drusen of the Optic Nerve Head

Characteristics

△ Often referred to as pseudopapilledema
△ Inherited in autosomal dominant irregular pattern with incomplete penetrance
△ Are bilateral in 70 percent
△ Occur primarily in whites
△ Occur in about 1 percent of the population
△ Calcium-like globular deposits anterior to the lamina cribrosa that become more apparent with age; appear to be calcifications of mitochondrial debris
△ In youth, present as only a swollen disc, but transilluminate as golden globs as the patient ages
△ The deposits can shear blood vessels, causing hemorrhage, and may precipitate development of juxtapapillary choroidal neovascularization
△ The deposits may alter axoplasmic flow, causing axonal death and progressive field loss
△ Autofluorescence with a barrier and excitor filter that aids in the differential diagnosis
△ Hyperfluorescence occurs throughout fluorescein angiography without leakage
△ Ultrasonography is very useful in differential diagnosis, especially when reducing gain because of high reflectivity, but is of questionable efficacy in young patients
△ If associated with retinitis pigmentosa, the drusen lie off the disc margin in the superficial retina

Management

△ Proper diagnosis and patient education
△ Baseline fields to monitor progression
△ Patient self-monitoring of vision
△ Routine yearly examinations
△ Always consider the possibility of associated systemic disorders, and if suspecting neurologic disorders, follow up for progression of visual field defects

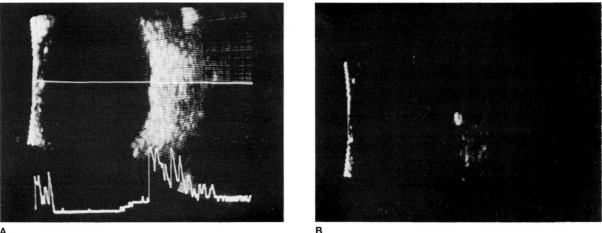

A   B

Figure 3–56. This illustrates a very valuable diagnostic tool to assist in determining the presence of buried drusen. **A.** Elevation of the nerve head (cursor) by B-scan ultrasonography. **B.** When the gain is reduced, solid structures, such as drusen and asteroid hyalosis, will continue to return signals to the transducer. The buried drusen becomes visible.

The astrocytic hamartoma is also highly reflective on reduced-gain B-scan ultrasonography. Baseline visual fields are of value in all suspected cases to provide a base to assess progression toward visual compromise. It is also important to educate patients about the condition so that they are prepared if field loss or hemorrhages occur. The patient should report immediately if any vision function changes are noted.

■ ■ ■ ■ ■ ■

Clinical Note: Drusen of the Optic Nerve Head Associated with Retinitis Pigmentosa

Drusen of the nerve head can arise in patients with retinitis pigmentosa. These drusen differ somewhat from the familial drusen in that they lie just off the disc margin in the superficial retina. There certainly will be the other fundus characteristics associated with retinitis pigmentosa, but the visual field defects can confound the diagnosis. Often, it is necessary to employ electrodiagnostic testing to confirm the diagnosis.

INHERITED FAMILIAL OPTIC ATROPHY

The hereditary aspect of optic atrophy can be misleading when consideration is given to the fact that atrophies may be of juvenile onset and may, in fact, progress. Hereditary optic atrophies include (1) autosomal dominant congenital optic atrophy, (2) autosomal recessive congenital optic atrophy, (3) autosomal dominant juvenile optic atrophy, (4) autosomal reces-

sive juvenile optic atrophy, (5) Leber's hereditary optic atrophy, and (6) Behr's optic atrophy. Differentiation of these conditions is best managed by referring to the clinical findings listed in Table 3–3. The more common hereditary optic atrophies are discussed briefly.

Autosomal Dominant Juvenile Optic Atrophy

Introduction and Description. Autosomal dominant juvenile optic atrophy is characterized by variable bilateral optic nerve pallor usually involving a temporal sector (Fig. 3–57). This characteristic is, however, variable from full pallor to no clinically observable pallor, and is usually the sole finding. There is a low correlation of optic nerve appearance and resultant acuity. The incidence is 1 in 50,000, with an autosomal dominant inheritance pattern.

Pearls

Autosomal Dominant Juvenile Optic Atrophy

Characteristics

△ Variable optic nerve pallor often temporal in presentation
△ Insidious loss of vision ages 4 to 12 years, with variable final acuity and fields that usually stabilize by age 30 years
△ Usually associated with a blue-yellow defect
△ Usually no nystagmus

Management

△ Rule out any neurologic cause
△ Patient education
△ Provision of best possible prescription
△ Routine yearly examinations
△ Genetic considerations

TABLE 3–3. INHERITED OPTIC ATROPHIES

Characteristic	Autosomal Dominant Juvenile Optic Atrophy	Autosomal Recessive Juvenile Optic Atrophy	Leber's Hereditary Optic Atrophy	Autosomal Dominant Congenital Optic Atrophy	Autosomal Recessive Congenital Optic Atrophy	Behr's Optic Atrophy
Inheritance pattern	Dominant	Recessive	Questionable, affects primarily males	Dominant	Recessive	Recessive
Age of onset	Insidious at 6–12 years	Insidious at 6–12 years	Acute at 10–40 years	Congenital	Congenital	1–9 years
Final acuity	20/20–1/60	Severe loss	1–/200	20/100 to severe	Severe loss	20/60–10/200
Nystagmus	No	No	No	Yes	Yes	Possible
Fundus picture	Temporal optic atrophy	Total optic atrophy	Optic disc edema followed by optic atrophy	Total optic atrophy	Total optic atrophy	Temporal optic atrophy
Visual fields	Relative centrocecal scotoma, inversion of peripheral color field	N/A	Central scotoma, normal peripheral fields	Constricted peripheral, possible scotoma	Constricted peripheral, possible scotoma	Central scotoma, normal peripheral fields
Color vision	Blue-yellow defect	N/A	Red-green defect	Red-green defect	Red-green defect	Red-green defect
Associated systemic signs and symptoms	N/A	Diabetes? Auditory problems?	Headaches, vertigo, nervousness	N/A	N/A	Increased deep tendon reflex, positive Romberg sign, ataxia, muscle rigidity, mental debilitation
Clinical course	Usually stabilizes but may present a slow progression	N/A	Acute loss that may regress or after years of delay may progress	May have slow progression	May have slow progression	Neurologic signs and symptoms evolve years after, then stabilize, optic atrophy stabilizes

There is a wide range of visual acuity in reports of autosomal dominant juvenile optic atrophy, from near normal to 1/60, but acuity usually ranges from 20/40 to 20/60. Near visual acuity may be better than distance acuity. Visual acuity may or may not be stable, but if progression occurs it is usually moderate. There is usually stability of acuity by age 30 years. The onset of visual loss is insidious, usually occurring in a 4- to 12-year-old. A blue-yellow defect often precedes the atrophy, and a wide range of field defects can occur. Most often there is a centrocecal scotoma. A Marcus Gunn pupil is usually absent because of bilaterality. Usually, electrodiagnostic tests and dark adaptation are unaffected. Diagnosis is often made after establishment of a pedigree. **See color plate 10.**

Management. The condition is usually stationary, but slight progressive loss of vision may occur. The clinician must make the correct diagnosis by ruling out potential neurologic causes. Patient education and genetic counseling are certainly in order. The patient with autosomal dominant juvenile optic atrophy can expect one half of the offspring to be affected, with equal sex distribution. It is important to provide the best possible prescription and low-vision rehabilitation if necessary.

Autosomal Recessive Congenital Optic Atrophy

Introduction and Description. Autosomal recessive congenital optic atrophy is very rare and is characterized by poor vision and nystagmus at birth. The condition is also known as early infantile recessive optic atrophy. The inheritance pattern implicates consanguinity of parents. The discs are usually very atrophic and may be deeply cupped. The vision is poor, at worse than 20/200, but does not usually progress.

Autosomal Recessive Congenital Optic Atrophy

Characteristics

△ Poor vision (20/200 and worse) and nystagmus at birth
△ Implication of parent consanguinity
△ Optic discs very atrophic and may be deeply cupped

Management

△ Rule out other causes of optic atrophy and blindness at birth
△ Genetic counseling
△ Routine eye examinations
△ Low-vision or blind rehabilitative efforts

Management. Management consists of ruling out other potential causes of optic atrophy, often necessitating a neurologic consultation. The differential of Leber's congenital amaurosis can be made by performing an electroretinogram (ERG), which will be depressed in Leber's congenital amaurosis but not in early infantile recessive optic atrophy. The pedigree should be generated and the family should be advised of the genetic implications. Routine eye examinations should be performed, and either blind rehabilitative or low-vision rehabilitative services should be provided.

Leber's Hereditary Optic Atrophy

Introduction and Description. Leber's hereditary optic atrophy is a bilateral disease of questionable etiology. The condition usually occurs as an acute to subacute disease in males between ages 15 and 30 years and less frequently in females in their 20s or 30s. In-

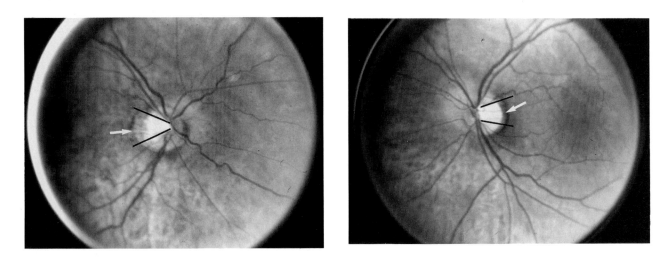

Figure 3–57. Classic presentation of autosomal dominant juvenile optic atrophy. There is a triangular sector (*arrows*) of temporal optic atrophy in both eyes.

Leber's Hereditary Optic Atrophy

Characteristics

△ Usually acute presentation at ages 15 to 30 years in males and in the 20s to 30s in females

△ Men affected 6.7 times more often than females

△ Optic disc edema accompanied by circumpapillary telangiectatic microvasculopathy that does not leak on fluorescein angiography as well as heightened opacification of the peripapillary nerve fiber layer

△ Severe optic atrophy ensues with severe loss of vision down to 20/200 and dense central and centrocecal scotomas with involvement of the fellow eye within months

△ May be associated systemic signs of headaches, vertigo, and nervousness

△ Diagnosis facilitated by analysis of mitochondrial DNA, which presents a mutation at position 11,778 in 50 to 60 percent of patients

△ Association with mitochondrial alterations of cardiac muscle creating cardiac conduction problems

Management

△ Proper differential diagnosis

△ Genetic counseling

Transmitted by females to manifest in 50 percent of sons

Transmitted by females to manifest in 10 percent of daughters

Transmitted in the carrier state by females to 100 percent of daughters

Not transmitted by males

△ Consultation with neurologist or neuro-ophthalmologist for possible medical intervention if in the acute stages

△ Consultation with cardiologist for patient and carrier family members

△ Provision of best possible refraction and low vision rehabilitation

---

heritance is a factor, but the precise pedigree fits no established pattern because of the fact that it is inherited with the mitochondrial DNA rather than the chromosomal DNA. Pedigree analysis is nevertheless important, as the disease is transmitted by females to 50 percent of their sons and 100 percent of daughters in the carrier state. Ten percent of females are expected to manifest the disease; males do not transmit it. At the onset of the acute attack, optic disc edema is often accompanied by circumpapillary telangiectactic microangiopathy that does not leak on fluorescein angiography as well as heightened opacification of the peripapillary retinal nerve fiber layer. Visual acuity quickly reduces to the 20/200 level. Both eyes are usually affected simultaneously, but this is not an absolute rule.

In some patients, there is a dropout of retinal nerve fibers, an alteration of the Farnsworth–Munsell 100-hue test, and altered visually evoked potential before the acute attack. During the active phase, there may be associated headaches, vertigo, and general nervousness.

As the condition progresses, the nerve heads become atrophic, resulting in dense central or centrocecal scotomas and color vision loss that progresses quickly over days to months. The fellow eye usually becomes affected within a few months. Stabilization of vision occurs in the 20/200 range.

Diagnosis of Leber's hereditary optic atrophy is now facilitated by analysis of mitochondrial DNA. There appears to be a mutation at the 11,778 position (50 to 60 percent of patients) and perhaps mutations at other locations. The mitochondrial assessment may be performed by special laboratories but is exceedingly expensive.

Management. The prognosis for Leber's hereditary optic atrophy is grim. There are reports of spontaneous recovery of vision as well as spontaneous further reduction in vision. Early recognition and the establishment of a pedigree are important in the management of Leber's hereditary optic atrophy. Genetic counseling is important, keeping in mind the following characteristics of the disease:

1. Men are affected 6.7 times more often than women.
2. The age of onset is 15 to 30 years in men, and 20 to 40 years in women.
3. Affected males cannot transmit the disease.
4. The sister of an affected male is a carrier.
5. Affected females have nonaffected fathers.
6. A heterozygous female can transmit the trait to a son (50 percent) and the carrier state (100 percent) to a daughter.

The metabolic abnormality suspected in the mitochondria is also present in the skeletal and cardiac muscle of Leber's patients and families, causing an increased incidence of cardiac conduction defects. The incidence of cardiac anomalies associated with the disease should be investigated in both the affected patient and in the carrier mother and sisters.

There are some advocates of medical intervention in this disease based on the hypothesis that the cause is a defect in cyanide metabolism. Although the issue of altered cyanide metabolism is controversial, there is evidence to support that a mitochondrial enzyme, rhodanese, is altered, allowing for the inability to detoxify cyanide. Rhodanese is decreased in the liver of patients with Leber's. It has been suggested that vitamin B_{12A} and vitamin B_{12} given 1 mg parenterally daily for 7 days may be effective in treatment of the acute phase. There is no proof as to its efficacy. Vitamin therapy is used in the treatment of Leber's hereditary optic atrophy because it cannot create a problem with toxicity (vitamin B variants are water soluble) and it may be beneficial.

The end result of Leber's atrophy becomes a problem best solved with an optimal ophthalmic prescription often accompanied by low-vision rehabilitation and vocational rehabilitation. Genetic counseling is also of tantamount importance as well as consideration of the potential cardiac anomalies.

ACQUIRED OPTIC NERVE DISEASE

Acquired optic nerve disease can be the result of numerous afflictions. Such terms as "optic neuritis" and "papilledema" have been applied erroneously in past discussions of optic neuropathy. This discussion considers all acquired diseases of the optic nerve under the terminology of "optic neuropathy." Terminology is applied that specifically defines the pathologic process. The suffix "itis" refers only to proven inflammatory processes, and the term "optic disc edema" refers to any swelling of the nerve fibers of the optic nerve. Table 3–4 summarizes the general categories of etiology of optic neuropathy, and Table 3–5 summarizes many of the causes of optic disc edema. Table 3–6 is a simplified summary of typical causes of optic neuropathy by age. The most common type of optic nerve head affectation, glaucomatous optic neuropathy, will be described first.

Glaucomatous Optic Neuropathy

Although many would consider glaucoma an anterior segment disease, enough confusion exists regarding the disease at this point in time that the topic of glaucomatous optic neuropathy will be covered as an acquired optic nerve head disease. There appears to be enough different presentations of glaucomatous optic neuropathy that vascular perfusion and alteration of axoplasmic flow has to play a part in the genesis of the disease process.

Evaluation of the Optic Nerve Head in Glaucoma. Evaluation of the optic nerve head is crucial in the as-

TABLE 3–5. SOME OF THE MORE COMMON CAUSES OF OPTIC DISC EDEMA

Anterior ischemic optic neuropathy	Orbital cellulitis
Carotid cavernous fistula	Papilledema secondary to intracranial mass or hemorrhage
Cavernous sinus thrombosis	
Central retinal vein occlusion	
Demyelinizing optic neuropathy	Papilledema secondary to benign intracranial hypertension
Diabetic papillopathy	Papillitis (inflammatory optic neuropathy)
Drusen of the nerve head	
Foster Kennedy syndrome	Papillophlebitis
Hemicentral retinal vein occlusion	Primary optic nerve tumors
Leukemic infiltrates of the optic nerve	Primary orbital tumors
	Thyroid eye disease

sessment of damage attributable to glaucoma. Unfortunately, there have been tremendous misunderstandings in terminology used to record nerve head variation as well as confusion in the methods used to observe the nerve head. Terms such as cup/disc (C/D) ratios have little meaning unless the observation technique is stereoscopic. It is believed that stereoscopic observation estimates of cup/disc ratios are about 50 percent larger than monocular estimates. Little attention has been given to the importance of asymmetrical disc presentation in optic nerve disease, much less in glaucomatous optic neuropathy. The optic nerve head is of paramount importance in the diagnosis of glaucoma. It has been stated that 35 to 50 percent of nerve fibers may be destroyed in glaucomatous optic atrophy prior to significant field loss. Although this may be slightly overstated, disc evaluation is crucial because it is the only objective technique currently available.

Basic Clinical Morphology of the Optic Nerve Head. When discussing glaucoma, the optic nerve head is considered to be the structure from the retinal surface to the start of myelination near the sclera. The optic nerve head is usually a vertical oval, with tremendous variation in size and shape. Usually, however, the nerve heads are a mirror image of one

TABLE 3–4. ETIOLOGY OF OPTIC NEUROPATHY

Glaucomatous optic neuropathy
Ischemic optic neuropathy
Demyelinizing optic neuropathy
Hereditary or familial optic neuropathy
Inflammatory optic neuropathy
Toxic optic neuropathy
Compressive optic neuropathy
Descending optic neuropathy secondary to retinal/choroidal disease

TABLE 3–6. TYPICAL CAUSES OF OPTIC NEUROPATHY CLASSIFIED BY AGE OF ONSET

Age (yr)	Typical Cause
1–10	Inflammatory optic nerve disease/hereditary optic neuropathy
11–20	Postinfectious optic nerve disease/Leber's in men
21–40	Demyelinizing disease/toxic optic neuropathy
40+	Glaucomatous optic neuropathy in blacks
50+	Glaucomatous optic neuropathy in whites
50–70	Ischemic optic neuropathy/toxic optic neuropathy
60–80	Giant-cell arteritic optic neuropathy

another, unless there are (1) congenital variations such as optic pits, nerve head colobomas, or optic nerve head hypoplasia; or (2) acquired nerve head changes such as glaucomatous optic atrophy, ischemic optic neuropathy, or optic disc edema. The "mirror image" concept is important to understand, because asymmetry is often the only early diagnostic clue that we may have in all optic nerve disease.

The central portion of the nerve head usually has a depression that is referred to as the "cup." Within the depression is an area of pallor that represents partial or complete absence of axons. In this area, the lamina is often visible. The pallor may be the same size of the "cup" except in diseased states. The cup will be larger when the disc/scleral canal is larger, and the larger cup is characteristic in various ethnic groups. Megalopapilla will often create an enlarged cup that may be asymmetrical and may confuse the issue of cup/disc analysis. The tissue between the "cup" and the disc margin is referred to as the neural retinal rim. The neural retinal rim is usually a variable saturation of red and contains the majority of axons, but color and contour may be very difficult to assess in conditions such as tilted or malinserted discs. Remember that in spite of anatomical variations, the rims should be mirror images of one another. This is often your only clue to a healthy set of optic nerve heads when there is disc tilting. The exception to this rule is the occurrence of congenital variations, which invariably present size differences between the two eyes.

The Cup (the Hole in the Donut). The cup size is determined by the size of the scleral canal and the amount of glial supportive tissue. Stereoscopic observation of the cup size gives approximately a 50 percent larger estimate of the cup than observation by direct ophthalmoscopy. Observation of the cup/disc (CD) ratio by stereo changes over time, or CD size difference between the two eyes, should be treated as a pathologic change suggesting glaucomatous optic atrophy until proven otherwise.

The cup size appears to have some genetic and ethnic predictability. Examination of other family members may be of benefit in suspect cases, but should only be used in the decision making as a part of the total picture. It has also been shown that CD ratios are consistently larger in blacks than in whites in healthy eyes.

Cup size enlarges and pallor intensifies with increasing age. This natural enlargement is barely perceptible with standard viewing techniques and is symmetrical in presentation. These changes may be secondary to an increase in the diameter of the optic nerve head with age.

There is always some concern in optic nerve head (ONH) evaluation when considering intraobserver

and interobserver consistency. Studies have pointed out that trained observers have excellent consistency both in interobserver and intraobserver trials with maximum performance attained using stereoscopic disc photographs. Other reports address the problem of tremendous variability in observation and recording of CD ratios. Cups also present different shapes. These shapes have been classified by Elschnig, but such variation occurs in the population that it is best to attempt to draw the characteristics rather than lump the variations into Elschnig classifications. Figures 3–58 and 3–59 represent a method of mapping the optic nerve head in conditions such as glaucoma. When using this method, the practitioner does not need to make the mental correction for the upside down and backwards view experienced with a typical fundus lens. Always remember that when you are looking at the CD you are looking at a void, a "hole" in the center of the donut. If the CD enlarges, it implies that the donut (neural retinal rim) is being eaten from the inside out. This observation is erosion (destruction) of the neural retinal rim. *A good rule to follow when observing suspicious discs is that glaucoma often shows cup changes early if the original CD was small. If the original CD was large, you may have to rely on visual fields to pick up the early changes of evolving glaucoma.*

Evaluation of the area of the neural retinal rim appears to be much more predictive of glaucomatous loss than evaluation of CD ratios. Unfortunately accurate repeatable measurement techniques for the area of the neural retinal rim are not yet available clinically. As a clinician, you must therefore make the observation and draw or photograph the disc.

Great care must be exercised when viewing the neural retinal rim, as the color may vary considerably with observation techniques and types of illumination, media opacities, and the incidence angle of observation. Perhaps the best example of this problem is the variation of disc color when viewing a patient with a cataract in one eye and an IOL in the other. The pink disc color will appear more desaturated in the pseudophakic eye. Again, stereoscopic viewing techniques become crucial when color evaluation is compromised.

Another common source of error in interpreting the neural retinal rim occurs when the ONH is tilted or obliquely inserted, as in myopia. As a clinician, you must observe color, contour, and asymmetry when evaluating the optic nerve head (Fig. 3–60).

Clinical Morphology of Glaucomatous Optic Atrophy. There are two basic schools of thought as to why patients lose viable optic nerve head tissue and thus portions of visual field secondary to increased intraocular pressure. The two basic theories are a vascular theory and a mechanical theory. The arguments

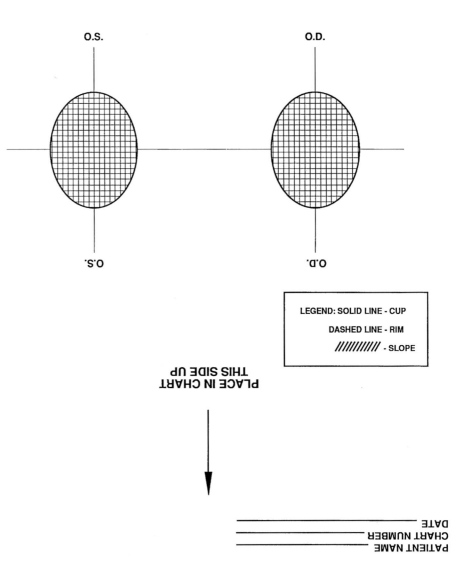

Figure 3–58. A map for drawing the optic nerve head characteristics as seen in a fundus lens. Alexander LJ Optom Clin 1991;1:19–102.

have no particular clinical relevance, but will be summarized to give the clinician a basic understanding of the pressure–perfusion concept.

In the discussion of glaucoma, the optic nerve head is considered to be the structure from the retinal surface to the start of the nerve fiber myelination near the sclera. Within this structure are approximately 1.2 million neurons grouped into about 1000 bundles that are supported by astrogliocytes. The nerve head is usually divided into four regions for clinical discussions: (1) the nerve fiber layer, (2) the prelaminar or glial region, (3) the lamina cribrosa and, (4) the retrolaminar optic nerve. The superficial nerve fiber layer consists of nonmyelinated nerve fibers entering from various parts of the retina. Usually, the different areas of the retina have corresponding specific loci on the nerve head. This distribution is especially relevant when analyzing visual field loss associated with excavation and/or atrophy of the optic nerve head. The fibers from the macular zone take a more direct course to the disc in the papillomacular bundle. The arcuate fibers, which occupy the superior and inferior notch zones of the disc, are most susceptible to damage. It should also be noted that peripheral fibers enter the disc nearer the disc margin, whereas the fibers originating nearer the optic nerve head run closer to the vitreous base and enter the disc more centrally.

It is useful to envision the nerve fibers as a conduit running from a synapse at the ganglion cell to a synapse at the lateral geniculate body. The nerve impulse travels in the walls of the conduit while the center is filled with a protoplasmic or axoplasmic flow

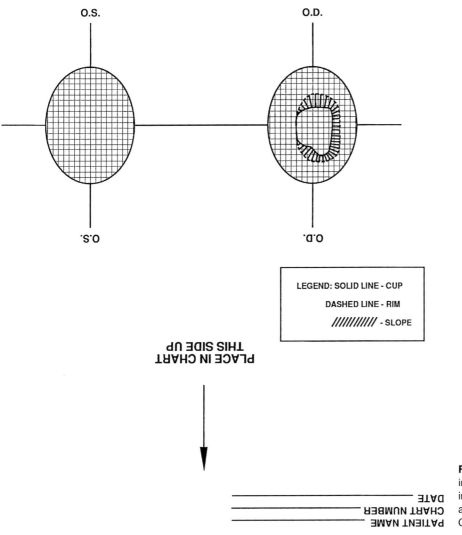

DRAW IN THE APPROPRIATE SPACE

THEN TURN THE PAGE OVER

O.S.   O.D.

LEGEND: SOLID LINE - CUP

DASHED LINE - RIM

/////////// - SLOPE

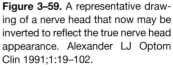

Figure 3–59. A representative drawing of a nerve head that now may be inverted to reflect the true nerve head appearance. Alexander LJ Optom Clin 1991;1:19–102.

that acts to supply nutrients to the nerve fiber. The prelaminar region is the supportive and nutritive zone for the nerve fibers as they make the turn into the optic nerve. Encircling this area is the border tissue of Elschnig, which is collagenous and very resistant. The lamina cribrosa is composed of sheets of connective tissue and elastic fibers that are continuous with and bridge the scleral canal. This seive-like structure has larger holes superiorly and inferiorly and supports the exit of the nerve fibers. The lamina can be visualized in about 35 percent of normal eyes at the base of the cup. The retrolaminar portion of the optic nerve is about twice the diameter of the intraocular portion because of the acquisition of myelin sheathing at the sclera.

The vascular supply has been discussed previ-

ously but a review regarding the relevance to glaucoma is important. The origin of the vascular supply is the ophthalmic artery. The central retinal artery pierces the nerve posterior to the globe and runs forward through the lamina. Most of the blood supply to the nerve head is from the short posterior ciliary arteries, the posterior ciliary arteries, and the pial artery. Small branches of the central retinal artery supply the most superficial layers of the optic nerve head.

The *vascular theory* of glaucoma attempts to explain some but certainly not all of the aspects of optic nerve head alteration in glaucoma. The vascular theory is supported by clinical observations that decreased blood flow in the anterior portion of the optic nerve head is the primary factor producing visual

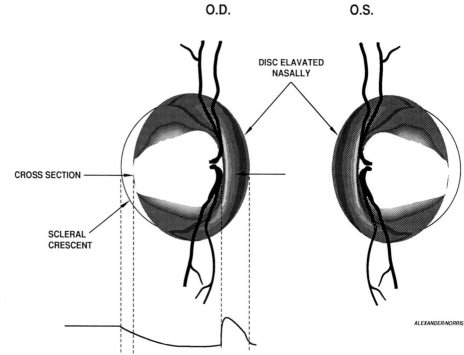

O.D.   O.S.

DISC ELAVATED
NASALLY

CROSS SECTION

SCLERAL
CRESCENT

ALEXANDER/NORRIS

Figure 3–60. A schematic illustrating the development of a scleral crescent and apparent temporal erosion that develops as the result of disc tilting. Alexander LJ Optom Clin 1991; 1:19–102.

field loss in glaucoma. These observations were made in relationship to the lowering of systemic blood pressure in patients who previously had no optic nerve alterations associated with IOP. Fluorescein angiographic studies also support the vascular theory by demonstrating persisting hypoperfusion or absolute filling defects (decreased blood flow and/or increased vascular permeability) that are characteristic of normotensive glaucoma. Other studies suggest that patients with normotensive glaucoma have a higher incidence of ischemic cerebral and cardiovascular disease, which may explain the ischemic optic nerve degeneration. It has also been reported that normotensive glaucoma patients have histories of diabetes, vascular hypotension, and major vascular crises, and have altered blood chemistries. A recent study, however, failed to demonstrate group differences for markers of atherosclerotic vascular disease between patients with high-tension and normotensive glaucoma. There is, however, little doubt that alteration of the vascular supply to the optic nerve head plays some role in the genesis of glaucomatous optic atrophy. Clinical observations support the theory that "vascularly ill" patients have more glaucomatous optic neuropathy than "vascularly well" patients.

Ischemic optic neuropathy (ION) creates a situation similar to glaucomatous optic atrophy. ION results in atrophy after optic disc edema. Eventually the atrophic area becomes somewhat eroded or cupped, mimicking glaucomatous optic atrophy (GOA). The major difference between GOA and ION is the se-

quence of events. In both conditions there is an alteration of the pressure–perfusion ratio—the balance of the blood pressure within disc vessels and the intraocular pressure. *In GOA, excavation typically precedes atrophy, whereas in ION atrophy typically precedes excavation.* In both cases, an alteration of this pressure results in destruction of disc/retinal tissue. The peripapillary choroidal blood supply is also affected by increased IOP. It appears that as blood flow decreases in the peripapillary choroidal circulation, there is a corresponding vascular insufficiency in the nerve head. This peripapillary change is getting much attention of late and will be discussed under clinical evaluation of the optic nerve head.

The *mechanical theory* of the genesis of glaucomatous optic atrophy is supported by the fact that loss of axonal tissue occurs early near the lamina cribrosa involving all axons. There seems to be greater involvement at the superior and inferior poles, where the fenestrations of the lamina are larger. It is hypothesized that the origin of axonal death in this region is secondary to the mechanical alteration (pinching) that fouls axoplasmic transport. The healthy eye has a flow of protein within the nerve fibers from the retinal ganglion cells to the lateral geniculate nucleus. With alterations in IOP, the slow phase of this protein flow (axoplasmic flow) is reduced. The rapid phase of the axoplasmic flow is altered as the IOP rises. This altered flow is thought to occur as the IOP increase pushes nerve fibers against a resistant structure such as the lamina creating an anatomic obstruction to flow.

Other studies that support the mechanical theory include the proponents of the proposition that the glial supportive network at the optic nerve head is affected by the increased IOP. It has been suggested that the glial tissue is altered by the increased IOP, resulting in exposure of the capillaries of the disc. The increased IOP then alters the capillaries, resulting in loss of vascular supply. Others have refuted this concept by pointing out that there is little loss of glial tissue in the optic nerve head associated with glaucomatous optic atrophy.

Perhaps the newest theory revolves around the contention that the earliest damage in glaucoma occurs within the retinal structure, specifically the ganglion cell layer. This theory is supported by observations of guttering in the nerve fiber layer and the recent recognition of depressed central thresholds in patients with glaucoma. It is thought that when the ganglion cell layer is altered, there is a retrograde atrophy of the nerve fiber layer through the optic nerve. Recent work directly ties retinal ganglion cell atrophy to visual field defects. It was shown that throughout the central 30 degrees of the retina, with a 20 percent loss of ganglion cells there was a 5-dB sensitivity loss in the visual field. With a 40 percent cell loss, there was a corresponding 10-dB decrease in sensitivity.

Once the destruction of the disc tissue begins, the cupping increases and the lamina cribosa bows backward. When this occurs, the nerve fibers passing through the pores of the lamina are subjected to increased mechanical stress, resulting in a further decrease of function. This is one of the reasons that more aggressive therapy of significant reduction of IOP is recommended as more disc erosion occurs.

The pathogenesis of glaucoma appears to be multifaceted and often confusing. Certainly it can be said that the damage in glaucoma is secondary to a nonphysiologic IOP. It is well recognized that increases in IOP are usually secondary to a restriction in the outflow of aqueous. The second factor to consider in glaucoma is the disease process of the optic nerve head or retinal ganglion cells. Whether the origin of glaucoma damage in the posterior segment is vascular or mechanical, the mainstay of treatment revolves around reduction of the intraocular pressure to a point that causes no further tissue destruction or visual field loss.

Both the vascular and mechanical theories present asymmetrical and progressive ONH changes. The following sections discuss generalized categories of ONH alterations associated with glaucoma.

Focal Enlargement. Focal enlargement of the cup is often referred to as polar notching, and usually occurs at the superior and inferior poles. Focal enlargement

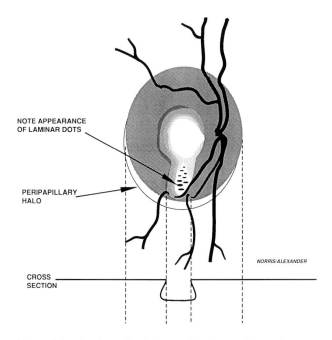

Figure 3–61. A schematic illustrating focal excavation of the neuroretinal rim in glaucomatous optic neuropathy. Alexander LJ Optom Clin 1991;1:19–102.

creates an altered cup/disc ratio vertically when compared to the horizontal. The focal enlargement usually starts as a small "bite" taken out of the rim, which may then enlarge and deepen (Figs. 3–61 and 3–62). The nasal aspect may also become undermined and indicates the last stage of erosion of the rim. The focal

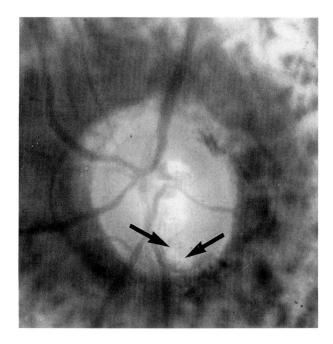

Figure 3–62. Inferior focal notching (*arrows*) of the neuroretinal rim in glaucomatous optic neuropathy.

O.D.   O.S.

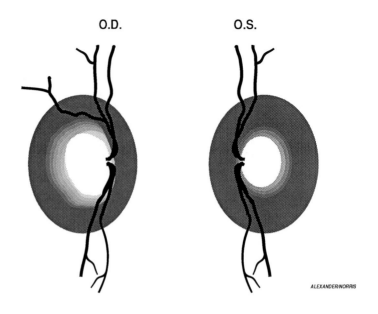

ALEXANDER/NORRIS

Figure 3–63. A schematic illustrating asymmetry of the neuroretinal rims characteristic of concentric enlargement in glaucomatous optic neuropathy. Alexander LJ Optom Clin 1991;1:19–102.

notch evolves toward the rim, where it becomes undermined, creating apparent breaks in vessels crossing at that point. Some clinicians believe that focal enlargement is associated with localized vascular ischemia. Focal enlargement is characterized by wedge-shaped scotomas that have a tendency to approach fixation and more dramatic nerve fiber layer dropout in darkly pigmented individuals.

Concentric Enlargement. Glaucoma may also cause cup enlargement in concentric circles. The circles may unfold in any direction, but usually progress toward the temporal rim. This alteration is often subtle and requires simultaneous disc comparison to detect early asymmetrical changes. Remember that cupping, or rim tissue erosion, usually precedes pallor.

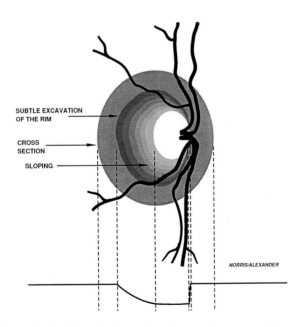

SUBTLE EXCAVATION OF THE RIM

CROSS SECTION

SLOPING

NORRIS/ALEXANDER

Figure 3–64. Schematic illustration of early-stage concentric enlargement of the temporal neuroretinal rim associated with the development of glaucomatous optic neuropathy. Alexander LJ Optom Clin 1991;1:19–102.

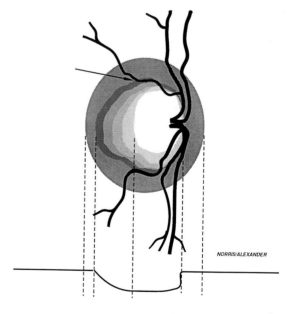

NORRIS/ALEXANDER

Figure 3–65. Schematic illustration of late-stage concentric enlargement of the temporal neuroretinal rim associated with the development of glaucomatous optic neuropathy. Alexander LJ Optom Clin 1991;1:19–102.

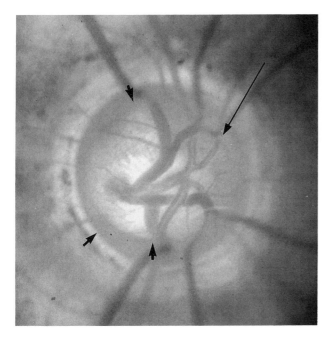

Figure 3–66. Concentric erosion of the temporal neuroretinal rim (*arrows*) associated with evolving glaucomatous optic neuropathy.

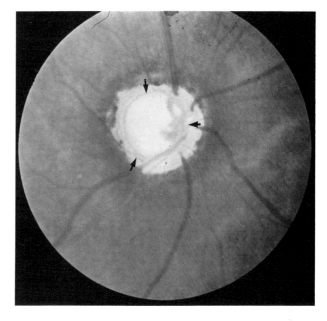

Figure 3–67. Generalized deepening of the cup (*arrows*) associated with developing glaucomatous optic neuropathy.

Disc erosion in concentric enlargement is shallow, in many instances giving a saucerized appearance. As the erosion progresses, the saucer deepens. In the area of saucerization, the color of the rim often desaturates, creating a "tinted hollow" appearance. As the neural retinal rim erodes, the area of the neural retinal rim decreases.

Concentric enlargement of the cup relates to diffuse axon loss. This diffuse axon loss may create any variation of visual field defect including generalized field depression. There may also be altered color vision as well as decreased contrast sensitivity. The nerve fiber layer dropout in these cases is more difficult to detect. Figure 3–63 illustrates an important feature of concentric enlargement, the asymmetry of disc erosion. Figures 3–64 to 3–66 demonstrate the temporal unfolding of the rim.

Generalized Deepening of the Cup. Although less prevalent, early glaucomatous optic atrophy may present as a generalized deepening of the cup. This may occur rapidly enough to allow the vessels to hover over the deepened cup for a while. This has been referred to as vessel overpass. As the disc tissue erodes, the lamina becomes more visible, indicating laminar and retrolaminar compromise (Fig. 3–67).

End-stage Glaucomatous Optic Atrophy. As glaucoma continues to develop there is further erosion of neural retinal rim tissue. Eventually the lamina is exposed and bows backward. At this point, the edge of the disc is undermined, creating the appearance of a

bowl with a lip. This appearance has been referred to as "bean-pot cupping." Although previously thought to be "characteristic glaucomatous optic atrophy," this stage of glaucomatous optic atrophy is in reality fairly rare.

Peripapillary Crescents and Halos. The presence of a peripapillary crescent correlates well with ONH damage in the patient with glaucoma. The precise etiopathogenesis is somewhat obscure, but appears to occur at a higher rate in patients with normotensive or low-tension glaucoma. It appears that as the erosion of the neural retinal rim approaches the edge of the disc, the likelihood of peripapillary atrophy increases. It must be remembered that halos and crescents also occur in other conditions and may be an entirely normal anatomic variation. Other than being another factor in assisting in differential diagnosis, peripapillary halos have no apparent prognostic significance.

Optic Nerve Head Hemorrhages. Splinter hemorrhages near the nerve head are considered by many to be a relatively common occurrence (33 percent) in damage to the optic nerve head. The hemorrhages occur most commonly in the inferior quadrant of the disc and are transient in nature. Splinter hemorrhages may precede neural retinal rim compromise, visual field defects, and nerve fiber layer defects. An optic nerve head hemorrhage is a sign of disc damage and may indicate poor control of the IOP, but does not significantly alter the rate of glaucomatous optic atrophy de-

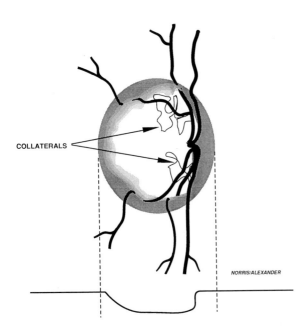

Figure 3–68. A schematic illustration of collateral vessel formation on the optic nerve head associated with chronic open-angle glaucoma. Alexander LJ Optom Clin 1991;1:19–102.

velopment. Again, it must be remembered that splinter hemorrhages occur in other diseased states of the optic nerve head such as the ischemic optic neuropathies and blood dyscrasias. Although the disc hemorrhage is important in the recognition of glau-

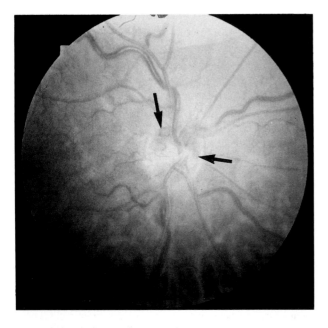

Figure 3–69. Collateral vessel formation on the optic nerve head (*arrows*) associated with chronic open-angle glaucoma.

comatous optic neuropathy, it should never become a sole determining factor in the diagnosis.

Collateral Vessel Formation on the Optic Nerve Head. As the retinal veins are very thin walled, increased intra-ocular pressure may compress the walls, creating an increased incidence of branch retinal vein occlusions and central retinal vein occlusions. Elevated intra-ocular pressure over a prolonged period may also cause stasis in the retinal vessels. This stasis may then produce collateral and shunt formation to assist in the recovery of poor perfusion. Collateral disc vessel formation is classically described as optociliary shunts in central retinal vein occlusion (CRVO). The difference between optociliary shunts in CRVO and collateral formation in chronic primary open-angle glaucoma (POAG) is the acuity level. In CRVO with shunts, the visual acuity level is decreased. Venous-to-venous anastomoses may also occur in cases of chronic POAG. Also remember that collaterals and shunts on the nerve head may be indicative of a retrobulbar compressive lesion. Figures 3–68 and 3–69 illustrate the formation of collateral vessels on the nerve head in chronic POAG.

Other Vessel Anomalies on the Optic Nerve Head. It has been suggested that the optic nerve head damage and resultant visual field loss is more prevalent in eyes with POAG and associated cilioretinal arteries. A recent study refutes this reporting that there is no significant correlation between glaucomatous damage and the presence of cilioretinal arteries.

Baring of the circumlimbal vessels has been considered a sign diagnostic of glaucoma. This refers to a situation in which vessels that outline the cup become separated from the margin of the cup. This may also occur in a nonglaucomatous eye as a normal anatomical variant.

Nasalization of the disc vessels was also once considered a major feature in the development of GOA. Nasalization of the disc vessels is actually a manifestation of erosion of the nasal neural retinal rim toward the nasal edge of the disc. Again, many congenital disc variations present with nasalized disc vessels, making the observation certainly questionable as a key feature of GOA.

Nerve Fiber Layer Changes. Striations in the retinal nerve fiber layer are a routine ophthalmoscopic observation. This observation can be enhanced by the use of various filters and by specialized photography. It has been shown that nerve fiber layer defects can be identified up to 5 years before visual field abnormalities appear. Over 90 percent of patients suspected of having glaucoma in one study had defects in the nerve fiber layer prior to the development of visual field defects. Nerve fiber layer defects are reported to precede

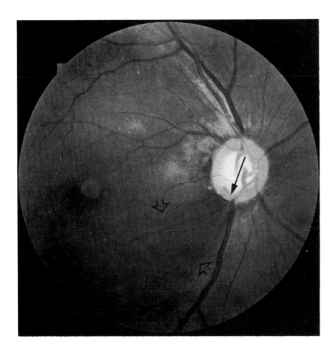

Figure 3–70. An illustration of a wedge defect of the nerve fiber layer in primary open-angle glaucoma. Note also the inferior notch of the neuroretinal rim (*arrow*).

enlargement of the cup/disc ratio in ocular hypertensive patients with optic disc hemorrhage. In view of the fact that nerve fiber layer loss probably precedes field cuts, it is advisable to at least attempt to enhance your view of the layer and carefully search for losses in that layer.

The striations are best seen (brightest) at the superior and inferior poles of the optic nerve head, where the nerve fiber layer is the thickest. The brightness of the reflections from the striations fades as the nerve fiber layer thins peripherally. The pattern is seen best in young patients and patients with heavily pigmented fundi.

When there is degeneration of the nerve fiber layer, there will be defects or alterations of the striations within 2 disc diameters of the optic nerve head. Defects within this zone are considered significant if they are wider than an arteriole and travel all the way back to the lip of the optic nerve head. The nerve fiber layer defects in glaucoma assume three specific patterns:

1. Slit defects, which usually are superior and inferior in the arcuate bundle zones and represent focal damage of the adjacent axons.
2. Wedge defects, which are narrow near the lip of the optic nerve head and spread out as they approach the periphery. Wedge defects represent a focal but expanding loss of axons, and are often associated

with a notch of the neural retinal rim. Figure 3–70 illustrates a wedge nerve fiber layer defect.

3. Diffuse defects, which are the most common but the most difficult to see. Diffuse defects are thinned striations most easily identifiable by comparing the superior and inferior striations. This follows the hemifield defect concept in the visual field analysis.

The Lamina Cribrosa. It has not been too many years since the observation of the variations in the lamina cribrosa were considered a key feature in the differential diagnosis of glaucomatous optic neuropathy. Although observation of the lamina cribrosa is common in the healthy optic nerve head, certain characteristic changes may occur in glaucomatous optic atrophy. As glaucoma worsens, the small round pores of the lamina become more horizontally oval, with vertical slits being evident in severe field loss. The largest pores of the lamina are arranged in a vertical hourglass pattern, with the greatest numbers in the superior and inferior zones of the OHN. The large pores conduct the nerve fibers of the arcuate fiber bundles. Fibers passing through these pores appear to be particularly susceptible to risk of damage. Fortunately, the clinician has more reliable methods of evaluating the optic nerve head for glaucomatous optic neuropathy. Refer to Figures 3–71 and 3–72 regarding laminar dot changes.

Technique of Viewing and Recording the Optic Nerve Head. Two crucial points must be addressed

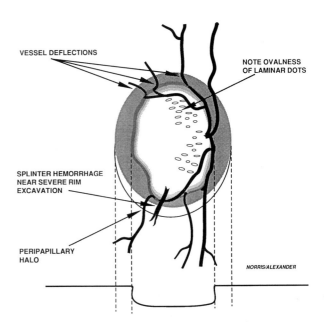

Figure 3–71. A schematic illustration of severe erosion of the neuroretinal rim in glaucoma associated with increasing evidence of the laminar dots. Alexander LJ Optom Clin 1991;1:19–102.

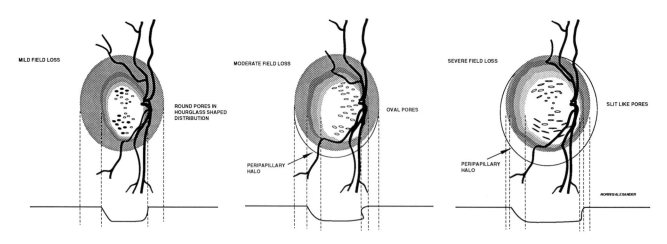

Figure 3–72. A schematic illustrating the progression of laminar dot changes associated with the development of unrelenting glaucoma. Alexander LJ Optom Clin 1991;1:19–102.

when viewing and recording the optic nerve head (ONH) for glaucomatous changes: (1) concentrate on asymmetry of disc size and asymmetry of neural retinal rim erosion and (2) use magnified stereoscopic viewing techniques. Asymmetry of disc size, and to some degree asymmetry of neural retinal rim erosion, can best be discerned by photography or a binocular indirect viewing technique described by LaRussa (1989), who suggests that simultaneous comparison of internal ocular structures is limited by iconic memory (memory stored in a visual form). He states that iconic memory lasts only about 1 second before it is cognitively processed and stored in short-term memory. When attempting to compare the right disc to the left, if the clinician takes more than 1 second to shift from one ONH to the other, he is comparing the cognitive image of the first ONH to the visual image of the second. To accomplish the shift within 1 second to maximize comparison, La Russa suggests the alternate fixation shift technique. This technique requires the use of the binocular indirect ophthalmoscope and specific fixation shifts by the patient. You must set fixation points in your examination room. If you have the patient recline, the fixation points must be placed on the ceiling. If you have the patient upright, the fixation points must be placed on the opposite wall.

Another method for simultaneous comparison is to use Polaroid disc photographs. Unfortunately, cost factors may be a limitation for widespread use. The other point in effective ONH evaluation in glaucoma is use of magnified stereoscopic viewing techniques. Mastery of stereoscopic disc evaluation is crucial, as erosion or excavation of disc tissue precedes atrophy in most cases of GOA. Several techniques for observation are available. Hruby lens or contact fundus lens

evaluation will give an erect nonreversed image. The clinician may record precisely what is viewed.

The most commonly used technique is fundus lens evaluation. A hand-held or mounted fundus lens is used to view the optic nerve head in stereo. A slit may be used to enhance the specific contours. Unfortunately, the image is upside-down and backwards; therefore the examiner must mentally correct for the image prior to recording or use the mapping process illustrated in Figures 3–58 and 3–59.

Digitized Imaging. Technical help is on the horizon to facilitate the ONH evaluation: digitized imaging, also called quantitative imaging. This type of processing is achieved by assigning depth and intensity values to points on the retina and optic nerve in stereo, running these numerical values through a computer and then recreating the image on screen or on a plotter. Graphical procedures in a computer are very complex and require considerable amounts of memory. Imaging devices to collect the data are also very complex, requiring scanning optical or nonoptical systems with the incorporation of laser technology. Because of the complexity of the instrumentation, the costs are astronomical.

By now you should realize that you already have the imaging system, your eyes. You have the computer, your brain. Unfortunately you cannot get your brain to store the information for perfect recall, to repeat the performance precisely 2 weeks from now, or to print out a hard copy for reference.

The potential value of digitized imaging in optic nerve head evaluation is incredible, especially when considering subtle disc erosion. Unfortunately, reproducibility, cost factors, and lack of clinical research data cast a shadow over the short term. The further development of digitized imaging is the next logical step to assist us in the differential of POAG.

Thyroid Eye Disease—Graves' Ophthalmopathy

Thyroid hormones increase protein synthesis in every bodily tissue and increase oxygen consumption by increasing activity of the Na-K ATPase pathway. Hyperactivity and hypoactivity of the thyroid system can create systemic metabolic and ocular signs and symptoms and are likely to present to the primary eyecare provider. The disease is complex, with hyperthyroidism being variably connected to the eye signs from a chronological standpoint. The eye signs can occur years before or years after the actual hyperthyroid event. It is important to realize that a high percentage of patients with Graves' disease develop eye signs, but it is equally important to realize that a low percentage of these patients ever develop serious impairment of visual function. It is equally important to understand that ophthalmopathy can present in the euthyroid state and that the ophthalmopathy may undergo spontaneous remission.

Hyperthyroidism is also referred to as thyrotoxicosis, toxic diffuse goiter, Graves' disease, Basedow's disease, toxic nodular goiter, and other terms. Graves' disease refers to toxic diffuse goiter and is thought to be an immunologic condition. Graves' disease presents as a goiter, exophthalmos, and pretibial myxedema, which is nonpitting infiltration of the ground substance in the pretibial area. The prominent eyes are the result of the retraction of the upper eyelid. There is also lid lag on downward gaze; proptosis, which may be either unilateral or bilateral; diplopia; and potential limitation of eye movements with infiltration and edema of the extraocular muscles (resistance on forced duction), as evidenced by an orbital CT scan. There may also be reduced blink rates, conjunctival injection near the sites of muscle insertion, resistance to retropulsion that is variable between the two eyes, eyelid swelling (edema), keratoconjunctivitis sicca, and exposure keratopathy with associated pain and photophobia and decreased vision. Optic nerve compression may produce pupillary signs, optic disc edema, and visual field and color vision changes. Intraocular pressure may also be elevated on upgaze because of the fibrosis of the inferior rectus muscle. Signs and symptoms are summarized in Table 3–7.

The classical signs of the infiltrative ophthalmopathy follow the NOSPECS acronym, which is summarized in Table 3–8. Class 0 indicates no signs or symptoms. Class 1 is the noninfiltrative stage, and is characterized by the upper lid retraction present in up to 90 percent of hyperthyroid patients. The lid retraction in the early stages is thought to be secondary to excessive adrenergic stimulation of Müller's muscle. With progression of the disease, there is overaction of

TABLE 3–7. SYSTEMIC SIGNS AND SYMPTOMS OF GRAVES' DISEASE ADRENERGIC EXCESS

Signs	Symptoms
Goiter	Nervousness
Widened pulse pressure	Increased sweating
Tremor	Hypersensitivity to heat
Ophthalmopathy	Palpitations
Tachycardia	Fatigue
Warm, moist skin	Frequent bowel movements
Atrial fibrillation	Increased appetite
Muscle wasting	Weight loss
	Tachycardia
	Insomnia
	Weakness

the levator muscle associated with excessive superior rectus stimulation attempting to overcome the fibrotic inferior rectus muscle coupled with ultimate fibrosis and restriction of the levator. Lid lag on looking down after extreme upgaze may also present in class 1 ophthalmopathy.

Class 2 is the first stage of infiltrative ophthalmopathy. This stage is characterized by lid swelling, orbital fat prolapse, lacrimal gland swelling, injection of the conjunctival vessels, inflammation near the insertion of the extraocular muscles, and conjunctival chemosis. Symptoms include foreign body sensation which precipitate lacrimation and photophobia.

Class 3 is characterized by proptosis, which is greater than 21 mm in approximately 67 percent of Graves' disease patients. The proptosis then creates a potential lagophthalmos situation resulting in worsening of keratoconjunctivitis sicca signs and symptoms. Exophthalmometry is necessary to make this diagnosis, with the upper limits of normal being 18 mm for orientals, 20 mm for whites, and 23 mm for blacks, and no more than 2 mm difference between the two eyes. Refer to Figure 3–73 for an illustration of thyroid proptosis.

Class 4 disease usually develops in up to 33 percent of patients with Graves' disease. This occurs most

TABLE 3–8. THE NOSPECS ACRONYM

Classification	Definition
0	**N**o signs or symptoms
1	**O**nly signs of upper lid retraction, stare, and lid lag on downgaze
2	**S**oft tissue involvement—swelling
3	**P**roptosis
4	**E**xtraocular muscle infiltration and fibrosis
5	**C**orneal changes manifest as exposure keratopathy
6	**S**ight loss, usually secondary to optic nerve involvement

Thyroid Eye Disease

Characteristics

Δ Eye signs may be separated in time from the hyperthyroidism

Δ High percentage of hyperthyroid patients develop eye signs, but a low percentage actually lose vision

Δ Systemic signs and symptoms related to adrenergic stimulation

Δ Eye signs and symptoms include:

> Lid retraction
> Lid lag on downgaze after upgaze
> The "stare"
> Lid swelling and orbital fat prolapse
> Injection of conjunctival vessels and chemosis
> Keratoconjunctivitis sicca with related symptoms
> Proptosis and lagophthalmos
> Mechanical restriction of extraocular muscles with diplopia and increase in IOP with upgaze
> Optic disc edema

Management

Δ Proper diagnosis, differential from other proptotic diseases and diplopic diseases

Δ Antithyroid drugs, RAI treatment, subtotal thyroidectomy

Δ Local ocular management (*see* Table 3–9 for management techniques)

Δ Routine follow up based on ocular/systemic status

often in females between the ages of 40 to 60 years, and is characterized by mechanical restriction of the extraocular muscles. The most common involvement is the inferior rectus, followed by the medial rectus and superior rectus. The increase of intraocular pressure on upgaze is a fair indicator of inferior rectus fibrosis.

Class 5 is corneal compromise secondary to exposure. Neurotrophic corneal ulceration is a threat in this stage. Class 6 is optic nerve involvement manifesting as optic disc edema.

Management. The basic management of ocular involvement in suspect thyroid disease is the diagnosis of the underlying condition with the subsequent treatment of the hyperthyroid condition. The initial screening for thyroid disease is usually accomplished by using serum T4 and T3U resin uptake, with serum T3 occasionally being required. From that point, laboratory testing becomes somewhat complex. Protein-bound iodine (PBI) estimates the circulating thyroid hormone level and may be useful in Hashimoto's thyroiditis. The serum total T4 (serum total thyroxine) is measured by radioimmunoassay (RIA) and is a direct measure of thyroxine, but a patient may be physiologically normal with an abnormal total T4 because of changes in the serum-binding protein levels. If there is a marked elevation of the thyroid stimulating hormone (TSH) level, this is considered a primary failure of the thyroid gland. Because of the complexity, the initial consultation should be with an internist or endocrinologist for specific diagnosis and initiation of appropriate treatment if indicated. Because of the variability of the disease, conservatism is usually the rule of thumb unless life- or vision-threatening situations exist.

Antithyroid drugs include propylthiouracil (PTU) at 100 to 150 mg every 8 hours or methimazole (MMI) at 10 to 15 mg every 8 hours, reducing the dosage with the euthyroid state at 6 to 12 weeks. Beta-adrenergic blocking agents are often used to control the accompanying sympathetic manifestations. Radioactive iodine (RAI) treatment is usually reserved for patients over age 30 and patients not anticipating or planning pregnancy within the next several months. Subtotal thyroidectomy is also used once the hyperthyroidism is under pharmacologic control.

Local ocular management is often necessary. The most menacing problem is the occurrence of ocular drying secondary to exposure. Modes of therapy include nonpreserved tear substitutes, nonpreserved ointments, collagen punctal implants, lid taping and shielding at night, and coverage with a nontoxic antibiotic ointment when there is the threat of infection. Because of the variability and possibility of spontaneous regression, permanent silicone punctal implants should be used with caution. If there is imminent threat to vision secondary to desiccation, tarsorrhaphy may be necessary.

The cosmetic effects of lid retraction may be managed at times by adrenergic blocking agents such as guanethidine and thymoximine. Thymoximine produces enough ocular irritation to prevent effective usage. Guanethidine is unpredictable and produces toxic corneal reactions, but may offer some relief over

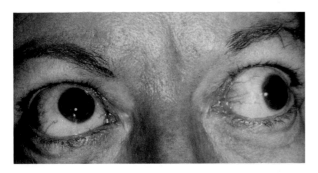

Figure 3–73. Thyroid eye disease illustrating lid retraction, proptosis, and extraocular muscle abnormalities.

TABLE 3–9. RECOMMENDED MANAGEMENT TECHNIQUES FOR GRAVES' OPHTHALMOPATHY

Class	Management Techniques
0	Routine follow-up
1	Methods to moisturize the eyes, topical adrenergic blocking agents for retraction, levator surgery, recession of Müller's muscle, cosmetic tinted lenses
2	Methods to moisturize the eyes, elevate head during sleep, systemic and periocular steroids
3	Methods to moisturize the eyes, lid taping, systemic and periocular steroids, tarsorrhaphy
4	Methods to moisturize the eyes, eye patching or prisms for diplopia, systemic steroids, botulinum toxin to muscles, muscle surgery
5	Methods to moisturize the eyes, systemic steroids, orbital decompression
6	Methods to moisturize the eyes, systemic and periocular steroids, orbital radiation, orbital decompression

a several-day period. After a prolonged period minimizing the likelihood for spontaneous regression, oculoplastic surgery may be considered to relieve the retraction.

With the advent of the infiltrative and edematous stages of the disease, the patient may need to sleep with the head elevated, especially in the presence of lid edema. Continue treatment for the exposure and consider the potential benefits of systemic and periocular steroid usage. Systemic adrenergic blocking agents may also be attempted for the proptosis but are typically of no benefit. Botulinum toxin injections may be attempted to assist in class 4 developments, but are clearly to be undertaken with caution.

Surgical intervention for extraocular muscle affectations as well as proptosis is clearly a last-ditch approach to the management of Graves' ophthalmopathy. Orbital decompression is indicated when there is a direct threat to vision secondary to optic nerve changes. The Kronlein approach (lateral orbital wall) is classical, but the Walsh and Ogura (1957) transantral approach (medial wall and floor of orbit) has a lower morbidity. Orbital radiation also offers some potential in the reduction of class 5 and 6 ophthalmopathy.

Follow-up of the patient with Graves' ophthalmopathy is dependent on the stage of evolution. Patients with severe changes must be followed on a routine basis, especially with the threat of vision loss secondary to exposure keratopathy and optic nerve edema. Patients with minimal exposure problems may be followed on a 3- to 6-month basis. Patients with fluctuating diplopia should have myasthenia gravis ruled out as a part of their treatment. Table 3–9 summarizes the management plan for the classes of Graves' ophthalmopathy.

Orbital Inflammatory Pseudotumor— Tolosa–Hunt Syndrome, Orbital Apex Syndrome, and Painful Ophthalmoplegia

Introduction and Description. Orbital inflammatory pseudotumor is an all-encompassing term describing a nonspecific orbital inflammatory disorder that may be acute or chronic and may demonstrate recurrence. The pediatric presentation may include fever, lethargy, and general malaise. The condition typically presents unilaterally as proptosis, restriction of ocular motility, or both, usually in middle age. Pain may also be a presenting feature that is quickly alleviated with a trial of systemic steroids. There may be lid and conjunctival edema, lacrimal gland enlargement, decreased vision, difficulty with retropulsion, elevated IOP, optic disc edema, and altered trigeminal sensitivity. Variable muscle palsies may also present. Many signs and symptoms mimic thyroid eye disease. The orbital CT scan demonstrates thickened posterior sclera, orbital fat and/or lacrimal gland involvement, and thickening of the extraocular muscles.

Pearls

Orbital Inflammatory Pseudotumor

Characteristics

△ Nonspecific orbital inflammatory disorder creating proptosis and/or ocular motility restriction
△ Signs and symptoms include:
  Unilateral presentation usually, but may be bilateral
  Pain
  Diplopia
  Lid or conjunctival edema
  Difficulty with retropulsion
  Elevated IOP
  Optic disc edema
  Trigeminal alteration
  Variable muscle palsies
  Thickened posterior sclera, thickened extraocular muscles

Management

△ Careful history for differential diagnosis
△ Complete ocular examination
△ Exophthalmometry
△ Ultrasonography
△ Orbital CT or MRI
△ Laboratory tests including ESR, CBC with differential, ANA, BUN, creatinine, fasting blood glucose
△ Orbital biopsy in cases not responding to oral steroids
△ Prednisone at 80 to 100 mg/day for 1 to 2 weeks, then taper
△ Low-dose radiation in recalcitrant cases
△ Monitor and manage IOP

If the condition is bilateral, there may be an elevated ESR and there is often an association with a systemic cause.

Management. The key to management is differential diagnosis. Neoplasia, infection, trauma, diabetic ophthalmoplegia, thyroid eye disease, and aneurysm are among the differentials. A careful history should be obtained, including previous episodes and associated systemic problems including cancer. An ocular examination should be performed, including motility, exophthalmometry, IOP, and stereoscopic nerve head examination. Evaluation should include ultrasonography, CT (axial and coronal), or MRI. Laboratory tests should include a Westergren ESR; a CBC with differential; ANA, BUN, and creatinine tests to rule out systemic vasculitis; and a fasting blood glucose test. Orbital biopsy may be necessary in difficult cases.

Treatment is almost diagnostic. Prednisone at 80 to 100 mg by mouth every day should create rapid regression. Low-dose radiation has also been recommended in recalcitrant cases verified as orbital inflammatory pseudotumor. Follow-up is crucial, with reevaluation recommended in 3 to 5 days. Patients responding to the oral steroids are maintained on the medication for 1 to 2 weeks and then tapered. The IOP, which is naturally elevated in the disease, must be monitored carefully and treated when necessary.

Inflammatory Optic Neuropathy

Introduction and Description. Inflammatory optic neuropathy presents initially as optic disc edema, with the possibility of accompanying hemorrhage, vascular changes, vitritis, and circumpapillary choroiditis. The affliction is an inflammatory reaction to an infection. The appearance of optic atrophy depends on the interval between genesis and therapeutic intervention. This condition usually occurs in younger patients (under 20 years) and is often referred to as "papillitis" (Fig. 3–74).

Papillitis is the most common form of optic neuropathy in children. Table 3–10 summarizes the common etiologic factors associated with optic neuropathy secondary to inflammatory processes. The vision loss in papillitis is similar to other forms of optic neuropathy in that there is a rapid decrease in acuity over the first 2 to 3 days, followed by stabilization over 7 to 10 days, ultimately resulting in a slight improvement. Optic atrophy usually occurs 4 to 8 weeks after the inflammation starts.

Two distinctive types of papillitis may occur. The papillitis associated with viral infections in children exhibits dirty-yellow globular exudates scattered throughout the papillomacular bundle. These exudates may coalesce to form a macular star or wing. Retinal edema often accompanies the process. The localized exudate variety of papillitis may resolve spontaneously without treatment.

The other variety of papillitis, neuroretinitis implying ganglion cell layer involvement, is characterized by a yellow, swollen disc obscuring vessels and spreading far into the retina. Linear hemorrhages may appear adjacent to the disc. This form usually results in poor vision, gliosis, perivascular sheathing, and optic atrophy. Posterior vitreous cells are often present in the neuroretinitis variety.

Inflammatory optic neuropathy occurs as a unilateral mild to severe loss of vision and visual field but

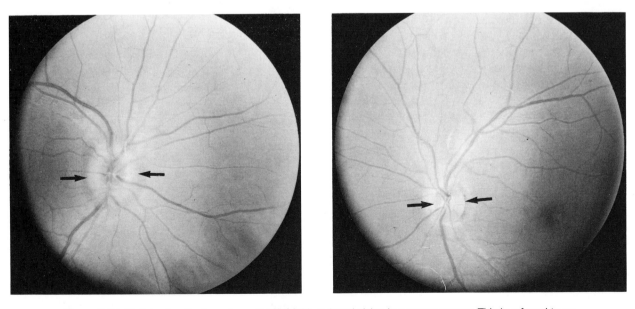

Figure 3–74. Unilateral optic disc edema (*arrows*) with reduced vision in a young person. This is referred to as inflammatory optic neuropathy, or papillitis.

TABLE 3–10. FACTORS ASSOCIATED WITH THE DEVELOPMENT OF INFLAMMATORY OPTIC NEUROPATHY

Acute encephalo-myelitis	Crohn's disease	Pharmacologic idio-syncrasies
Bacterial infections	Fungal infections	Post-vaccination reaction
Bee sting to the eye	Guillain–Barre syndrome	Presumed ocular histoplasmosis
Behçet's disease	Herpes simplex	
Birdshot chorioretinopathy	Herpes zoster	Reiter's disease
	Lyme disease	Syphilis
Brucella infection	Measles	Systemic lupus erythematosus
Cat-scratch fever	Meningitis	
Chickenpox	Mononucleosis (Epstein Barr virus)	Toxocariasis
Collagen vascular diseases	Mumps	Toxplasmosis
		Tuberculosis

may occasionally present bilaterally. Field defects vary depending on the location and severity of the inflammation. There is usually an associated Marcus Gunn pupillary defect as well as other signs of optic nerve conduction compromise, including a red desaturation defect. There may be ocular pain or tenderness as well as some pain on motion of the globe as well as antecedent upper respiratory infections or gastroenterologic disease that is often viral in origin. **See color plate 13.**

Management. Prognosis for inflammatory optic neuropathy varies considerably. Reduction of the inflammation by ACTH or steroid usage has proponents and opponents. Recent work has cast a cloud over the use of steroid in the treatment of optic neuritis of any kind. Diagnosis of the underlying causative agent or condition is crucial to specify the proper therapeutic intervention. The sooner the resolution, the better the prognosis for return of visual function.

The most important aspect of management of inflammatory optic neuropathy is rapid diagnosis, with emphasis placed on attempting to ascertain the etiology. Differential diagnoses include ischemic optic neuropathy, diabetic papillopathy, papillophlebitis, malignant hypertension, orbital or intracranial mass creating papilledema, Leber's optic neuropathy, and toxic optic neuropathy. Basic adjunct diagnostic tests should be run on patients and should be supplemented by others when a specific etiologic agent is suspected. Basic differential diagnostic tests should include blood pressure, careful threshold visual field examination, erythrocyte sedimentation rate (to rule out temporal arteritis), complete blood count (CBC), fluorescent treponemal antibody absorption test (FTA-ABS) (to rule out syphilis), collagen vascular screen including ANA, chest x-ray, computed axial tomography, or magnetic resonance imaging of orbits and brain in atypical cases or if the other tests are negative and the condition is not showing improvement. Supplementary tests may include specific antibody titer tests (such as toxoplasmosis titer) for infection. Visually evoked potentials are also useful in the differential diagnosis of any optic neuropathy displaying a delay in the conduction.

Therapeutic intervention must be applied as soon as the etiologic factor has been determined. The therapy may be insufficient in reducing the inflammation, necessitating incorporation of steroids into the treatment regimen. All arguments that support initiation of steroid or ACTH therapy must be tempered by the associated inherent risk factors.

Pearls

Inflammatory Optic Neuropathy

Characteristics

△ Optic disc edema, hemorrhage, vitritis, and peripapillary choroiditis usually in younger patients—possibility of pain and tenderness of globe especially on movement

  Viral variety, with dirty-yellow globular exudates in papillomacular bundle often forming macular star; reasonable prognosis

  Neuroretinitis, with yellow swollen disc spreading into posterior pole with linear hemorrhages; poor prognosis

△ Rapid decrease in vision over 2 to 3 days, followed by stabilization over 7 to 10 days. Optic atrophy occurs in 4 to 8 weeks

△ May be accompanying pain and tenderness of globe

△ Often a central scotoma, but visual field may be variable with overall depression on threshold perimetry

△ Associated optic nerve conduction defects (eg, Marcus Gunn pupil, color desaturation, contrast sensitivity reduction)

△ Associated with a wide variety of inflammatory processes

Management

△ Ascertain etiology

△ Basic testing

  Blood pressure

  Careful visual field testing

  Westergren erythrocyte sedimentation rate in older patients

  FTA-ABS

  Collagen vascular screen when indicated

  Chest x-ray

  Specific antibody titer tests such as toxoplasmosis

  CT or MRI of orbit in atypical cases or if all other tests are negative

△ Immediate consultation with neurology or neuro-ophthalmology for consideration of steroid usage

△ Follow up at least within 1 month, especially if the patient is on steroid therapy (IOP check)

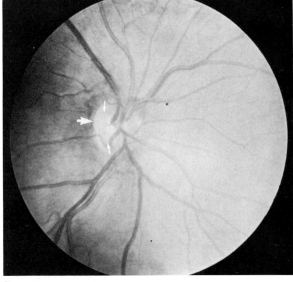
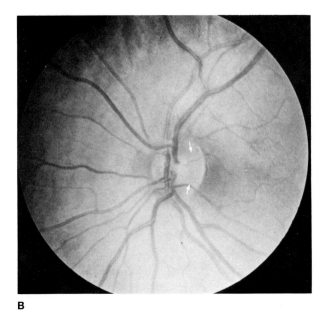

A   **B**

Figure 3–75. A. The large arrow points to a zone of optic atrophy secondary to demyelinizing optic neuropathy. The zone of atrophic neuroretinal retinal rim is difficult to discern unless one makes a simultaneous comparison to the fellow eye **(B).** The small arrows demarcate the zone for comparison.

Follow-up is dependent on the status of the condition, but should at least be within 1 month for the first visit. The practitioner must never forget that there may be an underlying severe neurologic problem.

Demyelinizing Optic Neuropathy

Introduction and Description. Demyelinizing optic neuropathy (Fig. 3–75) is best known as "retrobulbar neuritis" and is classically described as "the patient sees nothing and the doctor sees nothing." The patient presents with a sudden unilateral loss of vision. The patient with demyelinizing optic neuropathy is usually 18 to 45 years of age. Demyelinization is the most frequent cause of optic neuropathy, and multiple sclerosis (MS) is the most frequent cause of demyelinization. Optic neuropathy is the first symptom in about 20 percent of MS patients, and occurs in about 75 percent of MS patients at some time in the course of their disease.

Very often there are no appreciable ophthalmoscopic nerve head changes, but optic disc edema secondary to axoplasmic stasis may occur. After the acute process runs its course, optic atrophy (often very subtle) will appear.

The process is thought to be secondary to a reaction of the nerve fibers to a demyelinizing process. The fibers lose function because the nerve-conducting sheath is compromised, allowing for an escape of the electrical charge coursing down the nerve fiber.

The patient with demyelinizing optic neuropathy presents with an impairment of visual acuity from 20/20 to severe compromise, or visual field alterations that progress to a maximum loss at the end of about 1 week. Other signs and symptoms that may be associated with vision loss are pain or tenderness of the globe near the insertion of the superior rectus, pain on gross excursions of the eye, a Marcus Gunn pupil, color desaturation, light comparison variation, Pulfrich's stereo phenomenon, Uhthoff's and Lhermitte's symptoms, and an altered visually evoked potential. Systemic manifestations include Romberg's sign, which indicates cerebellar dysfunction, as well as other indications of poor balance evidenced on attempting tandem walking. Finger to finger and finger to nose testing may also be altered. The patient may complain of mobility problems associated with the onset of optic neuropathy that will be exacerbated by attempting to climb stairs or other physical activity. Uhthoff's sign can be elicited by asking patients if they feel uncomfortable taking a hot shower or a warm bath, sitting in a sauna, or overheating in a warm climate.

Visual field defects associated with demyelinizing optic neuropathy vary considerably. The majority of defects are central, but peripheral defects as well as generalized depressions can occur. It should be noted that these fields can fluctuate depending on the activity of the disease process and may actually vary with increased physical activity and overheating. **See color plate 14.**

Management. Prognosis for return of at least some vision function is good (occurring in 70 to 90 percent

Demyelinizing Optic Neuropathy

Characteristics

Δ Sudden unilateral loss of vision in the 20/20 to no light perception (NLP) range or visual field in 18- to 45-year-old patients; loss progresses to maximum in about 1 week

Δ Demyelinization is the most frequent cause of optic neuropathy and MS is the most frequent cause of demyelinization

Δ Associated optic nerve conduction defects such as Marcus Gunn pupil and color desaturation

Δ May have associated optic disc edema but often no ophthalmoscopic signs—"Patient sees nothing and doctor sees nothing"

Δ Other signs include pain and tenderness of globe near insertion of the superior rectus, pain on gross excursion, associated cerebellar signs, and reduced vision associated with overheating

Δ Visual acuity or fields start to improve in 2 to 3 weeks and stabilize in 4 to 5 weeks, often accompanied by some optic atrophy

Management

Δ Ascertain cause

    MRI is the definitive test for picking up plaques in the optic nerve

    May use evaluation techniques involving the cerebrospinal fluid

    Consider visually evoked potential

    Consider systemic workup including:

        Blood pressure

        CBC

        FTA-ABS

        Antinuclear antibodies

        Chest x-ray

        Westergren sedimentation rate

Δ Consult with neurology for diagnosis and potential institution of therapy; note that steroid therapy is very controversial

Δ Provision of best refraction

Δ Discussion of the situation with the patient including the necessity of communicating recurrences and any other signs or symptoms of demyelinizing disease

Δ Regular eye examinations

    Repeat visual fields at routine intervals to assess progression

    Follow up intraocular pressure if the patient is placed on steroids

tient as a "washing out" or desaturation of perception. Recurrences can occur (in up to 20 to 30 percent of cases) and usually cause a further reduction in acuity or an enlargement of the visual field defects. Each attack has the potential to produce additive irreversible optic atrophy.

Of acute importance is the differential diagnosis of cause. Although most optic neuropathy in the 18- to 45-year age category can be attributed to a demyelinizing disease, it is important that the clinician rule out other potential causes such as Guillain–Barré syndrome, carbon monoxide poisoning, optic nerve and/or orbital tumor, Leber's optic neuropathy, and toxic/metabolic factors. Systemic tests may include blood pressure, complete blood check, FTA-ABS, antinuclear antibodies, chest x-ray, and a Westergren sedimentation rate.

Multiple sclerosis does not always occur as a systemic manifestation after demyelinizing optic neuropathy. Reports in the literature vary from zero to 85 percent of cases of MS developing after a case of retrobulbar neuritis. Some of the discrepancy probably revolves around an inappropriate diagnosis of either demyelinizing optic atrophy or MS. Studies using MRI plaque imaging will improve our understanding of the association of optic neuropathy with future development of full-blown systemic MS.

The criteria for the diagnosis of MS are very controversial. The Medical Research Council Committee developed a set of criteria for MS classification shown in Table 3–11.

A CT scan may be of some assistance in discovering a cortical plaque, but MRI has been proven to be more effective. The short-time inversion recovery (STIR) sequencing in MRI shows bright plaques in 80 to 90 percent of patients with demyelinizing optic neuropathy. Cerebrospinal fluid evaluation may reveal changes such as light chains; oligoclonal bands and myelin basic protein may also be of assistance in

TABLE 3–11. DIAGNOSTIC CLASSIFICATION CRITERIA FOR MULTIPLE SCLEROSIS

Classification	Criteria
Proven	Pathologic proof
Clinically definite	Some physical disability, remissions and relapses greater than two episodes
Early or probable	Signs of lesions at two or more sites, age of onset 10–50 years, no better explanation, lesions predominantly in white matter, remissions and relapses, early single episode suggesting MS with signs of multiple lesions, slight or no disability

Modified from Alexander LJ. Diseases of the optic nerve. In: Bartlett JD, Jaanus SD, eds. *Clinical Ocular Pharmacology.* Boston: Butterworth; 1989.

of patients). Visual acuity or fields usually begin to improve within 2 to 3 weeks of the attack and stabilize in 4 to 5 weeks. Some patients improve rapidly to a moderate acuity level, stabilize, and then return to better vision over a more prolonged period of time. Unfortunately, there will always be some compromise of visual function that is actually perceived by the pa-

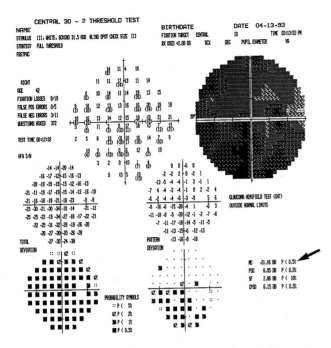

Figure 3–76. The visual field of a patient with demyelinizing optic neuropathy.

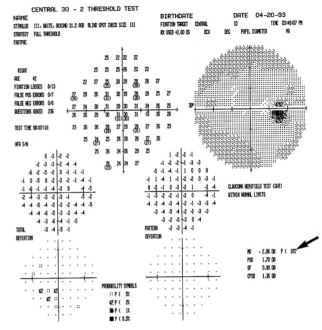

Figure 3–77. The same patient as in Figure 3–76 after therapeutic intervention with parenteral steroids.

the differential diagnosis. T-cell ratios, genetic markers, and HLA haplotypes may also offer some assistance in the future. Any patient suspected of having demyelinizing optic neuropathy should have a neurologic consultation to rule out other potential causes for the neuropathy. The neurologist will often hedge on the diagnosis, because MS conjures up images of severe disability that are often impossible to dispel. An isolated incident of optic neuropathy is often not even pursued until a second event or other systemic signs occur. The patient must realize the importance of reporting any future symptoms. Visual fields should be documented on a routine basis (e.g. every 6 months) to monitor for progress.

Reports of success in the treatment of the optic neuropathy and MS with interferon, plasmapheresis, and antimetabolites must be tempered until definitive controlled studies validate usage. Figures 3–76 and 3–77 show the benefit of therapeutic intervention.

The Optic Neuritis Treatment Trial has answered supporters and critics of steroidal therapeutic intervention in demyelinizing optic neuropathy. Randomized clinical trial assessed the effects of oral prednisone (1 mg/kg body weight/day for 14 days), intravenous (IV) methylprednisolone (250 mg every 6 hours for days) followed by oral prednisone (1 mg/kg body weight/day for 11 days), or an oral placebo. The oral prednisone and the oral placebo groups had essentially the same outcome at 6 months except the oral prednisone group had more recurrences than either the IV or placebo group. The IV methylprednisolone group had slightly better visual fields, contrast sensi-

tivity, and color vision than the oral prednisone or the placebo group, but not significantly better visual acuity than either at 6 months. The IV group also recovered vision function faster and had fewer recurrences than the placebo or oral prednisone group. It follows that the treatment of choice for optic neuropathy is IV methylprednisolone, followed by oral prednisone, but oral prednisone alone is not effective (Beck et al, 1992). There are associated side effects with IV methylprednisolone such as psychotic depression and acute pancreatitis, as well as common side effects such as sleep disturbances, mood changes, gastrointestinal distress, facial flushing, and weight gain.

In a follow-up on the trial after a year, visual acuity was 20/40 or better in 95% of the placebo group, 94% of the IV methylprednisolone group, and 91% of the oral prednisone group with recurrence rate significantly higher for the oral prednisone group. The conclusion is that the use of IV methylprednisolone is only of short term benefit and oral prednisone should not be used (Beck and Cleary, 1993).

■ ■ ■ ■ ■ ■
Clinical Note: Schilder's Disease

Schilder's disease (adrenoleukodystrophy; ALD) presents as cerebral demyelinization associated with Addison's disease and is inherited as a sex-linked disorder. ALD progresses to a severe form of spastic quadriparesis, whereas the milder form of adrenomyeloneuropathy (AMD) has a later onset in life with a milder progression.

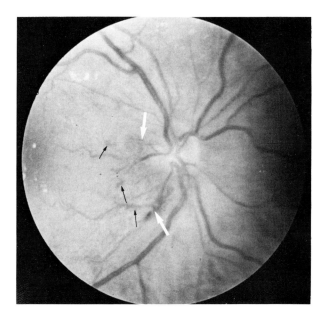

Figure 3–78. The white arrows demarcate the edematous zone of ischemic optic neuropathy. The black arrows point to flame-shaped hemorrhages.

■ ■ ■ ■ ■ ■

Clinical Note: Neuromyelitis Optica

Neuromyelitis optica (Devic's disease) is a demyelinizing disease occurring in children and young adults but that may present at any age. This disease is characterized by a rapid-onset bilateral loss of vision, poor prognosis for recovery, and accompanying transverse myelitis. Devic's disease is also associated with severe pleocytosis in the cerebrospinal fluid. The disease may be fatal but often results in survival with paraplegia.

Ischemic Optic Neuropathy

Ischemic optic neuropathy (ION) is a disease of sudden onset with variable vision and visual field loss (Figs. 3–78 and 3–79). There is usually an absence of identifiable inflammatory cause, an absence of demyelinization, and an absence of an identifiable cranio-orbital mass. The process associated with the development of ischemic optic neuropathy is thought to be secondary to an alteration of the blood supply to the optic nerve or as the result of toxic alteration of the metabolism of the neurons. Many classifications have been assigned to ischemic optic neuropathy, but this discussion categorizes the affliction into (1) nonarteritic anterior ION, (2) arteritic ION, and (3) diabetic ION. With the exception of diabetic ION, most ION occurs in patients over 50 years of age; there are isolated reports of the occurrence of ION in younger patients.

Nonarteritic Anterior Ischemic Optic Neuropathy

Introduction and Description. Nonarteritic anterior ION (also known as anterior ischemic optic neuropathy or idiopathic ischemic optic neuropathy) is a small-vessel disease of the optic nerve head creating an imbalance in the pressure–perfusion ratio. Sudden systemic hypotension and the occurrence of systemic hypertension are sometimes associated with nonarteritic anterior ION and lend credence to the hypothesis that there is an acute alteration of the pressure–perfusion ratio within the nerve head. The

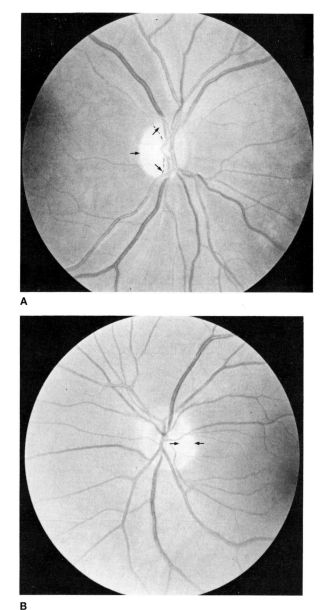

A

B

Figure 3–79. A. The small arrows point to the extent of the zone of atrophy in ischemic optic neuropathy. **B.** The fellow eye also has a smaller zone of atrophy of the neuroretinal rim.

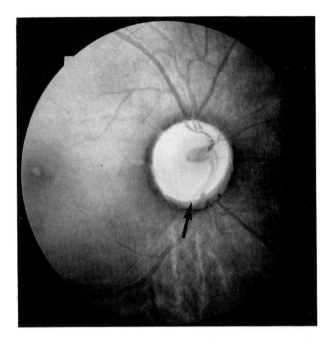

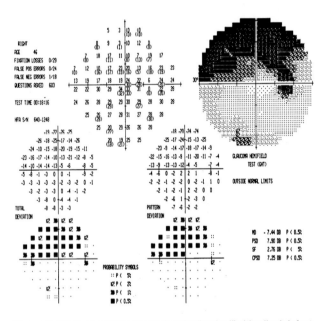

Figure 3–80. A visual field illustrating the "typical" altitudinal defect associated with ischemic optic neuropathy.

alteration also occurs in glaucoma (both chronic and low tension) only over a prolonged period of time. It should be noted that a patient with a chronically lowered pressure–perfusion ratio, as in glaucoma, has a greater chance of developing nonarteritic anterior ION. Likewise, it follows that the patient with diabetes with associated microvasculopathy would also be more prone to the development of ischemic optic neuropathy. Fluorescein angiography often confirms the presence of an occlusive disorder of the short posterior ciliary arteries. There is delayed to absent filling associated with this affliction; however, it is known that the vessels need not be totally occluded to produce the clinical picture of ischemic optic neuropathy. The occlusion usually affects only isolated sections of the nerve.

Nonarteritic anterior ION usually occurs in patients over 50 (ages 50 to 60) years of age, with men being affected more frequently than women. The condition may become bilateral after a time delay. Reports vary from 14 to 73 percent regarding bilaterality in nonarteritic anterior ION. The optic disc changes can be variable, from isolated sectoral optic disc edema to full-blown areas of disc swelling with coincidental variability in acuity and visual field defects. Small, linear, flame-shaped hemorrhages may occur on the disc margin. These hemorrhages disappear in 3 to 5 weeks. Eventually, acute activity subsides, and optic atrophy appears in about 3 months.

Prodromal signs and symptoms can occur with nonarteritic anterior ION (25 percent of patients). Prodromata consist of transient blurring of vision and sectors of visual field loss, very similar to transient monocular blindness of internal carotid disease. Orbital pain may precede the visual loss and is unassociated with eye movement. In addition, blurring, flashing, and flickering of vision may occur. With the onset of the attack, vision is decreased, and visual field loss may occur over 24 hours to 4 weeks without remission. Often the sudden decrease in vision is noted on awakening. A Marcus Gunn pupil can occur as well as other optic nerve conduction defects. The classic visual field defect is a variety of an altitudinal loss consistent with the termination of the nerve fiber layer at the horizontal raphe, and is usually inferior, but any field defect is possible (Fig. 3–80).

There is often a family history of hypertension or diabetes in the patient with nonarteritic anterior ION, but usually there is no strong history of transient ischemic attacks, cerebral infarction, or cardiac disease. Table 3–12 illustrates the differential diagnosis between ION and Foster Kennedy syndrome. **See color plates 15 through 18.**

Management. Visual acuity usually stabilizes at 20/60 or better in 45 to 50 percent of cases of nonarteritic anterior ION and is worse than 20/200 in about 40 percent. Recurrence in the same eye is uncommon, but the incidence of development in the fellow eye averages about 35 percent. The development in the fellow eye occurs more frequently in young patients and in vascularly compromised patients such as the diabetic. There is some concern about the possibility of secondary central and branch retinal artery occlusion, but this is not well documented. Cupping of the disc—that is, erosion of disc tissue—may occur secondary to

TABLE 3–12. DIFFERENTIAL DIAGNOSIS OF FOSTER KENNEDY SYNDROME AND ISCHEMIC OPTIC NEUROPATHY

Characteristic	Ischemic Optic Neuropathy	Foster Kennedy Syndrome
Onset	Sudden vision loss or field defect in one eye, followed by stabilization	Insidious progression of reduced vision with papilledema in fellow eye
Fields	Altitudinal hemianopsia, arcuate scotoma, central scotoma	Central scotoma in atrophic eye and enlarged blind spot in fellow eye
Fundus picture	Sector optic disc edema followed by sector atrophy	Uniform optic atrophy with optic disc edema in fellow eye
Associated systemic signs and symptoms	May be a family or personal history of hypertension, diabetes, or stroke	Hemiplegia, loss of smell, personality change

Modified from Alexander LJ. Diseases of the optic nerve. In: Bartlett JD, Jaanus SD, eds. *Clinical Ocular Pharmacology.* Boston: Butterworth; 1989.

the nonarteritic anterior ION, but always occurs after the presentation of atrophy. *This contrasts with glaucoma, where cupping precedes atrophy.*

In some instances, patches of chorioretinal degeneration may occur in the periphery after an incident of nonarteritic anterior ION. This chorioretinal breakdown may be physical evidence of further choroidal vascular compromise.

Of special interest is the phenomenon of the appearance of nonarteritic anterior ION during the cataract postoperative period. The presentation of ION associated with cataract surgery is thought to be secondary to an increased intraocular pressure in the immediate post-operative period. It has been documented that the patient presenting with the postoperative nonarteritic anterior ION is at greater risk in the fellow eye should surgery be performed. If cataract extraction is attempted in the fellow eye, presurgical reduction of intraocular pressure is crucial, with special attention to maintenance of reduced pressure in the immediate postoperative period. Intraocular pressure should be maintained at a low level for at least 1 week

postoperatively, and should be followed carefully thereafter.

Recognition and management of any underlying systemic condition is imperative. Table 3–13 lists some of the systemic diseases of concern. The primary workup in the case of an active presentation of nonarteritic anterior ION should include blood pressure, fasting blood glucose, a complete blood count with differential and platelets, and carotid auscultation. There is no strong correlation of nonarteritic anterior ION with carotid occlusive disease but the possibility does exist. The secondary workup should consider serum protein electrophoresis, a cardiovascular workup, duplex ultrasonography, and possibly fluorescein angiography if there is doubt as to the diagnosis. A STAT Westergren sedimentation rate is in order for all cases of suspect nonarteritic anterior ION.

When considering therapeutic intervention of nonarteritic anterior ION, two schools of thought exist, the treaters and the nontreaters. If treatment is employed, it is in the form of steroids or intraocular pressure-lowering drugs. Results of the optic neuritis treatment trial should be followed. Optic nerve decompression has also been reported to be of benefit in patients with progressive ION.

The successful treatment of nonarteritic anterior ION by steroids, if seriously considered by the clinician, depends on rapid diagnosis and immediate institution of therapy. It is proposed that the steroid reduces capillary permeability in the optic nerve, reducing swelling and improving circulation. This process, coupled with a reduction of intraocular pressure, improves the pressure–perfusion ratio to minimize atrophy. There are some reports that advocate initiation of anticoagulant or antiplatelet therapy as well, but there are no controlled studies to validate this proposed modality. *It is very important to understand that current belief is that no therapeutic intervention beyond management of any potential underlying systemic condition is of any benefit in the management of nonarteritic anterior ION. This is in contrast with the benefits in*

TABLE 3–13. SYSTEMIC ASSOCIATIONS WITH NON-ARTERITIC ISCHEMIC OPTIC NEUROPATHY

Allergic disorders	Intra-arterial chemotherapy
Blood loss	Intranasal anesthetic injections
Cardiac emboli	Lyme disease
Carotid artery disease(?)	Lymphoma
Cavernous sinus thrombosis	Mitral valve prolapse
Clotting disorders	Myocardial infarction
Diabetes	Polyarteritis Nodosa
Fabry's disease (carrier state)	Radiation therapy, especially head/neck
General surgery	
Generalized atherosclerosis	Relapsing polychondritis
Generalized autoimmune disorders	Renal transplantation
	Syphilis
Glaucoma (increased IOP)(?)	Systemic hypertension
Head and neck surgery	Systemic hypotension
Heart transplantation	Systemic lupus erythematosus
Hematologic disorders (polycythemia, sickle cell)	Tamoxifen therapy
	Vasomotor problems (migraine)
Herpes zoster	

Nonarteritic Anterior Ischemic Optic Neuropathy

Characteristics

△ Small-vessel disease of the optic nerve vascular supply indicating an imbalance in the pressure–perfusion ratio
  May occur in severe reduction in blood pressure
  May occur if IOP is relatively high and there is a moderate reduction in blood pressure
△ Usually occurs in patients aged 40 to 60 years and in men more frequently than women
△ Recurrence in the same eye is unusual, but incidence in the fellow eye averages about 35 percent. Recurrence is more common in younger patients and vascularly compromised patients
△ If nonarteritic anterior ION occurs postoperatively with cataract surgery it is typically secondary to postoperative rise in IOP, and the fellow eye is at severe risk with surgery if IOP is not kept low about 1 week postoperatively
△ Prodromal signs occur in about 25 percent of patients as transient blurring or transient field cuts, orbital pain without eye movement, and flashing or flickering vision
△ Optic disc edema, which may be sectoral or full disc, may be accompanied by hemorrhage in active phase, which eventually subsides with ensuing optic atrophy within about 3 months
△ Optic nerve conduction defects such as Marcus Gunn pupil occur as well as visual field compromise (often altitudinal), and possible severe vision reduction

△ Acuity stabilizes at 20/60 or better in about 50 percent of cases and is worse than 20/200 in about 40 percent of cases

Management

△ Attempt to ascertain underlying systemic disease
△ Primary workup
  STAT Westergren sedimentation rate
  Blood pressure
  Fasting blood glucose
  Complete blood count with differential and platelets
  Carotid palpation and auscultation
△ Secondary workup
  Rule out hyperviscosity syndromes
  Consider a cardiovascular workup
  Consider duplex ultrasonography
  Fluorescein angiography if doubts exist as to diagnosis
△ If resolved, educate patient about possibility of occurrence in other eye and use home monitoring
△ Reevaluate according to level of activity, but at least within 1 month, to assure that there is no progression
△ If active, consult with neuro-ophthalmology for possible initiation of steroid or other therapy (controversial)

---

the management of arteritic anterior ischemic optic neuropathy, in which there is a demonstrable rise in the Westergren sedimentation rate and/or a confirmed giant cell arteritis by biopsy.

The patient should be educated regarding the condition and should monitor the fellow eye for recurrence. If the condition is active, a neuro-ophthalmology consultation is in order to determine if intervention would be beneficial. A follow-up visit should be scheduled in 1 month if active or inactive to assure that there is no progression indicating neurologic disease.

Arteritic Ischemic Optic Neuropathy

Introduction and Description. Arteritic ION is an autoimmune disorder usually affecting patients over the age of 60 years, with females more often affected than males. It is a blood vessel disease of the optic nerve head creating an imbalance in the pressure–perfusion ratio in a fashion similar to nonarteritic anterior ION. The cause is unknown; the disease appears as inflammation of the elastic tissue in the media and adventitia of the arterial walls, leading to occlusion

(Fig. 3–81). Any large or medium-sized artery may be involved. In about 10 percent of patients, retinal arterial occlusion is the presenting sign. Concurrent occlusion of the ophthalmic and posterior ciliary arteries leads to sudden loss of function. Arteritic ION is an ocular emergency, necessitating immediate therapeutic intervention to prevent contralateral involvement, which occurs in about 75 percent of cases. It has been reported that if the second eye is not involved within 6 to 8 weeks, the prognosis is good for that eye.

The ophthalmoscopic picture at onset varies between two common presentations. In 50 percent of patients, the discs appear chalky white, with an apparent white mass lying deep in the disc with a circumpapillary white zone. Hemorrhages usually are absent in this variety. In 50 percent of the cases, the disc is edematous and pale pink. Edema spreads to the circumpapillary area, with superficial flame-shaped hemorrhages. When viewed with a fundus lens, a layer of pallor exists in the prelaminar region. Optic atrophy eventually presents secondary to the infarct.

Prodromal symptoms occur in approximately 75

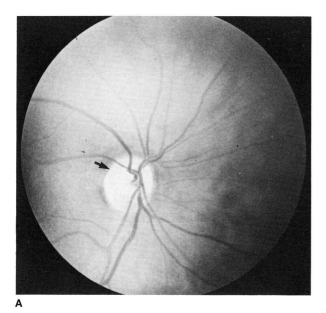

A

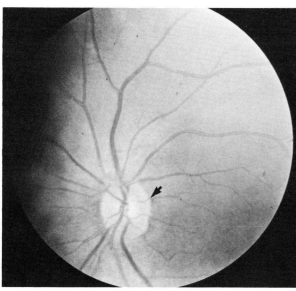

B

Figure 3–81. Example of total atrophy of the optic nerve head **(A)** compared to **(B)** in a case of temporal arteritic ischemic optic neuropathy.

percent of patients with arteritic ION about 1 to 2 weeks before the acute attack. These symptoms include trouble in focusing, loss of vision with return to normal, flashing or flickering, color disturbances, headaches (50 percent), weight loss, suboccipital neck pain, scalp tenderness on the affected side, and jaw aches (jaw claudication) associated with mastication (50 percent).

The attack of arteritic ION is heralded by an acute vision loss of 20/60 to no light perception (NLP), with poor vision being the rule. All nerve conduction defects are potentially present. As stated previously, arteritic ION can affect the fellow eye (up to 75 percent)

at variable intervals. I have seen onset occur within 2 days in the second eye in spite of massive doses of corticosteroids. The second eye is usually lost within 1 week if not treated promptly.

Leukocytosis, elevated erythrocyte sedimentation rate (ESR usually above 50 mm), and a palpable hard, nonpulsating temporal artery also present. The key feature, however, is sudden loss of vision in an elderly patient. The symptom complex of polymyalgia rheumatica may occur, consisting of pain and stiffness in the shoulders and neck and in the hips and thighs, marked morning stiffness, and pain increasing with motion (joint pain). **See color plate 19.**

Management. Visual acuity rarely improves with arteritic ION. In spite of long-term steroid therapy, loss

Arteritic Ischemic Optic Neuropathy

Pearls

Characteristics

△ Inflammation of the elastic tissue in the media and adventitia of the arterial walls
△ Considered to be an autoimmune process
△ Occurs in patients over 60, with strong possibility of bilaterality (up to 75 percent)
△ If second eye remains uninvolved within 6 to 8 weeks, prognosis is considered to be good
△ Prodromal symptoms may occur about 1 to 2 weeks prior to the attack and include
  Transient monocular blindness, trouble focusing
  Flashing or flickering, color vision disturbances
  Headaches, weight loss, neck pain
  Scalp tenderness and jaw aches with mastication
△ Attack is a sudden loss of vision 20/60 to NLP
  Pale swollen disc with or without hemorrhages
  Optic nerve conduction defects are present
  Strong chance of occurrence in fellow eye in 1 to 2 weeks without treatment
△ May have associated polymyalgia rheumatica

Management

△ STAT Westergren erythrocyte sedimentation rate
  Males = Age/2
  Females = (Age + 10)/2
△ Emergency neuro-ophthalmology or neurology consultation for immediate institution of steroid therapy
△ Temporal artery biopsy by a skilled individual within 1 week of initiation of therapy
△ Monitoring of steroid therapy with ESR
△ Careful follow up examinations including visual acuity and visual fields and constant communication with the neuro-ophthalmologist or neurologist

can occur in the fellow eye. From a management standpoint, it should be assumed that the fellow eye will become involved. Even if both eyes are involved to the point of loss of vision, discontinuing steroid therapy can allow for further compromise of visual field. Mortality rates associated with giant-cell arteritis average about 20 percent. Death is associated with complications of cerebrovascular disease. As would be expected, optic disc cupping occurs over a time in temporal arteritic ION.

In any elderly patient suspected of having ION, an immediate Westergren erythrocyte sedimentation rate determination should be ordered. Although reports vary concerning normal ranges for ESRs in elderly patients, it can be said that any patient suspected of having ION with an ESR above 40 mm in the first hour of a Westergren test should be considered as having giant-cell arteritis until proven otherwise. A general rule for normal values for the Westergren ESR is:

$$\text{Average for male} = \text{Age}/2$$

$$\text{Average for females} = (\text{Age} + 10)/2$$

An emergency neuro-ophthalmology or neurology consultation is necessary with any suspicion of arteritic ION.

Temporal artery biopsy is the definitive diagnostic test for arteritic ION. The biopsy should be performed within 1 week after starting therapy; a positive biopsy may even occur up to 1 month later. Biopsy of the temporal artery is difficult because the presentation of the granulomas is sporadic throughout the artery and should only be performed by someone experienced in the process. Therapy should not, however, be withheld while awaiting the results of the biopsy. Systemic steroids should be given immediately on suspicion of arteritic ION to prevent involvement in the contralateral eye. The steroids act as anti-inflammatory agents to decrease arterial inflammation. Often the best approach is to initiate therapy intravenously using methylprednisolone 250 mg every 6 hours for 12 doses. The patient may then be maintained on oral steroid. The initial dosages of oral steroids are high (80 to 120 mg/day). The dosage is adjusted downward according to signs, symptoms, and reduction of the ESR. Therapy is often continued at 5 to 10 mg/day for several years while the patient's ESR is monitored. Treatment usually is carried for at least 3 to 6 months but may be necessary for much longer.

The use of anticoagulants and vasodilators may be indicated if hematologic disorders accompany the giant-cell arteritis. Inherent risks in this therapy necessitate constant monitoring by a hematologist.

Follow-up in arteritic ION consists of crucial monitoring for the sedimentation rate as well as visual acuity and visual fields.

Diabetic Ischemic Optic Neuropathy (Diabetic Papillopathy)

Introduction and Description. Ischemic optic neuropathy can occur in any patient with diabetes, because diabetes is a small-vessel disease. Diabetic ION or diabetic papillopathy, however, refers to optic neuropathy in a young type 1 (IDDM) diabetic patient typically in their 20s to 30s, whereas the classic ION secondary to small-vessel disease occurs in older patients. Diabetic ION often presents bilaterally. Diabetic ION can be characterized as neither AION nor papilledema because it lacks some characteristics of both processes. Diabetic ION is considered to be the result of diffuse microangiopathy.

The clinical appearance of diabetic ION is optic disc edema that may be sectoral or total (Fig. 3–82). There may be associated circumpapillary superficial hemorrhages. There is usually associated background diabetic retinopathy, although disc neovascularization has been reported along with diabetic ION. **See color plate 20.**

There are often no reported signs or symptoms associated with diabetic ION. Visual field loss varies from enlarged blind spots to isolated scotomas. Vision loss may occur but is typically mild to moderate.

Management. Vision loss or visual field compromise usually resolves over a few months (up to 6 months) without therapeutic intervention. The disc swelling may, however, take up to 1 year to resolve.

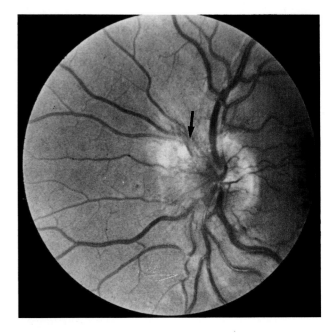

Figure 3–82. The arrow points to a nasal zone of disc edema in a case of diabetic ischemic optic neuropathy.

Diabetic Ischemic Optic Neuropathy

Characteristics

Δ Diabetic microangiopathy of the optic nerve head

Δ Occurs in young type 1 (IDDM) diabetic patients

Δ Optic disc edema that may be accompanied by hemorrhages

Δ May be bilateral

Δ Vision loss is typically minimal, but visual field loss may be variable

Δ Usually resolves over months without damage, but swelling may persist for 12 months

Management

Δ Rule out other causes of optic disc edema; a neuro-ophthalmology or neurology consultation

Δ Evaluate control of diabetes

Δ Standard eye examination follow-up assuring that there is no coincidental space-occupying lesion

If the condition is extensive, residual optic atrophy may occur. Proper diagnosis is crucial. The practitioner must rule out optic disc edema secondary to a space-occupying lesion as well as ruling out neovascularization of the disc. This usually necessitates a consultation with a neurologist or neuro-ophthalmologist. Fluorescein angiography will demonstrate leakage with both diabetic ION and neovascularization of the disc. Certainly, one must investigate the current status of control of the diabetes as well as the possibility of other types of hematologic or blood vessel disease.

In general, steroid therapy should be avoided in patients with diabetes because of the potentiation of the diabetes by these therapeutic agents.

The patient should be followed in at least 3 months to assure that a silent neurologic mass is not present that has not been discovered by routine testing.

Papillophlebitis

Introduction and Description. Papillophlebitis (Figs. 3–83 and 3–84) was previously considered to be a relatively minor affliction of the optic nerve occurring in otherwise healthy young adults 20 to 50 years of age. More recent reports point to the fact that the condition can be visually devastating especially when related to advancing age and associated systemic medical conditions. Males are affected about twice as often as females. The condition actually appears to be a variation of a central retinal vein inflammation in patients under the age of 50 years that leads to a partial occlusion. Papillophlebitis has been reported as benign retinal vasculitis, optic disc vasculitis, nonischemic CRVO, presumed phlebitis of the optic disc, and the big blind spot syndrome. The condition is almost exclusively unilateral in presentation.

Papillophlebitis appears as optic disc edema supposedly secondary to inflammatory occlusion of the central retinal vein. There are two distinctive ophthalmoscopic presentations: (1) gross unilateral optic disc edema with no retinal vascular changes and (2) unilateral optic disc edema with hemorrhages on and surrounding the disc, accompanied by grossly dilated and tortuous retinal veins. The retina may show small white dots in the edematous zone. Fluorescein angiography shows a prolongation of venous transit and some leakage at the nerve head.

A patient with papillophlebitis usually has visual acuity reduced to the 20/30 level but that may be re-

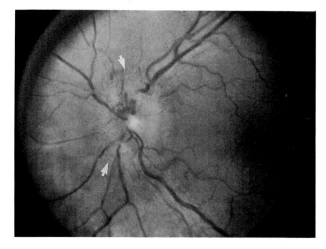

Figure 3–83. Optic disc edema, hemorrhage, and venous tortuosity in a case of papillophlebitis.

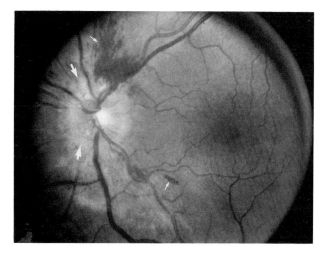

Figure 3–84. Variant of papillophlebitis characterized by scattered hemorrhaging.

Papillophlebitis

Characteristics

Δ Occurs in healthy young adults ages 20 to 50 years

Δ Affects males more than females

Δ Thought to be a variation of central retinal vein inflammation/occlusion

Δ Gross unilateral optic disc edema alone or with gross optic disc edema with dilated tortuous veins and possibly hemorrhage

Δ May be nonischemic or ischemic presentation

Δ Variable vision reduction and enlarged blind spots—big blind spot syndrome

Management

Δ Self-limited over a 6- to 18-month period; however, may result in severe vision loss

Δ Macular pigmentary changes, cystoid macular edema (CME), venous sheathing, iris neovascularization, neovascular glaucoma, and vitreous hemorrhage may occur

Δ Rule out potential associated diseases even though there is no strong association:
    Complete blood count with differential and platelets
    Antinuclear antibodies
    Chest x-rays
    CT or MRI
    FTA-ABS

Δ Panretinal photocoagulation in cases of iris neovascularization

Δ Possible therapeutic intervention, although there is no proven benefit

Δ Neuro-ophthalmology or neurology consultation is prudent when in doubt

---

duced to the light perception level. The complaint of reduced visual acuity, however, is often vague. There may be enlarged blind spots and variable central scotomas. At times papillophlebitis is seen following a viral syndrome.

Management. Papillophlebitis is considered self-limiting, with none of the sequelae commonly identified with central retinal vein occlusion, papilledema, inflammatory optic neuropathy, or ischemic optic neuropathy. The condition is a hybrid, resolving untreated over a 6- to 18-month period. Vision reduction may occur associated with macular pigmentary changes, with over 50 percent of patients recovering to better than 20/40. Up to approximately 15 percent of patients may, however, sustain vision reduction to the 20/400 level or worse. The degree of vision recovery is dependent on the extent of associated hypoxia (nonischemic versus ischemic vein occlusion). Cystoid macular edema perhaps with exudates, venous collateral formation, venous sheathing, iris neovascu-

larization, neovascular glaucoma, and vitreous hemorrhage are all potential sequelae of papillophlebitis. Younger age at presentation also offers a better visual prognosis.

Of primary concern in this disease is the elimination of other causes of optic disc edema. To rule out other causes of optic disc edema, the clinician may order skull films and CT scans, chest x-rays, blood work including complete blood count, lupus erythematosus (LE) preparation, antinuclear antibody (ANA), ESR, fluorescent treponemal antibody absorption (FTA-ABS), and possibly a lumbar puncture. Always remember, however, that in most cases of papillophlebitis these tests are nonproductive. In approximately 50 percent of cases of papillophlebitis there are no associated medical conditions. Hypertension, heart disease, gastrointestinal disease, hyperlipidemia, pulmonary disease, renal disease, arthritis, human immunovirus, and a smattering of other diseases have been reported to be associated with the development of papillophlebitis and are more common in patients over age 40 years. There is also only a rare presentation of associated ocular diseases such as glaucoma and vascular occlusive disease.

As with all other optic nerve diseases, management is controversial in papillophlebitis. Intervention with steroid therapy is advocated by some who point to the inflammatory nature of the disease. Opponents of therapy note the fact that the disease is basically benign and self-limited and institution of therapy may mask the true underlying cause. Platelet inhibitors have also been suggested as having potential benefit for treatment of the disease. Panretinal photocoagulation may offer some options for minimizing the risk of neovascularization in cases of ischemic presentation, whereas grid photocoagulation may benefit patients suffering from macular edema.

The neuro-ophthalmology or neurology consultation can best rule out the cause of unilateral optic disc edema. In the case of suspected papillophlebitis, the consultation is not an emergency as it is in arteritic AION.

■ ■ ■ ■ ■ ■

Clinical Note: Acute Idiopathic Blind Spot Enlargement

Acute idiopathic blind spot enlargement appears to be associated with retinal dysfunction similar to and possibly an extension of the multiple evanescent white dot syndrome. There is often the presentation of juxtapapillary white dots extending into the posterior pole. Paradoxically, there appears to be no associated optic disc edema. On fluorescein angiography, there appears to be a circumpapillary alteration of the retinal pigment epithe-

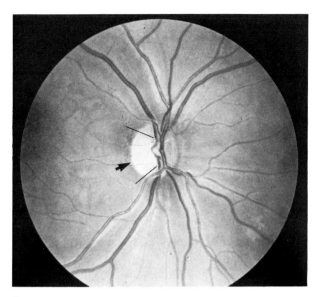

A

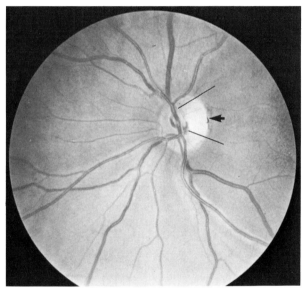

B

Figure 3–85. In both the right eye **(A)** and the left eye **(B),** there is a zone of optic atrophy secondary to alcohol toxicity.

lium appearing as hyperfluorescence. Acute idiopathic blind spot enlargement, like papillophlebitis, appears to be a disease of young patients. Photopsia may present in the affected zone initially, followed by enlargement of the blind spot with potential reduction in acuity and possible alteration of color vision.

Toxic Optic Neuropathy

Introduction and Description. Toxic optic neuropathy (Fig. 3–85) can occur as a result of nerve fiber reaction to toxins or deficiencies of nutrition. The atrophy occurs secondary to exogenous metabolic stimuli. The affectation of the nerve fibers appears to be the result of alteration in adenosine triphosphate (ATP)

formation. This alteration seems to cause a stasis of axoplasmic flow, with secondary optic disc edema and eventual axonal atrophy. **See color plate 21.** Initially, there may be optic disc edema with the possibility of splinter hemorrhages. As the condition progresses unchecked, optic atrophy occurs, with corresponding nerve fiber layer dropout most obvious in the papillomacular bundle.

With toxic optic neuropathy, there is a gradual, painless, often asymmetrical bilateral loss of visual acuity. Centrocecal scotomas are the classic presentation, but there is some variability. Concentric contraction of the visual fields occurs with tryparsamide poisoning. The field changes are progressive, but may be reversed with therapeutic intervention. There is apparent color vision loss as well. Toxic optic neuropathy is insidious in its onset and progression.

Management. Toxic optic neuropathy progresses to permanent irreversible vision loss if intervention does not occur. Even with intervention, permanent loss of vision or visual field may occur. The degree of vision loss may progress to severe levels but the patient never becomes totally blind.

Toxic optic neuropathy is reversible if the toxic agent or nutritional problem is discovered and eliminated. Table 3–14 lists some of the substances responsible for the genesis of toxic optic neuropathy. Certain drugs will alter zinc serum levels and precipitate optic atrophy. These include ethambutol, diiodohydroxyquin, and iodochlorhydroxyquin. Serum zinc levels

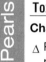

Pearls

Toxic Optic Neuropathy

Characteristics

△ Possible optic disc edema followed by optic atrophy (often in the temporal aspect of the nerve head)
△ The result of toxins or nutritional deficiencies
△ Gradual, painless, bilateral loss of vision with classic presentation of central scotomas, but visual fields may be variable
△ With significant ingestion of alcohol, vision loss may occur in hours to days
△ May result in severe vision loss but never total blindness

Management

△ If diagnosed early enough, possible to reverse the process by elimination of the toxic agent
△ Nutritional supplementation may be of some benefit but reports of success are often conflicting
△ Patients taking systemic medications known to be toxic should have routine eye examinations and should employ home monitoring to prevent irreversible changes

TABLE 3–14. DRUGS OR SUBSTANCES ASSOCIATED WITH THE DEVELOPMENT OF RETINAL CHANGES OR OPTIC NEUROPATHY

Alcohol	Cyproterone	Methotrexate
Barbiturates	acetate	Placidyl
Carbon monoxide	Digitalis	Phenothiazines
Chlorambucil	Diiodohydroxyquin	Steroid compounds
Chloramphenicol	Disulfiram	Streptomycin
Chloroquine	Ethambutol	Tamoxifen
Ciprofloxacin hy-drochloride	Ethchlorvynol	Tobacco
	Iodide compounds	Typarsamide
Cocaine	Isoniazid	Vitamin D
Corticosteroids	Hexamethonium	Vitamin A and
Cyanide	Lead	retinoids
Cyclosporine	Lithium	

should be evaluated in these patients, with 100 to 250 mg of zinc sulfate (three times a day) given if the initial signs of neuropathy develop. The dosage of oral zinc sulfate depends on the individual's ability to absorb the drug as well as the appearance of side effects, such as nausea, vomiting, diarrhea, and gastric bleeding. Zinc sulfate therapy is currently under investigation by the Food and Drug Administration for this condition as well as age-related macular degeneration.

Should isoniazid be implicated in toxic optic neuropathy, pyridoxine (vitamin B_6) may be used, with 25 to 100 mg per day as the standard dosage. This therapy has been recommended prophylactically in all patients placed on isoniazid therapy.

Toxic neuropathy secondary to tobacco or alcohol use is usually associated with vitamin B_{12} deficiencies if the abuse is chronic. With alcohol as the toxic substance, however, the vision loss may occur within hours to days depending on the amount and type of alcohol ingested. Treatment for this condition involves removal of the violating dietary agent and adjunctive vitamin therapy. Because there is often poor intestinal absorption of vitamin B_{12} in alcoholic conditions due to an alteration of the intrinsic factor, the therapy must be given intramuscularly. The standard dosage is 1000 µg of intramuscular hydroxo-cobalamin each week for 3 weeks, often supplemented by 300 µg of oral thiamine each week. It should be noted that vitamin B_{12} deficiency in association with folic acid deficiency may also cause megaloblastic anemia, which would appear as hemorrhages and cotton-wool spots in the posterior pole. A complete blood count will confirm the diagnosis of associated anemia. Serum folate levels may need to be checked as well as serum vitamin B_{12} levels.

In the management of toxic optic neuropathy, prevention is the most effective tool. Although prevention is not always possible because of the nature of the disease, prevention can be a part of the plan when known violating drugs are used in patients for therapeutic purposes. With the initiation of any drug therapy known to cause optic neuropathy, it is important to use routine eye examination as well as some form of patient home monitoring. The sooner the optic neuropathy is discovered, the better the potential for reversal.

Papilledema

Introduction and Description. Papilledema (Figs. 3–86 to 3–89) is best defined as optic disc edema secondary to increased intracranial pressure. Distension of the optic nerve sheaths, especially if bilateral, on ul-

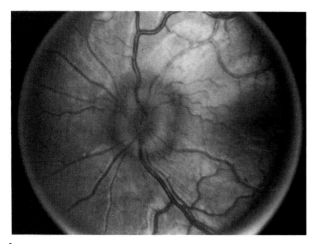

A

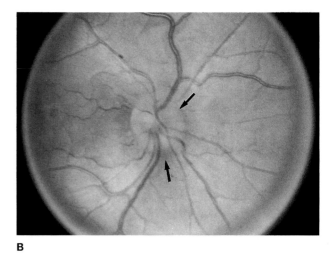

B

Figure 3–86. A. Considerable disc swelling is the characteristic in this left optic nerve head. This compensated papilledema was secondary to benign intracranial hypertension. **B.** The fellow eye, with moderate swelling confined to the areas of the disc (*arrows*).

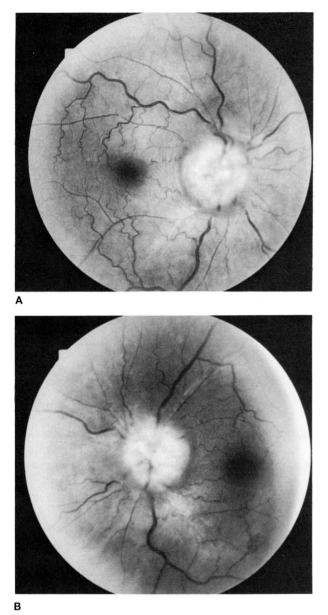

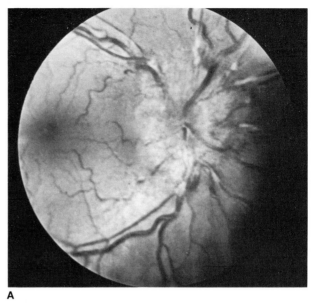

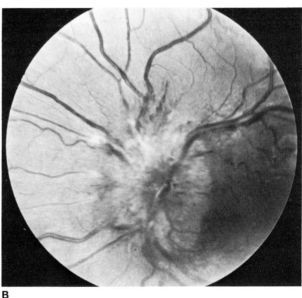

Figure 3–87. Bilateral compensated papilledema. Note the severe disc swelling and venous tortuosity but absence of hemorrhage and cotton-wool spots.

Figure 3–88. Bilateral noncompensated papilledema characterized by significant disc edema, venous tortuosity, flame-shaped hemorrhages, and cotton-wool spots.

trasonography or neurologic imaging, is a sure sign of increased intracranial pressure creating papilledema. The primary cause of disc swelling is the blockage of axoplasmic transport in the prelaminar portion of the ganglion cell axons. The blockage occurs at the lamina cribrosa, with accumulation of mitochondria and other axoplasmic particles in the nerve head. The nerve head swells forward into the vitreous as well as laterally, causing the retina to buckle inward at the temporal aspect of the nerve head. This buckling is known as Paton's folds and affects the function of the circumpapillary photoreceptors, creating the enlarged blind spot. The disc swelling in papilledema is

usually very dramatic, obscuring disc vessels as they cross the disc margin. The patient may notice metamorphopsia in the area of the blind spot as well. Figure 3–90 outlines the proposed etiopathogenesis of papilledema.

Optic disc edema is considered the first observable clinical sign of papilledema. The disc edema can occur 1 to 7 days after an increased intracranial pressure but even sooner (2 to 48 hours) as the consequence of abrupt intracranial hemorrhage. The swelling of the nerve fibers and subsequent debris accumulation occur initially in the inferior aspect of the disc, followed by the superior, nasal, and temporal as-

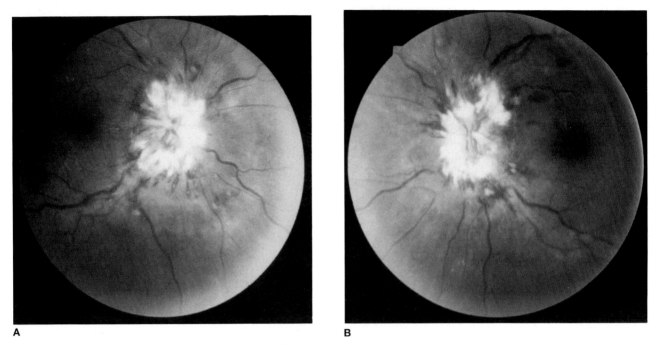

A   B

Figure 3–89. Bilateral noncompensated papilledema with a predominance of cotton-wool spots overlying severely swollen nerve heads.

pects. The swelling spreads into the surrounding retina. Disc vessel involvement may then occur. Papilledema is usually bilateral but may be asymmetrical. **See color plates 22 and 23.** Clinically, one may consider two distinct varieties of papilledema, compensated and noncompensated, as well as variations on the gradient. Acute noncompensated papilledema is representative of a rapid rise in intracranial pressure that does not allow for compensatory measures by the disc vasculature. This acute rise results in grossly swollen discs with flame-shaped hemorrhages and cotton-wool spots. Initially, vision is intact, but blind spots are enlarged. Chronic compensated papilledema

is characterized by gross disc-into-retina swelling with minimal vascular changes because the disc vessels have had time to compensate for the rise in pressure.

Absence of venous pulsation is of questionable value in differentiating papilledema from pseudopapilledema unless venous pulsation has been noted in a previous eye examination. Approximately 20 percent of normal individuals do not have spontaneous venous pulsation. The often reported sign of reddish disc coloration may be due solely to a smaller than average scleral canal. A hyperemic disc does not equate to acquired papilledema, in which the disc displays diffuse translucent swelling. As papilledema becomes more chronic, progressing toward optic atrophy, the hemorrhages and cotton-wool spots resolve, gliosis and sheathing of the papillary vessels occur, and shunt vessels may develop on and around the disc. In addition, bright masses, resembling but smaller than disc drusen, may appear on the nerve head. These masses probably represent deposits from the decompensating nerve fibers. Optic disc edema in a patient with chronic leukemia may also have associated infiltrations of the nerve head simulating optic disc drusen.

Transient obscurations, or 5- to 30-second blurring or loss of vision associated with postural changes, may occur as prodromal symptoms of papilledema. Visual symptoms are rare in the early phases of papilledema because axoplasmic stasis will not alter the transmission of the nerve impulse along the outer membrane of the nerve fibers. The visual symptoms do not appear until chronic swelling creates axoplasmic

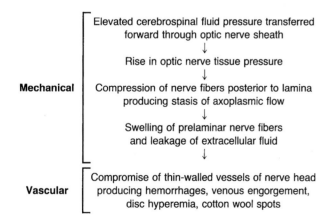

Figure 3–90. Mechanical theory of etiopathogenesis of papilledema.

stasis with subsequent destruction of the individual nerve fibers. There are no signs of optic nerve conduction defects such as the Marcus Gunn pupil or color desaturatrion until optic atrophy sets in. Reduction in vision may occur later in the process with ischemia secondary to compression of optic nerve vasculature.

Early visual field defects appear as an enlarged blind spot. The blind spot may then spread out to involve the macular area, giving the appearance of a projection emanating from the nerve head to the macular area. As nerve destruction continues, variable field defects occur.

Focal neurologic signs such as cranial nerve palsies, usually the sixth nerve, often present associated with increased intracranial pressure. Headache and vomiting without nausea but associated with straining or worse on awakening may present associated with papilledema. In addition, *benign intracranial hypertension (pseudotumor cerebri)* is another important cause of papilledema. Benign intracranial hypertension (BIH) is characterized by bilateral papilledema associated with headache that is often worse in the morning, transient obscurations, altered blind spot, sudden increased obesity, occasional diplopia caused by sixth-nerve palsy with the absence of frank neurologic signs, tinnitus, dizziness, nausea, vomiting, and depressed plasma corticosteroid levels. Benign intracranial hypertension occurs most frequently in females aged 10 to 50 years. Paradoxically, the CT or MRI may appear normal and the cerebrospinal fluid may be normal on lumbar puncture.

Benign intracranial hypertension is not life threatening, but optic atrophy can occur secondary to the long-standing disc edema and represents the primary morbidity factor in the disease. Benign intracranial hypertension may be secondary to pregnancy, otitis media, minor head injury, or such toxic conditions as hypervitaminosis A (especially in children), tetracycline, or nalidixic acid toxicity. In over 50 percent of the patients, the etiology of benign intracranial hypertension remains unknown. Severe malignant hypertension may also present a very dramatic optic disc edema similar to acute noncompensated papilledema.

Should vitamin A intoxication be suspected as the cause of papilledema, other signs may appear. Vitamin A intoxication is characterized by dry rough skin, fissuring of the angles at the mouth, loss of hair, migratory bone pain, headache, blurred vision or diplopia, and nausea with vertigo.

Complications of papilledema that may lead to reduction of visual acuity include choroidal neovascularization, preretinal macular hemorrhage, choroidal folds, and macular star formation. A sign of long-standing papilledema is the appearance of an optociliary shunt vessel on the nerve head occurring secondary to optic nerve compression. These shunt vessels are often associated with sphenoid ridge meningiomas.

Management. When managing papilledema, the clinician must realize that untreated papilledema can result in optic atrophy, but the underlying condition may cause death or severe disability. It is imperative that the cause of increased intracranial pressure be determined and eliminated or controlled. Even obscure causes such as spinal tumors must be considered in the differential diagnosis.

Pearls

Papilledema

Characteristics

△ Optic disc edema secondary to increased intracranial pressure

△ Distension of optic nerve sheaths on ultrasonography, CT, and/or MRI

△ Acute noncompensated papilledema occurs with acute rise in pressure and characterized by grossly swollen discs, hemorrhages, cotton-wool spots, and loss of spontaneous venous pulsation

△ Chronic compensated papilledema occurs with an insidious rise in pressure and characterized by swollen discs with minimal vascular response and loss of spontaneous venous pulsation

△ In both cases, in the early phase there is maintenance of vision, no nerve conduction defects, but enlarged blind spots

△ Transient obscurations may occur—5- to 30-second blurs of vision often associated with postural changes

△ May have other focal neurologic signs such as headache and vomiting on awakening or with physical straining, diplopia from sixth-nerve palsy

△ Benign intracranial hypertension is a cause of papilledema and is characterized by:
   Presentation predominantly in females
   Bilateral papilledema
   Headache
   Transient obscurations
   Sudden increase in obesity
   Depressed plasma corticosteroid levels
   Often normal CT/MRI/lumbar puncture

Management

△ Differentiation from pseudopapilledema

△ Consultation with neurosurgery or neurology to ascertain underlying cause

△ Surgical intervention may be necessary to prevent optic atrophy

△ Medical intervention when indicated

△ Follow up every 1 to 2 weeks until optic disc edema is under control, and coordinate care with tertiary specialist; repeat visual field tests are of value in monitoring the disease process

After differentiating papilledema from pseudo-papilledema, it is important to determine the cause of increased intracranial pressure (Table 3–15). The determination of the cause necessitates a neurologic consultation asking specifically for CT scans, MRI studies, or both. A lumbar puncture may be necessary to ascertain the intracranial pressure and presence of inflammatory or red blood cells. If the underlying cause cannot be determined readily, medical or surgical intervention must be undertaken to prevent continuing compromise resulting in optic atrophy. Surgical intervention may involve decompression techniques similar to those used for thyroid eye disease.

Medical treatment must be initiated only after ruling out space-occupying lesions, because papilledema may resolve but the causative agent may remain. Medical intervention is usually confined to cases of benign intracranial hypertension. Medical therapy is instituted to control or eliminate cerebral edema. Medical control can be achieved by using 2 to 4 g of acetazolamide plus 40 to 100 mg of oral steroids per day. Should this not achieve control, surgical intervention by lumbar puncture, neurosurgical shunting procedures, or optic nerve decompression must be employed. Surgical intervention can be compromised by infection and must be undertaken with great care.

Treatment of benign intracranial hypertension is determined by cause. Because benign intracranial hypertension is considered a self-limiting process, intervention is necessary only in cases of severe headaches or papilledema threatening to progress. There are advocates of the standard prednisolone–acetazolamide therapy and advocates of dehydration therapy. In any case, if increased intracranial pressure threatens vision, intervention must occur even to the point of neurosurgical shunting or optic nerve decompression.

Should a patient be suspected of having papilledema, take care to effect a careful differential diagnosis from other causes of optic disc edema.

TABLE 3–15. POSSIBLE CAUSES OF INCREASED INTRACRANIAL PRESSURE

Space-occupying lesion
Aqueductal stenosis
Obstruction of cerebrospinal fluid resorption
Intracerebral hemorrhage
Subarachnoid hemorrhage
Tumors of the spinal cord
Inflammatory polyneuritis
Infectious disease
Toxic metabolic diseases
Trauma
Lithium carbonate at therapeutic doses

Immediate consultation with neurology, neuro-ophthalmology, or neurosurgery is indicated to discern the cause of the papilledema and initiate therapy or surgical intervention as soon as possible. Careful follow up by the primary and tertiary-level provider is necessary and should occur initially every 1 to 2 weeks until resolution is obvious. Follow-up visual field tests are of value in monitoring the progression or regression of the disease. Table 3–16 provides a summary of the characteristics of optic neuropathy.

Optic Nerve Head Tumors

Both primary and secondary tumors may occur within the confines of the optic nerve. Primary tumors of the optic nerve head include vascular tumors, astrocytic hamartomas, melanocytomas, and medulloepitheliomas. Secondary tumors, such as retinoblastoma, uveal melanoma, metastatic carcinoma, and meningiomas, may extend into the optic nerve head. Differential diagnosis and clinical "pearls" for some of the more common tumors are listed in Table 3–17. Vascular tumors are discussed in the section on retinal vascular disease.

Melanocytoma

Introduction and Description. A melanocytoma of the optic nerve head is a benign primary tumor that occurs as an elevated black (may be gray to dark black) lesion on the nerve head that can involve the nerve fiber layer and present flayed edges similar to myelinated nerve fibers (Fig. 3–91). A melanocytoma can actually appear as the photographic negative of myelinated nerve fibers. The lesion arises from dendritic melanocytes and can occur anywhere within the uveal tract, conjunctiva, and sclera. Optic nerve melanocytoma is more prevalent in females than males, but there is no apparent hereditary pattern. Usually 50 percent or less of the disc is covered, but in approximately 10 percent of cases, most of the disc is covered. The melanocytoma may grow beyond the borders of the disc. In about 50 percent of melanocytomas there is a juxtapapillary benign choroidal melanoma and often is accompanying RPE degeneration. Growth can occur over 5 to 20 years, and there may be potential for malignant transformation. Optic disc edema, sheathing of retinal vessels, and subretinal edema may occur associated with the tumor. The space-occupying aspect of the lesion allows for compromise of vision and visual field; therefore even though it is benign, it carries a certain degree of morbidity. In many cases there is an enlarged blind spot that may be accompanied by other visual field defects.

Vision may become reduced with melanocytoma, but over 75 percent of eyes maintain an acuity of 20/15

TABLE 3–16. CHARACTERISTICS OF OPTIC NEUROPATHY

Characteristic	Inflammatory Optic Neuropathy	Demyelinizing Optic Neuropathy	Arteriosclerotic–Hypertensive Ischemic Optic Neuropathy	Temporal Arteritic Ischemic Optic Neuropathy	Diabetic Ischemic Optic Neuropathy	Papilledema
Age	Usually under age 20	20–40 years	50–70 years	60–80 years	Young diabetics	No specific age
Laterality	Usually unilateral in adults, may be bilateral in children	Unilateral initially	Unilateral but may become bilateral	Starts unilateral	Variable	Typically bilateral but asymmetrical
Vision loss	Moderate to severe	Variable but worsens with repeated attacks	Minimal to severe	Usually severe	None to minimal	Usually none
Visual field	Usually central scotoma	Variable but often central scotoma	Altitudinal, arcuate, central scotoma or generalized field constriction	Altitudinal, arcuate, central scotoma or field constriction	Enlarged blind spot	Enlarged blind spot
Pupillary findings	Positive Gunn sign	Positive Gunn sign	Positive Gunn sign	Positive Gunn sign	Usually normal	Normal
Fundus	Often exudates near disc; disc swelling and flame hemorrhages; optic atrophy occurs	Usually retrobulbar and nothing is seen; may have optic disc edema; optic atrophy is the end result	Segmental or diffuse disc swelling, splinter hemorrhages; optic atrophy segmental	Disc swelling and chalky appearance to disc; ultimately optic atrophy	Disc edema plus other signs of diabetes possible	Variable disc edema with flame hemorrhages and cotton-wool spots
Other signs	Pain on ocular movement in addition to a tender globe, plus orbit or brow ache	Pain on gross excursions, cerebellar signs, remissions, and exacerbations	Elevated blood pressure possible, diabetes possible, prominent temporal migraine possible, occlusive artery disease possible	Fever, weakness, muscle pain, head pain, jaw pain, weight loss, artery nonpulsatile and tender to palpation, transient blackouts	Type 1 diabetes	Headache, nausea, vomiting, transient obscurations
Treatment	Controversy, but possible steroid therapy; discern cause	Controversial, but possible steroid therapy	No specific treatment but monitor vascular status; steroid use often attempted	Aggressive steroid therapy	None, but assess systemic health and assure that there is no neurologic cause	Referral to neuro-ophthalmologist or neurosurgeon for further testing to uncover underlying etiology
Visual prognosis	Poor prognosis unless therapy instituted to prevent optic atrophy	Unpredictable and highly variable, with exacerbations	Poor prognosis for recovery	Poor prognosis with chance of fellow eye involvement	Usually returns to normal or near normal	Good vision if pressure is relieved

TABLE 3–17. OPTIC NERVE HEAD TUMORS—PEARLS

Tumor	Age of Onset	Laterality	Progression	Ophthalmoscopic Picture	Associated Systemic Conditions	Prognosis and Management
Angiomatosis retinae (autosomal dominant)	15–40 years	Bilateral in 50%	Yes	Reddish orange elevated, well circumscribed	25% with CNS hemangioblastomas; some have pheochromocytoma	Loss of vision, tough to photocoagulate, genetic counseling, neurology consultation
Cavernous hemangioma (possible autosomal dominance)	First to second decade	Unilateral	Rare	Grape clusters of aneurysmal dilations with preretinal membrane	Neurocutaneous or oculocutaneous lesions	Education, rare progression, genetic counseling
Melanocytoma	Variable	Unilateral	Common but rare loss of vision	Elevated gray to black lesion eccentric on the nerve head, flayed edges	None	May grow over the years to 2 disc diameters; monitor for conversion to malignancy
Astrocytic hamartoma	Congenital	Unilateral	Possible	Dirty white oval, smooth lesion; multilobullated mulberry yellowish lesion	Tuberous sclerosis, neurofibromatosis	Rule out systemic disease, patient education, possible field loss or reduced vision
Retinoblastoma (autosomal dominant)	0–4 years	Either	Yes	Retinomas (nonmalignant), elevated dull chalky lesion with evidence of calcium	Only subsequent possibility of metastasis to intracranial, bone, and liver	Deadly without intervention; 90% survival with intervention
Spread of diffuse choroidal melanoma	Variable	N/A	Yes	Subretinal yellowish brown area with optic nerve swelling and variable pigmentation	Metastasis to other organs	Five-year mortality rate of 75%; no effective intervention
Metastatic carcinoma	Variable	Bilateral in 20%	Yes	Swollen nerve head associated with yellowish structure; often choroidal metastases as well	Metastasis from breast, lung, stomach, sarcoma	Mean survival time 10 months; symptomatic treatment with radiation and chemotherapy
Leukemic nerve head infiltration	Variable, most often in acute cases	Variable	Yes, several	Optic disc edema, hemorrhage, surround of subretinal fluid	Leukemia	Survival rate usually less than 12 months; irradiation may delay vision loss

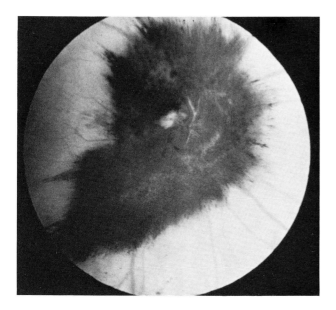

Figure 3–91. Melanocytoma of the optic nerve head spreading to involve the surrounding retina.

to 20/30. Melanocytomas occur in blacks as well as whites, but uveal melanomas are very rare in blacks. The fluorescein angiogram will differentiate the melanocytoma from a malignant melanoma. The fluorescein angiogram of a malignant melanoma will demonstrate hyperfluorescence because of the increased vascularity, whereas a melanocytoma will hypofluoresce throughout the course of the study because of the blockage of choroidal fluorescence by the polyhedral pigment cells.

Management. Management of melanocytoma of the optic disc consists of proper diagnosis and follow-up to ensure that there is no progression to malignancy. After the initial diagnosis, the lesion should be followed within 3 months to assure stability, and then followed thereafter according to stability.

Astrocytic Hamartoma

Introduction and Description. Astrocytic hamartomas are considered to be congenital and have variable presentation. Hamartomas are composed of tissue that is normal for the site in which they present but are malformed or mal-arranged. In the eye, the hamartoma arises from astrocytes in the optic nerve head and the nerve fiber layer. Astrocytomas may be bilateral and may present multiple lesions in one eye. The lesions are nonmetastasizing but grow associated and coincident with normal growth patterns. The lesions may appear anywhere in the retina but tend to occur on or near the optic nerve head. Astrocytic hamartomas have an association with tuberous scle-

rosis (Bourneville's disease) and, less commonly, neurofibromatosis (von Recklinghausen's disease). In fact, over 50 percent of patients with tuberous sclerosis have astrocytic hamartomas of the retina or optic nerve. Tuberous sclerosis presents other signs and symptoms to assist in the differential diagnosis, including adenoma sebaceum (butterfly-shaped angiofibromas on nose and cheeks), seizures, cutaneous patches, mental retardation, and intracranial calcifications. Neurofibromatosis presents café-au-lait spots, plexiform neuromas of the skin giving the dermatologic deformities, orbital and eyelid abnormalities giving proptosis, ocular neuromas, and fundus abnormalities.

The tumor may appear as a dirty white (translucent) lesion that is oval with a relatively smooth surface. This presentation may be a germinative stage of the tumor. It may also appear as a whitish yellow multilobulated mulberry lesion that may calcify with age. This calcification makes the lesion similar to buried drusen of the optic nerve head in the reflectance presented during B-scan ultrasonography. It has been suggested that the multilobulated lesion may be an aged version of the smooth variety. An astrocytic hamartoma may be one-half to several disc diameters in size. Associated retinal pigment epithelial alterations may be present both near and remote to the primary lesion. Figure 3–92 represents a significant retinal/optic nerve astrocytoma and Figure 3–93 is the B-scan of the eye, demonstrating significant re-

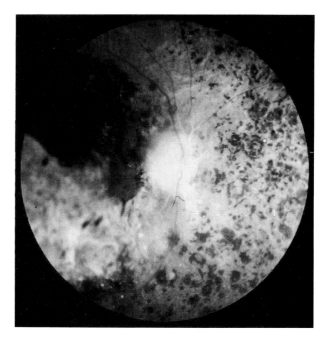

Figure 3–92. An astrocytic hamartoma of the optic nerve head and retina associated with tuberous sclerosis.

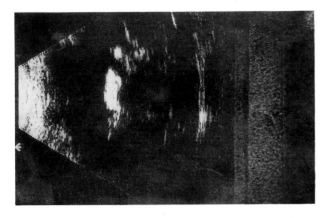

Figure 3–93. B-scan of the patient shown in Figure 3–90, illustrating the strong reflectivity of the astrocytic hamartoma.

flectance at low gain. The lesions may autofluoresce with appropriate barrier and excitor filters.

Vision may be decreased, and visual fields may be affected due to compression of the healthy optic nerve components. The lesion is very slow growing or may even remain stable. An astrocytic hamartoma is highly vascularized and hyperfluoresces in all stages of fluorescein angiography. The vascular component of the angiogram differentiates the hamartoma from buried drusen.

Management. The astrocytic hamartoma is composed of benign astrocytes, calcium, and collections of other materials. Management of an astrocytic hamartoma consists of ruling out systemic disease associated with the lesion, consecutive visual field tests to assess progression and to assure that it is not some manifestation of a neurologic disorder, and patient education about the condition. **See color plate 24.**

Combined Hamartoma of the Retina and Retinal Pigment Epithelium

Introduction and Description. Combined hamartoma of the retina and the retinal pigment epithelium is believed to originate from changes in the retinal pigment epithelium that are secondary to an intraretinal vascular hamartoma. The result is a dramatic pigmentary disturbance that has an increase in associated retinal vasculature, often with a prominent epiretinal membrane. Combined hamartomas may affect the optic nerve head as well as being an isolated finding in the retina. The lesions are usually unilateral and do not follow a hereditary pattern.

The combined hamartoma has characteristics of both a melanocytoma and an astrocytic hamartoma. There is usually a gray lesion partially overlying the disc with a feathered border extending into the retina. The surface is covered by an epiretinal membrane that

creates traction lines (usually in the 40s) in the surrounding retina. Because the lesion is thought to partially originate from the vascular network, there may be dilated vessels and the epiretinal membrane creates tortuosity in all associated vasculature.

Combined hamartomas near the nerve head are usually asymptomatic and are discovered on routine eye examinations. Visual field tests will demonstrate an enlarged blind spot or scotoma in the affected area. Combined hamartomas in the peripheral retina may present at an earlier age and are often more symptomatic, because the epiretinal membrane is more active, creating traction and visual morbidity. As would be expected because of the vascular component, fluorescein angiography demonstrates hypervascularity that may present leaking microaneurysms and telangiectatic vessels.

Management. Management includes correct differential diagnosis and a retinal consultation for possible surgical intervention if vision becomes threatened by the epiretinal traction and if leakage threatens macular function.

Retinoblastoma

Introduction and Description. Retinoblastoma is a malignant congenital tumor that is derived from the neural elements of the evolving fetal retina. The tumor may extend from the retina to occupy the optic nerve head, which is an ominous sign because of the possibility of intracranial spread. Retinoblastoma is the most common malignant intraocular tumor in infants and children, with about 30 percent of patients affected bilaterally. Retinoblastoma is a tumor of the young in that almost all cases are diagnosed before 4 years of age. The mean age of diagnosis is 18 months.

Some families with the inherited form (autosomal dominant with variable penetrance, which represents about 5 percent of cases) of retinoblastoma do not show high penetrance and demonstrate retinal lesions, called retinomas, that do not show progression. Retinomas are characterized by a translucent grayish mass protruding into the vitreous that may have cottage cheese calcifications or retinal pigment epithelium migration and proliferation. Virtually all (98 percent) bilateral cases of retinoblastoma are hereditary, whereas 10 to 15 percent of unilateral cases are hereditary. The majority of cases (95 percent) appear to arise through mutation and about 25 percent of these mutations may be transmitted to the next generation.

Retinoblastoma may be flat and diffuse, extending into the subretinal space with an associated non-rhegmatogenous retinal detachment. The tumor may also present an endophytic variety, which varies in appearance according to the stage of development. In the early stage the tumor appears as a gray elevation with associated vascular changes developing into a mushroom elevation that is whitish pink with superficial telangiectasia. The telangiectasia may leak and hemorrhage. Other vascular anomalies may also exist. With time, the tumor's blood supply necroses and the surface becomes calcified, creating a chalky appearance. The retinoblastoma of the optic nerve head is an elevated, dull, chalky lesion that usually is present also in the adjacent retina. The tumor has a high calcium content and is, therefore, very reflective on B-scan ultrasonography. Calcium deposits may be visible within the tumor. Fluorescein angiography shows hyperfluorescence throughout, indicating that the tumor is vascularized. Leukokoria, strabismus, and iris neovascularization are also common. Spread into the anterior chamber may create seeding, heterochromia, and hyphema.

Management. Early identification is crucial, because retinoblastoma can metastasize to the brain, bones, and liver through the optic nerve or the subarachnoid space. Metastasis may also occur through the blood and lymphatic system. About 15 percent of patients surviving bilateral retinoblastomas develop unrelated malignancies later in life. Enucleation is indicated when the lesion is unilateral and acuity is severely impaired. When bilateral, the lesions may be treated by irradiation, photocoagulation, or cryotherapy. Survival rates for patients with retinoblastoma are above 90 percent when the lesions are treated.

Pedigree analysis and genetic counseling are crucial in cases of retinoblastoma in spite of the fact that preditions from and about inheritance patterns are not that reliable.

Choroidal Melanoma

Introduction and Description. Choridal melanomas of the optic nerve head result from intrusion from the choroid. Choroidal melanomas are the most common primary malignancy in adults. The malignancy develops in uveal tissue, most often in the choroid (80 percent). Choroidal melanomas are more often unilateral and occur most frequently in persons over age 50 years. Choroidal melanomas are only rarely found in darkly pigmented races. The diffuse variety of choroidal melanoma may actively infiltrate the optic nerve area, especially when located in the posterior pole. The diffuse variety is more malignant than the circumscribed type and therefore offers a poorer prognosis. The 5-year mortality rate associated with this tumor approaches 75 percent.

The diffuse choroidal melanoma of the optic nerve head is a subretinal yellowish brown area with variable surface pigmentation. As the tumor invades, the optic nerve head swells as the result of the physi-

cal compression. Fluorescence with fluorescein angiography is variable depending on the degree of pigmentation, but usually demonstrates some form of hyperfluorescence because of the vascularity of the tumor.

Visual acuity and visual field findings are variable depending on the stage of development. Pain is not usually a factor in the melanomas presenting in the posterior pole. Venous occlusions may also occur because of the physical presence of the tumor.

Management. Management of diffuse choroidal melanoma of the optic nerve head is somewhat controversial owing to the fact that enucleation has a strong association with metastases and other forms of treatment offer no significant improvement in morbidity and mortality. Management of malignant choroidal melanomas elsewhere in the retina offers some improvement in morbidity and mortality. A consultation with a retinal oncologist is in order in all cases of suspect malignant melanoma invasion of the optic nerve head. In addition, if this is the primary tumor site, a consultation with an oncologist is in order to rule out metastases.

Metastatic Carcinoma

Introduction and Description. Carcinomas represent the most common malignancies of the eye, and usually metastasize to the choroid although occasionally the optic nerve head may be involved. The primary site may be anywhere but is usually in the breast in females and in the lungs in males. When a carcinoma metastasizes to the optic nerve head, it occurs bilaterally in almost 20 percent of patients. Often, there will be coincident choroidal metastases, which appear as placoid yellow or cream-colored subretinal masses with overlying retinal detachment that may have a mottled appearance due to altered retinal pigment epithelium (Figs. 3–94 and 3–95). Multiple lesions may present.

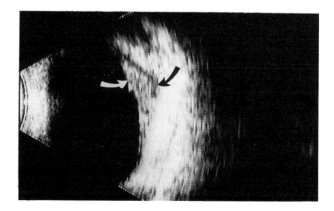

Figure 3–94. A metastatic carcinoma to the choroid (*arrows*).

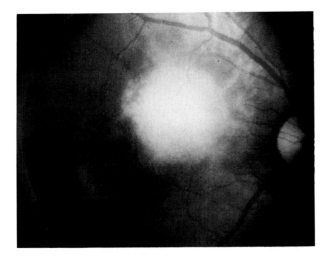

Figure 3–95. An example of a choroidal metastasis (carcinoma).

Carcinomas of the optic nerve head usually cause loss of vision (80 percent), an edematous nerve head, and a yellowish structure above normal anatomic structures. Venous tortuosity or central retinal vein occlusion are often present secondary to the physical compression within the nerve.

Management. The mean survival time after the metastasis to the nerve head is under 10 months. A consultation with a retinal oncologist is in order as well as assurance that the patient's oncologist is aware of the ocular situation. Radiation and chemotherapy may be of symptomatic benefit.

Leukemic Nerve Head Infiltration

Introduction and Description. There is a high rate of ocular involvement in patients who die of leukemia. Acute forms usually create more ocular involvement than do chronic forms. The choroid is the site of greatest involvement, and the optic nerve head is affected at about the same rate as it is with metastatic carcinoma. Optic nerve head involvement usually occurs only in acute cases (about one-third of those cases).

Leukemic infiltration of the nerve head occurs as optic disc edema and may have associated hemorrhaging. The optic disc edema may also be associated with the chronic steroid usage often associated with leukemia. In the early stages of infiltration, the optic disc may just appear swollen and pale; as the condition progresses, yellow deposits appear within the disc structure. Subretinal fluid may surround the infiltrated area. As the leukemic cells replace normal nerve tissue, vision drops significantly to a point where it is not amendable by therapy.

Management. Survival rates after nerve head infiltration are usually less than 12 months, but irradiation may

delay or abort nerve head destruction and vision loss. With any tumor or infiltrative process there may be associated orbital involvement giving rise to proptosis.

Choroidal Osteoma

Introduction and Description. A choristoma is a tumor mass arising from tissues foreign to the site of development, in direct contrast to a hamartoma. A choroidal osteoma is a bonelike tumor (ossification) arising in the choroid that may occur near the optic nerve head. This type of tumor occurs most frequently in young females.

The tumor may create optic disc edema if it develops near the optic nerve head. The osteoma is often a variation of orange and pink with a mottled surface and pigmentary disorganization. The margins are scalloped and well defined. There may be associated retinal changes such as hemorrhaging and neovascular formation often with scar formation. The fluorescein angiogram demonstrates the mottled hyperfluorescent pattern and vascular nature of the tumor.

Vision and visual fields are variable depending on location and extent of expansion. The tumor is highly reflective on B-scan ultrasonography and is also visible on CT scanning.

Management. Management is a consultation with a retinal oncologist with comanagement depending on the course of the disease and the treatment options.

Glioma of the Optic Disc

Introduction and Description. A glioma typically involves the optic nerve, but the optic disc will demonstrate the result of the involvement, optic atrophy. Most gliomas occur in females and usually present before age 20 years. The diagnosis is most often made between the ages of 4 and 8 years. In youth, the tumor is considered relatively benign, with the more malignant form, the glioblastoma, presenting in adults. A glioma may present on the optic nerve head as a smooth, elevated, whitish mass over the disc. The space-occupying lesion may also create venous occlusive disease and, as mentioned previously, optic atrophy.

Proptosis with minimal if any reduction in visual acuity is often the presenting symptom and sign. There may be associated limitation of eye movements. As with any proptosis, neurologic imaging is crucial.

Management. Surgical excision of the tumor is desirable, with radiologic intervention necessary in the older patient. In addition, it should be noted that over 50 percent of patients with optic nerve gliomas also have neurofibromatosis. This coincidence of neurofibromatosis necessitates neurologic studies limited not just to the orbital areas. In all cases of suspect optic nerve gliomas, a neurosurgical consultation is indicated.

Meningioma of the Optic Disc

Introduction and Description. A meningioma rarely presents initially on the optic disc. If there is direct involvement, it is seen as an elevated pale mass above the disc with hemorrhagic changes. The meningioma usually creates changes in the optic nerve by insidious progression and compression behind the eyeball. The signs and symptoms include a pale edematous disc, reduced visual acuity, and optociliary shunt vessels.

About half of meningiomas occur in patients over age 30 years (usually white females) and about half occur under age 20 years. The morbidity and mortality is much worse in the patients under age 20. There is typically an insidious but progressive reduction in vision, with the expected proptosis being a late sign. Diagnosis is achieved through neurologic scanning.

Management. Management of the suspected meningioma consists of a consultation with a neurosurgeon. The treatment is surgical excision and ruling out associated disorders such as neurofibromatosis.

REFERENCES

Congenital Macrovessel

Chronister CL, et al. Congenital retinal macrovessel. *Optom Vis Sci.* 1991;68:747–749.

Tilted and Malinserted Discs

Alexander LJ. The tilted disc syndrome. *J Am Optom Assoc.* 1978;49:1060–1062.

Apple DJ, et al. Congenital anomalies of the optic disc. *Surv Ophthalmol.* 1987;27:3–41.

Bass SJ, Sherman J. Visual evoked potential (VEP) delays in tilts and/or oblique entrance of the optic nerve head. *Neuro-ophthalmology.* 1988;8:109–122.

Brown GC, Tasman W. *Congenital Anomalies of the Optic Disc.* New York: Grune & Stratton; 1983.

Circumpapillary Staphyloma

Apple DJ, et al. Congenital anomalies of the optic disc. *Surv Ophthalmol.*1987;27:3–41.

Brown GC, Tasman W. *Congenital Anomalies of the Optic Disc.* New York: Grune & Stratton; 1983.

Fantes FE, Anderson DR. Clinical histologic correlation of human peripapillary anatomy. *Ophthalmology.* 1989;96:20–25.

Spalton DJ, Hitchings RA, Hunter PA. *Atlas of Clinical Ophthalmology.* London: Gower; 1984.

Yanoff M, Fine BS. *Ocular Pathology. A Text and Atlas.* Hagerstown, MD: Harper & Row; 1975.

Colobomas of the Optic Nerve and Retina

Apple DJ, et al. Congenital anomalies of the optic disc. *Surv Ophthalmol.* 1987;27:3–41.

Brown GC, Tasman W. *Congenital Anomalies of the Optic Disc.* New York: Grune & Stratton; 1983.

Cogan DG. Coloboma of optic nerve with overlay of peripapillary retina. *Br J Ophthalmol.* 1978;62:347–350.

Corbett JJ, Savino PJ, Schatz NJ, Orr LS. Cavitary developmental defects of the optic disc. *Arch Neurol.* 1980;37:210–213.

Spalton DJ, Hitchings RA, Hunter PA. *Atlas of Clinical Ophthalmology.* London: Gower; 1984.

Steahly LP. A colobomatous optic disc anomaly and associated retinal detachment. *J Pediatr Ophthalmol Strabismus.* 1977;14:103–105.

Theodossiadis G. Evolution of congenital pit of the optic disc with macular detachment in photocoagulated and nonphotocoagulated eyes. *Am J Ophthalmol.* 1977;84:620–631.

Morning Glory Disc

Apple DJ, et al. Congenital anomalies of the optic disc. *Surv Ophthalmol.* 1987; 27:3–41.

Beyer W, et al. Morning glory syndrome. *Ophthalmology.* 1982;89:1362–1367.

Brown GC, Tasman W. *Congenital Anomalies of the Optic Disc.* New York: Grune & Stratton; 1983.

Spalton DJ, Hitchings RA, Hunter PA. *Atlas of Clinical Ophthalmology.* London: Gower; 1984.

Steinkuller PG. The morning glory disc anomaly: Case report and literature review. *J Pediatr Ophthalmol Strabismus.*1980;17:81–87.

Congenital Pits of the Optic Nerve Head

Apple DJ, et al. Congenital anomalies of the optic disc. *Surv Ophthalmol.* 1987;27:3–41.

Brown GC, Augsburger JS. Congenital pits of the optic nerve head and retinochoroidal colobomas. *Can J Ophthalmol.* 1980;15:144–146.

Brown GC, Shields JA, Goldberg RE. Congenital pits of the optic nerve head, II. Clinical studies in humans. *Ophthalmology.* 1980;87:51–65.

Brown GC, Tasman W. *Congenital Anomalies of the Optic Disc.* New York: Grune & Stratton; 1983.

Fantes FE, Anderson DR. Clinical histologic correlation of human peripapillary anatomy. *Ophthalmology.* 1989; 96:20–25.

Javitt JC, et al. Acquired pits of the optic nerve. Increased prevalence in patients with low-tension glaucoma. *Ophthalmology.* 1990; 97:1038–1044.

Spalton DJ, Hitchings RA, Hunter PA. *Atlas of Clinical Ophthalmology.* London: Gower; 1984.

Steahly LP. A colobomatous optic disc anomaly and associated retinal detachment. *J Pediatr Ophthalmol Strabismus.* 1977;14:103–105.

Theodossiadis G. Evolution of congenital pit of the optic disc with macular detachment in photocoagulated and nonphotocoagulated eyes. *Am J Ophthalmol.* 1977;84:620–631.

Congenital Optic Nerve Hypoplasia

Bjork A, et al. Bilateral optic nerve hypoplasia with normal visual acuity. *Am J Ophthalmol.* 1978;86:524–529.

Kim RY, et al. Superior segmental optic hypoplasia: A sign of maternal diabetes. *Arch Ophthalmol.* 1989; 107:1312–1315.

Lambert SR, et al. Optic nerve hypoplasia. *Surv Ophthalmol.* 1987;32:1–9.

Ouvrier R, Billson F. Optic nerve hypoplasia: A review. *J Child Neurol.* 1986:1:181–188.

Pinkert RB. Superior segmental optic hypoplasia. *Clin Eye Vis Care.* 1991;3:187–189.

Roberts-Harry J, et al. Optic nerve hypoplasia: Associations and management. *Arch Dis Child.* 1990;65:103–106.

Romano PE. Simple photogrammetric diagnosis of optic nerve hypoplasia. *Arch Ophthalmol.* 1989;107:824–826.

Stromland K. Ocular abnormalities in the fetal alcohol syndrome. *Acta Ophthalmol.* 1985;171(suppl):1–50.

Zeki SM. Optic nerve hypoplasia and astigmatism: A new association. *Br J Ophthalmol.* 1990;74:297–299.

Zeki SM, Dutton GN. Optic nerve hypoplasia in children. *Br J Ophthalmol.* 1990;74:300–304.

Buried Drusen of the Optic Nerve Head

Brown GC, Tasman W. *Congenital Anomalies of the Optic Disc.* New York: Grune & Stratton; 1983.

Clarkson JG, Altman RD. Angioid streaks. *Surv Ophthalmol.* 1982;26:235–246.

Grand MG, et al. Angioid streaks associated with pseudoxanthoma elasticum in a 13-year-old patient. *Ophthalmology.* 1987;94:197–200.

Harris MJ, et al. Hemorrhagic complications of optic nerve drusen. *Am J Ophthalmol.* 1981;92:70–76.

Hoover DL, et al. Optic disc drusen in children. *J Pediatr Ophthalmol Strabismus.* 1988;25:191–195.

Lowder CY, et al. Visual loss from pituitary tumor masked by optic nerve drusen. *Neurosurgery.* 1981;8:473–476.

Mustonen E. Pseudopapilledema with and without verified optic disc drusen: A clinical analysis, I. *Acta Ophthalmol.* 1983;61:1037–1056.

Mustonen E, et al. Neurological findings in patients with pseudopapilledema with and without verified optic disc drusen. *Acta Neurol Scand.* 1983;68:218–230.

Rosenberg MA, Savino PJ, Glaser JS. A clinical analysis of pseudopapilledema, I. Population, laterality, acuity, refractive error, ophthalmoscopic characteristics, and coincident disease. *Arch Ophthalmol.* 1979;97:65–70.

Savino PJ, Glaser JS. Pseudopapilledema versus papilledema. *Int Ophthalmol Clin.* 1977;17:115–137.

Savino PJ, Glaser JS, Rosenberg MA. A clinical analysis of pseudopapilledema. II. Visual field defects. *Arch Ophthalmol.* 1979;97:71–75.

Sibony PA, et al. Intrapapillary refractile bodies in optic nerve sheath meningioma. *Arch Ophthalmol.* 1985;103:383–385.

Spalton DJ, Hitchings RA, Hunter PA. *Atlas of Clinical Ophthalmology.* London: Gower; 1984.

Spencer WH. *Ophthalmic Pathology. An Atlas and Textbook.* Philadelphia: Saunders; 1986.

Tso MOM. Pathology and pathogenesis of drusen of the optic nerve head. *Ophthalmology.* 1981;88:1066–1079.

Wise GN, et al. Optic disc drusen and subretinal hemorrhage. *Trans Am Acad Ophthalmol Otolaryngol.* 1974;78:212–219.

Leber's Hereditary Optic Atrophy

Brown GC, Tasman W. *Congenital Anomalies of the Optic Disc.* New York: Grune & Stratton; 1983.

Francois J. Hereditary optic atrophy. *Int Ophthalmol Clin.* 1968;8:1016–1054.

Glaser JS. The eye and systemic disease. In: Goldberg ME, ed. *Goldberg's Genetic and Metabolic Eye Disease.* Boston: Little, Brown; 1986.

Hotta Y, et al. Diagnosis of Leber's optic neuropathy by means of polymerase chain reaction amplification. *Am J Ophthalmol.* 1989;108:601–602.

Hoyt CS. Autosomal dominant optic atrophy. *Ophthalmology.* 1980;87:245–250.

Kline LB, Glaser JS. Dominant optic atrophy. *Arch Ophthalmol.* 1979;97:1680–1686.

Seedorff T. Leber's disease, IV. *Acta Ophthalmol.* 1969;47:813–821.

Seedorff T. Leber's disease, V. *Acta Ophthalmol.* 1970;48:186–213.

Singh G, et al. A mitochondrial DNA mutation as a cause of Leber's hereditary optic neuropathy. *N Engl J Med.* 1989;320:1300–1305.

Uemura A, et al. Leber's hereditary optic neuropathy: Mitochondrial and biochemical studies on muscle biopsies. *Br J Ophthalmol.* 1987;71:531–536.

Walsh FB, Hoyt WF. *Clinical Neuro-ophthalmology.* 3rd ed. Baltimore: Williams & Wilkins; 1969.

Yanoff M, Fine BS. *Ocular Pathology. A Text and Atlas.* Hagerstown, MD: Harper & Row; 1975.

Glaucomatous Optic Neuropathy

Alexander LJ. Diagnosis and management of primary open angle glaucoma. *Optom Clin.* 1991;1:19–102.

Bengtsson B, et al. Disc hemorrhage and glaucoma. *Acta Ophthalmol.* 1981;59:1–7.

Buus DR, Anderson DR. Peripapillary crescents and halos in normal-tension glaucoma and ocular hypertension. *Ophthalmology.* 1989;96:16–19.

Chi T, et al. Racial differences in optic nerve head parameters. *Arch Ophthalmol.* 1989;107:836–839.

Fulk GW, VanVeen HG. How to photograph and evaluate the retinal nerve fiber layer. *J Am Optom Assoc.* 1986;57:760–763.

Iwata K. Ophthalmoscopy in detection of optic disc and retinal nerve fiber layer changes in early glaucoma (summary). *Surv Ophthalmol.* 1989;33(suppl):447–448.

LaRussa F. Ophthalmoscopic comparison of the discs: The alternate fixation shift technique. *S J Optom.* 1989;7:19–21.

Lewis TL, Fingeret M. *Primary Care of the Glaucomas.* Norwalk, CT: Appleton & Lange; 1992.

Lindenmuth KA, et al. Significance of cilioretinal arteries in primary open angle glaucoma. *Arch Ophthalmol.* 1988;106:1691–1693.

Litwak, AB. Evaluation of the retinal nerve fiber layer in glaucoma. *J Am Optom Assoc.* 1990;61:390–397.

Luxenberg MN. Collateral vessel formation in the optic disc in glaucoma. *Arch Ophthalmol.* 1987;105:1287.

Miller KM, Quigley HA. The clinical appearance of the lamina cribrosa as a function of the extent of glaucomatous optic nerve damage. *Ophthalmology.* 1988;95:135–138.

Quigley HA. Glaucoma's optic nerve damage: Changing clinical perspectives. *Ann Ophthalmol.* 1982;14:611–612.

Shields MB, et al. Reproducibility of topographic measurements with the optic nerve head analyzer. *Am J Ophthalmol.* 1987;104:581–586.

Shihab ZM, et al. The significance of disc hemorrhage in open-angle glaucoma. *Ophthalmology.* 1982;89:211–214.

Tielsch JM, et al. Intraobserver and interobserver agreement in measurement of optic disc characteristics. *Ophthalmology.* 1988;95:350–356.

Webb RH, et al. Confocal scanning laser ophthalmoscope. *Appl Optom.* 1987;26:1492–1499.

Thyroid Eye Disease

Anderson RL, Linberg JV. Transorbital approach to decompression in Graves' disease. *Arch Ophthalmol.* 1981; 99:120–124.

Bullock JD, Bartley GB. Dynamic proptosis. *Am J Ophthalmol.* 1986;102:104–110.

Dallow RL. Ultrasonography of the orbit. *Int Ophthalmol Clin.* 1986;26:51–76.

Dixon RS, et al. The use of thymoxamine in eyelid retraction. *Arch Ophthalmol.* 1979;97:2147–2150.

Dunn WJ, et al. Botulinum toxin for the treatment of dysthyroid ocular myopathy. *Ophthalmology.* 1986;93: 470–475.

Fells P, McCarry B. Diplopia in thyroid eye disease. *Trans Ophthalmol Soc UK.* 1986;105:413–423.

Frueh BR, et al. Exophthalmometer readings in patients with Graves' eye disease. *Ophthal Surg.* 1986;17:37–40.

Gamblin GT, et al. Prevalence of increased intraocular pressure in Graves' disease—Evidence of frequent subclinical ophthalmopathy. *N Engl J Med.* 1983;308:420–424.

Gasser P, Flammer J. Optic neuropathy of Graves' disease. A report of a perimetric follow-up. *Ophthalmologica.* 1986;192:22–27.

Gay AJ, Wolkstein MA. Topical guanethidine therapy for endocrine lid retraction. *Arch Ophthalmol.* 1966;76:364–367.

Hornblass A, et al. Orbital lymphoid tumors located predominantly within extraocular muscles. *Ophthalmology.* 1987;94:688–697.

Hurbli T, et al. Radiation therapy for thyroid eye disease. *Am J Ophthalmol.* 1985;99:633–637.

Leib MC. Computed tomography of the orbit. *Int Ophthalmol Clin.* 1986;26:103–121.

Leone CR. The management of ophthalmic Graves' disease. *Ophthalmology.* 1984;91:770–779.

Putterman AM, Fett DR. Muller's muscle in the treatment of upper eyelid retraction: A 12-year study. *Ophthal Surg.* 1986;17:361–367.

Ravin JG, et al. Orbital radiation for the ocular changes of Graves' disease. *Am J Ophthalmol.* 1975;79:285–288.

Riddick FA. Update on thyroid diseases. *Ophthalmology.* 1981;88:467–470.

Rush JA, Older JJ. Graves' orbitopathy and the thyrotropin-releasing hormone (TRH) test. *J Clin Neuro-ophthalmol.* 1981;1:219–224.

Sergott RC, Glaser JS. Graves' ophthalmopathy. A clinical and immunologic review. *Surv Ophthalmol.* 1981;26:1–21.

Spencer CA. Clinical utility of sensitive TSH assays. *Thyroid Today.* 1986;9:1–8.

Surks MI. Assessment of thyroid function. *Ophthalmology.* 1981;88:476–478.

Walsh TE, Ogura JH. Transantral orbital decompression for malignant exophthalmos. *Laryngoscope.* 1957;67:544–568.

Werner SC. Modification of the classification of the eye changes of Graves' disease. *Am J Ophthalmol.* 1977;83: 725–727.

Orbital Inflammatory Pseudotumor

Atkin SR. Orbital pseudotumor, differential diagnosis. *Optom Vis Sci.* 1990;67:840–844.

Friedberg MA, Rapuano CJ. *Wills Eye Hospital Office and Emergency Room Diagnosis and Treatment of Eye Disease.* Philadelphia: Lippincott; 1990.

Newman NM, ed. *Neuro-ophthalmology. A Practical Text.* Norwalk; CT: Appleton & Lange; 1992.

Inflammatory Optic Neuropathy

Boghen D, et al. Paraneoplastic optic neuritis and encephalomyelitis. *Arch Neurol.* 1988;45:353–356.

Fraunfelder FT, Roy FH. *Current Ocular Therapy.* Philadelphia: Saunders; 1980.

Gupta DR, Strobas RJ. Bilateral papillitis associated with Cafergot therapy. *Neurology.* 1972;22:793–797.

Newman NM. *Neuro-ophthalmology. A Practical Text.* Philadelphia: Lippincott; 1992: chaps 4 and 5.

Nikoskelainen E. Symptoms, signs, and early course of optic neuritis. *Acta Ophthalmol.* 1975;53:254–271.

Parmley JVC, et al. Does neuroretinitis rule out multiple sclerosis? *Arch Ophthalmol.* 1987;44:1045–1048.

Perkin GD, Rose FC. *Optic Neuritis and Its Differential Diagnosis.* New York: Oxford University Press; 1979.

Smith JL. *The Optic Nerve.* Miami: Neuro-Ophthalmology Tapes; 1977.

Spalton DJ, Hitchings RA, Hunter PA. *Atlas of Clinical Ophthalmology.* London: Gower; 1984.

Spencer WH. *Ophthalmic Pathology. An Atlas and Textbook.* Philadelphia: Saunders; 1986.

Spoor TC. *Modern Management of Ocular Diseases.* Thorofare, NJ: Slack; 1985.

Walsh FB, Hoyt WF. *Clinical Neuro-ophthalmology.* 3rd ed. Baltimore: Williams & Wilkins; 1969.

Yanoff M, Fine BS. *Ocular Pathology. A Text and Atlas.* Hagerstown, MD: Harper & Row; 1975.

Demyelinating Optic Neuropathy

Beck RW, Cleary PA, Anderson MM, et al. A randomized, controlled trial of corticosteroids in the treatment of acute optic neuritis. The Optic Neuritis Study Group. *N Engl J Med.* 1992;326:581–588.

Beck RW, Cleary PA. The Optic Neuritis Study Group. Optic Neuritis Treatment Trial. *Arch Ophthalmol.* 1993;111: 773–775.

Chrousos GA, Kattah JC, Beck RW, et al. Side effects of glucocorticoid treatment. Experience in the optic neuritis treatment trial. *JAMA.* 1993;269:2110–2112.

Dutton JJ, et al. Autoimmune retrobulbar neuritis. *Am J Opththalmol.* 1982;94:11–17.

Goldstein JE, Cogan DG. Exercise and the optic neuropathy of multiple sclerosis. *Arch Ophthalmol.* 1964;72:168–170.

Griffin JF, Wray SH. Acquired color vision defects in retrobulbar neuritis. *Am J Ophthalmol.* 1978;86:193–201.

Hammond SR, et al. The epidemiology of multiple sclerosis in three Australian cities: Perth, Newcastle, and Hobart. *Brain.* 1988;111:1–26.

Killian JM, et al. Controlled pilot trial of monthly IV cyclophosphamide in multiple sclerosis. *Arch Neurol.* 1988;45:27–30.

Miller DH, et al. MRI of the optic nerve in optic neuritis. *Neurology.* 1988;38:175–179.

Newman NM. *Neuro-ophthalmology. A Practical Text.* Philadelphia: Lippincott; 1992: chaps 4 and 5.

Nikoskelainen E. Symptoms, signs and early course of optic neuritis. *Acta Ophthalmol.* 1975;53:254–271.

Perkin GD, Rose FC. *Optic Neuritis and Its Differential Diagnosis.* New York: Oxford University Press; 1979.

Perkin GD, Rose FC. Uhthoff's syndrome. *Br J Ophthalmol.* 1976;60:60–63.

Rizzo JF, Lessell S. Risk of developing multiple sclerosis after uncomplicated optic neuritis. *Neurology.* 1988;38:185–190.

Rudick RA, et al. Relative diagnostic value of cerebrospinal fluid kappa chains in MS: Comparison with other immunoglobulin tests. *Neurology.* 1989;39:964–968.

Slamovits TL, et al. What to tell the patient with optic neuritis about multiple sclerosis. *Surv Ophthalmol.* 1991;35:47–50.

Sokol S. The Pulfrich stereo-illusion as an index of optic nerve dysfunction. *Surv Ophthalmol.* 1976;20:432–434.

Spalton DJ, Hitchings RA, Hunter PA. *Atlas of Clinical Ophthalmology.* London: Gower; 1984.

Spencer WH. *Ophthalmic Pathology. An Atlas and Textbook.* Philadelphia: Saunders; 1986.

Spoor TC. *Modern Management of Ocular Diseases.* Thorofare, NJ: Slack; 1985.

Walsh FB, Hoyt WF. *Clinical Neuro-ophthalmology.* 3rd ed. Baltimore: Williams & Wilkins; 1969.

Yanoff M, Fine BS. *Ocular Pathology. A Text and Atlas.* Hagerstown, MD: Harper & Row; 1975.

Nonarteritic Anterior Ischemic Optic Neuropathy

Boghen DR, Glaser JS. Ischemic optic neuropathy. *Brain.* 1975;98:689–708.

Boke W, Voigt CJ. Circulatory disturbances of the optic nerve. *Ophthalmologia.* 1980;180:88–100.

Flaharty PM, Sergott RC, Lieb W, et al. Optic nerve sheath decompression may improve blood flow in anterior ischemic optic neuropathy. *Ophthalmology.* 1993;100:297–302.

Hayreh SS. *Anterior Ischemic Optic Neuropathy.* New York: Springer-Verlag; 1975.

Hayreh SS. Anterior ischemic optic neuropathy, III. Treatment, prophylaxis, and differential diagnosis. *Br J Ophthalmol.* 1974;58:981–989.

Miller NR. Anterior ischemic optic neuropathy: Diagnosis and management. *Bull NY Acad Med.* 1980;56:643–654.

Quigley H, Anderson DR. Cupping of the optic disc in ischemic optic neuropathy. *Trans Am Acad Ophthalmol Otolaryngol.* 1977;83:755–762.

Spoor TC, McHenry JG, Lau-Sickon L. Progressive and static nonarteritic ischemic optic neuropathy treated by optic nerve sheath decompression. *Ophthalmology.* 1993;100:306–311.

Spoor TC. *Modern Management of Ocular Diseases.* Thorofare, NJ: Slack; 1985.

Arteritic Ischemic Optic Neuropathy

Behn AR, et al. Polymyalgia rheumatica and corticosteroids: How much for how long? *Ann Rheumat Dis.* 1983;42:324–328.

Boghen DR, Glaser JS. Ischemic optic neuropathy. *Brain.* 1975;98:689–708.

Boke W, Voigt CJ. Circulatory disturbances of the optic nerve. *Ophthalmologia.* 1980;180:88–100.

Fraunfelder FT, Roy FH. *Current Ocular Therapy.* Philadelphia: Saunders; 1980.

Hayreh SS. *Anterior Ischemic Optic Neuropathy.* New York: Springer-Verlag; 1975.

Hayreh SS. Anterior ischemic optic neuropathy, III. Treatment, prophylaxis, and differential diagnosis. *Br J Ophthalmol.* 1974;58:981–989.

Huston KA. Temporal arteritis: A 25 year epidemiological, clinical and pathological study. *Ann Int Med.* 1978;88:162–167.

Miller NR. Anterior ischemic optic neuropathy: Diagnosis and management. *Bull NY Acad Med.* 1980;56:643–654.

Mosher HA. The prognosis in temporal arteritis. *Arch Ophthalmol.* 1959;62:641–644.

Nikoskelainen E. Symptoms, signs and early course of optic neuritis. *Acta Ophthalmol.* 1975;53:254–271.

Rosenfeld SI, et al. Treatment of temporal arteritis with ocular involvement. *Am J Med.* 1986;80:143–145.

Spalton DJ, Hitchings RA, Hunter PA. *Atlas of Clinical Ophthalmology.* London: Gower; 1984.

Spencer WH. *Ophthalmic Pathology. An Atlas and Textbook.* Philadelphia: Saunders; 1986.

Diabetic Ischemic Optic Neuropathy (Diabetic Papillopathy)

Appen RE, et al. Diabetic papillopathy. *Am J Ophthalmol.* 1980;90:203–209.

Boghen DR, Glaser JS. Ischemic optic neuropathy. *Brain.* 1975;98:689–708.

Hayreh SS. *Anterior Ischemic Optic Neuropathy.* New York: Springer-Verlag; 1975.

Perkin GD, Rose FC. *Optic Neuritis and Its Differential Diagnosis.* New York: Oxford University Press; 1979.

Papillophlebitis

Appen RE, et al. Optic disc vasculitis. *Am J Ophthalmol.* 1980;90:352–359.

Ellenberger C, Messner KH. Papillophlebitis: Benign retinopathy resembling papilledema or papillitis. *Ann Neurol.* 1978;3:438–440.

Fletcher WA, et al. Acute idiopathic blind spot enlargement. A big blind spot syndrome without optic disc edema. *Arch Ophthalmol.* 1988;106:44–49.

Fong ACO, et al. Central retinal vein occlusion in young adults (papillophlebitis). *Retina.* 1991;11:3–11.

Fraunfelder FT, Roy FH. *Current Ocular Therapy.* Philadelphia: Saunders; 1980.

Frucht J, et al. Central retinal vein occlusions in young adults. *Acta Ophthalmol.* 1984;62:780–786.

Gittinger JW. Unilateral blurred vision and dilated veins. *Surv Ophthalmol.* 1987;31:270–276.

Hamed LM, et al. Protracted enlargement of the blind spot in multiple evanescent white dot syndrome. *Arch Ophthalmol.* 1989;107;194–198.

Hayreh SS. Optic disc vasculitis. *Br J Ophthalmol.* 1972;56: 652–670.

Laibovitz RA. Presumed phlebitis of the optic disc. *Ophthalmology.* 1979;86:313–319.

Rosenberg ML, et al. Idiopathic unilateral disc edema: The big blind spot syndrome. *J Clin Neuro-Ophthalmol.* 1984;14: 181–184.

Singh K, et al. Acute idiopathic blind spot enlargement. *Ophthalmology.* 1991;98:497–502.

Wakakura M, Furuno K. Bilateral slowly progressive big blind spot syndrome. *J Clin Neuro-Ophthalmol.* 1989;9: 141–143.

Toxic Optic Neuropathy

Fraunfelder FT. *Drug-induced Ocular Side Effects and Drug Interactions.* 2nd ed. Philadelphia: Lea & Febiger; 1982.

Hayreh MS, et al. Methyl alcohol poisoning, III. Ocular toxicity. *Arch Ophthalmol.* 1977;95:1851–1858.

Knox DL, et al. Nutritional amblyopia, folic acid, vitamin B_{12} and other vitamins. *Retina.* 1982;2:287–293.

Leopold IH. Optic nerve: Drug-induced optic atrophy. In: Fraunfelder FT, Roy FH, eds. *Current Ocular Therapy.* Philadelphia: Saunders; 1980.

Leopold IH. Zinc deficiency and visual impairment? *Am J Ophthalmol.* 1978;85:871–878. Editorial.

Lessel S. Toxic and deficiency optic neuropathies. In: Smith JL, ed. *Neuro-ophthalmology.* St. Louis: Mosby; 1973.

Martin-Amat G, et al. Methyl alcohol poisoning, II. Development of a model for ocular toxicity in methyl alcohol poison using the rhesus monkey. *Arch Ophthalmol.* 1977;95:1847–1850.

Papilledema

Bird AC, Sanders MO. Choroidal folds in association with papilledema. *Br J Ophthalmol.* 1973;57:89–97.

Boddie HG, Banna M, et al. "Benign" intracranial hypertension: A survey of the clinical and radiological features, and long-term prognosis. *Brain.* 1974;97:313–326.

Corbett JJ. Problems in the diagnosis and treatment of pseudotumor cerebri. *Can J Neurol Sci.* 1983;10:221–229.

Corbett JJ, Thompson HS. The rational management of idiopathic intracranial hypertension. *Arch Neurol.* 1989;46:1049–1051.

Eggers HM, Sanders MD. Acquired optociliary shunts vessels in papilloedema. *Br J Ophthalmol.* 1980;64:267–271.

Freidberg MA, Rapauno CJ. Neuro-ophthalmology. In: *Wills Eye Hospital Office and Emergency Room Diagnosis and Treatment of Eye Disease.* Philadelphia: Lippincott; 1990.

Galvin R, Sanders MD. Peripheral retinal hemorrhages with papilloedema. *Br J Ophthalmol.* 1980;64:262–266.

Guiseffi V, et al. Symptoms and disease associations in idiopathic intracranial hypertension (pseudotumor cerebri): A case control study. *Neurology.* 1991;41:239–244.

Guy J, et al. Treatment of visual loss in pseudotumor cerebri associated with uremia. *Neurology.* 1990;40:28–32.

Hayreh SS. Optic disc edema in raised intracranial pressure. *Arch Ophthalmol.* 1977;95:1553–1565.

Ireland B, et al. The search for causes of idiopathic intracranial hypertension: A preliminary case-control study. *Arch Neurol.* 1990;47:315–320.

Jamison RR. Subretinal neovascularization and papilledema associated with pseudotumor cerebri. *Am J Ophthalmol.* 1978;85:78–81.

Jefferson A, Clark J. Treatment of benign intracranial hypertension by dehydrating agents with particular reference to the measurement of the blind spot area as a means of recording improvement. *J Neurosurg Psychiatry.* 1976; 39:627–639.

Johnson I, Paterson A. Benign intracranial hypertension, I. Diagnosis and prognosis. *Brain.* 1974;97:289–300.

Johnson I, Paterson A. Benign intracranial hypertension, II. CSF pressure and circulation. *Brain.* 1974;97:301–312.

Lobo A, Pilek E, et al. Papilledema following therapeutic dosages of lithium carbonate. *J Nerv Ment Dis.* 1978;166: 526–529.

Matzkin DC, et al. Disc swelling: A tall tail? *Surv Ophthalmol.* 1992:37:130–136.

Newman NM. *Neuro-ophthalmology. A Practical Text.* Philadelphia: Lippincott; 1992: chaps 4 and 5.

Rosenberg MA, Savino PJ, et al. A clinical analysis of pseudopapilledema, I. Population, laterality, acuity, refractive error, ophthalmoscopic characteristics, and coincident disease. *Arch Ophthalmol.* 1979;97:65–70.

Savino PJ, Glaser JS. Pseudopapilledema versus papilledema. *Int Ophthalmol Clin.* 1977;17:115–137.

Savino PJ, Glaser JS, et al. A clinical analysis of pseudopapilledema, II. Visual field defects. *Arch Ophthalmol.* 1979; 97:71–75.

Spalton DJ, Hitchings RA, et al. *Atlas of Clinical Ophthalmology.* London: Gower; 1984.

Spencer WH. *Ophthalmic Pathology. An Atlas and Textbook.* Philadelphia: Saunders; 1986.

Spoor TC. *Modern Management of Ocular Diseases.* Thorofare, NJ: Slack; 1985.

Swanson MW. Spontaneous regression of pregnancy-associated papilledema. *S J Optom.* 1991;9:26–31.

Walsh FB, Hoyt WF. *Clinical Neuro-ophthalmology.* 3rd ed. Baltimore: Williams & Wilkins; 1969.

Wirtschafter JD, Rizzo FJ, et al. Optic nerve axoplasm and papilledema. *Surv Ophthalmol.* 1975;20:157–189.

Yanoff M, Fine BS. *Ocular Pathology. A Text and Atlas.* Hagerstown, MD: Harper & Row; 1975.

Optic Nerve Tumors

Albers GW, et al. Treatment response in malignant optic glioma of adulthood. *Neurology.* 1988;38:1071–1074.

Alvord C, Lofton S. Gliomas of the optic nerv or chiasm: Outcome by patient's age, tumor site and therapy. *J Neurosurg.* 1988;68:85–98.

Archdale TW, Magnus DE. Melanocytoma of the optic disc. *J Am Optom Assoc.* 1993;64:98–103.

Brown GC, Shields J. Tumors of the optic nerve head. *Surv Ophthalmol.* 1985;4:239–262.

Brown GC, Tasman W. *Congenital Anomalies of the Optic Disc.* New York: Grune & Stratton; 1983.

Clark WC, et al. Primary optic nerve sheath meningiomas. *J Neurosurg.* 1989;70:37–40.

Kennerdell JS, et al. Management of optic nerve sheath meningiomas. *Am J Ophthalmol.* 1988;106:450–457.

Kritzinger EE, Beaumont HM. *A Colour Atlas of Optic Disc Abnormalities.* London: Wolfe Medical; 1987: chap 7.

Walsh FB, Hoyt WF. *Clinical Neuro-ophthalmology.* 3rd ed. Baltimore: Williams & Wilkins; 1969.

Wright JE, et al. Optic nerve glioma and the management of optic nerve tumours in the young. *Br J Ophthalmol.* 1989; 73:967–974.

Wright JE, et al. Primary optic nerve sheath meningioma. *Br J Ophthalmol.* 1989;73:960–966.

Chapter Four ■ ■ ■ ■ ■ ■

*R*etinal Vascular Disorders

RETINAL VASCULAR ANATOMY AND PHYSIOLOGY

The retinal tissue has the highest consumption of oxygen by weight of any tissue in the human body. The outer third of the retina is supplied by the choroidal–choriocapillaris system, and the inner two thirds of the retina is supplied by branches of the central retinal artery system. The choroidal system is characterized by fenestrated vessels that allow for a free exchange of fluids, creating a spongelike tissue layer. This system is nutritive but also serves as a cooling system for the retina. The retinal circulation is characterized by vessels that do not leak readily except in diseased conditions.

Basic Embryologic Development

The hyaloid vascular system supplies the eye structures until the fourth month. At that stage, spindle (mesenchymal) cells of Bergmeister's papilla form vascular channels that grow into the nerve fiber layer. This cellular proliferation continues toward the ora serrata in the form of endothelial cords. Clefts then develop in these cords by endothelial cell proliferation. These clefts expand into a profusion of very small vascular channels that spread throughout the retina. The channelization reaches the nasal ora at about the same time as it reaches the temporal equator.

As development continues, larger-caliber vessels are created by redirection of blood flow combined with selective atrophy of a large number of endothelial cords. There remains a vascular-free zone around the larger vessels in adulthood, wider around arteries than around veins. The retinal vasculature is the last of retinal structures to develop and does not stop until about 3 months after full gestation. Retinal capillaries do not attain maturity for several years, as evidenced by the fact that intramural pericytes only begin to appear at birth.

The Arteries

The central retinal artery along with a cilioretinal artery (25 percent of the population) serves as the blood supply to the inner retina. The central retinal artery is a branch of the ophthalmic artery derived from the internal carotid system. The central retinal artery has a smooth muscle layer as it passes through the optic nerve, and can be affected by diseases of other muscular arteries, such as cranial arteritis. The central retinal artery loses the internal elastic lamina as it passes into the retina. Arteriosclerosis that involves intimal and endothelial hyperplasia may occur within the optic nerve and retinal portion of the arteries. As the artery passes through the lamina cribrosa, there is a focal constriction that can serve as a site for embolic occlusion.

As mentioned previously, the arteries within the retina are devoid of elastic lamina but have well-developed smooth muscle. The vessels diminish in caliber toward the retinal periphery to come within about 1.5 mm of the ora. Throughout the retinal tissue, the arteries maintain a strong barrier to perfusion of blood components. Diseased vascular states alter this tight-walled construction, allowing for leakage and intraretinal edema. Intraretinal arteries are not affected by either sympathetic or parasympathetic innervation.

Arteries lie in the nerve fiber or ganglion cell layer, with strong connections to the internal limiting membrane. This strong adhesion may become an important factor in the genesis of retinal hemorrhage. The arteries are insulated from retinal tissue by the glial perivascular limiting membrane of Kruckmann.

Grossly, the arteries appear less tortuous and of a smaller diameter than the veins. The blood column is a brighter red because of the oxygenation of the blood. The central retinal artery typically enters nasally to the central retinal vein and bifurcates above the nerve head. Arteries typically cross over veins and find their deepest penetration into retinal tissue at this point. There are supposedly no arteriovenous shunts in the retina, and with the exception of the congenital macrovessel, the arteries and veins usually do not cross the horizontal raphe.

The Veins

The veins are all thin walled with abundant elastic tissue, and are very subject to compression by any outside source. Near the nerve head, the vein walls contain muscle cells that disappear toward the periphery, being replaced by pericytes. The lack of definitive wall structure allows for the variable appearance (sausaging and distention) in diseased conditions. The veins have isolated attachments to retinal structure, contributing to the serpentine appearance in vaso-occlusion. The same glial insulating structure exists with veins as with arteries. An anatomic variation may occur in which the central retinal vein bifurcates retrolaminarly and enters the intraocular region as two separate vessels. This anatomic variation is thought to be one explanation for hemicentral retinal vein occlusions.

The central retinal vein represents the drain for the retinal vascular watershed. When this drain is closed at the lamina or retrolaminarly, a shunt may develop between the central retinal vein and the choroidal system, which is known as an optociliary shunt. At the lamina, as with the central retinal artery, there is compression of the vein or a stricture during passage. This compression is an area for potential turbulence and thrombus deposition, with the possibility of development of a central retinal vein occlusion.

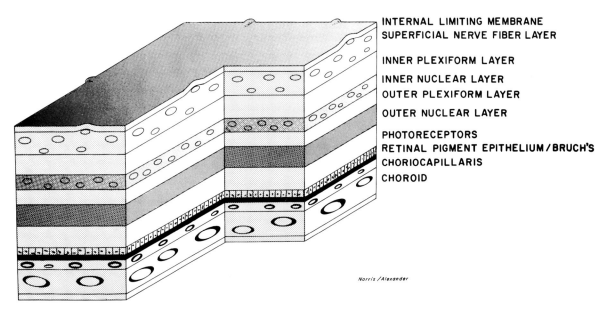

INTERNAL LIMITING MEMBRANE
SUPERFICIAL NERVE FIBER LAYER

INNER PLEXIFORM LAYER
INNER NUCLEAR LAYER
OUTER PLEXIFORM LAYER
OUTER NUCLEAR LAYER

PHOTORECEPTORS
RETINAL PIGMENT EPITHELIUM/BRUCH'S
CHORIOCAPILLARIS
CHOROID

Norris / Alexander

Figure 4–1. A schematic cross section of the normal retina with representation of vascular locations.

At artery–vein crossings, there is a merging of arterial adventitia and venous glial coverings. This sharing of tissue results in compression of the vein wall when the arterial wall develops atherosclerotic changes. The compression is variously interpreted as artery–vein crossing changes, with the ultimate example being branch retinal vein occlusion. The venous system extends to within about 1.5 mm of the ora serrata.

The Capillaries

The capillaries spread throughout the retina in two networks. The superficial network runs in the superficial nerve fiber layer and the ganglion cell layer. The superficial network is of a loose arrangement and is considered the postarteriolar network. The superficial network is most often affected in arterial-based diseases. The deep network runs primarily in the inner nuclear layer, is tightly packed, and is considered prevenular. The deep capillary layer is most often affected in congestive venous-based diseases such as diabetes and vein occlusions (Fig. 4–1). Three zones of the retina are known to vary from this basic scheme. In the circumpapillary zone, there may be four capillary layers, the most superficial of which is the radial peripapillary capillaries, which originate from precapillary retinal arterioles and drain into intraretinal venules on the nerve head. These capillaries are long and pursue a straight path along the superior and inferior temporal arcades out 2 disc diameters but not involving the macula. Figure 4–2 demonstrates the distribution pattern of the radial peripapillary arteries. There is no anastamosis of the radial peripapillary bed with other capillary beds, implying that infarction

in this area could create a scotoma. The radial peripapillaries have been implicated in the genesis of glaucomatous field defects, flame-shaped hemorrhages, and cotton-wool spots. In the zone near the ora and in the perifoveal region, the capillary net thins to one layer.

Three areas of the retina are devoid of capillaries. Near the ora serrata, there are no capillaries. This anatomical fact plays strongly in the development of peripheral neovascular development. There is a capillary-free zone 0.5 mm wide centered at the fovea. There is also a capillary-free perivascular zone throughout the retina that is larger around the arteries.

The basic capillary structure is that of endothelial cells, intramural pericytes, and basement membrane.

RADIAL PERIPAPILLARY DISTRIBUTION

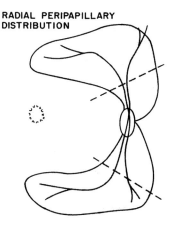

Figure 4–2. A schematic representing the proposed distribution pattern of the superficial radial peripapillary arteries.

Even with a simplistic structure, the walls form a tight barrier to passage of fluids (blood–retinal barrier) such that metabolic transfer is achieved through pinocytotic vesicle transfer. The pericytes display necrosis in some ischemic vascular disorders, such as diabetes. This loss of pericytes may be the initiating step in microaneurysm formation and possibly shunt formation, especially in the genesis of diabetic retinopathy.

With age, peripheral vessels lose endothelial cells and pericytes. When both are compromised, the capillary shuts down. Dilatation of adjacent capillaries, shunts, and microaneurysms occur as a normal aging process in the peripheral retina secondary to capillary death. Often this will appear as isolated hemorrhaging in the aged peripheral retina.

The Choroid and Choriocapillaris

Any discussion of the choroid–choriocapillaris complex must include the retinal pigment epithelium and Bruch's membrane.

Retinal Pigment Epithelium. The retinal pigment epithelium (RPE) is a single layer of heavily pigmented cuboidal cells extending from the optic nerve head to the ora serrata. Anterior to the ora, the layer continues but becomes the pigmented epithelium of the ciliary body. The density of the intracellular melanin determines the relative degree of pigmentation. There is a space between the RPE and the photoreceptors filled with mucopolysaccharide glue that can be altered by liquefied vitreous, allowing for a breakdown of the structure. The RPE is loosely adherent to the overlying sensory retina. The pigment cells are tightly adherent to one another in an area known as the zonula occludens. Breaks in the zonnula occludens allow fluid to leak upward underneath the retina from the choroid choriocapillaris structure. The basement membrane of the RPE and the fibers of the inner collagenous zone of Bruch's membrane form a very strong bond.

The RPE serves as a barrier between the sensory retina and the choroid. It processes metabolites for the retina and absorbs and neutralizes the potential toxic effects of short-wavelength light. A break in the RPE can cause sensory retinal detachments.

Bruch's Membrane. Bruch's membrane extends from the optic nerve head to the ora serrata as a multilayered structure. It continues beyond the ora with modification characterized by absence of the elastic layer. The innermost layer is the basement membrane of the RPE. The inner collagenous zone is the thickest layer covered by the elastic layer. The outer collagenous zone becomes continuous with the choroidal zone to become a structural framework for the cho-

riocapillaris. The basement membrane of the choriocapillaris envelops the structure. With age, Bruch's membrane develops vesicles, holes, and calcific foci that may allow leakage into the zone under the sensory retina or may allow for the development of choroidal neovascular membranes.

Choriocapillaris. The choriocapillaris is the capillary bed of the choroidal system. The vessels are of larger caliber than retinal capillaries and are fenestrated, which creates a wet sponge effect under Bruch's membrane. The short posterior ciliary arteries, the recurrent branches of the long posterior ciliary arteries, and branches of the anterior ciliary arteries feed this system. Drainage of the system is provided by venules that eventually drain into the vortex vein ampulla scattered about the equator.

The greatest hemodynamic activity in the retina occurs at the foveal area. As a result, the choriocapillaris is densest in this area. It is important to realize that the choriocapillaris blood supply in this area is compartmentalized as it is in the periphery. A feeder vessel supplies a particular zone, and there is limited anastomoses of the vascular system. An infarct of this vessel creates a window defect of the retinal pigment epithelium and loss of photoreceptor function because of the loss of the nutrient supply. This infarct is known as Elschnig spots (Fig. 4–3). Elschnig spots reflect acute hypertensive alterations of the choroidal vascular system, especially in younger patients whose blood vessel system is not yet sclerotic enough to resist spikes in blood pressure. Siegrist's streaks are radially oriented chains of pigmented spots along scle-

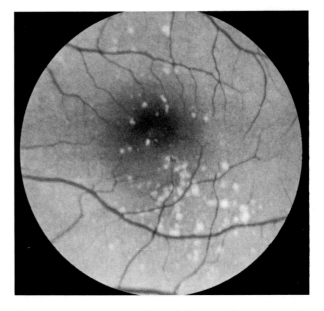

Figure 4–3. Photograph of focal infarcts of the choriocapillaris (Elschnig spots).

rosed choroidal vessels emanating from the disc and usually confined to the posterior pole. These linear RPE disruptions are associated with the choroidal vascular sclerosis in spiking hypertensive events creating tissue alterations. The histopathologic equivalent in the peripheral retina is primary chorioretinal atrophy, or pavingstone degeneration.

Choroid. The choroid proper is composed of larger blood vessels, nerves, melanocytes, immune system cells, and extensions of the collagenous supporting tissue of Bruch's membrane. The larger blood vessels are branches of feeder arteries and drainage veins that support the choriocapillaris. Again, as with the choriocapillaris, there is limited anastomosis of vessels. There is a nervous supply to this vascular system that has been identified as sympathetic-like cells. The immunologic cells represent a source for the genesis of inflammatory retinal disease, such as presumed ocular histoplasmosis.

The choroid supplies nutrition to the RPE and outer third of the retina and serves as a method of dispersion of heat generated by light absorption of the RPE and metabolic activity of the retina.

Basic Physiology of Retinal Vessels

The ophthalmic artery has sympathetic innervation up to the eye, but there is no sympathetic retinal vessel control within the eye. Retinal vascular changes occur secondary to local metabolic regulation. Adult retinal vessels are narrowed when exposed to excessive oxygen, whereas vasodilatation and hemorrhaging occur at low oxygen concentrations.

The flow of blood within the vessels is faster at the center of the vessels than at the walls. In veins, the blood returning from the periphery flows along the walls, whereas blood from the posterior pole flows through the center of the vein. This gives rise to the laminar flow apparent in fluorescein angiography.

Venous pulsation is present in most adult eyes, and its incidence increases with age because of increased intraocular pressure as well as increased systemic blood pressure. Venous pulsation is determined by the ventricular rate, and can therefore show alterations during cardiac arrythmia. Venous pulsation may be diminished or absent with (1) decreased intraocular pressure, (2) central retinal vein occlusion, (3) mechanical elevation of venous pressure, (4) increased intracranial pressure, and (5) any localized external pressure at the wall of the central retinal vein.

Arterial pulsation is an unusual finding in the adult eye. For arterial pulsation to occur, intraocular pressure must be raised above ophthalmic artery pressure (glaucoma) or ophthalmic artery pressure must be lowered below intraocular pressure (internal carotid stenosis). In any case, arterial pulsation at the nerve head is often indicative of an underlying disease condition. A serpentine pulsation—rhythmic lateral arterial movements—may be seen in retinal vessels and is not necessarily indicative of vascular disease.

THE BASICS OF PHOTOCOAGULATION

General Principles

Laser (*light amplification by stimulated emission of radiation*) photocoagulation is used to treat retinal vascular disease by its effect on the alteration of ocular tissue. The tissue is altered by varying wavelength and intensity of radiation and is dependent on the absorption characteristics of the retinal tissue and the scatter of that light by the ocular media. The effects on tissue include photochemical effects, thermal effects, thermal relaxation, vaporization, and optical breakdown. With the photochemical effect, there is ultraviolet and visible light absorption, which converts the absorbing molecule into toxic molecules such as free radicals. The excimer laser cuts tissue by directly breaking organic molecular bonds. Thermal effects result from visible and infrared absorption by tissue pigment that denatures the protein in the absorbing tissue. Pigment absorbers in the retina are shown in Table 4–1.

Thermal relaxation results as heat created by a laser burn is dissipated away from the burn. The larger the spot, the more heat is created. Usually when doubling the spot size, the power only needs to be increased by a factor of two because of the thermal relaxation. Vaporization of tissue is the result of a microexplosion occurring when water achieves the boiling point. This occurs when using the carbon dioxide laser or in a very heavy argon burn. Optical breakdown results from the application of the neodynium:yttrium-aluminum-garnet (Nd:YAG) laser,

TABLE 4–1. ACTIONS OF PIGMENT ABSORBERS IN THE OCULAR TISSUE

Pigment Type	Actions
Xanthophyll	Located in the inner and outer plexiform layers. Maximally absorbs blue light
Hemoglobin	Oxyhemoglobin has poorer red absorption than deoxyhemoglobin. Hemoglobin absorbs blue, green, and yellow (best absorption)
Melanin	Located in melanosomes of retinal pigment epithelium and in melanocytes of choroid. Absorbs most of the visible wavelengths

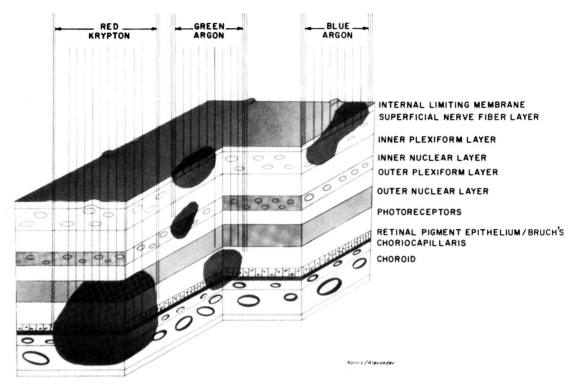

Figure 4–4. Tissue penetration by laser light of various wavelengths (shading indicates the site of the burn).

creating plasma formation leading to a shock wave that physically disrupts the tissue.

High-energy (short-wavelength) photons in the laser dissociate or ionize, disrupting DNA and RNA, which leads to cell death. Photons in the longer wavelengths (low energy) cause vibration and bending of molecules and thermal changes, resulting in cell death. Visible wavelength photons cause thermal damage to the incident cell, resulting in vaporization of intracellular and extracellular fluid and cell death. In all wavelengths, the surrounding tissue is spared as the thermal change is localized, and heat

TABLE 4–2. CHARACTERISTICS OF LASERS USED IN OPHTHALMIC DISEASES

Commonly Used Lasers in Retinal Vascular Disease	Wavelength	Molecule and Tissue Absorption Characteristics	Clinical Use
Green argon	514.5 nm	Hemoglobin	Penetration of media and retina without thermal damage
		Oxyhemoglobin	Minimal xanthophyll absorption
		Melanin	Problem with blood vessel absorption
		Pigment epithelium	Used in hemorrhagic retinal disease
			Retinal tears and holes
			Retinoschisis
Blue argon	488 nm	Vitreous	Used to treat retinal hemorrhagic disease
		Crystalline lens	Retinoschisis
		Hemoglobin	Retinal tears or holes
		Oxyhemoglobin	
		Melanin	
		Pigment epithelium	
		Xanthophyll pigment	
Red krypton	647.1 nm	85% choroid	Penetrates cataracts and cloudy media
		15% retinal pigment epithelium	Passes through hemorrhage and retinal vessels
			Passes through xanthophyll
			Treatment of choroidal neovascularization
			Treatment of retinal tears

dissipates rapidly when proper burns have been applied.

Pulsed laser energy is also effective in altering structure because a dramatic increase in tissue temperature occurs over a short time frame. The target tissue is treated without altering the surrounding structures. Optical breakdown is the microexplosion that results from pulsed photocoagulation. This can create tissue destruction without thermal change and protein destruction.

Proper photocoagulation depends on effective transmission through the ocular media. It is well known that in the aging eye, transmission in all wavelengths is severely depressed. This reduction in transmission is especially apparent in the shorter wavelengths. To offset the scattering and achieve therapeutic effect at the retinal site, the laser intensity and spot size must be increased. Any time a spot size is increased, however, there is the chance of damaging surrounding retinal tissue that is not intended to be treated. This is of special importance near the fovea, because the presence of the yellowish xanthophyll pigment naturally attracts blue wavelengths, enhancing the chances of photochemical and thermal damage to the photoreceptors.

Absorption of the laser wavelengths assists in the therapeutic effect. Most absorption occurs within the melanin-containing retinal structures and blood vessels containing different hemoglobins. Figure 4–4 summarizes absorption characteristics of different lasers within the retina. Table 4–2 summarizes the characteristics of the lasers used in retinal work. Figures 4–5 through 4–7 illustrate the characteristics of the tissues affected by the application of laser to the retina. New work in dye lasers offers the possibility of improved success rates in laser treatment.

Types of Lasers

The development of lasers is difficult to follow. However, the following types represent the current state of the art. Argon blue-green lasers represent a spectrum of wavelengths from 457.9 to 528.7 nm but are about 70 percent blue (488 nm). The blue-green argon is absorbed by the inner retina, hemoglobin, and melanin. Because of the dominance of the blue, there is considerable scatter by the media, especially with aging. There is also considerable damage to the surrounding retina due to retinal scattering and xanthophyll pigment absorption of the blue wavelengths.

Argon green laser has a wavelength of 514.5 nm, which is well absorbed by melanin and hemoglobin but only minimally absorbed by the inner retina. Because of the minimal effect on xanthophyll pigment within the macular area, use of this wavelength is popular for lesions near the fovea.

Krypton red laser has a wavelength of 647.1 nm and is well absorbed by melanin but minimally absorbed by hemoglobin (hemorrhages) and xantho-

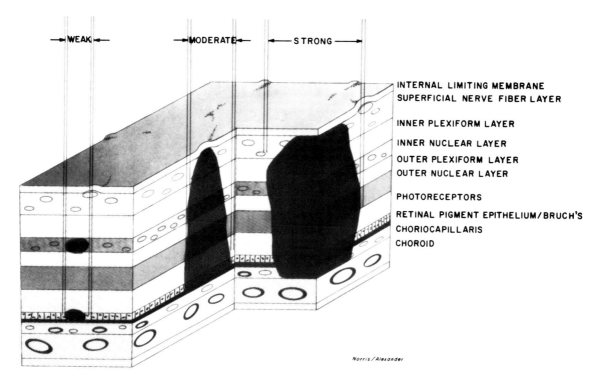

Figure 4–5. Retinal tissue effects of varying intensities of blue-green argon laser burns.

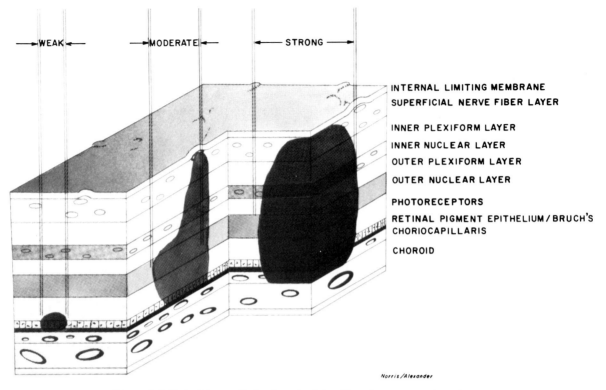

Figure 4–6. Retinal tissue effects of varying intensities of green argon laser burns.

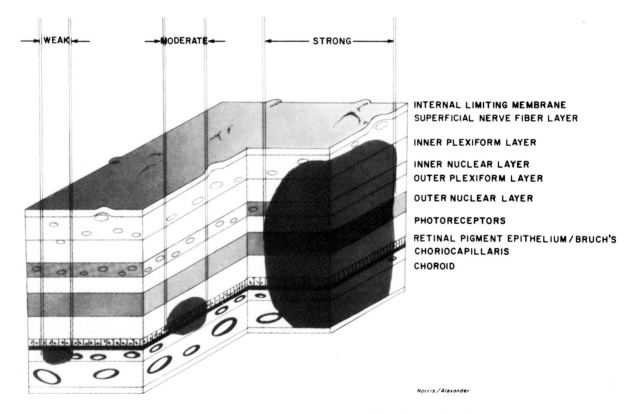

Figure 4–7. Retinal tissue effects of varying intensities of krypton laser burns.

phyll (minimal thermal effect near the fovea). The minimal absorption by hemoglobin and xanthophyll make this wavelength especially useful for treating choroidal neovascular membranes near the fovea. Krypton is also useful in hazy media because it is only minimally scattered. Unfortunately, the krypton laser can create problems in the choroid, such as choroidal hemorrhage, because of its ease of penetration.

The dye laser (tunable wavelengths) transmits a yellow 560 to 580 nm) or orange (580 to 610 nm) wavelength. The yellows are absorbed by oxyhemoglobin, deoxyhemoglobin, and melanin but are minimally scattered and are not absorbed by xanthophyll. The orange range penetrates hemorrhage, and is less painful than the red krypton, but may lead to retinal damage close to the fovea. The current usage is usually limited to panretinal photocoagulation when a vitreous hemorrhage creates problems for the blue and green spectrum lasers.

Effects of Lasers on Specific Conditions

Lasers may be used to treat a variety of ocular conditions and the effect varies among the conditions. When applied to retinal vascular anomalies the laser actually heats the lesion, resulting in clotting and thrombosis of the tissue leading to scarification.

Scatter photocoagulation results in a direct destruction of ischemic (hypoxic) retina. This destruction is thought to suppress the vasoproliferative stimulus, resulting in prevention or regression of neovascularization in the uveal structure. Another theory is that the photocoagulation results in a release of a neovascularization inhibitor found in the retinal pigment epithelium.

Photocoagulation to create a regression of macular edema is based on direct closure of specific leaking vascular structures such as telangiectasia or microaneurysms or on alteration of retinal structure such as that created by a grid pattern. The grid application of photocoagulation is thought to result in the removal of dysfunctional RPE cells, resulting in an enhanced blood retinal barrier system, or the alteration in inner retinal oxygen demands, which creates vasoconstriction limiting vascular leakage. The reason for the success of grid application is evasive; nevertheless, it works.

The success of photocoagulation in idiopathic central serous choroidopathy (ICSC) is the result of either direct photocoagulation of a defined site of leakage creating an RPE sealing effect, or indirect effects creating a channel for the drainage of subretinal fluid into the choriocapillaris.

Photocoagulation of choroidal neovascular membranes enjoys variable success. The membrane may be directly treated, resulting in coagulation and destruction of the membrane. The feeder vessels may also be treated to minimize development of the membrane and in some cases cause regression. As with ICSC, there may be resorption of the subretinal fluid through the RPE.

Photocoagulation of retinal breaks creates chorioretinal scarring around the break. This seals the retina from the vitreous cavity. The total scarification takes several weeks, and activity should be limited in the reparative phase.

In all cases of photocoagulation, it must be remembered that there is the threat of complication as there is tissue destruction, especially in the RPE–Bruch's membrane area, allowing for future development of dry or wet breakdown of the retina in this zone. The patient is also in pain in many instances, has had retrobulbar block, and needs to be on mild analgesics. If severe pain occurs postoperatively, the patient must be seen immediately because of the threat of angle closure glaucoma. The patient's activities must also be limited to avoid bleeding from the compromised tissue until scarification occurs. The patient should be followed closely over the first 2 months in the case of photocoagulation near the macular zone, because of the threat of further development of revascularization or neovascularization.

CLINICOPATHOLOGIC BASIS OF RETINAL VASCULOPATHY

Retinal Hemorrhages

Retinal hemorrhages are not an ocular disease process but rather an ocular manifestation of underlying vascular or blood disease. Hemorrhages are a sign to the clinician that an evaluation of the systemic health of the patient is indicated.

Retinal hemorrhages are discussed here with specific emphasis on cause and management. The practitioner should always remember that the superficial capillary layer in the retina is considered to be postarteriolar, and as such is most often affected by artery-based diseases. Superficial hemorrhages, such as flame-shaped and preretinal hemorrhages, may then be considered as arterial-based hemorrhages. The deeper capillary bed is considered prevenular and is affected most often by vein-based or congestive diseases. Dot-blot hemorrhages are deep in the retina and are considered to be related to congestive retinal diseases, such as central retinal vein occlusion.

Preretinal Hemorrhages. Preretinal hemorrhages (Figs. 4–8 to 4–12) lie just under the internal limiting membrane and in front of the nerve fiber layer. **See color plate 23.** The hemorrhages arise from the superficial capillary system or the radial peripapillary

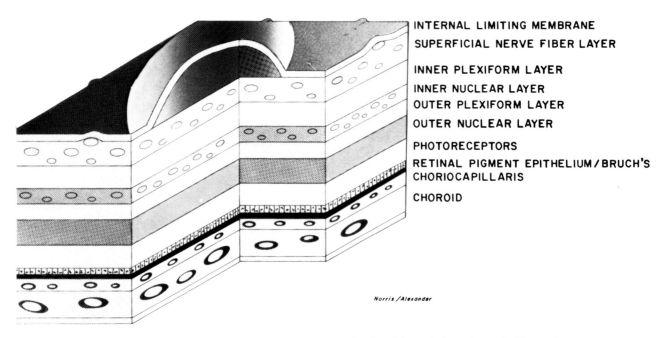

INTERNAL LIMITING MEMBRANE
SUPERFICIAL NERVE FIBER LAYER

INNER PLEXIFORM LAYER
INNER NUCLEAR LAYER
OUTER PLEXIFORM LAYER
OUTER NUCLEAR LAYER

PHOTORECEPTORS
RETINAL PIGMENT EPITHELIUM / BRUCH'S
CHORIOCAPILLARIS

CHOROID

Norris / Alexander

Figure 4–8. Schematic cross section of the retina demonstrating the clinicopathology of preretinal hemorrhages.

system. Preretinal hemorrhages typically occur in the posterior pole and create a positive scotoma. Vision may be severely reduced if preretinal hemorrhages occur in front of the macula. The typical preretinal hemorrhage is about 1 to 2 disc diameters in size, with gravity affecting the appearance. Gravity causes the blood to settle, resulting in darker blood at the bottom of the D-shape or keel-shape and a horizontal clear line demarcating the top of the hemorrhage.

With resolution, the thinner layer at the top clears first. Resolution demonstrates a very specific color change, going from red to yellow to white, and often leaving no trace of the hemorrhage and no compromise of retinal function. The rapidity of resolution depends on the amount of blood within the pocket. The hemorrhage will appear black on a background of choroidal hyperfluorescence with fluorescein angiography.

Preretinal Hemorrhages

Characteristics

Δ Occur between internal limiting membrane and nerve fiber layer
Δ Create a positive scotoma
Δ Gravity creates D-shape
Δ Change red to yellow to white on resorption
Δ Usually related to arterial-based diseases
Δ May occur associated with a posterior vitreous detachment
Δ Do not leak

Management

Δ Ascertain the underlying cause
Δ Allow time for resorption
Δ MUST DETERMINE UNDERLYING SYSTEMIC CAUSE

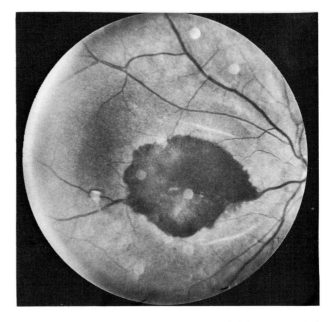

Figure 4–9. Black-and-white photograph of a large preretinal hemorrhage nasal to the optic nerve head.

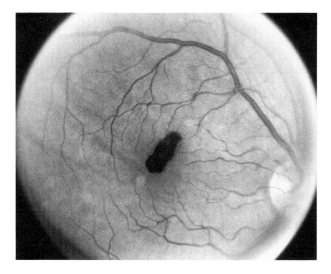

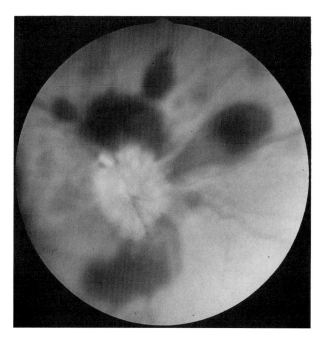

Figure 4–10. Black-and-white photograph of a small preretinal hemorrhage over the macula creating 20/200 vision. The hemorrhage cleared, with resultant 20/20 visual acuity.

A variation of preretinal hemorrhage occurs in what has been called a "thumbprint" pattern, in the posterior pole and about 1 disc diameter in size. It is darkest centrally, with flayed edges and a small central reflex that moves with the viewing angle. Although not specific to any disease, the thumbprint hemorrhage is often associated with pernicious anemia.

Preretinal hemorrhages may be caused by many factors, and it is important to determine the precipitating factor because of systemic disease associations. Table 4–3 shows common causes of preretinal hemor-

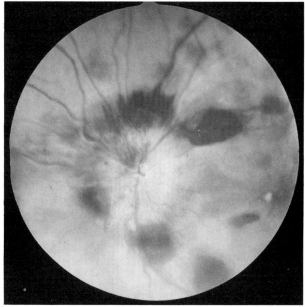

Figure 4–12. Bilateral preretinal hemorrhages surrounding the optic nerve head secondary to a subarachnoid hemorrhage dissecting forward through the optic nerve sheath.

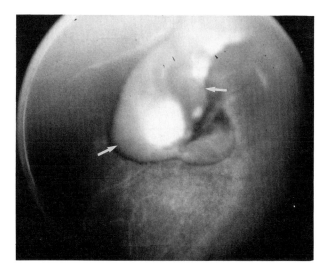

Figure 4–11. A large preretinal hemorrhage (*arrows*) in the stage of color change.

rhages. Determination of the cause is the primary treatment for the preretinal hemorrhage.

Superficial Flame-shaped Hemorrhages. Superficial flame-shaped hemorrhages (Figs. 4–13 and 4–14) originate from the postarteriolar superficial capillary bed or the radial peripapillary capillary system. The flayed or flame-shaped edges result from the blood seeking lines of least resistance in the contour of the

TABLE 4–3. TYPICAL CAUSES OF PRERETINAL HEMORRHAGES

Posterior vitreous detachment, near optic nerve head
Subdural hemorrhage in children
Subarachnoid hemorrhage in adults and children
Pernicious anemia, thumbprint
Hypertension
Diabetes
Emboli
Blood dyscrasias
Anemias
Leukemias
Bacterial endocarditis
Trauma
Idiopathic

Superficial Flame-shaped Hemorrhages

Characteristics

Δ From the postarteriolar superficial capillary bed
Δ Possible radial peripapillary capillary bed
Δ Occur in nerve fiber layer in posterior pole
Δ Usually related to arterial-based diseases—hypoxia
Δ Do not leak

Management

Δ Ascertain the underlying cause
Δ Allow time for resorption
Δ Observe for other signs of hypoxia
Δ MUST DETERMINE UNDERLYING SYSTEMIC CAUSE

nerve fiber layer. These hemorrhages vary in size, configuration, and color. Often they have a white center and are called Roth's spots. Superficial flame-shaped hemorrhages are short-lived, lasting but a few weeks, and have no particular effect on vision. During resorption, there is a color change to dull red, with fragmentation and disappearance. A scotoma will occur at threshold levels if carefully investigated. The hemorrhage appears black on fluorescein angiography.

Superficial flame-shaped hemorrhages usually are confined to the posterior pole, most commonly occurring in the radial peripapillary distribution area. These hemorrhages represent an area of localized retinal hypoxia as the oxygenated arterial supply is compromised. As such, the hemorrhage may be a sign that neovascularization is a potential problem.

Roth's spots represent hemorrhage surrounding a white center. This white center may represent any of the following: (1) focal accumulations of white blood cells in inflammatory vascular disease, (2) cotton-wool spots surrounded by hemorrhage, (3) leukemic cell foci surrounded by hemorrhage, or (4) fibrin surrounded by hemorrhage. As with superficial hemorrhages, the clinician must attempt to ascertain the cause of the arterial capillary compromise. Table 4–4 lists the common causes of superficial flame-shaped hemorrhages, and Table 4–5 outlines the diseases associated with white-centered flame-shaped hemorrhages. **See color plate 26.**

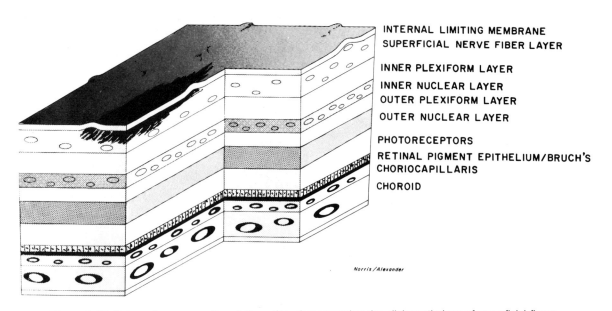

INTERNAL LIMITING MEMBRANE
SUPERFICIAL NERVE FIBER LAYER

INNER PLEXIFORM LAYER
INNER NUCLEAR LAYER
OUTER PLEXIFORM LAYER
OUTER NUCLEAR LAYER

PHOTORECEPTORS
RETINAL PIGMENT EPITHELIUM/BRUCH'S
CHORIOCAPILLARIS
CHOROID

Norris/Alexander

Figure 4–13. Schematic cross section of the retina, demonstrating the clinicopathology of superficial flame-shaped hemorrhages.

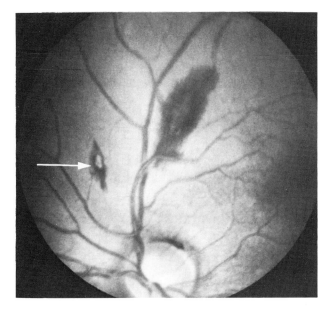

Figure 4–14. Black-and-white photograph of a flame-shaped hemorrhage and a white-centered flame-shaped hemorrhage (*arrow*). These hemorrhages were secondary to bacterial endocarditis.

Dot-blot Hemorrhages. Dot-blot hemorrhages (Figs. 4–15 and 4–16) are also known as deep retinal hemorrhages. Dot-blot hemorrhages occur in the inner nuclear layer, outer plexiform layer, and at times outer nuclear layer. Dot-blot hemorrhages originate from the prevenular deep capillary bed, and as such are most often associated with venous-based congestive disease. Dot-blot hemorrhage configuration results from the compression deep in the retina, confining the hemorrhages to specific localities. Dot-blot hemorrhages typically follow vertical lines of cleavage within the retina. Retinal structure is displaced in the area of the hemorrhage, but there is no necrosis of tissue. A dot-blot hemorrhage usually is indicative of deep retinal edema, although this is difficult to appreciate clinically. The deep retinal edema is usually a by-product of deep retinal vascular stasis.

Dot-blot hemorrhages may persist longer than a superficial flame-shaped hemorrhage, but eventually disappear, leaving no evidence of their existence. A visual compromise in the form of threshold field defects

TABLE 4–4. CONDITIONS COMMONLY ASSOCIATED WITH SUPERFICIAL FLAME-SHAPED HEMORRHAGES

Ocular	Systemic
Papilledema	Hypertension
Papillitis	Diabetes
Ischemic optic neuropathy	Blood dyscrasias
Papillophlebitis	Anemias
Low-tension glaucoma	Leukemias, large fan-shaped
Glaucoma	Oral contraceptives
Branch retinal vein occlusion	Idiopathic
Central retinal vein occlusion	

TABLE 4–5. SYSTEMIC DISEASES ASSOCIATED WITH ROTH'S SPOTS

Diabetes	Disseminated lupus erythematosus
Leukemias	Dysproteinemia
Bacterial endocarditis	Aplastic anemia

may occur in areas with dot-blot hemorrhages, or vision reduction can occur if the hemorrhages occur in the macula. The vision compromise is, however, a manifestation of the stasis in the involved retina rather than directly related to the hemorrhage. The hemorrhage is an indicator of intraretinal compromise. Dot-blot hemorrhages do not leak into the retina. **See color plate 25.**

Dot-blot hemorrhages may be isolated in such conditions as localized diabetic retinopathy. They may, however, involve a total sector of the retina, as in branch retinal vein occlusion (BRVO), or the entire retina out to the periphery, as in central retinal vein occlusion (CRVO). The hemorrhages are easy to distinguish from microaneurysms, because most microaneurysms are smaller than the resolution power of the direct ophthalmoscope. The differential from macroaneurysms is more difficult, and the clinician may have to rely on observation or fluorescein angiography for differential diagnosis. On fluorescein angiography, dot-blot hemorrhages block background choroidal fluorescence, whereas microaneurysms and macroaneurysms typically leak. Microaneurysms are almost always present when there are dot-blot hemorrhages.

Management of dot-blot hemorrhages can become a complicated matter. It is important to ascertain the underlying cause (Table 4–6). The clinician must remember that the dot hemorrhage is a sign of venous stasis and retinal edema. Should this edema and hemorrhage appear in the macular area or encroach on the macular area, fluorescein angiography is indicated to determine if photocoagulation can be applied to assist in regression of the edema.

Pearls

Dot-blot Hemorrhages

Characteristics

△ Occur in inner nuclear to outer nuclear layer
△ Originate from prevenular deep capillary bed
△ Associated with deep retinal edema but do not leak
△ Most often a sign of venous stasis retinopathy

Management

△ Ascertain cause
△ MUST DETERMINE UNDERLYING SYSTEMIC CAUSE
△ Fluorescein angiography if encroaching on or within the macula

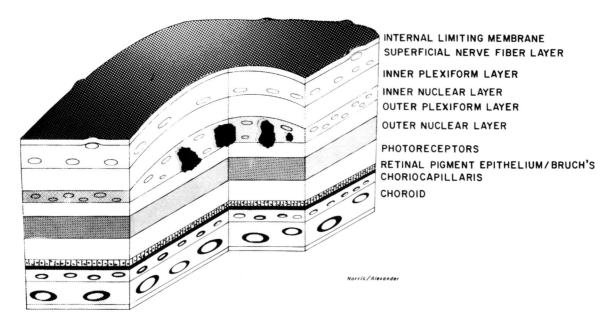

INTERNAL LIMITING MEMBRANE
SUPERFICIAL NERVE FIBER LAYER

INNER PLEXIFORM LAYER

INNER NUCLEAR LAYER
OUTER PLEXIFORM LAYER

OUTER NUCLEAR LAYER

PHOTORECEPTORS
RETINAL PIGMENT EPITHELIUM/BRUCH'S
CHORIOCAPILLARIS

CHOROID

Norris/Alexander

Figure 4–15. Schematic cross section of the retina demonstrating the clinicopathology of dot-blot hemorrhages.

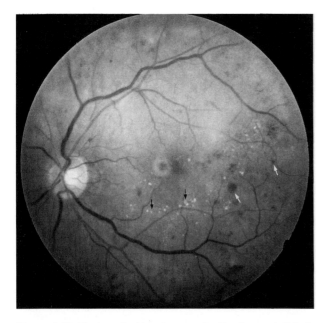

Figure 4–16. Black-and-white photograph of background diabetic retinopathy, with white arrows pointing to dot-blot hemorrhages and black arrows pointing to hard exudates.

TABLE 4–6. CONDITIONS ASSOCIATED WITH DOT-BLOT HEMORRHAGES

Diabetes
Retinal venous occlusive disease
Hypertension
Juxtafoveal telangiectasia
Coats' disease
Ipsilateral internal carotid stenosis (equatorial)
Retinal vascular tumors
Choroidal neovascular membranes
Blood dyscrasias and hypercoagulability
Estrogen-based pharmaceutical agents

Subretinal Hemorrhages. Most subretinal hemorrhages in the clinical population are secondary to choroidal neovascular membranes (Figs. 4–17 and 4–18). Subretinal hemorrhages can, however, occur as an extension of deep retinal hemorrhages breaking through to lie underneath the retina. This development can occur in conditions such as Coats' disease, sickle-cell disease, leukemia, retinopathy of prematurity, angiomatosis retina, and severe diabetic retinopathy.

Subretinal hemorrhages secondary to retinal vascular disease appear between the retinal pigment epithelium and sensory retina. They usually occur in the posterior pole, are large, and have lobulated borders. When the hemorrhages are fresh, they are usually

Pearls

Subretinal Hemorrhages

Characteristics

Δ Usually secondary to a ruptured choroidal neovascular network
Δ Often large with lobullated borders
Δ If subretinal, the hemorrhages are red
Δ If sub-RPE, the hemorrhages are gray-green, as the RPE acts as a filter for the color red
Δ Visually devastating when in the posterior pole

Management

Δ Fluorescein angiography must be obtained to ascertain the cause and to determine if it is beneficial to photocoagulate
Δ Retinal consultation should be considered

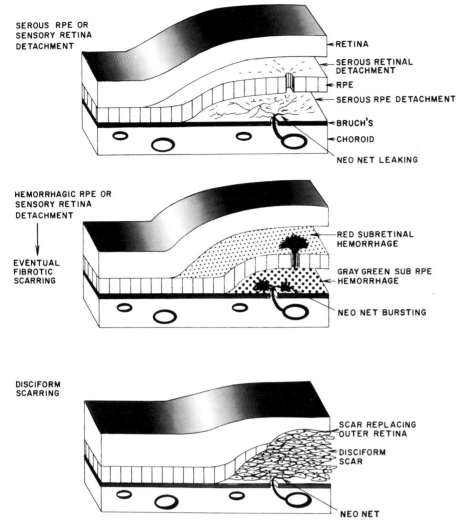

SEROUS RPE OR
SENSORY RETINA
DETACHMENT

←RETINA

SEROUS RETINAL
DETACHMENT

←RPE

←SEROUS RPE DETACHMENT

←BRUCH'S

←CHOROID

NEO NET LEAKING

HEMORRHAGIC RPE OR
SENSORY RETINA
DETACHMENT

↓

EVENTUAL
FIBROTIC
SCARRING

RED SUBRETINAL
HEMORRHAGE

GRAY GREEN SUB RPE
HEMORRHAGE

NEO NET BURSTING

DISCIFORM
SCARRING

SCAR REPLACING
OUTER RETINA

DISCIFORM
SCAR

NEO NET

NORRIS/ALEXANDER

Figure 4–17. Possible consequences of choroidal neovascularization.

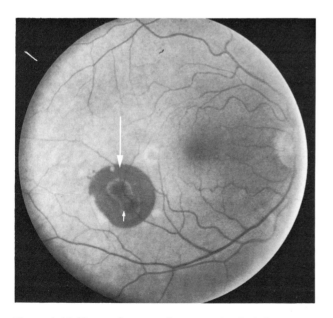

Figure 4–18. The small arrow points to a subretinal pigment epithelial hemorrhage, which is gray-green in color. The overlying subretinal hemorrhage (*long arrow*) is red.

dark red, often darker at the bottom. With age, subretinal hemorrhages show yellowish exudative accumulations eventually being replaced by scar tissue and pigment mottling. They resorb from the area of thinnest hemorrhage, which is often superior. Subretinal hemorrhages are very destructive, resulting in permanent scotomas with vision loss. Subretinal pigment epithelial hemorrhages are gray-green in color, with the same devastating effects.

Should a subretinal hemorrhage occur, the clinician must ascertain the cause. If the cause is choroidal neovascularization, laser photocoagulation may be beneficial. Control of any associated systemic condition may prevent involvement of the fellow eye. Photocoagulative intervention may be beneficial if the macula is not involved. If the macula is involved, little can be done to reverse the process and restore vision. **See color plates 59 to 61.**

Vitreous Hemorrhage. Vitreous hemorrhage (Figs. 4–19 and 4–20) can occur either out into the vitreous body or between the detached vitreous face and the

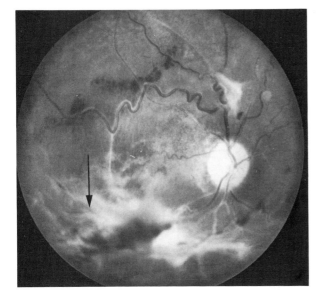

Figure 4–19. Black-and-white photograph of a resolving vitreous hemorrhage. The arrow points to the gray glial sheaths coursing out into the vitreous cavity.

Vitreous Hemorrhage

Characteristics

Δ Two basic forms: retrovitreous and intravitreous
Δ Usually secondary to rupture of neovascular net or development of a retinal tear associated with a vitreous detachment
Δ ALWAYS LOOK FOR A NEOVASCULAR FORMATION OR A RETINAL DETACHMENT
Δ Often visually devastating
Δ If long standing, feathery white sheets into inferior vitreous

Management

Δ Ascertain cause—usually secondary to a retinal tear or a ruptured retinal or optic nerve head neovascular formation
Δ Strongly consider a retinal consultation, as new evidence attests to the efficacy of early intervention in some cases

internal limiting membrane (retrovitreous). The blood in the vitreous is the result of a break in the internal limiting membrane, allowing for retinal or disc bleeding to flow forward. This process may occur in diseases with associated periphlebitis, allowing for inflammatory breakdown of the overlying internal limiting membrane, or in situations such as a retinal break with destruction to associated vasculature. This bleeding can also occur from a fragile neovascular network emanating from the optic nerve head where there is no true internal limiting membrane, or from preretinal neovascularization with inherent compromise to the internal limiting membrane.

The appearance of a vitreous hemorrhage depends on extent and elapsed time since the event. In the early phase of a hemorrhage out into the vitreous body, the retina may not be visible. The red blood cells may persist for a few weeks if the hemorrhage is small, or may remain for years. With time, the hemorrhage will settle to the inferior retina. Large clumps of blood remain, with clear zones, whereas in the inferior periphery, large feathery whitish sheets appear. These sheets may persist for years and can create occasional complaints of floaters in an especially syneretic vitreous.

Management of the vitreous hemorrhage consists of first determining the cause and then possible therapeutic intervention once the hemorrhage has cleared enough to assess the retina. Early intervention with vitrectomy is indicated in some cases secondary to diabetic retinal disease. Combined procedures of photocoagulation, vitrectomy, and at times scleral buckling may be necessary to effect a cure. Common causes of vitreous hemorrhage include diabetes, retrolental fibroplasia, sickle-cell disease, Eales' disease, hypertension, trauma, and retinal tears. Vitreous hemorrhage is discussed in greater detail in the section on the vitreous and peripheral retina.

Retinal Exudates and Cotton-wool Spots

The discussion of retinal exudates is limited to cotton-wool spots in the superficial nerve fiber layer and lip-

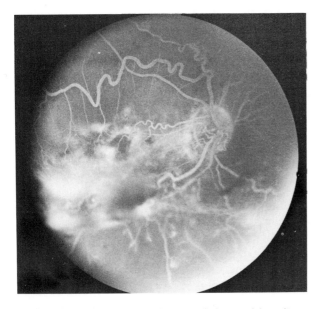

Figure 4–20. Fluorescein angiogram of the resolving vitreous hemorrhage shown in Figure 4–19.

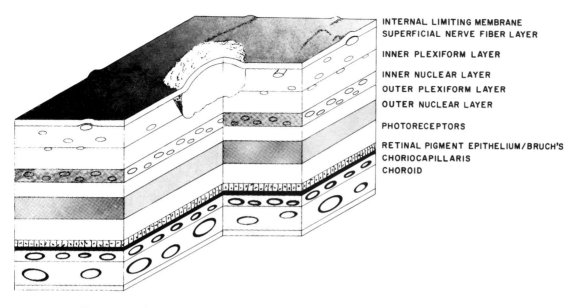

INTERNAL LIMITING MEMBRANE
SUPERFICIAL NERVE FIBER LAYER
INNER PLEXIFORM LAYER
INNER NUCLEAR LAYER
OUTER PLEXIFORM LAYER
OUTER NUCLEAR LAYER
PHOTORECEPTORS
RETINAL PIGMENT EPITHELIUM/BRUCH'S
CHORIOCAPILLARIS
CHOROID

Figure 4–21. Schematic cross section of the retina demonstrating the clinicopathology of cotton-wool spots.

id deposition in the deeper retinal layers, known as hard exudates. As with deep hemorrhages, lipid exudates are related to venous congestive retinal diseases. Cotton-wool spots are similar to superficial flame-shaped hemorrhages in that they are related to arterial-based retinal diseases.

Cotton-wool Spots. The retina is a tissue with a very high oxidative capacity and high glycolytic activity. As such, the tissue is very susceptible to hypoxia, which can occur immediately with arterial occlusive disease such as an embolic branch artery occlusion, or as a sequela to long-standing venous occlusive disease. With venous occlusive disease, hypoxia results when arterial blood supply to a region meets with inflow resistance secondary to edema.

With hypoxia, the retinal capillary endothelium is compromised, leading to edema. The retinal cells destroyed by lack of oxygen lyse, releasing macromolecules that further increase the edema, which ultimately close down the capillaries. The nuclei and nerve fibers may survive a brief bout with hypoxia, but with long-standing reduction in oxygen, the neurons will be lost and the nerve fibers will degenerate.

Cotton-wool spots (Figs. 4–21 and 4–22) are a manifestation of ischemia within the nerve fiber layer. Cotton-wool spots are microinfarcts from arteriolar–capillary occlusion. They usually occur in an area of the retina within about 3 disc diameters from the disc except in the foveal avascular zone. This zone corresponds to an area of the nerve fiber layer richly supplied by the superficial capillary network. The capillaries within the cotton-wool spot are usually devoid of blood, with loss of endothelial cells and intramural pericytes. On resolution of the cotton-wool spot, the infarcted area becomes revascularized. In the area of the cotton-wool spot, the ganglion cell and nerve fiber layers are swollen by the cytoid body-containing lesion. This swelling and debris accumulation may be the result of interruption in axoplasmic flow. **See color plates 28 to 30.**

In the early stages of development, cotton-wool spots appear above the retinal vessels in a fuzzy non-

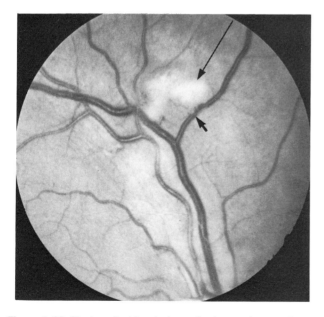

Figure 4–22. Black-and-white photograph of a very large cotton-wool spot (*arrows*).

Cotton-wool Spots

Characteristics

Δ Ischemia within nerve fiber layer resulting from arteriolar infarcts

Δ Usually within 3 disc diameters of optic nerve head

Δ Edema secondary to interruption of axoplasmic flow

Δ A definite sign of retinal hypoxia

Δ Typically disappear in 5 to 7 weeks assuming the condition is brought under control

Management

Δ Ascertain the underlying cause

Δ MUST DETERMINE UNDERLYING SYSTEMIC OR OCULAR CAUSE

Δ Allow time for resorption

Δ Watch for other signs of hypoxia

Δ Follow the patient at least every 3 months

descript shape. If they become dense enough, cotton-wool spots can produce a scotoma at threshold and can minimally block background choroidal fluorescence. The size varies and cotton-wool spots are transient, disappearing in 5 to 7 weeks. With resolution, cotton-wool spots fade to a gray color and become granular. When the spots disappear, retinal function resumes in the area with no apparent sequelae.

Many different disease processes can manifest cotton-wool spots in the retina. Table 4–7 lists the more common conditions associated with cotton-wool spots. It is absolutely imperative that the clinician determine the cause of cotton-wool spots, because they are a sign of underlying retinal hypoxia. Any retinal vascular disease that creates low oxygen concentration can manifest cotton-wool spots. Retinal hypoxia is the immediate precursor of neovascularization, which occurs to create an alternative oxygen supply to the retina. Control of the underlying systemic disease or internal carotid stenosis should be questioned in retinal vascular disease with cotton-wool spots. Patients with cotton-wool spots must be followed at routine intervals of 3 months or less.

TABLE 4–7. CONDITIONS COMMONLY ASSOCIATED WITH COTTON-WOOL SPOTS

Hypertension	Anemias	Papilledema
Diabetes	Leukemias	Papillitis
Systemic lupus erythematosus	Septicemias	Papillophlebitis
	Dysproteinemias	Ischemic optic
Blood dyscrasias	Venous occlusive	neuropathy
Dermatomyositis	disease	Acquired
Scleroderma	Internal carotid	immunodeficiency
Purtscher's retinopathy	stenosis	syndrome (AIDS)

Lipid (Hard) Exudates. Lipid exudates (Figs. 4–23 and 4–24) represent a distinctive sign of retinal vascular compromise, because they are the by-products of breakdown of retinal vessels and liberation of blood-bound lipids. Hard exudates are characteristic of venous-based congestive diseases more often affecting the deeper capillary beds (prevenular). Hard exudate formation is also characteristic in the leakage associated with choroidal neovascular membrane formation. The hard exudates deposit in the outer plexiform layer throughout the retina and Henle's layer in the macular area, but may extend from the internal limiting membrane to the outer nuclear layer. Most of the time, hard exudates are confined to the posterior pole, except in the case of Coats' disease and retinal vascular tumors such as angiomatosis retina, when the exudates may be deposited peripherally. It should be noted that in Coats' disease the exudates dominate and can totally occupy the retina, extending into the subretinal space and causing moundlike non-rhegmatogenous detachments of the sensory retina.

The genesis of hard exudates is controversial but is thought to be associated with microglial tissue macrophages that are derived from mesodermal tissue or blood monocytes. These macrophages are

Lipid Exudates

Characteristics

Δ Occur in venous stasis diseases in deep retina

Δ Associated with deep retinal edema

Δ Usually confined to posterior pole, except in conditions such as Coats' disease and retinal vascular tumors, where the exudates become very space occupying

Δ Often present associated with choroidal neovascular membranes

Δ Result of macrophages attempting to remove lipid deposits from within the retina and migrating to the extent of the edema, where they deposit the debris in a ring formation

Δ Form a ring around intraretinal edema often created by leaking microaneurysms and telangiectatic vessels

Management

Δ Ascertain cause

Δ MUST DETERMINE UNDERLYING OCULAR/SYSTEMIC PROCESS

Δ If encroaching on or within ⅓ disc diameter of macula, fluorescein angiography and retinal consultation are indicated

Δ If away from macula, document, educate, and follow up according to underlying disease process and specific causative factors, but certainly every 6 months

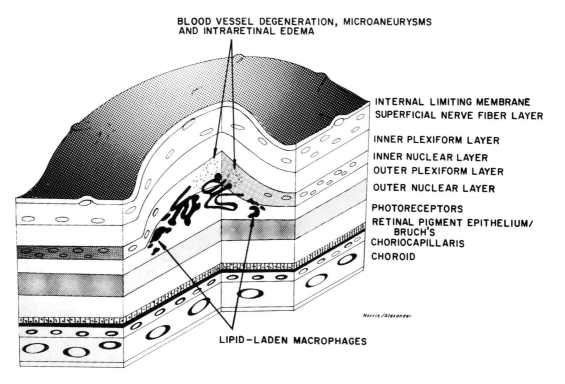

BLOOD VESSEL DEGENERATION, MICROANEURYSMS AND INTRARETINAL EDEMA

INTERNAL LIMITING MEMBRANE
SUPERFICIAL NERVE FIBER LAYER

INNER PLEXIFORM LAYER
INNER NUCLEAR LAYER
OUTER PLEXIFORM LAYER
OUTER NUCLEAR LAYER

PHOTORECEPTORS
RETINAL PIGMENT EPITHELIUM/
BRUCH'S
CHORIOCAPILLARIS
CHOROID

Norris/Alexander

LIPID—LADEN MACROPHAGES

Figure 4–23. Schematic cross section of the retina demonstrating the clinicopathology of hard exudate formation.

resistant to hypoxia but are destroyed by anoxia. Macrophages function to remove extravascular blood, exudates, and cellular debris from vascular breakdown. The combination of ingredients of the vascular breakdown forms a lipid soup. The macrophages

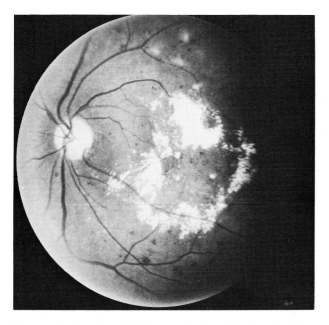

Figure 4–24. Photograph of severe hard exudate formation surrounding the macula in diabetic retinopathy.

laden with lipid then remain in the outer plexiform layer. The lipid-laden macrophages along with free lipids migrate to the outer reaches of the diseased edematous retinal area. This "circling of the wagons" serves as a clinicopathologic boundary for identification of intraretinal microvasculopathy. Often, this forms a circle, oval pattern, or partial arcs and is dictated by fluid dynamics in a confined area. This pattern may remain after resolution—either normal or induced by photocoagulation—of the intraretinal disease, much as a ring is left around the bathtub when the water is drained. In the macular area, the pattern may be that of a radiating star because of the absence of an outer plexiform layer, which is replaced by a tightly bound Henle's layer. The absence of hard exudates in retinal ischemic disease, such as branch retinal arterial disease, may be secondary to microglial (macrophage) death from anoxia. **See color plate 31.**

Clinically, hard exudates are dense, with color varying from whitish yellow to gold but most often waxy yellow. Long-standing fatty exudates assume a glittering gold color because of the accumulation of cholestrin crystals. The material is space occupying, pushing aside retinal elements already compromised by deep retinal edema and often dot-blot hemorrhages. More often than not, microaneurysms or macroaneurysms can be demonstrated by fluorescein angiography near the hard exudates in the developmental phase. These microaneurysms are often

TABLE 4–8. CONDITIONS ASSOCIATED WITH INTRARETINAL HARD EXUDATES

Diabetes: Circular	Retinal macroaneurysms
Hypertension: Star	Leber's miliary aneurysms
Coats' disease: Dense peripheral	von Hippel–Lindau— angiomatosis retinae
Coats' response in exudative maculopathy	Papillitis: Macular wing
Venous occlusive disease	Papilledema

TABLE 4–9. RETINAL DISEASES ASSOCIATED WITH MICROANEURYSM FORMATION

Diabetes	Eales disease
Venous occlusive disease	Sickle-cell disease
Coats' disease	Hypertension (severe)
Blood dyscrasias	Dysproteinemias
Leukemias	Leber's disease
Peripheral retina in aged	

secondary to an obliterated capillary bed. Edema, whether deep in such diseases as diabetes or superficial in such diseases as hypertension, is a necessary precursor to exudate formation.

Exudates are a sign of retinal or choroidal vasculopathy and in and of themselves require no treatment. It is well known that hard exudates in the fovea are a poor prognostic sign for recovery of vision. This is only because the retina in that area had to be edematous for a long period of time for the development of the exudates. Long-term macular edema creates permanent malfunction of at least some of the tightly packed photoreceptors. When a hard exudate formation is observed, it is a clinicopathologic sign of retinal edema, either present or past, that may be amendable to photocoagulative intervention. If this edema is threatening the macular area, fluorescein angiography is indicated to determine the desirability of photocoagulation. If the exudate pattern is not encroaching on the macula, it is important to determine the underlying cause of the edema, ascertain the control of the systemic disease, and follow the patient on at least a 12-month basis, barring extenuating circumstances. Table 4–8 lists conditions often associated with intraretinal hard exudates. **See color plate 28.**

RETINAL BLOOD VESSEL ANOMALIES AND ALTERATIONS

Retinal Microaneurysms

Retinal microaneurysms are omnipresent in retinal congestive diseases (Table 4–9). Microaneurysms are 50 to 100 microns in size, and are therefore difficult to resolve by direct ophthalmoscopy but become readily apparent on fluorescein angiography. Microaneurysms glow like miniature Christmas tree lights on performing fluorescein angiography. Larger microaneurysms are visible by ophthalmoscopy, especially when they occur in the center of active retinal microvasculopathy or when they become hyalinized with age. Microaneurysms occur in cases of retinal hypoxia when there is associated microcapillary obliteration. The vascular alterations develop most often

near the venous side of the deep capillary structure.

Capillary microaneurysms appear as saccules on the wall of the vessel, often in clusters directed toward the areas of capillary obliteration. Within the wall, there is a proliferation of endothelial cells. Initially, these cells leak, but with age the wall becomes hyalinized, sealing the leakage. The hyalinized microaneurysms may persist 1 to 2 years.

The precise etiopathogenesis of the endothelial proliferation in response to the hypoxia of capillary obliteration is unknown. There are proponents of a theory that the ballooning occurs in response to lipid infiltration of the endothelial walls. Some clinicians believe that microaneurysms are aborted attempts at neovascularization or revascularization of previously atrophied channels. This theory gains support with the realization that peripheral retinal microaneurysms are common with aging, because capillary structure normally closes down in the periphery with age. In diabetes alone, there is a selective loss of intramural pericytes that could weaken the capillary wall, allowing for aneurysmal formation. This does not, however, explain the genesis of microaneurysms in other retinal vascular diseases. The only substantiated fact is that microaneurysms occur in areas of hypoxia secondary to capillary obliteration where the endothelium is still viable.

It is important to recognize retinal diseases that may have associated microaneurysms. The microaneurysms leak, creating intraretinal edema with resulting potential acuity, field loss, or both. Although microaneurysms are not routinely observable, there are signs of their presence. Any disease creating stasis microvasculopathy probably will have associated microaneurysms. The signs of these diseases include dot-blot hemorrhages, intraretinal edema, and hard exudates. Any time dot-blot hemorrhages or hard exudates are visible, it is safe to assume that microaneurysms are present or have been present in the recent past. Fluorescein angiography will confirm the presence of microaneurysms.

If microaneurysmal leakage occurs in the macular area, there is a significant threat to vision. The microaneurysms are, however, amendable to photocoagula-

Retinal Microaneurysms

Characteristics

Δ Usually related to conditions creating venous stasis

Δ Often nonresolvable by direct ophthalmoscopy, but signs of presence such as intraretinal edema, hard exudates, and hemorrhages may be present

Δ Vascular response to a weakening of the capillary wall

Δ Leak profusely and are best seen by fluorescein angiography

Management

Δ Ascertain cause, both ocular and systemic

Δ If indication of encroachment within macula, order fluorescein angiography and consider retinal consultation

Δ If distant from macula, educate and follow up in at least 12 months. Modify follow-up according to overall status of the retina and systemic health

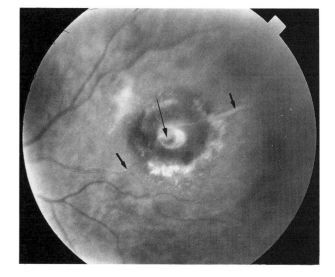

Figure 4–25. A retinal macroaneurysm secondary to sustained uncontrolled systemic hypertension. The macroaneurysm has hemorrhaged under the RPE and under the sensory retina and was pulsating necessitating an urgent retinal consultation. The long arrow points to the macroaneurysm while the two small arrows point to the ingress and egress vessels.

tion to arrest the leakage. It is important to recognize conditions associated with microaneurysms, perform fluorescein angiography to determine their presence, and intervene with photocoagulation when the microaneurysms are a threat to vision. All management must be underscored by the importance of maximal control of the underlying systemic condition.

Retinal Macroaneurysms

Introduction and Description. A retinal macroaneurysm is an isolated dilated area of a major retinal vascular branch. The condition is associated with systemic hypertension, arteriosclerosis, and retinal emboli, and results from focal damage to the vessel wall. Similar lesions may be seen in central nervous system vasculature. The associated microvasculopathy of capillary obliteration that one finds with microaneurysms is generally absent, yet there is edema, exudation, and hemorrhage secondary to the macroaneurysm (Fig. 4–25).

Macroaneurysms of the retinal arterial tree typically occur in patients aged 50 to 80 years, with an increased incidence in females. Of these patients, about 50 percent have systemic hypertension and 25 percent demonstrate a high 5-year postdiscovery mortality rate associated with systemic cardiovasculopathy. **See color plate 40.**

Clinical diagnosis is made in the early phase by observation of an isolated ballooning of the vessel,

usually within the radius of the first three branchings of the arteries, most often superotemporally. The macroaneurysm may be multifocal but is usually unilateral. As the macroaneurysm leaks, retinal edema allows for intraretinal and subretinal hemorrhage and intraretinal and subretinal lipid exudate deposition. Should this process occur in the macular area, there is a definite threat to severe vision loss. Once bleeding occurs, the macroaneurysm usually becomes sclerosed. Branch artery and vein occlusions may accompany the retinal arterial macroaneurysm. As would be expected, the macroaneurysm fills in the arterial phase of fluorescein angiography with late stage leakage.

Management. Besides the systemic implications and the necessity for a cardiovascular physical examination, it is important to realize that localized ocular treatment may be of benefit. Asymptomatic macroaneurysms need only be observed at 6-month intervals, with the patient monitoring vision at home. These asymptomatic macroaneurysms are characterized by an absence of exudation and hemorrhage. Localized exudation and hemorrhage that is not threatening macular function may be followed at 1- to 3-month intervals with patient self-monitoring.

Photocoagulation should be applied if there is a persistence of macular edema or exudate without a spontaneous self-sealing of the macroaneurysm after 3 months of observation. Spread of the effects of the

Retinal Macroaneurysms

Characteristics

Δ Isolated dilatation of major arterial branch usually within the radius of third branching, usually unilateral but may be multifocal

Δ Associated with hypertension, arteriosclerosis, retinal emboli, and cardiovascular disease

Δ No microvasculopathy but edema, exudation, and hemorrhage, which can affect macular function

Δ Hemorrhage may be intraretinal or subretinal

Management

Δ **Minimal systemic health workup**
  Blood pressure and pulse rate
  Fasting blood sugar
  Complete blood count with differential and platelets
  Fasting lipid profile
  Palpation/ausculation of the carotid system—ophthalmodynamometry (ODM)? with a strong consideration of DUPLEX ULTRASOUND
  Cardiology consultation
    Echocardiography
    Blood chemistries
    Holter monitor

Δ Photocoagulation if threat to vision, if lesion pulses, or if lesion spreads

Δ If asymptomatic, 6-month follow-up and home monitoring

Δ If localized exudation and hemorrhage that is not threatening macular function, may follow at 1- to 3-month intervals with self-monitoring. If persistence of macular edema or exudate without a spontaneous self-sealing, must consider photocoagulation

Note: Venous system macroaneurysm may occur often in the zone of a branch or central retinal vein occlusion, and should be handled in the same manner as the arterial variety once the occlusive area is managed with photocoagulation

macroaneurysm on serial observations is also an indication for photocoagulation. Another indicator for photocoagulative intervention is the observation of pulsation of the macroaneurysmal wall, which suggests a very thin wall that is subject to rupture. The recommended methods of photocoagulation include direct treatment with argon green and/or dye yellow. Vitrectomy may be necessary for nonresolving vitreous hemorrhage causing visual loss.

A note should be made regarding the occurrence of retinal venous macroaneurysms. Venous macro-aneurysms are usually found in areas of branch, hemicentral, or central retinal vein occlusions. The appearance is the same as retinal arterial macroaneurysms except that they arise from the venous system. The sequelae are similar to the arterial variety. The photocoagulative treatment should involve the area of the associated vein occlusion as well as focal treatment of the macroaneurysm if vision is decreased secondary to the associated retinal changes.

Idiopathic Juxtafoveal (Parafoveal) Retinal Telangiectasia

Introduction and Description. Idiopathic juxtafoveal retinal telangiectasia has the appearance of Coats' disease and is thought to represent a variation of the process. Juxtafoveal retinal telangiectasia may be a cause of macular edema and reduced visual acuity. The telangiectasia is a developmental anomaly, with aneurysms of the capillaries involving several retinal areas.

Unilateral congenital juxtafoveal telangiectasia occurs only in men and is usually asymptomatic until after age 40 years. The condition involves a 1 to 2 disc-diameter area often temporal to the fovea (Fig. 4–26). The leakage from the compromised vessels may encroach into the macular zone, creating a reduction in vision but not usually below 20/40. The clinical picture may be similar to a retinal macroaneurysm, and fluorescein angiography is necessary to make the proper differential diagnosis.

Bilateral idiopathic acquired parafoveal telangiectasia may occur in either sex, often in the later years (40s to 60s). The presentation is bilateral and often symmetrical, involving less than 1 disc diameter. The clinical picture includes intraretinal edema, retinal white punctate opacities, a one third disc-diameter round yellow foveal lesion, RPE hyperplasia, and often choroidal neovascularization. Hard exudates are not a characteristic of the bilateral presentation and vision is usually not worse than 20/30 at presentation.

Management. Management of juxtafoveal telangiectasia should be underscored with the term *conservatism*, as most patients experience little to no progressive loss of vision. Photocoagulation with grid argon green or krypton red should only be considered if there is significant progression of vision loss. The foveal avascular zone should always be avoided. Should choroidal neovascularization be discovered, appropriate management techniques must be applied. There is no strong relationship of juxtafoveal retinal telangiectasia to systemic diseases in spite of the fact that the clinical appearance makes it difficult to not consider systemic conditions such as diabetes.

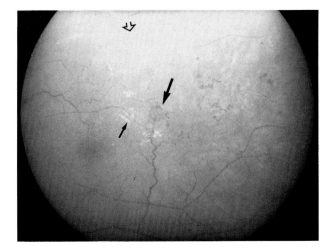

Figure 4–26. Parafoveal or juxtafoveal retinal telangiectasia creating some moderate hemorrhaging and hard exudate formation. The large black arrow points to the telangiectatic vessels, the small black arrow points to hard exudates, and the open arrow points to a sheathed vein associated with a prior coincidental BRVO.

It is important to educate the patient and follow up according to the severity of threat to vision loss.

Retinal Collateralization

Retinal collaterals are blood vessels that develop within the framework of the existing vessel network, usually near or adjacent to areas of nonperfusion of the capillary bed. These areas of collateralization may be contrasted with neovascularization, which occurs in zones of the retina that are normally avascular. Initially, collaterals are capillary in nature but may evolve into vein-to-vein collaterals after venous occlusion, artery-to-artery collaterals after branch arterial occlusion, and occasionally artery-to-vein collaterals after capillary bed obstruction. Artery-to-vein communications without associated capillary bed obstructions are called *shunts,* and may occur isolated as congenital variations or may be acquired in conditions such as retinal angiomatosis and Coats' disease.

Collaterals are beneficial to the health of the retina and optic nerve, because they drain venous blood or shunt arterial blood around an area of compromised retinal or optic nerve head vascular bed. These channels occur as the blood seeks a new route. The walls of the channels develop, and the lumen of the vessel enlarges to take on more blood. With en-

Pearls

Idiopathic Juxtafoveal (Parafoveal) Retinal Telangiectasia

Characteristics

Δ Unilateral

Occurs only in men and is asymptomatic until after age 40

1 to 2 disc-diameter area temporal to fovea

Leakage into macula may create visual acuity decrease to 20/40

If severe, may need photocoagulative intervention, but the best approach is conservative monitoring of patient

Δ Bilateral

Either sex in the 40s to 60s

Often symmetrical, involving 1 disc-diameter areas including intraretinal edema, white punctate retinal opacities, a ⅓ disc-diameter yellow foveal lesion, RPE hyperplasia, and possible choroidal neovascularization

Often presents with 20/30 vision but should be monitored for progression

Management

Δ Photocoagulation indicated if progression is a severe threat to vision or the development of choroidal neovascularization

Δ Follow up patient at routine intervals

Pearls

Retinal Collateralization

Characteristics

Δ Develops near zones of capillary nonperfusion and often near areas of cotton-wool spot formation

Δ Develops within the framework of existing vessel network

Δ Acts as a detour to shunt blood around a closed area in vaso-occlusive disorders and situations of vascular nonperfusion of the optic nerve head, such as chronic open-angle glaucoma

Δ May leak in the early phases with fluorescein angiography

Δ IRMA requires fluorescein angiography to determine stage of development

Δ An optociliary shunt is a sign of past central retinal vein occlusion, and shunt vessels at the disc are a characteristic of long-standing chronic open-angle glaucoma

Δ IRMA indicates retinal hypoxia and is a strong indication for a retinal consultation to consider measures to prevent progression to neovascular development

largement, the channels become visible to ophthalmoscopy. These collaterals may be multiple or single and ultimately assume a similar structure to the occluded vessel. Collaterals lie within the retina or on the surface of the optic nerve head and typically do not leak fluorescein. At times, the occluded vessel will become patent and the collateral will recede; other times, the occluded vessel will become sheathed (vein) and the collateral will assume responsibility for the affected retinal area (Fig. 4–27).

A variation of the retinal collateral is the occurrence of optociliary shunt vessels at the optic nerve head associated with central retinal vein occlusion that may be secondary to thrombosis or to pressure exerted on the vein by an orbital mass. These serve to shunt venous blood from the retina to the optic nerve choroidal vasculature, bypassing the occluded central retinal vein (Fig. 4–28). Another variation of collaterals on the optic nerve head occurs in chronic open-angle glaucoma in response to compromise of nerve vascular perfusion. These collaterals also function to shunt the blood flow around compromised areas.

Collateral formation is an important aspect of resolution of retinal vascular disease. Rapid, extensive collateralization can effectively supply or drain blood to an area of retinal vascular compromise, averting total sensory retinal loss. Identification of collaterals indicates present or past regional retinal vascular disease. It is important to ascertain the underlying systemic cause of this disease and manage it appropriately. Collaterals are never to be photocoagulated. If there is confusion about whether the vascular alter-

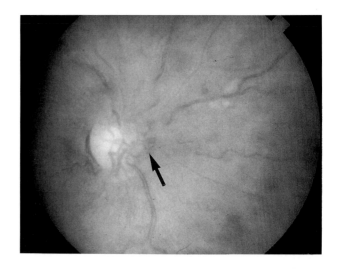

Figure 4–28. An optociliary shunt (*arrow*) created secondary to a central retinal vein occlusion. The shunt connects to the choroidal vascular system within the optic nerve head.

ations are collaterals or neovascularization, fluorescein angiography will effectively differentiate the two. Collaterals typically do not leak on fluorescein angiography, but neovascularization does in the early arterial phase.

Intraretinal microvascular abnormalities (IRMA) describe a variation of shunt (collateral) formation and dilated capillaries in areas of nonperfusion in diabetic retinopathy. IRMA looks like intraretinal neovascularization and is actually similar to new vessels in that the structure is composed of endothelium with only a few intramural pericytes (Fig. 4–29). IRMA may leak fluorescein in the early phases of development. It does leak on fluorescein angiography as neovascularization develops in the area. IRMA is considered to be the germination bed for retinal neovascularization, and fluorescein angiography is indicated in most cases to determine the stage of development. The presence of IRMA is a dangerous prognostic sign indicating retinal hypoxia and the distinct immediate potential for the development of neovascularization. Should IRMA be obvious, fluorescein angiography and a retinal consultation are indicated. **See color plate 48.**

Neovascularization

Neovascularization is a complex reaction to a simple stimulus—lack of oxygenated blood. Any retinal vascular disease that creates hypoxia can have the associated development of neovascularization. Retinal neovascularization typically occurs in avascular zones of the ocular structure, to attempt to supply oxygenated blood to a hypoxic retinal or uveal area. The attempt is noble, but the new vessels are very fragile

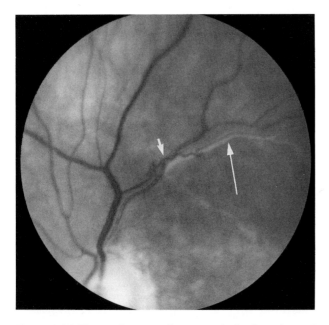

Figure 4–27. The small arrow points to a retinal collateral vessel formed in response to a branch retinal vein occlusion. The large arrow points to the sheathed retinal vein.

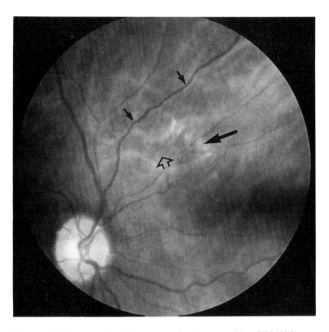

Figure 4–29. Intraretinal microvascular abnormalities (IRMA) (*open arrow*), which serve as the germination bed for the genesis of neovascularization elsewhere. The large black arrow points to associated cotton-wool spots and the two small black arrows point to venous beading, another sign of retinal vascular hypoxia.

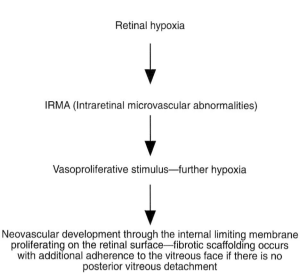

Figure 4–30. Proposed etiology of neovascularization elsewhere in diabetic retinopathy.

and subject to leakage, fibrosis, and hemorrhage. The fibrotic scaffolding that accompanies neovascularization sets up potential retinal traction when the fibrosis contracts. By definition, retinal neovascularization develops from and is contiguous with the preexisting viable retinal vascular bed.

The etiopathogenesis of retinal or optic disc neovascularization is somewhat controversial, but the effects and proper management are universally accepted. Several theories of genesis of retinal neovascularization exist; two are shown in Figures 4–30 and 4–31. It is important to recognize that viable retinal tissue or optic nerve head tissue is necessary to support new vessel growth. Anoxic retinal areas will not grow new vessels; that is why it is a bit unusual (but not impossible) to see retinal and disc neovascularization in central retinal arterial occlusions. Likewise in ischemic central retinal vein occlusion there is limited viable retinal and optic disc tissue that will support the development of vessel growth; therefore the stimulus for neovascular development courses through the uvea and creates the vasoproliferative stimulus in the iris tissue. Table 4–10 lists some conditions associated with development of peripheral neovascularization.

Retinal neovascularization (Fig. 4–32) is thought to be a proliferation of the endothelium of the capillaries and veins. An arterial association is also proposed. The lumen in retinal neovascularization is usu-

ally larger than a capillary, and is also differentiated from a capillary by the profuse leakage of intravascular fluid. All new vessels may be accompanied by fibrotic scaffolding, but some may be characterized by a profusion of lacy tortuous vessels, with fibrosis occurring after the network has aged.

As mentioned previously, the new vessels may form on the retinal surface, but they may also emanate from the optic nerve head and the iris vascular network. When neovascularization occurs at the optic nerve head (Fig. 4–33), the new vessels penetrate easily into the vitreous body because of the lack of a true internal limiting membrane at this location. The possible location for the development of neovascularization in diseases with retinal hypoxia has some degree of predictability. The neovascularization usually will occur within or very near the identified hypoxic zone or on the disc in an area that would face the hypoxic retina. The neovascularization in choroidal membrane formation also often faces the demonstrable

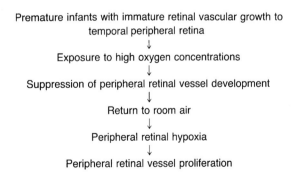

Figure 4–31. The proposed etiology of neovascularization in retinopathy of prematurity.

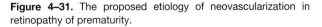

TABLE 4–10. DISEASES KNOWN TO BE ASSOCIATED WITH PERIPHERAL NEOVASCULARIZATION

Disease	Age of Onset	Possible Locations	Heredity
Branch retinal vein occlusion	50s–60s	Area of nonperfusion	N/A
Diabetes	Variable usually after 20 years	Entire fundus	N/A
Retinopathy of prematurity	Birth through first year	Temporal periphery	N/A (Prematurity)
Eales disease	Teens through 30s	Area of involved vein	N/A
Thick blood syndromes	Variable	Periphery	N/A
Sarcoidosis	Variable	Periphery	N/A
Retinal telangiectasia (Coats' disease)	Teens through 30s	Entire fundus	N/A
Familial exudative vitreoretinopathy	Variable	Periphery	Autosomal dominant
von Hippel–Lindau (angiomatosis retinae)	Teens through 40s	Periphery	Autosomal dominant
Hemoglobinopathies, eg, sickle-cell disease	Variable	Temporal periphery	Autosomal
Aortic arch syndrome	After 20 years	Entire fundus	N/A

area of hypoxia. **See color plate 32.**

Retinal and optic nerve head neovascularization represent a direct threat to maintenance of visual function. The new vessels can leak, creating edema; can hemorrhage into the vitreous; or can cause retinal traction associated with the fibrotic scaffolding. **See color plate 33.** It is important to ascertain the underlying cause of the neovascularization. Table 4–11 lists some of the diseases associated with retinal neovascularization. Fluorescein angiography should be performed to differentiate neovascularization from collateral formation and the early stages of IRMA. Photocoagulation is indicated to eliminate the hypoxic stimulus and cause regression of the neovascularization, but these indications are disease specific and reference to each condition should be made prior to initiation of treatment.

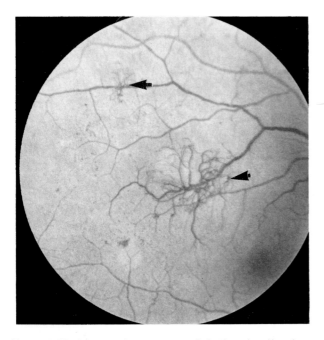

Figure 4–32. Arrows point to neovascularization elsewhere in a case of diabetic retinopathy.

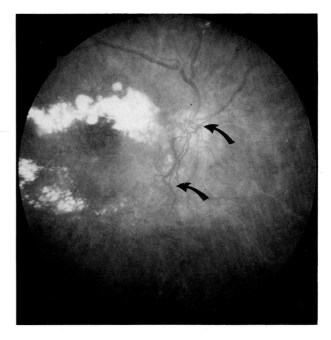

Figure 4–33. An illustration of disc neovascularization with a strong propensity for hemorrhage and fibrotic proliferation. The two curved arrows point to neovascularization. The hard exudates are secondary to a choroidal neovascular net.

Neovascularization

Characteristics

Δ A response to ocular uveal hypoxia
Δ The response may be chemical or may be just the relative hypoxia
Δ Retinal, disc, iris, and choroidal forms
Δ Vessels are fragile, leak, and may be accompanied by fibrotic scaffolding
Δ Develops from viable preexisting vascular bed
Δ Strong association with IRMA
Δ Direct threat to vision
　　Hemorrhage into vitreous
　　Fibrotic scaffolding leading to traction retinal detachment

Management

Δ Check the status of the underlying systemic condition that is precipitating the problem
Δ Perform fluorescein angiography and determine if amendable by photocoagulation
Δ Retinal consultation is indicated if active regardless of the associated systemic/ocular precipitating cause

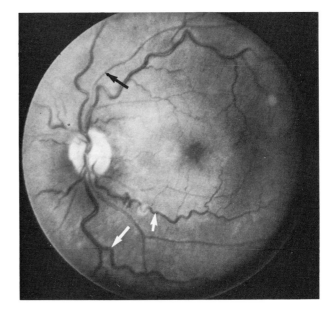

Figure 4–34. The black arrow points to a straight retinal artery; the white arrows point to acquired venous tortuosity.

Specific guidelines for intervention are outlined in subsequent sections on diseases associated with new vessel growth. It is important to realize that neovascularization can, at times, regress with removal of the hypoxic stimulus, but a conservative approach for all retinal neovascularization would be a retinal consultation. Also remember that the presence of the neovascularization indicates retinal hypoxia and is strongly associated with systemic disease and probable poor control of the systemic vascular situation. The systemic workup associated with the presence of neovascularization is disease specific. An example would be the strong association of proliferative neovascular retinopathy in diabetes, the elevation of glycated hemoglobin levels, and the presence of microalbuminuria.

Retinal Vessel Tortuosity

Tortuosity of retinal vessels, specifically veins, can be an important diagnostic sign (Fig. 4–34). Acquired venous tortuosity usually occurs in conditions of retinal hypoxia. The most common vascular tortuosity is,

TABLE 4–11. DISEASES COMMONLY ASSOCIATED WITH RETINAL NEOVASCULARIZATION

Diabetic retinopathy	Eales' disease
Branch retinal vein occlusion	Sarcoidosis
Hemicentral retinal vein occlusion	Pulseless disease
Central retinal vein occlusion	Behçet's disease
Sickle-cell retinopathy	Hemoglobinopathies
Retinopathy of prematurity	

Retinal Vessel Tortuosity

Characteristics

Δ Congenital
　　Involving all quadrants
　　Symmetrical in both eyes
　　Vein tortuosity associated with arterial tortuosity
Δ Acquired venous tortuosity
　　Previously documented normalcy
　　Sectoral involvement may occur
　　Associated darkening and thickening of the blood column
　　Indicator of hypoxia
　　May have associated localized retinal vascular anomaly
　　Venous beading is a variation
　　Note: Inherited venous beading is characterized by marked bilateral retinal venous beading, conjunctival beading, vascular retinopathy similar to diabetes, and a variable systemic status
Δ Acquired arterial tortuosity
　　Rare
　　Usually associated with localized retinal vascular conditions such as sickle-cell retinopathy, ROP, and preretinal membrane formation

Management

Δ Monitor carefully after ascertaining local and systemic cause
Δ Schedule for routine eye examinations in congenital tortuosity situations

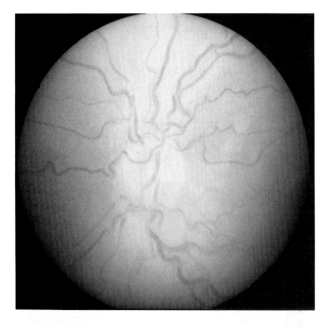

**TABLE 4–12. DISEASES ASSOCIATED WITH
ACQUIRED ARTERY AND VEIN TORTUOSITY**

Congenital heart disease
Retinopathy of prematurity
Leber's miliary aneurysms
Coats' disease
Racemose angioma

thy of prematurity, and sickle-cell retinopathy when outside traction factors create retinal wrinkling and subsequent arterial tortuosity. Tortuosity of the veins in just one sector or tortuosity in previously normal channels is of diagnostic significance. There is usually dilatation of the vein and a darkening of the blood column in the affected region. Increased vein tortuosity is indicative of venous stasis, retinal hypoxia in the immediate area, or any form of localized occlusion from blood disease. It is likely that tortuosity in a vein is related to the distensibility of the vein related to increases in internal pressure. The veins do have localized periodic attachments to the retinal tissue. With dilatation, the veins remain attached at certain points, while the vessel swells, creating a serpentine form. **See color plate 30.**

Retinal vascular tortuosity is important because it is an indicator of blood sludging in the presence of hypoxia. Isolated areas of tortuosity appear as venous beading and have the same diagnostic/prognostic significance as overall tortuosity. The hypoxia then acts as a neovascular stimulus. The clinician must attempt to uncover the underlying disease retinal and systemic disease process as well as carefully follow the affected retina for signs of further developments. Tables 4–12 and 4–13 list diseases commonly associated with acquired vascular tortuosity.

Figure 4–35. Right and left eyes illustrating congenital vascular tortuosity. Note the tortuosity of both veins and arteries as well as the similarity (mirror image) of the two eyes.

however, congenital. Extreme tortuosity involving all quadrants, tortuosity of the same degree symmetrical in both eyes, or vein tortuosity with associated arterial tortuosity is characteristic of congenital vascular tortuosity (Fig. 4–35). Congenital vascular tortuosity has no significant implications. Comparison of both eyes, looking for symmetry, is valuable in all potentially congenital conditions including congenital vascular tortuosity.

Isolated arterial tortuosity is rare except in conditions like preretinal membrane formation, retinopa-

■ ■ ■ ■ ■ ■

**Clinical Note: Inherited Retinal
Venous Beading**

Inherited retinal venous beading has been reported as an autosomal dominant condition consisting of marked bilateral retinal venous beading accompanied by minimal conjunctival venous beading. The patients reportedly have associated vascular retinopathy simulating diabetic retinopathy, including the proliferative forms. The patients cited in this report had leukocytopenia, hereditary nephritis, but the majority were purportedly in good health. The patients with hereditary retinal venous beading presenting with vision-threatening conditions should be managed in a similar fashion to patients with diabetic retinopathy.

TABLE 4–13. DISEASES ASSOCIATED WITH ACQUIRED VEIN TORTUOSITY

Ipsilateral internal carotid artery disease

Diabetic retinopathy

Blood dyscrasias

Sickle-cell disease

Branch retinal vein occlusion

Central retinal vein occlusion

Hemicentral retinal vein occlusion

Vascular Sheathing

Retinal blood vessel walls are usually invisible by ophthalmoscopic examination. The blood vessel appearance is actually the visualization of the blood column. Retinal blood vessel walls only become visible when altered by an acquired disease or when congenital sheathing is present. When there is an acquired uniform change of the vessel wall, it is often most visible lateral to the blood column, because the thickness of the viewed wall is greater laterally (Fig. 4–36). Management of all vascular sheathing consists of diagnosis and management of the underlying systemic or retinal disease, as there is no particular management for the localized condition (Fig. 4–37).

Congenital vascular sheathing is a common occurrence in both retinal arteries and veins. This sheathing is usually continuous with and within 2 disc diameters of the optic nerve head. The vascular change is usually densest at the disc, tapering in density toward the periphery. Congenital vascular sheathing is more commonly associated with veins and may be present with persistence of the hyaloid vasculature. It is presumed that there is some connection between congenital vascular sheathing and the

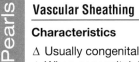

Vascular Sheathing

Characteristics

Δ Usually congenital

Δ When congenital, is continuous with and within 2 disc diameters of optic nerve

Δ Veins are most often affected and the sheathing appears along with other hyaloid remnants

Δ Venous

Halo sheathing is secondary to venous obstructive disease

Phagocytized RPE and fat have an affinity for vein walls in many localized retinal conditions

May occur in periphlebitis (MS), Eales' disease, sarcoidosis, toxoplasmosis, retinoschisis, and pars planitis

Δ Arterial

Typical sheathing associated with arteriosclerosis—copper to silver wire

With increasing severity, yellow reflex at bifurcations of large arteries

Management

Δ Ascertain underlying cause, whether localized retinal/optic nerve or systemic, and treat accordingly

Δ No specific localized management techniques for the sheathing

Δ Continue to monitor patient at routine intervals

residual tissue of the hyaloid vascular network.

Most of the time, venous sheathing is a collagenous or lipohyaline thickening of the venous walls, appearing hazy white. Venous sheathing often occurs secondary to long-standing venous obstructive disease. This type of sheathing is uniform and is known

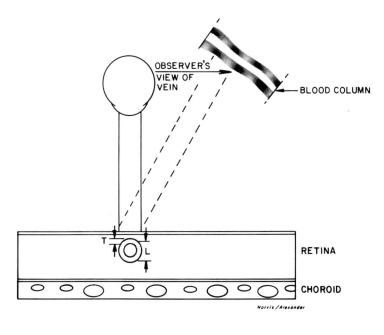

Figure 4–36. Top view of a sheathed retinal vein wall. Section L is thicker and more visible than section T.

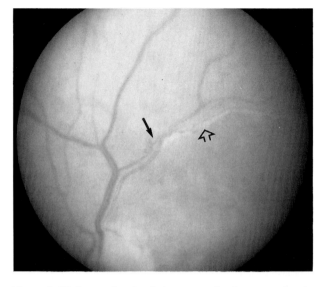

Figure 4–37. A vascular sheath (*open arrow*), often secondary to prior venous occlusion. The black arrow points to a collateral or shunt vessel in this long-standing BRVO.

as "halo" sheathing. When halo sheathing occurs, the vein may still be patent but may have a slightly reduced lumen.

It is important to note that phagocytized retinal pigment and free fat have an affinity for venous walls. This is most apparent in the condition of pigmented paravenous retinochoroidopathy as well as several other inflammatory retinal conditions.

Venous sheathing may occur in 10 to 25 percent of patients with multiple sclerosis (MS). The sheath-

ing in MS usually occurs away from the posterior pole. In the active inflammatory phase, a fuzzy white perivenous cuffing of the vein occurs. This stage is known as periphlebitis (Fig. 4–38), and may come and go with cyclical MS attacks. If prolonged periphlebitis occurs, permanent sheathing of the veins may occur. Periphlebitis can occur with other retinal and systemic diseases, such as Eales' disease, sarcoidosis, toxoplasmosis, acquired retinoschisis, pars plantis, and generalized posterior uveitis. There may be other vascular irregularities, such as hemorrhage associated with vein wall inflammation (periphlebitis) and pigment accumulation with chorioretinal inflammation.

Sheathing of both the arteries and veins may occur near the disc associated with prolonged papillitis, papillophlebitis, and papilledema. This should be easy to differentiate from congenital sheathing by the presence of other signs of nerve head disease.

Arterial sheathing occurs secondary to many systemic conditions that can have a negative impact on arterial wall structure. Early arteriosclerotic changes appear as a broadening of the central white reflex of an artery. This increases to the point where fine white lines may occur along the artery wall. Continued sclerosis of the vessel wall will lead to the classic copper wire appearance of the vessel, which is nothing more than an enhanced arterial wall reflex. Sclerosis of the arterial wall can lead to artery and vein crossing changes and, ultimately, branch retinal vein occlu-

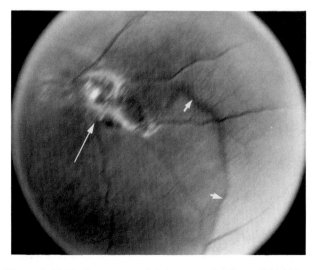

Figure 4–38. The long arrow points to a zone of active periphlebitis. The small arrows demarcate a zone of white without pressure.

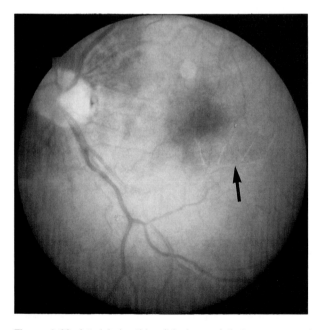

Figure 4–39. Arterial sheathing (*black arrow*) that was unassociated with systemic disease but was presumed instead to be of congenital origin.

TABLE 4–14. TRIGLYCERIDE LEVEL IN RELATION TO RETINAL APPEARANCE

Grade of Lipemia Retinalis	Triglyceride Level (mg%)	Fundus Appearance
I	2500–3500	Creamy thin peripheral vessels
II	3500–5000	Creamy thin peripheral vessels, abnormal color in vessels of posterior pole but veins and arteries distinguishable
III	> 5000	Fundus salmon colored, veins and arteries creamy and difficult to distinguish at disc

Modified and reprinted with permission from Alexander LJ. Ocular signs and symptoms of altered blood lipids. *J Am Optom Assoc.* 1983;54:123–126.

sions. With an increase in severity, the sclerosis of vessels may be random but will predominantly affect larger vessels. At the bifurcations of larger arteries, a yellow reflex often develops with crystalline reflections that spread into surrounding areas. There may be associated focal constrictions. The longer the patient survives, the more the sheathing may extend symmetrically to involve smaller vessels. These severely compromised arteries are still patent but represent a life-threatening underlying systemic disease process. The author has also seen a situation where the arteries were sheathed in a zone and all ocular and systemic findings were negative (Fig. 4–39).

Lipemia Retinalis

Lipemia retinalis refers to the ophthalmoscopic picture in which the retinal blood vessels assume a salmon or creamy color secondary to elevated serum triglyceride levels. A grading system for lipemic vessels has been suggested that distinguishes the fundus appearance related to the serum triglyceride levels. Table 4–14 outlines the grading system.

The retinal picture varies with the systemic triglyceride level. The first sign of lipemia retinalis is a creamy appearance to the peripheral retinal vessels (Fig. 4–40). As the triglyceride level increases, the vessels of the posterior pole become affected, ultimately leading to the point where arteries and veins become indistinguishable in color at the optic nerve head.

Lipemia retinalis is classically recognized as being non-vision-threatening. However, there have been reports of isolated complications, such as macular edema, retinal detachment, and hemorrhages secondary to the increased viscosity and decreased oxygen-carrying capacity of the affected blood. Other reports have suggested a retinal involvement similar to Coats' disease, with multiple hemorrhages and lipid infiltration. Certainly, the consistency of the

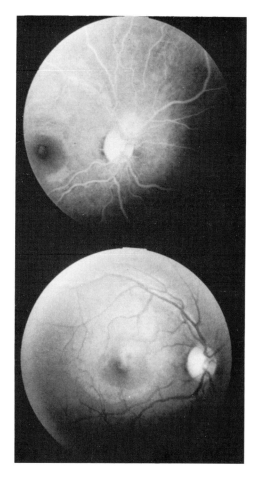

Figure 4–40. Top. Lipemic vessels associated with extremely high triglyceride levels. **Bottom.** Same patient after the triglyceride levels have been controlled.

Pearls

Lipemia Retinalis

Characteristics

△ Salmon or creamy colored retinal arteries and veins, varying in presentation with the triglyceride level

△ Retinal involvement may include retinal vaso-occlusive diseases as well as other manifestations of retinal hypoxia

Management

△ Assess for the presence and type of hyperlipoproteinemia

△ Tremendous concern because of the cardiovascular implications

△ A cardiology consultation and a nutritional consultation are in order

△ Follow at routine intervals dependent on both the localized ocular status and the systemic status

TABLE 4–15. THE HYPERLIPOPROTEINEMIAS: CLINICAL LABORATORY AND OCULAR SIGNS

Type of Hyperlipoproteinemia	Clinical Laboratory Signs	Ocular Signs
Type 1 chylomicronemia	Increased cholesterol Increased chylomicrons (triglycerides)	Lipemia retinalis, palpebral xanthomas, corneal arcus, xanthelasma
Type 2 hyperbeta-lipoproteinemia	Increased cholesterol Mild to moderately increased triglycerides	Corneal arcus, xanthelasma
Type 3 abnormal beta-lipoproteins and elevated triglycerides	Variable excesses in cholesterol and triglycerides	Possible corneal arcus, possible xanthelasma, palpebral xanthomas, lipemia retinalis
Type 4 hyperbeta-lipoproteinemia and elevated triglycerides	Variable excesses in cholesterol and triglycerides	Palpebral xanthomas, lipemia retinalis
Type 5 hyperchylomicronemia and hyperbeta-lipoproteinemia (type 1 and type 4)	Increased variable cholesterol and increased chylomicrons (triglycerides)	Palpebral xanthomas, lipemia retinalis

Modified and reprinted with permission from Alexander LJ. Ocular signs and symptoms of altered blood lipids. *J Am Optom Assoc.* 1983;54:123–126.

blood with such elevated triglyceride levels lends to vaso-occlusive disease.

Management. Of utmost importance in the management of lipemia retinalis is the realization of the impact of the elevated triglyceride levels on the cardiovascular system. The highly viscous blood coupled with the decreased oxygen-carrying capacity creates a situation of potential severe hypoxia. The patient should have a complete physical examination with emphasis on differential diagnosis of the hyperlipoproteinemias with serum electrophoresis. Under dietary control and possibly with pharmacologic intervention, the triglyceride level can be controlled, causing total resolution of the lipemic retinal picture. In certain instances, the nutritional consultation is as important as the cardiology consultation. Table 4–15 summarizes the clinical and ocular signs of hyperlipoproteinemias. **See color plate 35.**

Lipemia retinalis is often associated with diabetes, but the one condition does not automatically imply the other. The overall compromised systemic status, especially the fragility of the lipid metabolism, in diabetes does allow for the complications such as lipemia to manifest more easily.

Retinal Emboli

Introduction and Description. Often emboli eroding from remote vascular locations may occur within the retinal vasculature. Theoretically, any foreign substance introduced into the system could travel to the retinal system. The most frequent sites of genesis of retinal emboli are eroding carotid sinus lesions, eroding cardiac vegetations, and self-injected emboli associated with drug usage. Regardless of the source or clinical appearance, there is a strong association of retinal emboli with significant systemic cardiovascular disease.

The clinical picture of retinal emboli varies with the type and extent of the embolus. The embolus may be nothing more than a glowing intravascular plug or may cause vascular occlusion (Fig. 4–41). Table 4–16 summarizes the characteristics of commonly encountered retinal emboli. Further discussion of some of the effects of retinal emboli and thrombi are presented in the section on retinal vaso-occlusive disease later in the chapter. **See color plate 36.**

Identification of Hollenhorst plaques with or without symptoms has long been considered the equivalent of a retinal stroke or a sign of retinal ischemia and as such a warning for an impending cerebrovascular embolism. More recent reports, however, suggest that Hollenhorst plaques as an isolated phenomenon have a poor predictive value for further embolic events. A review of the literature reveals that the

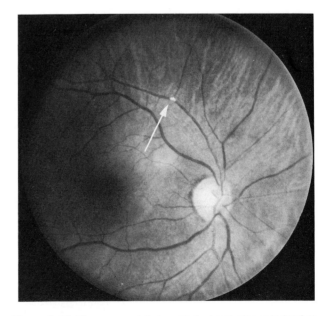

Figure 4–41. The arrow points to a Hollenhorst plaque lodged at an arterial bifurcation.

TABLE 4–16. CHARACTERISTICS OF EMBOLI AND THE RETINAL VASCULAR SYSTEM

Type of Embolus	Color	Location	Source	Retinal Prognosis
Cholesterol	Shiny yellow-orange	Often at bifurcations, may be mobile	Atheromas of carotid and of other vessels	No infarction unless multiple
Calcium	Gray-white	Unbranched arterioles, usually nonmobile	Eroding cardiac atheromas, artificial heart valves	Branch retinal artery occlusion
Platelets	Dull white long plugs	Arterioles but may readily break up	Carotid atheromas and thrombocytopenia	May lead to branch retinal artery occlusion
Fibrin	Not readily observed	Often laminar location, creating occlusion of central retinal artery	Thromboemboli after acute mitral insufficiency	Arterial occlusions
Talc or cornstarch	Shiny red-yellow	Capillaries of posterior pole	Self-injected in drug users	Microinfarcts in capillaries (cotton-wool spots)

proper approach to Hollenhorst plaques has yet to be discovered.

Emboli were first described in small and medium-sized arteries from atheromatous plaques, and were first observed as retinal artery plaques associated with ipsilateral disease of the internal carotid artery. Hollenhorst then described bright refractile plaques in retinal vessels in many patients with cerebral vascular insufficiency, assuming these to be common in carotid artery disease. A 1973 study by Pfaffenbach and Hollenhorst reported the morbidity and survivorship of patients with retinal emboli. The results for 208 patients (median age 64 years, range 46 to 84 years) are presented in Table 4–17. The causes of death for the 135 patients are presented in Figure 4–42. Table 4–18 lists the incidence of concurrent systemic disease or findings with the presentation of retinal emboli.

Survivorship rates have been assessed in patients presenting with central retinal artery occlusion (CRAO), branch retinal artery occlusion (BRAO), and retinal emboli. The survivorship rates with the retinal

ischemic events were less than an age- and sex-matched population and became statistically significant after 3 years (Savino et al, 1977). The survivorship rates between the control group and patients with visible retinal emboli was even greater than for those without visible retinal emboli. The report also demonstrated a four- to fivefold increase in stroke mortality rates. Figure 4–43 presents the causes of death encountered. In this report there is an increased prevalence of generalized vasculopathy (especially cardiac disease) in patients who develop retinal ischemia. This finding has been confirmed in other studies.

Early reports suggested that the presence of a retinal arterial embolus is an absolute indicator for extracranial arteriography, and that when ipsilateral ulcerative disease is found, carotid endarterectomy is indicated. More recent reports certainly temper this aggressive treatment. In fact, risk to vision as well as to life is significantly associated with the performance of carotid endarterectomy. A report published in 1990 found that the incidence of new Hollenhorst plaques

TABLE 4–17. MORBIDITY AND SURVIVORSHIP OF PATIENTS WITH EMBOLIC CHOLESTEROL CRYSTALS IN THE OCULAR FUNDUS

Years After Observation of Retinal Embolus	Death Rate (%)
1	15
3	29
7	54

From Pfaffenbach DD, Hollenhorst RW. Morbidity and survivorship of patients with embolic cholesterol crystals in the ocular fundus. *Am J Ophthalmol.* 1973;75:66–72.

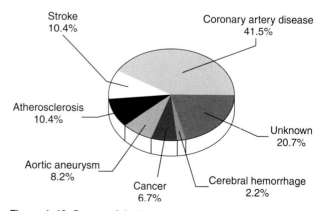

Figure 4–42. Causes of death associated with retinal emboli. *(Reproduced with permission from Alexander LJ. Variations in physician response to consultation requests for Hollenhorst plaques: A pilot study. J Am Optom Assoc. 1992;63:326–332.)*

TABLE 4–18. PREVALENCE OF VASCULAR DISEASE AMONG 208 PATIENTS WITH RETINAL CHOLESTEROL EMBOLI

Systemic Vascular Disease	Incidence of Concurrence With Retinal Artery Emboli (%)
Atherosclerosis	47.6
Angina or abnormal ecg	52.9
Carotid occlusive disease	47.6
Stroke	54.3
Myocardial infarction	60.1
Transient ischemic attacks	27.4
Amaurosis fugax	13.0
Retinal arterial occlusion	14.9
Arterial embolus in fellow eye	10.6

Pfaffenbach DD, Hollenhorst RW. Morbidity and survivorship of patients with embolic cholesterol crystals in the ocular fundus. *Am J Ophthalmol.* 1973;75:66–72.

(16.6 to 5.4 percent), new complaints of amaurosis fugax (4.2 to 0 percent), and new strokes (8.3 to 5.4 percent) was greater in patients with carotid endarterectomy than in those patients treated medically (Schwarcz et al, 1990). This group also noted that more than one third of patients with asymptomatic Hollenhorst plaques had normal internal carotid arteries as demonstrated by duplex ultrasonography, suggesting that the emboli originated elsewhere. Concomitant medical conditions in this study group are shown in Table 4–19. This report recommends no carotid endarterectomy with the presentation of an asymptomatic Hollenhorst plaque, but does recommend a thorough medical evaluation. Bunt (1986) found that a Hollenhorst plaque is a retinal embolic event that may have been present for several months and is not highly correlated with significant carotid disease. He does add that the patient should have a thorough medical evaluation. Other clinicians have emphasized that should visual symptoms also be present, arteriography and perhaps endarterectomy are in order.

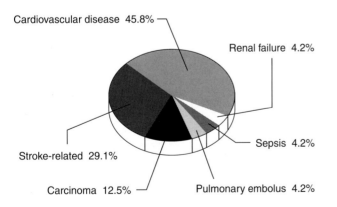

Figure 4–43. Causes of death associated with retinal ischemia. *(Reproduced with permission from Alexander LJ. Variations in physician response to consultation requests for Hollenhorst plaques: A pilot study. J Am Optom Assoc. 1992;63:326–332.)*

TABLE 4–19. CONCOMITANT MEDICAL CONDITIONS ASSOCIATED WITH HOLLENHORST PLAQUES

Systemic Vascular Disease	Incidence of Concurrence With Retinal Artery Emboli (%)
Hypertension	70.0
Diabetes mellitus	45.0
Cardiac disease	41.0
Elevated cholesterol levels	59.0
Carotid stenosis ipsilateral	55.2

Schwarcz TH, et al. Hollenhorst plaques: Retinal manifestations and the role of carotid endarterectomy. *J Vasc Surg.* 1990;11:635–641.

Further analysis of reports confirms the confusion that exists in the interpretation of ocular signs of potential cardiovascular disease. Very often the reports use differing methodology, making it even more difficult to interpret results. Berguer (1985) found that vascular lesions could also be present in the ophthalmic arteries and the posterior ciliary arteries in retinal ischemia syndromes, confirming the fact that the clinician must look deeper than just the carotid system. Berguer looked at 20 patients averaging 63 years in age (range, 47 to 91 years) with retinal ischemia syndromes (35 percent central retinal artery occlusion, 20 percent retinal artery embolus, 15 percent amaurosis fugax, 15 percent ischemic optic neuropathy, 10 percent cilioretinal artery occlusion, and 5 percent venous stasis retinopathy). He found that 60 percent of the patients had ipsilateral carotid occlusion and 50 percent contralateral occlusions. Table 4–20 presents concomitant medical conditions in his patient cohort. Other investigators have found a weak correlation between retinal ischemic syndromes and carotid disease, but did suggest that the presence of a Hollenhorst plaque is more likely to be a marker for a stenotic or ulcerated plaque. The group also found that migraines and/or cardiac sources for the transient ischemic attacks must be considered. Bruno (1990) reviewed 24 patients with persistent monocular vision loss secondary to retinal ischemia. Carotid disease was found in 80 percent of patients in whom infarction had occurred during wakefulness and in 50

TABLE 4–20. CONCOMITANT MEDICAL CONDITIONS ASSOCIATED WITH RETINAL ISCHEMIC SYNDROMES

Systemic Vascular Condition	Incidence of Concurrence With Retinal Ischemic Syndromes (%)
Hypertension	55.0
Coronary Artery Disease	40.0
Diabetes	25.0
Elevated erythrocyte sedimentation rate	15.0
Lipid/cholesterol abnormality	15.0

Berguer R. Idiopathic ischemic syndromes of the retina and optic nerve and their carotid origin. *J Vasc Surg.* 1985;2:649–653.

TABLE 4–21. CONCOMITANT MEDICAL FINDINGS IN PATIENTS WITH RETINAL INFARCTS

Systemic Vascular Condition	Incidence of Concurrence With Retinal Infarcts (%)
Hypertension	62.5
Diabetes	20.8
Carotid disease	62.5
Cardiac source of embolus	8.3

From Bruno A, et al. Retinal infarction during sleep and wakefulness. *Stroke.* 1990;21:1494–1496.

percent in whom infarction had occurred during sleep. In patients under age 50 years, carotid studies were all normal. Concomitant medical conditions found in Bruno's patients are listed in Table 4–21. Bruno and associates also found in a later study (1992) the correlation of Hollenhorst plaques to hypertension, cigarette smoking, ischemic heart disease, and echolucent carotid plaques.

Trobe (1987) summarized the most recent data regarding the risk of stroke related to "specific patient groups" (Fig. 4–44). As late as 1990, the introductory statement in a report by Bruno concerning the risk of stroke is "More than 90% of patients with Amaurosis Fugax have abnormal carotid angiograms." The confusion still exists.

A retinal arterial embolus is an indication of associated systemic vascular disease. Both morbidity and survivorship are diminished associated with the appearance of a retinal embolus. The primary cause of death associated with a retinal embolus is coronary artery disease. The primary cause of death associated with retinal ischemia is cardiovascular disease. The risk of stroke also increases with the appearance of retinal arterial emboli.

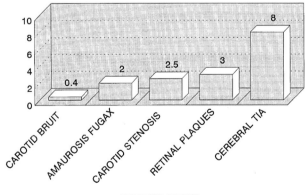

AVERAGE ANNUAL UNTREATED STROKE RISK(%)

PATIENT GROUP

Figure 4–44. Physical findings associated with increased risk for the development of stroke. TIA, transient ischemic attack. *(Reproduced with permission from Alexander LJ. Variations in physician response to consultation requests for Hollenhorst plaques: A pilot study. J Am Optom Assoc. 1992;63:326–332.)*

Retinal Emboli

Characteristics

Δ Strong association with systemic diseases such as internal carotid stenosis and cardiovascular disease

Δ Manifest in many different forms

Δ May precipitate vaso-occlusive retinal disease

Management

Δ Ascertain underlying systemic cause. Comprehensive physical examination including:
  1. Real time ultrasound evaluation of carotids
  2. Arteriography only if necessary
  3. Stress electrocardiography
  4. Echocardiography
  5. Blood chemistries/lipid profiles as indicated
  6. In-depth assessment of hypertension
  7. Counseling for cigarette smokers

Management. When considering concomitant medical conditions associated with retinal emboli and retinal ischemic syndromes, hypertension, coronary artery disease (abnormal ECG), and diabetes dominate the picture along with carotid artery disease.

In view of both morbidity characteristics and concomitant medical conditions, it appears that investigation of both the carotid system and the cardiac system is indicated. The basis of the workup must be a comprehensive physical examination. Certainly, real-time ultrasound evaluation of the carotid system is indicated in cases of both symptomatic and asymptomatic Hollenhorst plaque. It has been shown that real-time ultrasonography demonstrates a 95 percent agreement with angiography in identifying carotid stenosis of greater than 50 percent. Although angiography is diagnostic, it carries a significantly higher morbidity and mortality rate than ultrasonography. Because of the strong relationship to cardiac disease and the potential for emboli dislodging from cardiac valves, both electrocardiography and echocardiography may be indicated. Although ECG is insensitive as an indicator of cardiac disease, stress ECG and a thallium graduated exercise test may be more effective. Echocardiography, although not documented in the literature as an effective test in the workup of a Hollenhorst plaque, deserves consideration because of the potential association of valvular disease and circulatory emboli. Fasting lipid levels are of limited value except from the standpoint of the strong relationship of elevated cholesterol levels to coronary artery disease. Blood chemistry values, specifically of cardiac enzymes, would give some indication of active underlying systemic cardiovascular disease.

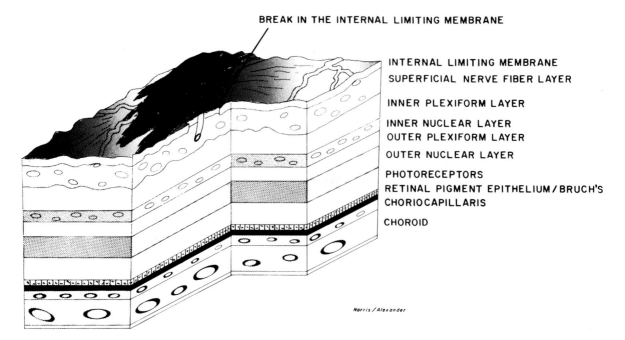

BREAK IN THE INTERNAL LIMITING MEMBRANE

INTERNAL LIMITING MEMBRANE
SUPERFICIAL NERVE FIBER LAYER

INNER PLEXIFORM LAYER

INNER NUCLEAR LAYER
OUTER PLEXIFORM LAYER

OUTER NUCLEAR LAYER

PHOTORECEPTORS
RETINAL PIGMENT EPITHELIUM/BRUCH'S
CHORIOCAPILLARIS

CHOROID

Norris/Alexander

Figure 4–45. Schematic cross section demonstrating the clinicopathology of preretinal membrane formation.

Preretinal Membrane Formation

Introduction and Description. Preretinal membrane formation includes premacular fibroplasia, preretinal gliosis, epiretinal membrane, macular pucker, preretinal macular fibrosis, and surface-wrinkling retinopathy. Preretinal membrane formation (Figs. 4–45 to 4–48) is discussed in this section of the text because the genesis is often associated with retinal vasculopathy.

Preretinal membrane formation is an anatomic alteration that can result from a variety of precipitating factors. The condition is often placed in the category of venous and capillary obstructive diseases, because the advanced stages are similar to the retinal reaction seen after the obstruction of a macular draining vein. There also seems to be a relationship between diabetes and preretinal membrane formation, especially in the ab-

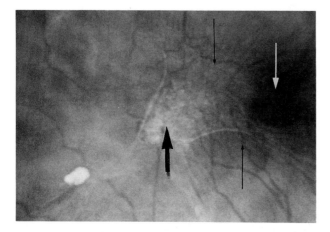

Figure 4–46. Photograph demonstrating a gathered pleat variety of preretinal membrane. The white arrow points to the macula, the large black arrow points to the bulk of the membrane, and the small black arrow points to the tugging of the membrane. *(Modified and reprinted with permission from Alexander LJ. Pre-retinal membrane formation. J Am Optom Assoc. 1980; 51:567–572.)*

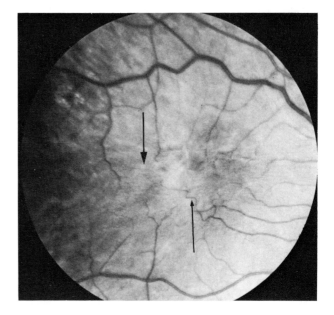

Figure 4–47. A preretinal membrane *(large arrow)* creating vascular tortuosity *(small arrow)*.

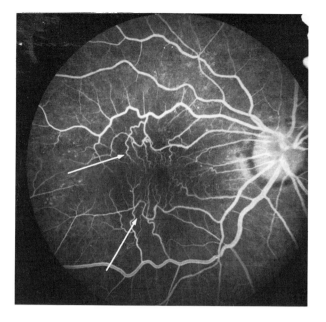

Figure 4–48. Angiogram of the eye shown in Figure 4–47, demonstrating the vascular tortuosity that results from a preretinal membrane.

sence of diabetic retinopathy. Preretinal membrane formation is often associated with surgical procedures for retinal detachment, becoming a significant postsurgical complication in some instances and being referred to as *proliferative vitreoretinopathy* in those cases. Preretinal membrane formation may been seen with photocoagulation, trauma, macular holes, and inflammation of ocular tissue. Idiopathic preretinal membrane formation also occurs as a separate entity, predominantly in patients over 50 years of age with no demonstrable etiology. It has been proposed and demonstrated histologically that the glinting reflex of the fundus described in patients with retinitis pigmentosa is the result of preretinal membrane formation.

Preretinal membranes have been classified into three grades according to appearance. Grade 0 is cellophane maculopathy, which appears as a translucent membrane without distortion of the inner retinal surface. Grade 1 occurs as a translucent membrane with the underlying retina gathered into a series of small folds. The underlying vessels may be indistinct, and surrounding small vessels may be slightly tortuous. In grades 0 and 1, visual acuity may be compromised but metamorphopsia is characteristic. Grade 2 appears as a semitranslucent membrane that may obscure the underlying vessels of the retina. Retinal hemorrhages and localized serous detachment may accompany grade 2. At this stage, there is evidence of dye leakage with fluorescein angiography. Visual acuity in grade 2 is often compromised.

The etiology of preretinal membrane formation is controversial. Histologic studies support the theory that preretinal membranes occur as the result of proliferation of retinal glial cells on the internal limiting membrane that have escaped through breaks in the internal limiting membrane. This is supported by the appearance of membranes in retinal vascular diseases in which vasculitis contributes to a break in the internal limiting membrane. Trauma and retinal detachment also have the potential to compromise the internal limiting membrane. It should be noted that the membranes often are pigmented in postsurgical retinal detachment procedures.

Subjective complaints related to preretinal membrane formation vary according to associated conditions that precipitate the formation. Should the membrane be idiopathic, there may be a visual loss, but more often metamorphopsia is the complaint. Fewer than 5 percent of patients with only preretinal membranes have a visual loss to 20/200 or worse, and fewer than 20 percent have involvement of the fellow eye. More often there are no subjective complaints and preretinal membranes are found on routine examination. The earliest sign is described as a glinting reflex seen on the retinal surface with an ophthalmoscope. This may be accentuated by using the red-free filter. Deviation of retinal vessels (increased localized tortuosity) is also present. These vessels acquire a corkscrew pattern that is especially enhanced with fluorescein angiography. In approximately 25 percent of cases, traction on the retinal vessels from the preretinal membrane will alter vessel physiology, leading to leakage that may cause a further reduction of acuity because of resultant macular edema.

Preretinal Membrane Formation

Pearls

Characteristics

△ Associated with a break in the internal limiting membrane and proliferation of cells on its surface

△ Volcano and gathered pleat variety

△ Create underlying vascular tortuosity, often corkscrew vessels

△ May create metamorphopsia, macular edema, and vision reduction

△ Often benign and self-limited process

Management

△ If vision severely compromised or if fresh, consider a retinal consultation

△ If long-standing or removed from macula, educate patient and monitor yearly

△ Postvitrectomy correction may necessitate prescription of prism for monocular diplopia and iekonic lens considerations

The larger preretinal membranes are visualized more easily with stereoscopic examination techniques and red-free filters. They may become more translucent with age and typically have either a volcano pattern like puckered plastic wrap or a gathered pleat appearance.

Management. In general, preretinal membranes are benign, self-limited processes, but may cause significant reduction in vision if they have an impact on the macular area. Should vision be severely compromised or if the membrane is relatively fresh, a retinal consultation is indicated. There has been some success with vitrectomy in fresh cases of preretinal membranes, especially in diabetic retinopathy. There are, however, the potential side effects of long-standing macular edema and anatomically induced aniseikonia in patients who have had vitrectomy. Often monocular diplopia results from vitrectomy intervention necessitating implementation of prism correction added to iekonic lens prescription to overcome the untoward effects. **See color plate 37.** Recent reports cite visual improvement with intervention in 43 percent of cases in 6 to 12 months, with a 58 percent success rate over 5 years. Complications from vitrectomy for preretinal membranes may approach 13 percent. Factors determining long-term success with surgery include preoperative visual acuity, preoperative lens status, duration of symptoms, and the occurrence of intraoperative complications.

RETINAL VASO-OCCLUSIVE DISEASE

Retinal vaso-occlusive disease is the second most prevalent retinal vascular disease seen in clinical practice today. The process occurs more commonly in the elderly, but may occur in younger patients as well, as there is a strong relationship to the systemic vascular status. In younger patients, the vascular occlusion is more often related to situations of increased blood viscosity. Recent advances and modification of management protocol have, however, brought improvement in the prognosis of these disease processes. All basic principles regarding hemorrhages, exudates, and retinal vascular alterations discussed previously may be applied in developing an understanding of the five types of retinal vaso-occlusive disease: branch retinal vein occlusion, central retinal vein occlusion, hemicentral retinal vein occlusion, branch retinal artery occlusion, and central retinal artery occlusion.

Branch Retinal Vein Occlusion

Introduction and Description. Branch retinal vein occlusion (BRVO) has been reported to be the second most prevalent of the retinal vascular diseases seen in

---

Pearls

Branch Retinal Vein Occlusion

Δ Strong association with systemic disease

Characteristics

Δ Occurs most frequently at arteriovenous crossings and is the result of a thickened artery pressing on a thin-walled vein
Δ Nonischemic BRVO characterized by dot-blot hemorrhages and lipid infiltrates in the involved sector
Δ Ischemic (Hypoxic) BRVO characterized by dot-blot hemorrhages, lipid infiltrates, cotton-wool spots, and flame-shaped hemorrhages
Δ Collaterals may form to drain the affected area and should not be confused with neovascularization
Δ Twenty-five to thirty percent chance of neovascularization of disc or retina
Δ Visual fields will cross over the horizontal raphe secondary to spread of edema

Management

Δ Ascertain underlying systemic disease
Δ Rule out glaucoma
Δ **Primary workup**
    Blood pressure and pulse evaluation
    Fasting blood glucose
    Lipid profile
    Complete blood count with differential and platelets
    Carotid palpation and auscultation (ODM?)
Δ **Secondary workup**
    Rule out hyperviscosity—serum electrophoresis
    Prothrombin and partial thromboplastin times
    Erythrocyte sedimentation rate
    Antinuclear antibodies and rheumatoid factor
    Consider a cardiovascular workup with a chemistry profile, especially with hypertension
    Consider a carotid screening (duplex ultrasound)
Δ Fluorescein angiography indicated if threat of edema to macular area, indications of retinal nonperfusion, and indications of neovascularization secondary to hypoxia
Δ Follow carefully for the resolution of macular edema or the development of neovascularization every 1 to 2 months initially then every 3 to 12 months after
Δ Follow every 4 months postphotocoagulation, looking for the resolution of edema or the regression of neovascularization
Δ Follow 1 month post-grid photocoagulation for the threat of choroidal neovascularization
Δ When in doubt, a retinal consultation is indicated
Δ Some suggest that topical timoptic may increase retinal volumetric flow rate and may decrease the external pressure on the artery vein crossing

eyecare practice (diabetic retinopathy is first). There is little disagreement about the ophthalmoscopic characteristics of BRVO that assist in the diagnosis. There is, however, considerable controversy surrounding the etiology and management of patients with BRVO. There are also different types of BRVO that occur in clinically different ways, further adding to the confusion. Branch retinal vein occlusion is often classified in three categories: (1) major BRVO, which involves at least 5 disc diameters of the retina; (2) secondary BRVO, which involves at least 2 but not more than 5 disc diameters of the retina; and (3) tertiary or tributary BRVO, which involves fewer than 2 disc diameters of the retina.

From an epidemiologic standpoint, the peak incidence of BRVO is in the fifth to sixth decades of life, with no racial or sexual predilection. There appears to be an approximately 4 to 5 percent incidence of bilaterality. BRVO has also been related to diabetes, hyperopia, hypertension, and other vascular diseases as well as the suggestion that it occurs more frequently in glaucoma or with intraocular pressures in the 21 to 29 mm Hg range. The increase in intraocular pressure purportedly increases the pressure on the already thin-walled veins actually causing stress on the system. This is the basis for the recommendation of the implementation of topical antiglaucoma agents in the management of BRVO.

Although the specific microscopic events surrounding BRVO are somewhat obscure, a few broad statements can be made regarding the clinical process. Arterial disease plays a part in the process, but it is not possible to state that this is the sole initiating factor in the condition. It can be stated that BRVO has a strong association with systemic-based diseases (57 percent of patients). Hypertension, glucose intolerance, hyperlipidemia, and hypercholesterolemia have all been implicated. Recent work implicates platelet coagulation activities in early thrombosis formation in retinal vein occlusion. Table 4–22 summarizes some of the systemic factors common in BRVO. **See color plates 34, 38, and 39.**

The association with systemic disease points to the importance of diagnosis and appropriate management of any underlying systemic vascular condition. Patients with BRVO should have the following minimal screening tests performed: blood pressure and pulse, fasting blood glucose, lipid profile, complete blood count (CBC) with differential and platelet count, and carotid palpation and auscultation. Other tests should be to rule out hyperviscosity syndromes, especially in younger patients: prothrombin and partial thromboplastin times, erythrocyte sedimentation rate, antinuclear antibodies (systemic lupus erythematosus), the rheumatoid factor, and a chest x-ray. It is also prudent to consider a cardiovascular workup and internal carotid screening with the possible consideration of duplex carotid ultrasonography.

Branch retinal vein occlusion can occur as two distinct clinical entities, nonischemic retinopathy and ischemic retinopathy. The distinction is not, however, always clear-cut and often must be made with fluorescein angiography to ascertain areas of capillary nonperfusion. The ischemic variety implies hypoxia with the subsequent possibility of development of neovascularization. The distinction is a clinical impression depending on the degree of superficial hemorrhage, cotton-wool spots, and associated arterial changes, but is truly best determined by fluorescein angiography. The superior temporal veins are affected most often, this being attributed to the fact that there are more arteriovenous crossings in the superior temporal retina than elsewhere.

The clinical picture varies considerably depending on the site of the occlusion, degree of ischemia created, and elapsed time since the occlusion (Figs. 4–49 to 4–55). Often a prodromal sign (Bonnet's sign) will

TABLE 4–22. SYSTEMIC FACTORS COMMON IN BRANCH RETINAL VEIN OCCLUSION

Carotid artery disease	von Hippel–Lindau's disease
Hypertension	Coats' disease
Diabetes	Eales disease
Hyperlipidemia and hypercholesterolemia	Phlebitis
Altered platelet function	Cavernous sinus thrombosis
Estrogens	Elevated serum immunoglobulins
Chronic lung disease	Elevated intraocular pressure
Trauma	

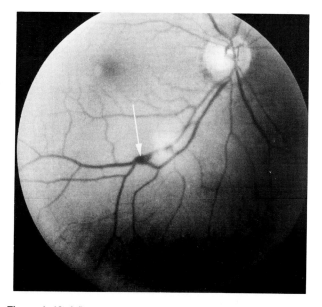

Figure 4–49. A flame-shaped hemorrhage (Bonnet's sign) at an arteriovenous crossing, the sign of a possible impending branch retinal vein occlusion at the site.

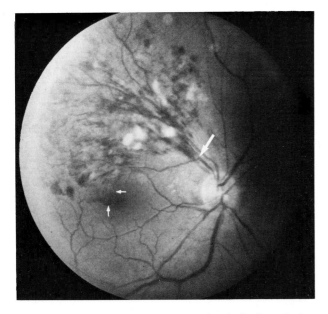

Figure 4–50. A full-blown ischemic branch retinal vein occlusion. The large arrow points to the site of the occlusion; the small arrows outline the ingress of edema into the macular area.

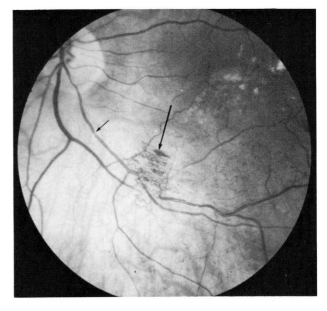

Figure 4–52. Black-and-white photograph illustrating the aftermath of a branch retinal vein occlusion. The small arrow points to the affected vein, and the large arrow points to a conglomerate of collaterals. *(Reprinted with permission from Alexander LJ. The implications and management of retinal vaso-occlusive disease. S J Optom. 1986;2:20–34.)*

occur as small splinter hemorrhages around an area of arteriovenous nicking (Fig. 4–49). Should an occlusion occur either at an arteriovenous crossing or elsewhere, the classical BRVO develops. Figure 4–56 demonstrates the factors involved in the genesis of the

occlusion. The clinical picture is that of dilated tortuous veins and dot-blot hemorrhages from the site of the obstruction out to the retinal periphery in the sector of the retina normally drained by the affected vein. Retinal ischemia and increases in venous pressure cre-

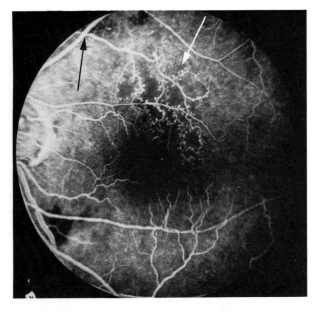

Figure 4–51. Early-phase fluorescein angiogram with the black arrow pointing to the site of the vein occlusion and the white arrow pointing to the area of microaneurysmal formation. These microaneurysms will leak, creating edema in the macula.

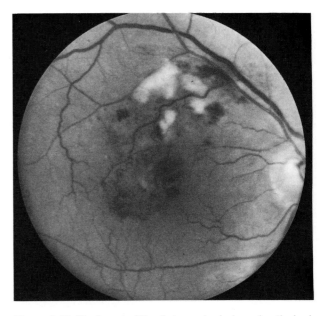

Figure 4–53. Black-and-white photograph of a branch retinal vein occlusion in the macular area.

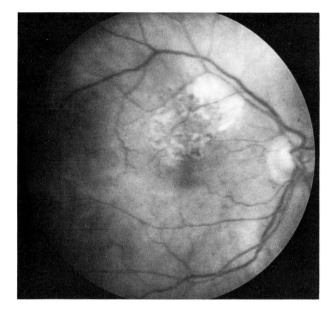

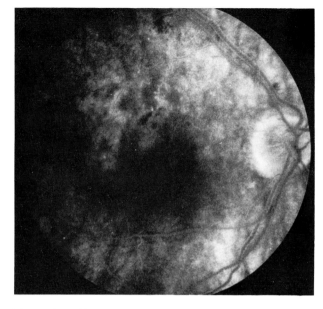

Figure 4–54. Black-and-white photograph of postphotocoagulation scars of branch retinal vein occlusion shown in Figure 4–53.

Figure 4–55. Fluorescein angiogram of the eye shown in Figure 4–54, demonstrating total absence of edema after photocoagulation.

ate perifoveal capillary endothelial damage, leakage, collateral formation, poor capillary perfusion, and ultimately signs of hypoxia with the possible end result being neovascularization. Microaneurysms also occur in the affected area, leaking and creating retinal edema. As more retinal hypoxia is created, cotton-wool spots and flame-shaped hemorrhages are added to the picture. Lipid infiltrates often occur near the site of the occlusion about 2 months after onset. Figure 4–57 is a schematic representation of the edema and sequelae. If the macular area is not adequately drained, partial or full macular edema (48 to 56 percent of cases) may develop, leading to visual compromise. It is important to understand that edema in the macula is one cause of vision loss in BRVO. Other causes of vision loss in BRVO include foveal hemor-

rhages, foveal retinal pigment epithelial hemorrhages, capillary nonperfusion in the foveal area, macular traction secondary to neovascularization, and the remote possibility of vitreous hemorrhage. As the BRVO progresses, collateral channels open to shunt blood around the occluded zone. The development of effective collaterals is crucial in the prognosis for recovery (Fig. 4–52). Collaterals observed temporal to the macula crossing the horizontal raphe are pathognomonic of an old BRVO.

Should the affected retinal area not drain properly, increased resistance to incoming oxygenated blood occurs. If this oxygenated blood is not allowed sufficient access to the retinal tissue, hypoxia results. If the hypoxia is sufficient, a vasoproliferative stimulus is created, precipitating the development of neo-

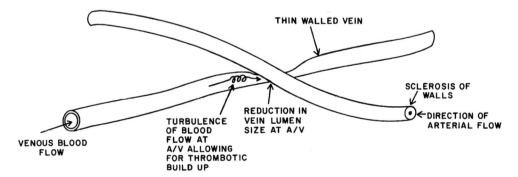

Figure 4–56. Schematic demonstrating the factors involved in the occlusion of a retinal vein. *(Reprinted with permission from Alexander LJ. The implications and management of retinal vaso-occlusive disease. S J Optom. 1986;2:20–34.)*

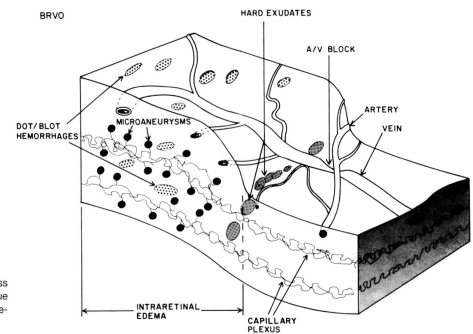

Figure 4–57. Schematic retinal cross section demonstrating the tissue changes secondary to the stasis created by a retinal vein occlusion.

vascularization. This neovascularization may occur in the preretinal form, the disc form, and has even been reported at the iris margin. Vitreous hemorrhage or retinal traction may then occur. It appears that neovascularization may occur in approximately 25 to 30 percent of patients with BRVO. Often this neovascularization is hidden by the overlying hemorrhage and becomes apparent only by fluorescein angiography after some resolution of the hemorrhage.

When retinal occlusive disease occurs, there appear to be changes in the vitreous overlying the process. When the vitreous is totally attached to the retina in eyes with BRVO, the vitreous adjacent to and overlying the area becomes liquefied. In the early stages, the gel exhibits white degenerative opacities that become larger with resorption of the retinal hemorrhage. Vitreous detachment also has an effect on the development of complications. The status of the vitreous as it relates to complications is summarized in Table 4–23.

TABLE 4–23. EFFECT OF THE STATE OF THE VITREOUS ON VISION-THREATENING FACTORS IN BRANCH RETINAL VEIN OCCLUSION

State of Vitreous	No Vitreous Detachment (%)	Partial Vitreous Detachment) (%)	Complete Vitreous Detachment (%)
Neovascularization	16	64	0
Vitreous hemorrhage	12	64	7
Macular edema	54	56	29

Reprinted with permission from Alexander LJ. The implications and management of retinal vaso-occlusive disease. *S J Optom.* 1986;2:20–34.

Another interesting variety of BRVO can be very visually devastating because of the location and the exquisite sensitivity of the macula to edema. Macular branch retinal vein occlusion (MBRVO) or tributary occlusion results from an occlusion of a small tributary branch near the macula. There is an 85 percent incidence of macular edema associated with MBRVO.

One additional finding that may assist in the diagnosis is the effect of venous occlusive disease on intraocular pressure (IOP). It has been found that 80 percent of patients have a decrease in IOP in the eye with venous occlusive disease. There is a greater decrease in central retinal vein occlusion (CRVO) than BRVO, a greater decrease in ischemic CRVO versus nonischemic CRVO, and a greater decrease in patients with relatively high IOPs in the fellow eye. There appears to be no significant effect in MBRVO. The decrease of the IOP is likely secondary to poor vascular perfusion to the ciliary body, creating a decrease in the production of aqueous. The duration of the hypotensive effect is 3 months in ischemic CRVO, 18 months in nonischemic CRVO, and 24 months in BRVO. Visual field defects may cross over the horizontal raphe due to the spread of edema, which has no firm anatomic boundaries.

Fluorescein angiographic findings are very important in the diagnostic process of BRVO and can be divided into signs of the acute and chronic phases (Table 4–24).

Much of the controversy surrounding the management of BRVO stems from the controversy surrounding the natural course of the disease. If untreated, patients often have results very similar to results in patients treated medically or surgically. Cer-

TABLE 4–24. FLUORESCEIN ANGIOGRAPHIC FINDINGS IN STAGES OF BRANCH RETINAL VEIN OCCLUSION

Acute Stage	Chronic Stage
1. Delayed filling of occluded vein, with possible leakage from wall	1. Appearance of collateral channels and shunt vessels
2. Focal hyperfluorescence near spot of occlusion	2. Microaneurysms and macroaneurysms
3. Obscuration of background choroidal fluorescence by hemorrhage	3. Areas of capillary dropout
4. Alterations in the perifoveal capillary net and areas of capillary nonperfusion	4. Macular edema
	5. Neovascularization (disc and elsewhere)
5. Diffuse intraretinal leakage of fluorescein	6. Neurosensory retinal detachment

Reprinted with permission from Alexander LJ. The implications and management of retinal vaso-occlusive disease. *S J Optom.* 1986;2:20–34.

tain factors are, however, well documented. In general, studies report visual acuities of 6/12 (20/40) or better in 53 to 60 percent of untreated BRVO patients who have been followed for at least 1 year. This neglects, however, the percent who do not improve.

Complications develop, including neovascularization, vitreous hemorrhages, macular edema, macroaneurysms, chronic fibrosis, rhegmatogenous retinal detachment, and possibly neovascular glaucoma. Prognostic indicators are outlined in Table 4–25.

Management. Management of BRVO is the area of greatest controversy, which exists because of the relatively good prognosis associated with the natural course of the disease. One uncontroversial aspect is the need to investigate each patient for the presence of associated systemic diseases. Every patient should have a complete physical examination, including blood pressure and pulse determination, blood glucose testing, lipid profile, CBC with differential and platelet count, and carotid palpation and auscultation (ophthalmodynamometry [ODM]?). Secondarily, the practitioner should rule out hyperviscosity syndromes especially in young patients, considering prothrombin and partial thromboplastin times, erythrocyte sedimentation rate, antinuclear antibodies, the rheumatoid factor, and a chest x-ray. A cardiovascular consultation asking for blood chemistries may be in order especially if hypertension is a factor or if there are signs or symptoms of internal carotid stenosis.

Several medical management approaches have been advocated for BRVO. Low-molecular-weight dextran in combination with papaverine hydrochloride, anticoagulants, fibrinolytic agents, antithrombotic agents, steroids, and vasodilators has been tried, but no proof exists as to its efficacy.

TABLE 4–25. PROGNOSTIC INDICATORS IN BRANCH RETINAL VEIN OCCLUSIONS

Factors	Impact on Prognosis
Location of occlusion	The nearer the disc, the more area involved
	The nearer the macula, the greater the likelihood of macular edema
Caliber of vessel	The larger the caliber (except macular BRVO) the poorer the prognosis
Degree of obstruction	Total obstruction creates poorer prognosis
Intensity and duration of macular edema	86% of patients with macular edema over 6 months and visual acuity of 20/50 or worse fail to improve
Degree of capillary closure: Either fluorescein angiography changes or sheathing of arterioles	The greater the area of capillary closure, the more likely the development of neovascularization
Status of perifoveal capillary net by fluorescein angiography	If perifoveal capillary net unbroken, better resultant vision
Presence of intact venule between obstructed vein and macula	Drainage of macula prevents threat of vision loss secondary to macular edema
Initial visual acuity	If 20/40 or better, excellent prognosis. If 20/200 or worse, poor prognosis
General systemic health	Blood, vessel, and coagulation status help determine rate of recovery

Ticlopidine has been evaluated for its action as a platelet aggregation inhibitor in the treatment of BRVO and has been shown to be effective if the occlusion is fresh. Ticlopidine has shown similar results in the treatment of central retinal vein occlusion.

Topical antiglaucoma medications are often recommended to decrease the intraocular pressure in order to reduce the external pressure on the artery/vein crossing. The topical beta blockers are also thought to positively effect the volumetric flow in the vessels, but this is controversial. A provocative question would be the possible efficacy of a topical beta blocker to abort or prevent the possible occlusion in the case of an impending occlusion as evidenced by a Bonnet's sign.

Photocoagulation has a place in the management of BRVO. The rationale for photocoagulation of non-proliferative BRVO is threefold: (1) the scar tissue formed in photocoagulation acts as a barrier to prevent retinal edema from spreading to the fovea, (2) areas of leakage are sealed to prevent further leakage, and (3) destruction of the capillary bed reduces the input of arterial blood to obstructed areas, which reduces edema and allows the intact bed to drain more effectively.

BRVOs threatening macular vision deserve a consultation with a competent retinal specialist, especially if the macular edema is persistent, causing vision of 20/40 or worse. Fluorescein angiography is indicated in all cases of macular edema once the retinal hemorrhages have cleared to produce a blueprint for the proper application of the photocoagulation. Grid photocoagulation is used in these instances, using green argon or red krypton applied in mild to moderate burns placed a burn width apart in the area of capillary leakage. The treatment may extend from the major vascular arcades to the edge of the foveal avascular zone. As with scatter, photocoagulation over a retinal hemorrhage is contraindicated. These patients must be followed up at 4-month intervals until stability occurs. Additional treatment is considered if visual loss from the edema persists at the 4-month follow-up.

The fresher the macular edema, the better the prognosis; however, it is recommended that laser intervention not be applied within the first 3 months postocclusion, because there may be spontaneous regression. If hemorrhage is present in the fovea, laser intervention is of questionable benefit, because clearing of the hemorrhage may result in improved acuity. There is a significantly more favorable prognosis (2:1) in patients treated by these criteria than in those left untreated. Regardless of criteria, which may change monthly, a BRVO threatening macular function requires a consultation with a retinal specialist. One of the possible results of grid photocoagulation is the appearance of choroidal neovascularization. The neo-

vascularization may appear early postintervention, and the patient should be examined within the first month for this complication.

Any retinal or disc neovascularization deserves a retinal consultation. Prophylactic scatter photocoagulation in the involved sector of a BRVO does not seem to be of benefit in the prevention of neovascularization. Scatter photocoagulation in the nonperfused area is, however, of benefit once neovascularization occurs. Regression of neovascularization is important to prevent the possibility of a devastating vitreous hemorrhage or the complication of macular traction. The preferred wavelength for scatter is argon green, but krypton red may be of benefit with cataracts and intraretinal and vitreous hemorrhage. Follow-up on these patients must be at least every 4 months until regression is documented. Additional treatment should be considered if the neovascularization persists at the 4-month follow-up.

There has been some suggestion that vitrectomy with surgical decompression of an arteriovenous crossing may be of benefit in the treatment of BRVO. Unfortunately, sufficient evidence does not yet exist to make an across-the-board recommendation for this type of intervention.

If photocoagulation is not indicated, patients with BRVOs should be followed very carefully, with routine assessment of visual acuity, Amsler grid (use the home Amsler grid), and careful dilated fundus examination every 1 to 2 months initially and then every 3 to 12 months depending on the retinal status. Fluorescein angiography should be performed when the fundus becomes suspect or when there is indication of the possibility of nonperfusion. It is important not to disregard the fact that there is probably an underlying systemic disease process that deserves careful investigation.

Central Retinal Vein Occlusion

Introduction and Description. Central retinal vein occlusion (CRVO) is a very destructive retinal condition with a strong association with systemic diseases or situations that can cause undue pressure on the optic nerve. The pressure within or without can easily compress the thin-walled central retinal vein. In addition, about 20 percent of patients with CRVO have chronic open-angle glaucoma. The association with POAG is logical when one realizes that the excessive intraocular pressure will compress the thin-walled central retinal vein at the lamina cribrosa. CRVO occurs more frequently in men, with the age of onset usually after age 50. Vision is invariably compromised in the total CRVO but may return in the incomplete variety (75 to 80 percent of occurrences), and in certain instances the eye is totally lost secondary to intractable neovascular glaucoma, which usually occurs

TABLE 4–26. SYSTEMIC FACTORS IN CENTRAL RETINAL VEIN OCCLUSION AS RELATED TO AGE OF ONSET

Age	Causes
Under 50 years	Head injuries
	Hyperlipidemia
	Estrogen-containing preparations
Over 50 years	Hypertension
	Abnormal glucose tolerance test
	Hyperlipidemia
	Chronic lung disease
	Elevated serum IgA
All ages	Hyperviscosity syndromes
	Cryofibrinogenemia

Modified from Alexander LJ. Diseases of the retina. In: Bartlett JD, Jaanus SD, eds. *Clinical Ocular Pharmacology.* Boston: Butterworth; 1989.

within 3 to 5 months and is sometimes called 90-day glaucoma. The incomplete variation of CRVO, in which there is the characteristic dot-blot hemorrhage distribution in the equatorial retina to the posterior pole often without reduction in vision, is often referred to as vascular hypoperfusion syndrome. This syndrome, like CRVO, is often linked to ipsilateral internal carotid compromise.

The etiology of CRVO varies considerably, but can be categorized as to age of onset. Table 4–26 summarizes the typical causes by age. The practitioner should understand that any condition that can create pressure on the central retinal vein has potential to cause closure of the vein at the lamina cribrosa. Table 4–27 lists some predisposing factors of CRVO, and Table 4–28 lists reported causes for CRVO. Any condition that allows for a thrombus buildup at the lamina, where the central retinal vein must constrict for passage through the pores of the lamina cribrosa, can create a potential CRVO. Turbulence occurs at this stricture (apply the principles of fluid dynamics), allowing debris in the blood to deposit on the wall be-

TABLE 4–27. PREDISPOSING FACTORS IN CENTRAL RETINAL VEIN OCCLUSION

Glaucoma
Papilledema
Subdural hematoma
Optic nerve hemorrhage
Drusen of the optic nerve
Cardiovascular and cerebrovascular disease
Diabetes
Hypertension
Leukemia
Thrombocytopenia
Sclerodermatous vascular disease
Reye's syndrome
Systemic lupus erythematosus
Trauma

Reprinted with permission from Alexander LJ. The implications and management of retinal vaso-occlusive disease. *S J Optom.* 1986;2:20–34.

TABLE 4–28. REPORTED CAUSES OF CENTRAL RETINAL VEIN OCCLUSION

Carotid artery disease
Antithrombin deficiency
Secondary to hemodialysis
Increase in platelet aggregability
Elevation of thrombocyte aggregation
Hypercholesterolemia
Hyperlipidemia
Hypertriglyceridemia
Mitral valve prolapse

cause of increased turbulence, which slows blood flow. Figure 4–58 illustrates this principle of the turbulence at the stricture. This deposition can eventually lead to a partial (nonischemic) or total (ischemic) closure of the central retinal vein.

As with BRVO, the strong association with systemic diseases, especially carotid artery disease, necessitates a thorough investigation for underlying systemic diseases. **See color plates 41 and 42.** The minimal screening workup should include blood pressure and pulse, fasting blood glucose, CBC with differential and platelet count, serum protein electrophoresis in younger patients to rule out hyperviscosity syndromes, FTA-ABS, antinuclear antibodies (ANA) and palpation/auscultation of the carotid system (ODM?). Secondarily, the clinician may consider hemoglobin electrophoresis, prothrombin and partial thromboplastin times, erythrocyte sedimentation rate, cryoglobulins, chest x-ray, carotid screening-duplex ultrasound, and a cardiovascular workup.

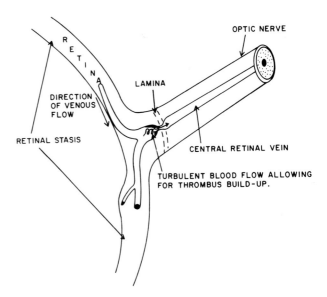

Figure 4–58. Schematic illustrating the turbulent blood flow and buildup of a thrombus at the stricture of the central retinal vein as it passes through the lamina cribrosa. *(Reprinted with permission from Alexander LJ. The implications and management of retinal vaso-occlusive disease. S J Optom. 1986;2:20–34.)*

Should there be a suspicion of an orbital mass, scans of the orbit are indicated. Human immunodeficiencyvirus (HIV) has also been associated with CRVO.

CRVO can occur as two distinct clinical entities from an ophthalmoscopic standpoint. There is not always, however, a clear distinction, because there may be an in-between variation that is a part of the continuum. The clinical categories are (1) nonischemic retinopathy (venous stasis retinopathy or incomplete CRVO) and (2) ischemic retinopathy (hemorrhagic or complete CRVO), which is characterized by at least 10 disc diameters of retinal capillary nonperfusion. The discovery of the retinal hypoperfusion requires the performance of fluorescein angiography. The primary difference involves the presence of significant retinal hypoxia or ischemia created by the totality of blockage of the lumen at the lamina cribrosa. In either case, CRVO can occur with the prodromal symptom of transient obscurations (brief blurring of vision associated with postural changes) and the prodromal sign of a yellowish hue in the posterior pole when comparing one eye to the other. The prodromata may last months, with the active phase being heralded by dot-blot hemorrhages extending to the periphery, accompanied by intraretinal edema. Evidence of capillary dilatation may occur near the optic disc or temporal vascular arcade as seen by fluorescein angiography. The vision loss that occurs is of relatively sudden onset, because the macular area is very susceptible to intraretinal edema.

The two types of CRVO have specific characteristics, prognoses, and management procedures. The thrombus forms, leading to retinal ischemia and increased venous pressure with leakage and optic disc collateral formation. It should be noted that optic disc

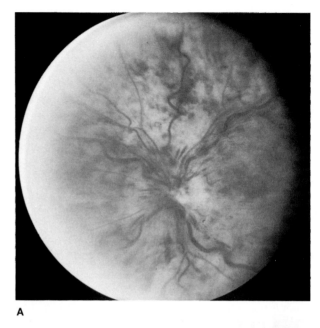

A

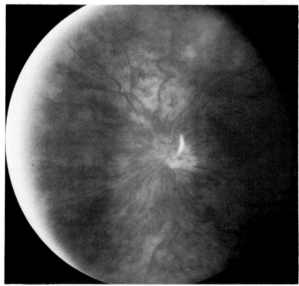

B

Figure 4–60. Illustration of the progression of severity of a CRVO. **A.** Initial view. **B.** After a 2-week period, ischemic CRVO.

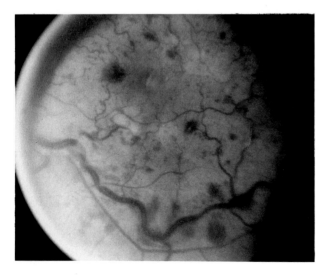

Figure 4–59. Nonischemic CRVO characterized by dot-blot hemorrhages throughout the retina accompanied by reduced visual acuity.

collaterals also form in chronic open-angle glaucoma secondary to the poor disc vessel perfusion. Nonischemic CRVO is characterized by dot-blot hemorrhages, intraretinal edema, and various degrees of macular edema and optic disc edema (Fig. 4–59). Ischemic (nonperfusing) CRVO occurs as dot-blot hemorrhages, superficial flame-shaped hemorrhages, cotton-wool spots, silver wire or sheathed arteries, gross intraretinal and macular edema, and often more significant optic disc edema (Fig. 4–60). Another clinical finding that accompanies the acute portion of the occlusion is a lowering of IOP. There is a greater initial reduction of IOP in ischemic CRVO than in nonischemic CRVO, and both of these have a greater reduction than do branch occlusions.

Fluorescein angiographic findings in CRVO vary considerably, depending on the types of occlusion as well as the elapsed time. The fluorescein is crucial in determining the degree of nonperfusion. Initially, there is blockage of background choroidal fluorescence by the intraretinal and flame-shaped hemorrhages. The retina will be stained because of intraretinal vascular leakage, and the macula will demonstrate varying degrees of edema. It is possible that neovascularization may develop with its classic fluorescein angiography picture.

The visual prognosis of CRVO is not promising, but one can expect better results in nonischemic than in ischemic CRVO. Although recovery of visual acuity is variable, it is well established that neovascular glaucoma is an identified complication in 14 to 20 percent of all CRVO cases. Recent work has refined further this expected complication rate, indicating that the risk of neovascular glaucoma is even higher (60 percent) in ischemic CRVO. Neovascularization at the iris occurs secondary to retinal hypoxia, which stimulates neovascularization. However, there is little to no viable retinal germinative capillary tissue in the area of vasostasis. As a result, the stimulus travels through the uveal network in an attempt to find a source for neovascular development. The iris tissue is the only available viable vascularized tissue, and new vessels sprout in this location. This leads to physical blockage of the trabecular meshwork and the development of increased IOP. It is reported that the incidence of chronic open-angle glaucoma in patients with CRVO is increased over the norm. Disc and retinal neovascularization do not represent the same kind of threat in CRVO as in BRVO because of the retinal capillary endothelial death that occurs in CRVO. With capillary death, the germinative tissue is not present that is necessary to support the development of neovascularization. Table 4–29 lists the estimated rate of the complication of neovascularization associated with the various forms of veinous occlusive disease.

Management. Diagnosis and management of the underlying systemic disease process associated with the CRVO is of critical importance. If oral contraceptives are in use, they should be discontinued. The intraocular pressure should be lowered if elevated and the clinician may even consider a topical beta blocker to increase the retinal volumetric blood flow rate (controversial) and likewise decrease the external pressure on the thin-walled central retinal vein. Management of the acute CRVO process is somewhat controversial. Anticoagulants will not dissolve a thrombus once it has formed, but it is thought that this therapy will limit the propagation of the thrombus. Monitoring of the blood levels of clottability (prothrombin times) is, however, an important aspect of any anticoagulant therapy. It has been suggested that anticoagulation therapy gives slightly better results than no therapy at all and that it lessens the development of neovascular glaucoma. An internist or hematologist should supervise all use of anticoagulants because of the inherent risk to the vascular system. Oral steroid therapy has been suggested to minimize the inflammatory component of the disease, but no clinical proof has been presented to substantiate the use of this treatment modality. Recent work has indicated that isovolemic hemodilution improves the visual outcome of patients with CRVO and does offer some hope. As mentioned previously, ticlopidine (a platelet aggregation inhibitor) may offer some hope in the management of CRVO. Recent work indicates that enzymes such as streptokinase may prove valuable, but again no controlled studies substantiate the treatment.

One indisputable mode of therapy is the use of panretinal photocoagulation to treat or prevent the development of neovascular glaucoma. Argon green or krypton red are the preferred wavelengths applied in a minimum of 1800 to 2200 burns, avoiding photocoagulation over a hemorrhage when possible be-

TABLE 4–29. ESTIMATED RATE OF THE COMPLICATION OF NEOVASCULARIZATION ASSOCIATED WITH RETINAL VENOUS OCCLUSIVE DISEASE

Diagnosis	Iris Neovasc (%)	Neovasc Glaucoma (%)	Neovasc of the Disc (%)	Neovasc Elsewhere (%)
Ischemic CRVO	58	47	5	8
Nonischemic CRVO	3	1	0	0
Ischemic Hemi-CRVO	13	3	29	42
Nonischemic Hemi-CRVO	0	0	0	0
Major BRVO 2	0	12	24	
Macular BRVO	0	0	0	0

CRVO = central retinal vein occlusion; BRVO = branch retinal vein occlusion; Neovasc = neovascularization.

From Hayreh SS, et al. Ocular neovascularization with retinal occlusion, III. Incidence of ocular neovascularization with retinal vascular occlusion. *Ophthalmology*. 1983;90:488–506.

Central Retinal Vein Occlusion

Characteristics

Δ Strong association with systemic disease
Δ May be secondary to localized optic nerve compression
Δ Occlusion occurs at the lamina cribrosa
Δ Nonischemic variety
  Dot-blot hemorrhages to the periphery
  Variable macular edema
  Dilated tortuous veins
  Optic disc edema
  Minimal threat to neovascular glaucoma (NVG)
Δ Ischemic variety
  Dot-blot hemorrhages to the periphery
  Dilated tortuous veins
  Variable macular edema
  Cotton-wool spots and flame-shaped hemorrhages
  Arterial changes
  Sixty percent chance of neovascular glaucoma

Management,

Δ Nonischemic variety
  Ascertain underlying cause
  Rule out glaucoma
  Possible use of IOP lowering drugs
  Possible need for anticoagulation
  Fluorescein angiography
  Retinal consultation to determine degree of ischemia
  Follow every 4 weeks for conversion to ischemia

Δ Ischemic variety
  Ascertain underlying cause
  Rule out glaucoma
  Possible use of IOP-lowering drugs
  Possible need for anticoagulation
  Fluorescein angiography
  Retinal consultation for possible panretinal photocoagulation
  Follow every 3 to 4 weeks for 6 months for development of neovascular glaucoma
Δ **Primary workup**
  Blood pressure and pulse evaluation
  Fasting blood glucose
  Complete blood count with differential and platelets
  Serum protein electrophoresis in younger patients
  FTA-ABS
  Antinuclear antibodies
  Carotid palpation and auscultation (ODM?)
Δ **Secondary workup**
  Hemoglobin electrophoresis
  Prothrombin and partial thromboplastin times
  Erythrocyte sedimentation rate
  Cryoglobulins
  Chest x-ray
  Carotid screening—duplex ultrasound
  Consider a cardiovascular workup
  If evidence of orbital mass, scan orbits

cause of unpredictability secondary to spread of the energy. The patients should then be followed in 3 to 4 weeks until regression of the neovascularization of the iris occurs. Visual outcome is not necessarily improved by photocoagulation, but the chance of further development of neovascular glaucoma is minimized by elimination of retinal hypoxia. It must be noted that panretinal photocoagulation has little effect in nonischemic CRVO unless it is secondary to ipsilateral carotid artery occlusion, whereas it is of significant benefit in ischemic CRVO. The application of photocoagulation minimizes the vasoproliferative stimulus created by the hypoxic retina, which then reduces the likelihood of iris neovascularization. It should be noted that retinal neovascularization may recur even after panretinal photocoagulation has been applied. Application of photocoagulation has yet to show any improvement in the status of the macular edema in cases of ischemic or nonischemic CRVO. It should also be noted that in the event that media opacities preclude effective viewing for photocoagulation, cryotherapy may be of benefit.

If nonischemic CRVO appears to be progres-

sively worsening and there is associated orbital pain, bypass surgery of the carotid system may produce beneficial results. Patients with neovascular glaucoma but without an obvious precipitating fundus condition should be suspected of having ipsilateral carotid artery disease until proven otherwise.

The patient with either an ischemic or nonischemic central retinal vein occlusion should have a consultation with a retinal specialist to ascertain the degree of ischemia and to provide photocoagulation when indicated. Fluorescein angiography is often the only method available to assess the degree of retinal capillary destruction. Should the primary care practitioner be asked to follow the patient after the consultation, the consideration of the development of neovascular (90-day) glaucoma should always be foremost in the mind. The patient with the ischemic variety of CRVO should be followed every 3 to 4 weeks for the first 6 months. If nonischemic, the patient should be followed every 4 weeks for the first 6 months, watching for a turn toward ischemia. Any attempt at anticoagulation must be undertaken by a physician experienced in the area of therapy.

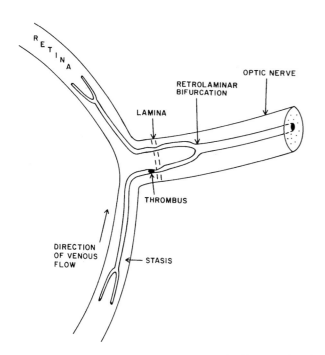

Figure 4–61. Schematic illustrating a hemi-CRVO. Note that the central retinal vein bifurcates retrolaminarly and thus exits the nerve head as two separate branches. This sets up the possibility that only one vein may occlude at the stricture in the lamina cribrosa. *(Reprinted with permission from Alexander LJ. The implications and management of retinal vaso-occlusive disease. S J Optom. 1986; 2:20–34.)*

Hemicentral Retinal Vein Occlusion

Introduction and Description. Hemicentral retinal vein occlusion (hemi-CRVO) has also been referred to as an altitudinal branch retinal vein occlusion or a

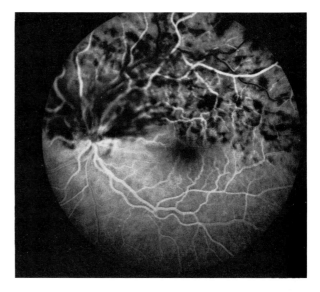

Figure 4–63. An early-stage angiogram of Figure 4–62. The significant amount of intraretinal hemorrhage effectively blocks background choroidal fluorescence.

dual branched retinal vein occlusion. The condition must be considered as a distinct entity, however, because it has characteristics of both CRVO and BRVO. The occlusion occurs at the stricture of the vein as it passes through the lamina in a manner similar to a CRVO. The etiopathogenesis is similar to that of a CRVO, including the positive association with glaucoma. The primary difference between the two entities is the anatomic characteristic of the central retinal vein. The central retinal vein in a hemi-CRVO does not become a single vessel until after it passes through the lamina. Figure 4–61 illustrates this principle of a dual

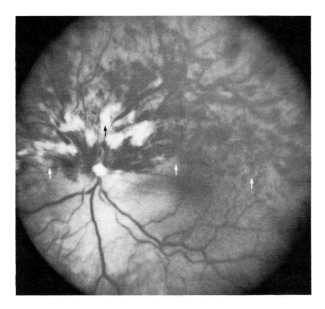

Figure 4–62. Black-and-white photograph of a hemi-CRVO. The white arrows point to the limitations of intraretinal hemorrhage; the black arrow points to a cotton-wool spot.

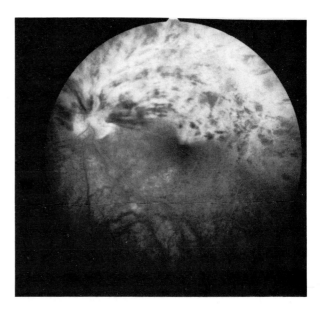

Figure 4–64. Late-stage angiogram of Figure 4–62, demonstrating staining of the intraretinal edema.

Hemicentral Retinal Vein Occlusion

Characteristics

Δ Strong association with systemic disease

Δ Occlusion at lamina cribrosa in one branch of the central retinal vein

Δ Maximal threat to neovascularization of disc and retina in the ischemic form

Δ Nonischemic variety (half of retina involved)
  Dot-blot hemorrhages to the periphery
  Variable macular edema
  Dilated tortuous veins
  Optic disc edema possible
  Minimal threat to neovascular glaucoma (NVG) and retinal/disc neovascularization

Δ Ischemic variety (half of retina involved)
  Dot-blot hemorrhages to the periphery
  Dilated tortuous veins
  Variable macular edema
  Cotton-wool spots and flame-shaped hemorrhages
  Arterial changes
  Optic disc edema possible
  Strong tendency for disc/retinal neovascularization and threat for neovascular glaucoma (NVG)

Management

Δ Nonischemic variety
  ASCERTAIN UNDERLYING CAUSE
  Rule out glaucoma
  Possible use of IOP-lowering drugs
  Possible need for anticoagulation
  Fluorescein angiography
  Retinal consultation to determine degree of ischemia
  Follow every 4 weeks for conversion to ischemia

Δ Ischemic variety
  ASCERTAIN UNDERLYING CAUSE
  Rule out glaucoma
  Possible use of IOP-lowering drugs
  Possible need for anticoagulation
  Fluorescein angiography
  Retinal consultation for possible photocoagulation of affected area
  Follow every 3 to 4 weeks for 6 months for development of neovascular glaucoma or retinal/disc neovascularization

Δ **Primary workup**
  Blood pressure and pulse evaluation
  Fasting blood glucose
  Complete blood count with differential and platelets
  Serum protein electrophoresis in younger patients
  FTA-ABS
  Antinuclear antibodies
  Carotid palpation and auscultation (ODM?)

Δ **Secondary workup**
  Hemoglobin electrophoresis
  Prothrombin and partial thromboplastin times
  Erythrocyte sedimentation rate
  Cryoglobulins
  Chest x-ray
  Carotid screening—duplex ultrasound
  Consider a cardiovascular workup

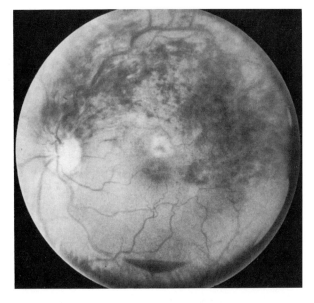

Figure 4–65. Black-and-white photograph of a superior hemi-CRVO with an inferior preretinal hemorrhage. *(Reprinted with permission from Alexander LJ. The implications and management of retinal vaso-occlusive disease. S J Optom. 1986;2:20–34.)*

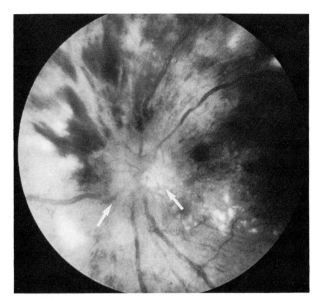

Figure 4–66. Disc neovascularization *(arrows)* secondary to the hypoxia created by a hemi-CRVO.

TABLE 4–30. COMPARISON OF CENTRAL, HEMICENTRAL, AND BRANCH RETINAL VEIN OCCLUSION

Features	CRVO	Hemi-CRVO	BRVO
Site of occlusion	In optic nerve at lamina	In optic nerve at lamina	Usually at arteriovenous crossing
Type of retinopathy	Nonischemic 80% Ischemic 20%	Nonischemic 67% Ischemic 33%	Primarily ischemic
Retinal collaterals	Absent	Present	Invariably present

Prognosis	Nonischemic: vision loss
	Ischemic: vision loss and 60%
	   chance neovascular
	   glaucoma
		Vision loss with macular
		  edema, retinal and disc
		  neovascularization
		  possible
			Vision loss with macular edema,
			  retinal and disc neovasculariza-
			  tion possible

vein system exiting the lamina cribrosa. Occlusion in one branch creates a picture similar to a BRVO. Once occlusion occurs, there is retinal ischemia, increased venous pressure, and leakage into the retina. As with the CRVO there is a strong tendency for the development of macular edema. In addition, there is the development of optic disc collaterals and the possibility of optic disc edema. Because an entire half of the fundus is nonperfused, there is a strong tendency toward macular edema and hypoxia. With the ischemic variety, there are also cotton-wool spots and arterial changes. Hypoxia in one half of the retina coupled with a viable capillary bed in the other half contributes to the development of neovascularization of the retina. **See color plates 43 and 44.**

The hemi-CRVO can appear either as ischemic or nonischemic (approximately 67 percent of the occurrences) (Figs. 4–62 to 4–66). Prognosis depends on the development of macular edema or the development of neovascularization. The vision prognosis in the nonischemic variety is better than in the ischemic variation, but is unpredictable. Neovascularization is not expected as frequently in the nonischemic variety but may develop in the ischemic variety within 6 months. Neovascularization develops in response to the retinal hypoxia occurring in half of the retina.

Management. Management involves the prevention of neovascularization of the disc and retina and the possibility of the subsequent neovascular glaucoma. Fluorescein angiography is necessary in all cases of hemi-CRVO to ascertain the degree of capillary nonperfusion. The fluorescein angiogram then becomes the map for the application of photocoagulation if it is necessary. The photocoagulation is usually applied in a scatter pattern in the affected area in an attempt to eliminate the hypoxic stimulus. Macular edema may also regress in response to photocoagulation. It is important to investigate carefully for the inevitable associated underlying systemic disease. The minimal screening workup should include blood pressure and pulse, fasting blood glucose, CBC with differential

and platelet count, serum protein electrophoresis in younger patients to rule out hyperviscosity syndromes, FTA-ABS, antinuclear antibodies (ANA), and palpation/auscultation of the carotid system (ODM?). Secondarily, the clinician may consider hemoglobin electrophoresis, prothrombin and partial thromboplastin times, erythrocyte sedimentation rate, cryoglobulins, chest x-ray, carotid screening—duplex ultrasound, and a cardiovascular workup.

Table 4–30 summarizes the comparisons of the clinical and pathogenic features of CRVO, hemi-CRVO, and BRVO.

Branch Retinal Artery Occlusion

Introduction and Description. Both branch retinal artery occlusion (BRAO) and central retinal artery occlusion (CRAO) are the result of emboli dislodged from vasculature elsewhere in the body that travel through the system until they reach a vessel caliber too narrow for passage. There is often an associated history of transient monocular blindness (amaurosis fugax). With arterial occlusion comes anoxia as the result of an absence of oxygenated blood. This anoxia results in a loss of inner retinal layers, including the nerve fiber layer, ganglion cell layer, inner plexiform layer, and the inner portion of the inner nuclear layer.

BRAO differs from CRAO only because the embolus was small enough to pass through the stricture of the central retinal artery as it traversed the laminar region. The embolus then moved into retinal circulation. The source of the emboli in both cases is essentially identical, but BRAO emboli are often the result of self-injected emboli associated with drug use or abuse.

BRAO occurs most frequently in the superior temporal region of the retina and may be produced by multiple emboli. Single cholesterol emboli (Hollenhorst plaques) usually will not create an occlusion but in sufficient numbers will shut the vessel down. Figure 4–67 illustrates the principle of a BRAO. Visual acuity and visual field loss are dependent on location of the occlusion as well as the extent of blockage. Re-

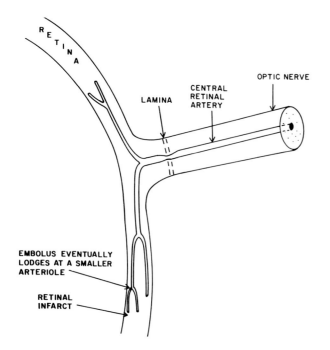

Figure 4–67. Schematic illustrating the etiology of a BRAO. The embolus is small enough to pass the stricture of the central retinal artery at the lamina but eventually becomes lodged in the smaller-caliber retinal arteries. *(Reprinted with permission from Alexander LJ. The implications and management of retinal vasco-occlusive disease. S J Optom. 1986;2:20–34.)*

call that the arterial supply to the hemiretina stops at the temporal horizontal raphe, which then creates a very classical sharp margined visual field defect ceasing at the horizontal. The visual field defect is very similar to that created by ischemic optic neuropathy

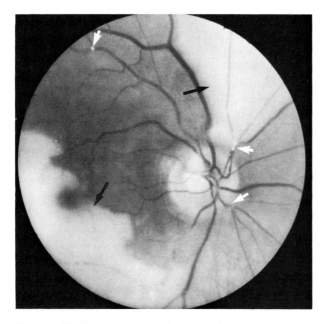

Figure 4–68. Photograph illustrating areas of retinal infarct (*black arrows*) secondary to emboli (*white arrows*) in a BRAO. *(Photo courtesy of W. Jones.)*

and low-tension glaucoma. Likewise, nerve conduction defects may be present depending on the extent of the occlusion. The ophthalmoscopic appearance is dependent on the elapsed time from the occlusion (Fig. 4–68). Initially, the affected arteries narrow and the retina becomes hazy. Over a few hours, the retinal tissue whitens because of the infarct. Descending segmental optic atrophy may develop in the affected region. **See color plates 45 and 46.**

Management. Prognosis depends on rapid institution of therapy. If there is more than a 1- to 2-hour lag,

Branch Retinal Artery Occlusion

Pearls

Characteristics

Δ Strong association with systemic disease, especially internal carotid and cardiac disease
Δ Secondary to embolus lodged in retinal artery
Δ Results in total anoxia of the retina, white retina in the area of distribution of the artery
Δ May have associated cotton-wool spots
Δ May have multiple visible emboli stacked or may have a relatively invisible blockage
Δ May have multiple emboli secondary to self-injection of drugs including Ritalin
Δ Visual field defect altitudinal respecting the horizontal raphe

Management

Δ Attempt to dislodge embolus by physical massage of the eyeball and immediate consultation with a retinal specialist
Δ Fluorescein angiography to ascertain type of damage
Δ Consider ocular paracentesis if damage is fresh and devastating to vision
Δ **Systemic health workup**
   Erythrocyte sedimentation rate if elderly
   Blood pressure and pulse rate
   Fasting blood sugar
   Complete blood count with differential and
      platelets
   Fasting lipid profile
   Prothrombin and partial thromboplastin times
   Antinuclear antibodies and rheumatoid factor
   FTA-ABS
   Palpation/ausculation of the carotid system
      (ODM?) with a strong consideration of
      duplex ultrasound
   Serum and hemoglobin electrophoresis
   Cardiology consult
      Echocardiography
      Blood chemistries
      Holter monitor
   Drug screen in younger patients
Δ Follow up in 3 to 6 months depending on health and ocular status

the likelihood of return of vision or visual field is minimal. The initial concern in BRAO is to attempt to reverse the occlusion if it severely affects vision. The next concern is to attempt to diagnose and manage the underlying systemic cause. If vision is severely compromised, aggressive therapy should be instituted immediately. This therapy should parallel that described in the next section on CRAO. Some clinicians advocate pentoxifylline, 300 to 600 mg per day over a 3-month period, to prevent retinal or intravitreal neovascularization caused by retinal ischemia. However, this mode of prophylaxis is still investigational.

The author has seen branch retinal artery occlusions that are only partial and have been reversed with aggressive therapy or even with the performance of the obligatory fluorescein angiography. A consultation with a retinal specialist is indicated in all but long-standing cases of BRAO.

Of greatest importance is the strong association of BRAO to systemic diseases, especially carotid and cardiovascular disorders. The major disorders associated with retinal arterial occlusions are listed in Table 4–31. The primary screening workup should include an immediate erythrocyte sedimentation rate if the patient is elderly (over 55 years), blood pressure and pulse rate, fasting blood sugar, complete blood count with differential and platelets, fasting lipid profile, prothrombin and partial thromboplastin times, antinuclear antibodies, rheumatoid factor, FTA-ABS, palpation and auscultation of the carotid system (ODM?) with a strong consideration for duplex ultrasound, and serum and hemoglobin electrophoresis in younger patients. All patients with retinal emboli should have a cardiology consultation with the request for an echocardiogram, blood chemistries, and consideration for a Holter monitor. In especially young patients, a drug screen may be necessary as self-injected emboli may create the BRAO picture. The patient should then be followed every 3 to 6 months after the total workup.

Central Retinal Artery Occlusion

The etiology of central retinal artery occlusion (CRAO) is presented in Table 4–31. The emphasis regarding etiology should be placed on the incidence of increased vascular resistance (carotid artery disease) in this disease process. The condition has a strong association to systemic conditions that produce emboli. Figure 4–69 illustrates the embolus lodged at the stricture created in the central retinal artery as it passes through the lamina. Occlusion of the ophthalmic artery can produce a similar clinical picture, with the exception that the cherry red spot characteristic of the CRAO is not present.

CRAO occurs as a sudden (occurs over seconds) painless loss of vision in an eye that is otherwise dis-

TABLE 4–31. REPORTED ETIOLOGIC FACTORS IN RETINAL ARTERIAL OCCLUSIONS

Emboli from ulcerated atheromatous plaques of the internal carotid artery

Increased vascular resistance (internal carotid disease)

Emboli from cardiac lesions, including atrial myxoma

Mitral valve prolapse

Emboli from artificial cardiac valves

Emboli from subacute bacterial endocarditis

Thrombi secondary to giant cell arteritis, syphilis, fungal sinus infections

Oral contraceptives

Polyarteritis nodosa

Occlusion secondary to methylprednisolone injections of the head and neck soft tissue

Cardiac catherization and other similar diagnostic procedures

Self-injected emboli

Migraine

ease free. There is often a loss of direct pupillary response associated with the vision loss. If a cilioretinal artery (choroidal vascular origin) is present, a variable island of vision will remain that corresponds to the geography of the vascular supply. This geographic area will be readily identifiable on ophthalmoscopy by the presence of perfusion of the blood supply.

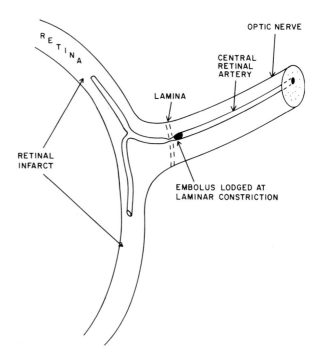

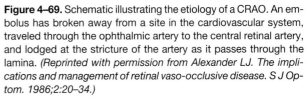

Figure 4–69. Schematic illustrating the etiology of a CRAO. An embolus has broken away from a site in the cardiovascular system, traveled through the ophthalmic artery to the central retinal artery, and lodged at the stricture of the artery as it passes through the lamina. *(Reprinted with permission from Alexander LJ. The implications and management of retinal vaso-occlusive disease. S J Optom. 1986;2:20–34.)*

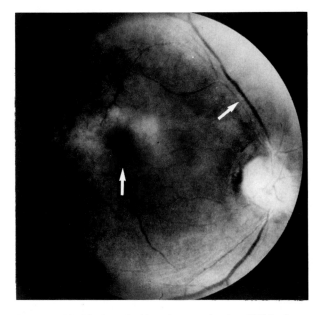

Figure 4–70. Black-and-white photograph of a CRAO. Arrows point to the macula, which becomes more visible in contrast to the opaque retina and the attenuated retinal arteries. *(Reprinted with permission from Alexander LJ. The implications and management of retinal vaso-occlusive disease. S J Optom. 1986; 2:20–34.)*

The clinical picture depends on the elapsed time since the occlusion (Fig. 4–70). Early changes involve narrowing of the retinal arteries and a haziness of retinal tissue. Within hours, this haziness of the retina becomes whitish, contrasting with the choroidal macular vascular supply—thus the cherry red spot. The veins then become distended and can exhibit segmentation, which is referred to as "boxcarring." It is also possible to occasionally see emboli in the arterioles. Ultimately, the infarcted retina is replaced by glial tissue, and the arterial tree assumes a more normal appearance except for some irregular narrowing. Descending optic atrophy can occur, but neovascular glaucoma is rare in CRAO. If neovascular glaucoma should occur associated with CRAO, the patient may have an ocular ischemic syndrome. **See color plate 47.**

Management. Visual prognosis depends on immediate initiation of therapy. Diagnosis and management of the underlying systemic condition are also of immediate concern. Occlusions caused by emboli may be partially reversible if therapy is instituted within 1 to 2 hours, although there are suggestions that attempts should be made up to 24 hours after the reported event. Digital massage of the globe through the eyelid may assist in dislodging the embolus. This, coupled with inhalation of carbogen for 15 minutes followed by 15 minutes of room air, and repeating the cycle over a 6- to 12-hour period, may be of some value. Recent studies, however, show carbogen ther-

apy to be of questionable value. The logic of carbogen inhalation is not very convincing to this clinician as the disease is more of a mechanical obstruction at the lamina than anything else, and it is impossible to dilate the pores of the lamina with any agent except for physical alteration.

It seems apparent that attempts at vasodilatation would offer little or no help in managing CRAO. The embolus is lodged at the stricture in the artery as it

Pearls

Central Retinal Artery Occlusion

Characteristics

△ Strong association with systemic disease, especially internal carotid and cardiac disease
△ Sudden-onset (within seconds), painless loss of vision
△ Embolus lodged at lamina cribrosa is implicated
△ Narrowing of arteries, haziness of retinal tissue secondary to total anoxia
△ Boxcar segmentation of veins is possible
△ "Cherry red" spot in macular area indicating intact choroidal circulation
△ If cilioretinal artery present, may have island of perfused retina in area of supply by the artery
△ May see an arteriolar embolus but this is not inevitable

Management

△ Attempt to dislodge embolus by physical massage of the eyeball and immediate consultation with a retinologist
△ Fluorsecein angiography to ascertain type of damage
△ Consider ocular paracentesis if damage is fresh and devastating to vision
△ Maintain lowered IOP over a period of time
△ **Systemic health workup**
  Erythrocyte sedimentation rate if elderly
  Blood pressure and pulse rate
  Fasting blood sugar
  Complete blood count with differential and platelets
  Fasting lipid profile
  Prothrombin and partial thromboplastin times
  Antinuclear antibodies and rheumatoid factor
  FTA-ABS
  Palpation/ausculation of the carotid system (ODM?) with a strong consideration of duplex ultrasound
  Serum and hemoglobin electrophoresis
  Cardiology consultation
    Echocardiography
    Blood chemistries
    Holter monitor
△ Follow up in 3 to 6 months depending on systemic and/or ocular status

passes through the lamina. Manipulation of the lamina to facilitate passage of the embolus is a much more logical approach, because the laminar passage will not enlarge with vasodilatation. Paracentesis of the anterior chamber may create enough hypotony to dislodge the embolus. This is typically performed with a 30-gauge short needle on a tuberculin syringe entering the eye at the temporal limbus with the bevel of the needle pointing up. The fluid is withdrawn until the anterior chamber shallows slightly (0.1 to 0.2 cc of fluid). The eye is then covered with a broad-spectrum antibiotic and the IOP must then be maintained at a low level for several days. The reduction of IOP is accomplished by using acetazolamide 250 mg every 6 hours in addition to using a topical beta blocker unless contraindicated because of compromised cardiac or pulmonary status. Retrobulbar injections of acetylcholine, atropine, and 25 mg of tolaxoline also may be beneficial. Papaverine plus heparin via the infraorbital artery has been attempted. Although there is no proof as to the efficacy of any treatment modality, any attempt is worthwhile, because the prognosis is so grim. Again, antiembolic enzymes such as streptokinase may offer some promise in the treatment of arterial occlusions.

Of greatest importance is the strong association of CRAO with systemic diseases, especially carotid and cardiovascular disorders. Major disorders associated with CRAO are listed in Table 4–31. The primary screening workup should include an immediate erythrocyte sedimentation rate if the patient is elderly (over 55 years), blood pressure and pulse rate, fasting blood sugar, complete blood count with differential and platelets, fasting lipid profile, prothrombin and partial thromboplastin times, antinuclear antibodies, rheumatoid factor, FTA-ABS, palpation and auscultation of the carotid system (ODM?) with a strong consideration for duplex ultrasound, and serum and hemoglobin electrophoresis in younger patients. All patients with retinal emboli should have a cardiology consultation with the request for an echocardiogram, blood chemistries, and consideration for a Holter monitor.

HYPERTENSIVE RETINOPATHY

Introduction and Description. In an advanced culture it is difficult to believe that a patient would have hypertension severe enough to create hypertensive retinopathy (HR). Unfortunately, several million hypertensive patients go untreated or mismanaged each year. In addition, there are several disease processes such as kidney disease or diabetes that contribute to poorly controlled hypertension, allowing for the development of HR. It is often difficult to distinguish diabetic and hypertensive retinopathy as the two are usually combined. HR is often asymptomatic and presents bilaterally. It seems to be a condition that presents sooner and at a younger age in blacks than in whites. There is a generalized narrowing of the arterioles, arteriovenous crossing changes, copper or silver wire artery sheath changes, cotton-wool spots, flame hemorrhages, intraretinal edema (into macular area if severe), some minor degrees of optic disc edema, possible retinal macroaneurysms, and the classic macular star configuration of hard exudates. Malignant hypertension will have all of the above signs with the addition of significant optic disc edema. Certainly any retinal vascular complication such as vitreous hemorrhage may occur. An HR appearance can present in other conditions such as diabetic retinopathy, venous occlusive disorders, collagen vascular conditions such as systemic lupus erythematosus, anemias, and radiation retinopathy. Figures 4–71 and 4–72 illustrate the variation in HR presentation. **See color plate 52.**

Management. The primary concern in HR is the discovery of the underlying cause of the process. If it is uncontrolled essential hypertension, more aggressive therapy must be instituted. It is imperative to consider other diseases such as diabetes, collagen vascular disorders, radiation retinopathy, anemias, or the combination of several disorders. This may also occur in the

---

Pearls

Hypertensive Retinopathy

Characteristics

△ Often asymptomatic and bilateral
△ Narrowing of arterioles
△ Arteriovenous crossing changes
△ Artery sheath changes
△ Cotton-wool spots
△ Flame-shaped hemorrhages
△ Intraretinal edema
△ Minor to severe (malignant hypertension) optic disc edema
△ Macular star configuration of hard exudates

Management

△ Ascertain and control underlying cause with a consultation to internal medicine or cardiology—at times an immediate consultation
△ If the patient is a kidney patient, an immediate consultation with the nephrologist
△ Follow up every 1 to 3 months depending on severity and have patient monitor with home Amsler grid
△ Consult with a retinal specialist if there is a threat of macular edema or hypoxic complications

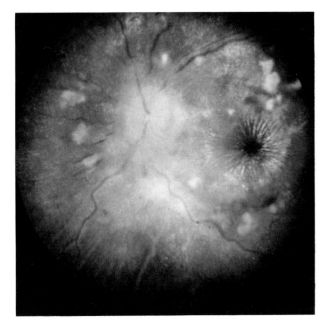

Figure 4–71. Example of bilateral malignant hypertensive retinopathy in a patient on dialysis with uncontrolled hypertension.

form of malignant hypertension and is related to kidney dysfunction and dialysis. The ocular signs are often not amendable by localized treatment, with the rare exception of the possibility of remediation of macular edema with grid photocoagulation. Often the

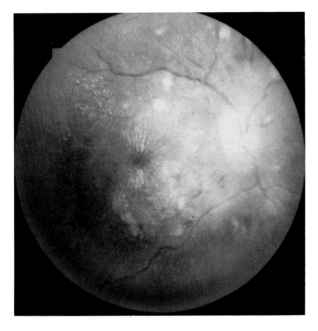

Figure 4–72. The fellow eye to that shown in Figure 4–71, illustrating severe malignant hypertensive retinopathy.

severity of the hypertension is such that immediate attention by an internist or cardiologist is of utmost importance, with the recommendation that kidney function be evaluated. If the patient is a kidney patient, the nephrologist should be notified immediately. A kidney patient on dialysis is far more susceptible to the development of hypertensive retinopathy at a lower blood pressure level than a nondialysis patient. The patient should initially be followed every 1 to 3 months depending on the severity, and then every 6 to 12 months.

RELATIONSHIP OF RETINAL VASO-OCCLUSIVE DISEASE TO CEREBROVASCULAR DISEASE

The patient with retinal vaso-occlusive disease should be a strong suspect for concurrent cerebrovascular disease (Fig. 4–73). There are two basic vascular supply systems to the brain, the internal carotid system and the vertebrobasilar system. Diseases of the internal carotid system are more intimately related to retinal vaso-occlusive disease than are vertebrobasilar occlusions. Vertebrobasilar occlusions are more likely related to bilateral, nonhomonymous visual field defects or bilateral visual phenomena.

Awareness of the possible association of retinal vaso-occlusive disease and cerebrovascular disease is a crucial part of management of these patients. The clinician must be well versed in the clinical signs and symptoms of impending stroke syndromes.

Stroke

The third leading cause of death in the United States is stroke. Often the patient with impending stroke presents with visual symptoms to the primary care practitioner, and this patient must be appropriately managed.

In 1986 over 147,800 Americans died from stroke. During that year, 2,020,000 people were alive who had survived a stroke. Approximately 500,000 persons suffer stroke each year. According to 1985 mortality statistics of major cardiovascular diseases, stroke ranks second behind heart attack, with 260,000 years of potential life lost. Seventy percent of stroke victims are over age 65 years, and the risk for stroke is 30 percent higher for men than women. The risk for death and disability from stroke is 60 percent higher in blacks. On the positive side, the death rate from stroke has declined from 88.8 per 100,000 in 1950 to 32.8 per 100,000 in 1985, largely attributed to better control of systemic hypertension.

Stroke mortality rates differ substantially by state. In 1980, 11 states had age-adjusted stroke mortality rates that were over 10 percent higher than the national average. Ten of the 11 states were in the

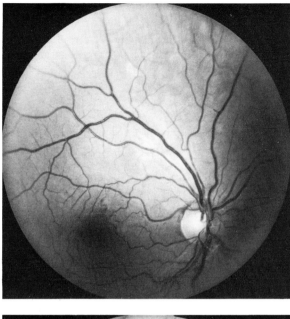

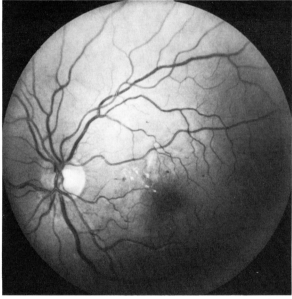

Figure 4–73. Black-and-white photographs illustrating asymmetrical retinopathy. In any patient with asymmetrical hemorrhages, exudates, cotton-wool spots, peripheral hemorrhages, or asymmetrical venous tortuosity, internal carotid stenosis should be suspected.

Southeast, forming a "stroke belt." Table 4–32 ranks the stroke-belt states' age-adjusted stroke mortality with estimates for 1986.

Stroke is also specifically related to race. Nationally, it is known that stroke death rates are higher for blacks than whites. This pattern also holds in the "stroke belt" states. Table 4–33 illustrates the age-adjusted stroke death rates per 100,000 population in the stroke belt states for 1980.

Death rates from stroke are declining in the

TABLE 4–32. RANKING OF STROKE BELT STATES' AGE-ADJUSTED STROKE MORTALITY RATES (1980 AND 1986)

	Ranking	
State	1980	1986
South Carolina	1	1
Georgia	2	2
Mississippi	3	6
Louisiana	4	12
Alabama	5	4
Tennessee	6	5
North Carolina	7	3
Arkansas	8	8
Indiana	9	9
Kentucky	10	11
Virginia	10	7
Oklahoma	14	10

From Division of Vital Statistics, National Center for Health Statistics, and Centers for Disease Control. MMWR. 1989;38(12):193.

United States, with an overall drop of about 40 percent between 1970 and 1980. The decline occurred in all race and sex groups: white men (41 percent), nonwhite men (40 percent), white women (38 percent), and nonwhite women (45 percent). It appears that the decline in stroke mortality rates are consistent even within the stroke belt, with isolated areas showing an increase. The primary factor involved in the decline was the more effective control of hypertension.

Risk factors for stroke include hypertension, smoking, being overweight, heart disease (which doubles the risk, and is also directly related to elevated blood lipid levels), high red blood cell count, transient ischemic attacks, age (the older, the higher the risk), sex (30 percent higher for men), diabetes, prior stroke,

TABLE 4–33. AGE-ADJUSTED STROKE DEATH RATES PER 100,000 POPULATION IN STROKE BELT STATES (1980)

	White Men	Nonwhite Men[a]	White Women	Nonwhite Women[a]
United States	41.4	69.4	34.9	55.8
Alabama	50.2	90.4	39.6	70.3
Arkansas	47.1	95.9	39.0	73.0
Georgia	53.1	106.9	**43.7**	**82.4**
Indiana	50.3	71.9	41.6	54.9
Kentucky	49.6	82.5	40.9	62.9
Louisiana	50.8	89.2	39.7	64.7
Mississippi	49.9	91.5	39.7	64.6
North Carolina	49.9	97.6	39.5	66.1
South Carolina	53.0	**115.2**	40.8	80.1
Tennessee	**53.4**	96.2	42.1	72.4
Virginia	44.5	80.7	38.0	64.3

[a]In the stroke belt the nonwhite category consists predominantly of blacks.

From Division of Vital Statistics, National Center for Health Statistics.

family history, asymptomatic carotid bruit, geographic location, climate and season (strokes occur more during periods of extreme temperatures), elevated lipid levels, excessive alcohol use, obesity, physical inactivity, use of oral contraceptives concurrent with smoking, and being black (60 percent higher).

Definition of Stroke. Stroke is a form of vascular disease that affects the blood vessels of the central nervous system. Stroke occurs when a blood vessel to the brain is compromised by hemorrhage or a clot. The lack of oxygenated blood creates the signs and symptoms associated with stroke. There are four types of stroke. Cerebral thrombosis and cerebral embolism are the most common, accounting for 70 to 80 percent of all strokes. These two types have the strongest relationship to ocular vascular signs and symptoms. Cerebral hemorrhage and subarachnoid hemorrhage occur less frequently but have a higher fatality rate. These variations would not be seen as frequently in the primary care office.

Cerebral thromboembolism is a blood clot of an artery that has usually been damaged by atherosclerosis. This type of stroke usually occurs at night or first thing in the morning. The attack is often preceded by transient ischemic attacks (TIAs). About 10 percent of strokes are preceded by TIAs; however, of those who have had one or more TIA, about 36 percent will later have a stroke. TIAs usually last less than 5 minutes, but can last for several hours. In about 50 percent of cases of TIA, the stroke occurs within 1 year of the attack, and in about 20 percent within 1 month. TIA symptoms are listed in Table 4–34.

Another type of stroke is a *cerebral embolism.* Emboli account for 5 to 14 percent of strokes. The embolus is formed elsewhere in the cardiovascular system, breaks away, and travels to the cerebral circulation to lodge in an artery and precipitate a stroke. Atrial fibrillation, which creates incomplete expulsion of blood from the heart, allowing for pooling of blood and subsequent clotting, accounts for the most common

source of emboli. Approximately 15 percent of all strokes occur in people who have atrial fibrillation. Atrial fibrillation is best discovered by physical examination including a comparison of the radial pulse to the auscultated heart sounds. This type of stroke is usually not preceded by a TIA.

Subarachnoid hemorrhages account for about 7 percent of all strokes and are often the result of a rupture of a cerebral aneurysm at the circle of Willis. The hemorrhage surrounds the brain. *Cerebral hemorrhage* also results from a ruptured microaneurysm in a blood vessel, but the bleed is directly into the brain tissue. About 10 percent of strokes are the result of a cerebral hemorrhage. In 50 percent of cerebral hemorrhages, the patients die because of increased intracranial pressure. Table 4–35 summarizes the general effects of stroke damage to both the right and left side of the brain.

Eye Signs of Stroke or Impending Stroke. There are two basic blood flow patterns to the brain, the carotid system and the vertebrobasilar system. The carotid system provides a dual supply to the anterior and lateral portions of the brain, ultimately terminating in the cortical areas. The ophthalmic artery is a branch of the internal carotid that supplies blood flow to the eye. The carotid system is unilateral in its supply—that is, affectations of this system result in monocular or unilateral symptomatology. Table 4–36 summarizes some of the signs and symptoms of carotid stenosis that may present during a routine eye examination.

The vertebrobasilar system supplies the posterior portion of the brain. The vertebral arteries join to form the basilar artery, which is the primary blood source for the occipital cortex. When there is an alteration of blood supply to this region, both sides of the body and both visual fields are affected. Table 4–37 summarizes some of the signs and symptoms of vertebrobasilar disease, emphasizing the bilaterality of presentation. Note that the clinician should always be suspicious of an elderly patient complaining of headaches, as these

TABLE 4–34. TRANSIENT ISCHEMIC ATTACKS: SIGNS AND SYMPTOMS

Sudden numbness or weakness of the face, arm, and/or leg on one side of the bodyTemporary loss of speech or difficulty in speaking

Temporary difficulty in understanding speech, particularly with right-sided weakness

Temporary dimness or loss of vision in only one eye for up to 2 hours, but always returning to normal—also known as amaurosis fugax or transient monocular blindness

Reprinted with permission from Alexander LJ. National health care issues: Stroke. *J Am Optom Assoc.* 1992;63:361–364.

TABLE 4–35. GENERAL EFFECTS OF STROKE DAMAGE TO THE RIGHT AND LEFT HEMISPHERES

Right Brain Damage	Left Brain Damage
Paralyzed left side of the body	Paralyzed right side of the body
Spatial, perceptual deficits	Speech, language deficits
Behavioral style is quick and impulsive	Behavioral style is slow and cautious
Memory deficits occur in performance	Memory deficits occur in language

Reprinted with permission from Alexander LJ. National health care issues: Stroke. *J Am Optom Assoc.* 1992;63:361–364.

TABLE 4–36. CAROTID ARTERY DISEASE: SIGNS AND SYMPTOMS

Sign or Symptom	Characteristic
Transient monocular blindness (amaurosis fugax)	Sudden unilateral blindness that lasts a short period of time but always returns to normal
Migraine symptoms	Unilateral transient alteration of function with or without accompanying headache
Frontal headache	Headache that may or may not be associated with other transient ischemic attack symptoms
Unilateral numbness or weakness	Unilateral loss of function or paresthesias of limbs
Aphasia	Dysfunctional speech due to stenosis of blood supply to dominant hemisphere
Cholesterol, platelet, or calcific emboli lodged in retinal circulation	Ipsilateral plaques from eroding carotid sinus or from cardiac vegetations. MUST ORDER AN ELECTROCARDIOGRAM AND ECHOCARDIOGRAM
Retinal arterial occlusions	Central or branch retinal artery occlusions characterized by opaque retina secondary to eroded emboli
Retinal vein occlusions	Central or branch retinal vein occlusions reflecting underlying systemic vascular disease
Asymmetrical retinal vasculopathy	Any sign of retinal vascular disease present or more dramatic in one eye but not in the other (eg, Cotton-wool spots in one eye). Indicates unilateral hypoxia.
Equatorial dot-blot hemorrhages	Dot-blot hemorrhages in the equatorial retina, especially unilateral and in a patient with no other apparent retinal vascular disease
Ocular ischemic syndrome	Unilateral red eye, cells, and flare in the anterior chamber, retinal/disc neovascularization, retinal arterial occlusion
Unilateral vision loss in bright light	Equivalent of macular photostress recovery test due to hypoxia and reduced retinal metabolic activity

Reprinted with permission from Alexander LJ. National health care issues: Stroke. *J Am Optom Assoc.* 1992;63:361–364.

TABLE 4–37. VERTEBROBASILAR TERRITORY SYNDROME: SIGNS AND SYMPTOMS

- Bilateral presentation that may be asymmetrical and may be variable
- Visual field defects that affect both fields. May be forms of homonymous or altitudinal defects
- Visual field defects that may present as tunnel vision. Central field is usually spared because of the gross distribution of macular fibers. Must rule out hysterical fields, syphilitic optic neuropathy, and buried drusen of optic nerve head
- Cortical blindness (rare). No apparent vision in spite of a healthy retina and optic nerve head
- Numbness, loss of sensation, or parasthesias that are often bilateral but may switch from side to side
- Weakness or paralysis of four extremities that may change from side to side during different attacks
- Loss of leg function resulting in falls (drop attacks)
- Altered hearing that may be bilateral or unilateral
- Transient confusion and recent memory problems
- Occipital headaches—"new" headaches that are nonorganic are rare in the elderly population
- Usual maintenance of consciousness
- Consider the subclavian steal syndrome, which is a loss of function associated with prolonged use of the arm in exercise "stealing blood flow" from the vertebrals, which are a branch of the subclavians. Toscanini's fumble

Reprinted with permission from Alexander LJ. National health care issues: Stroke. *J Am Optom Assoc.* 1992;63:361–364.

may be a sign of vascular insufficiency. Migraine headaches often mimic organic headaches, and often the only way to get a definitive diagnosis is to ask for a neurologic consultation. Table 4–38 summarizes some of the more common differential diagnostic criteria for headaches.

The patient with any signs or symptoms of either carotid or vertebrobasilar territory stroke should have a workup by either a neurologist or a neurovascular surgeon. This work up should include carotid duplex ultrasound, scans of the brain when indicated, cardiac evaluation when emboli are suspected, and a thorough systemic health evaluation similar to that ordered for venous and arterial occlusive disorders.

Ocular Ischemic Syndrome

Introduction and Description. The ocular ischemic syndrome (OIS) deserves special mention related to stroke syndromes because of the uniqueness of the characteristics. The disease is secondary to reduced oxygenated blood supply to the eye, and occurs most frequently in carotid disease with significant stenosis. OIS may also occur in pulseless disease, giant-cell arteritis, collagen–vascular diseases, endarteritis, and aortic arch syndromes, and typically occurs in elderly men.

TABLE 4–38. VARIOUS TYPES OF HEADACHES: SIGNS AND SYMPTOMS

Type	Symptoms	Cause/Cure
Organic/aneurysm	Early mimic migraine or cluster: Sudden unbearable headache, double vision, visual field defects, nuchal rigidity, unconsciousness—often fatal	Usually present from birth, or may be secondary to hypertension/Surgery if caught early enough
Organic/brain tumors	Morning pain, headaches worsening over time, projectile vomiting, speech and/or personality changes, visual field defects, problems with coordination, seizures	Cause unknown/Surgery, radiation, chemotherapy
Temporal arteritis	Prodromal symptoms including transient monocular blindness, flashes, focusing problems, headaches, weight loss, nuchal pain, scalp tenderness, and jaw aches on one side, sudden onset of vision loss	Cranial arteritis (granulomatous inflammation of arterial walls), often associated with polymyalgia rheumatica/Immediate ESR, biopsy—treat with corticosteroids stat
Migraine/common	Throbbing pain, which may include nausea, vomiting, tremor, unbalance, cold extremities, super sensitivity to stimuli	Usually hereditary but may have triggers such as food, oral contraceptives, stress, menstruation/Treat with life-style changes, vasoconstrictors, beta blockers
Migraine/classic	Prodromal symptoms (aura) which may include light flashes, field defects, numbness in extremities, auras, hallucinations, and headaches that follow. Headaches are throbbing, often with nausea and vomiting	Usually hereditary but may have triggers such as food, oral contraceptives, stress, menstruation/Treat with life-style changes, vasoconstrictors, beta blockers. May abort at aura stage
Migraine/cluster	Starts as excruciating pain surrounding or behind one eye, with tearing of that eye, nasal congestion, and facial flushing on that side. Pain radiates backward and attacks come in "clusters," eventually disappearing, then returning	Usually a migraine-type association often with alcohol or smoking/Treat with pain relievers or beta blockers
Migraine/exertion	Throbbing pain associated with physical exertion such as running, sex, bowel movement, coughing	Usually a migraine variant that is treated with pain relievers or beta blockers but may be mimiced by aneurysms or tumors
Temporomandibular joint headache	Sharp, stabbing pain (Charlie horse-like) accompanying jaw manipulation. May be a clicking sound in the jaw	Associated with stress (jaw clenching) and often malocclusion/Treat by relaxation, Tegretol, dental consultation
Sinus headache	Pressure or pain around sinuses, often localized to the eye. Often nasal congestion, runny nose, and lacrimation	Associated with history of allergies and recurrent sinus infections/Treat with decongestants, antibiotics, antihistamines, and ENT consultation
Caffeine withdrawal headache/may also occur with renewed consumption	Throbbing pain that occurs in heavy caffeine consumers when skipping usual dose	Caffeine is a vasoconstrictor, and when removed vasodilation creates headache much like a migraine/Treat by gradually reducing caffeine consumption
Hangover headache	Throbbing pain and even nausea associated with consumption of alcohol	Alcohol causes vasodilation and irritation of vessels of the brain/Treat by avoidance of alcohol or consumption of fructose to burn off alcohol
Hypoglycemia headache	Varying head pain associated with missed meals	Low blood sugar associated with rebound vasodilation/Treat by advising of benefits of regular meals
Stress/tension headache	Varying dull pain, usually encircling head in bands, focal golfball pain, tightness in scalp or neck	Stress, anxiety, depression/Treat with pain relievers, stress management, psychological or psychiatric counseling
Eyestrain headache	Varying pain often frontal associated with use of the eyes	Uncorrected refractive error, binocular vision problem/Treat by spectacles, prism, vision training

The ocular signs may include a unilateral red or injected eye with corneal edema, Descemet's folds, aqueous flare, iris atrophy, rubeosis iridis and/or neovascular glaucoma, hypotony, and rapidly developing cataract. There may be reduced vision early, ocular and periorbital pain, photophobia and prolonged vision recovery with exposure to light, and a history of unilateral transient monocular blindness or amaurosis fugax. Ophthalmoscopically, there is often unilateral venous dilation, narrowed retinal arteries, at times equatorial dot-blot hemorrhages, and often disc or retinal neovascularization with all of the potential

Ocular Ischemic Syndrome

Pearls

Characteristics

△ A variation of a "carotid stroke syndrome," and directly related to systemic disease
△ Unilateral in presentation
△ Unilateral red or injected eye
△ Corneal edema and Descemet's folds
△ Flare in the anterior chamber and iris atrophy
△ Rubeosis and neovascular glaucoma are a strong probability
△ A rapidly developing cataract is characteristic
△ Ocular and periorbital pain
△ Photophobia and prolonged photostress recovery
△ History of unilateral transient monocular blindness
△ Unilateral vein dilation and arterial attenuation
△ Possible equatorial hemorrhages, but hemorrhaging is rare
△ Disc/retinal neovascularization

Management

△ Retinal consultation with fluorescein angiography to determine the degree of retinal perfusion problems
△ Panretinal photocoagulation or cryopexy to minimize the hypoxia
△ Possible goniophotocoagulation
△ Control IOP with any possible technique
△ **Medical workup**
   Erythrocyte sedimentation rate if elderly
   Blood pressure and pulse rate
   Fasting blood sugar
   Complete blood count with differential and platelets
   Fasting lipid profile
   Prothrombin and partial thromboplastin times
   Antinuclear antibodies and rheumatoid factor
   FTA-ABS
   Palpation/ausculation of the carotid system (ODM?) and duplex ultrasound
   Carotid arteriography in surgical candidates
   Cardiology consultation
   Follow up in 3 to 6 months depending on retinal status, status of the anterior chamber, and level of control of the IOP

---

sequelae (Fig. 4–74). Optic disc edema is rare. Retinal arterial emboli may be present. ODM diastolic is usually significantly reduced and there is often spontaneous arterial pulsation because it is so low. Fluorescein angiography will demonstrate both a decreased dye transit time and a tremendous time differential between the two eyes. The entire sign and symptom package evolves because of the unilateral stenosis of the carotid supply system. The anterior reaction is a combination of ischemia and the shutdown in the internal carotid system, allowing for a shunting of the blood through the external carotid system—the unilateral red eye develops from external carotid engorgement. The hypoxia builds, creating a situation of retinal and anterior segment oxygen starvation, which stimulates disc, retinal, or iris neovascularization.

Management. The most important management strategy is to attempt to treat the underlying causative factor. Again, the same approach should be taken as with retinal vaso-occlusive diseases. The primary screening workup should include an immediate erythrocyte sedimentation rate if the patient is elderly (over 55 years), blood pressure and pulse rate, fasting blood sugar, complete blood count with differential and platelets, fasting lipid profile, prothrombin and partial thromboplastin times, antinuclear antibodies, rheumatoid factor, FTA-ABS, palpation and auscultation of the carotid system (ODM?), and duplex ultrasound. Carotid arteriography is sometimes indicated in the patient that is to have carotid surgery. All patients with retinal emboli deserve a cardiology consultation. Once the cause has been determined, some attempt may be made at managing the underlying disease.

The management of the ocular complications is straightforward yet frustrating, as the condition is difficult to halt. A retinal consultation with fluorescein angiography is a prudent first move. Panretinal photocoagulation is usually applied to minimize retinal hypoxia, which should then control the development of disc, retinal, and iris neovascularization. Cryotherapy and goniophotocoagulation may also be of benefit in controlling the neovascular development. Unfortunately, the development of the neovascular glaucoma often progresses, and appropriated mea-

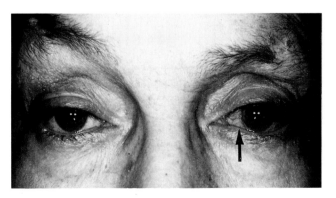

Figure 4–74. Example of engorgement of the scleral vessels and anterior uveitis associated with total occlusion of the left internal carotid artery. There was associated disc neovascularization secondary to hypoxia in an ocular ischemic syndrome.

sures must be used to control the pressure. Paradoxically, the author has seen the development of rubeosis recede with a subsequent reduction in IOP without intervention. The cause may be the fact that so little oxygenated blood is reaching the eye that both the neovascularization "dries up" and the perfusion at the ciliary body is reduced to the point that production of aqueous is minimized.

DIABETIC RETINOPATHY

I wish they did not. I wish we could say no to diabetic cataracts and retinopathy. I wish diabetes was not the leading cause of new blindness in our country. I wish I did not have to see another blind or significantly visually impaired diabetic patient—no more white canes, no more seeing-eye dogs.
—Marvin E. Levin, MD,
 Diabetes Spectrum 1991;4:118

Today, finding medical care is a multifaceted challenge. First, you must find a doctor who practices in an area you can drive or walk to and get an appointment with. It's nice, too, if you find a doctor you can talk to, someone you feel comfortable with, someone you trust. But when you have diabetes, you need more. Diabetes is not an easy disease to manage, and as such, you are entitled to medical care requiring special knowledge and experience. You are also entitled to quality medical care.
—Bruce Zimmerman, MD and Janice T. Radak
 ADA Advanced Information Series—Standards of Care
 for Patients With Diabetes Mellitus

Diabetes: The Disease

Glucose is an important nutrient for the human body, being the preferred source of energy for the blood cells and brain. Glucose supplies are provided through gluconeogenesis, occurring primarily in the liver. The liver is the central organ involved in providing glucose under fasting conditions. Many factors are involved in proper glucose production and use, including glucagon, cortisol, epinephrine, and insulin. Insulin is the primary factor in the control of glucose, and the liver is very sensitive to insulin levels. The peripheral sites of use of glucose are less sensitive to changes in insulin levels.

Diabetes is a disease of improper glucose production and use. The malfunction may be the result of absence of insulin, reduced supplies of insulin, or inability or reduced ability for receptor sites to use insulin. Insulin-dependent diabetes mellitus (IDDM) is the result of an absence of insulin. Tables 4–39 and 4–40 outline the common ocular and systemic signs and symptoms of type 1 (IDDM) diabetes. The triggering factors for type 1 diabetes are obscure, but it is

TABLE 4–39. INSULIN-DEPENDENT DIABETES MELLITUS (TYPE 1): COMMON SYSTEMIC SIGNS AND SYMPTOMS

Fatigue[a]	Cardiovascular disease
Excessive thirst[a]	Neurologic disease
Excessive hunger[a]	Impotence
Excessive urination[a]	Ketoacidosis
Weight loss	Hyperosmolar coma
Recurrent infections (vaginitis)[a]	Oral disease, periodontal Podiatric disease
Ketone (fruity) breath	
Nephropathy, responsible for death in 40%	

[a] Early.

known that the afflicted individual has a multigenetic predisposition.

Type 2 diabetes has many names, but is classically described as noninsulin-dependent diabetes mellitus (NIDDM). Patients with type 2 (NIDDM) diabetes may have a relative or partial deficiency of insulin. First-phase insulin secretion is markedly reduced in type 2 diabetes. Paradoxically, many type 2 diabetic patients must use insulin to properly control their disease. Type 2 diabetes also may be the result of resistance to insulin action. This resistance may be the result of an intracellular defect or alteration of insulin receptors. Type 2 diabetes usually develops in the following manner: (1) obesity creates insulin resistance and decreased insulin production, and (2) postreceptor defects occur, leading to glucose intolerance. Table 4–41 lists the common systemic and ocular signs and symptoms of type 2 diabetes. There are other variations of diabetes, such as gestational diabetes and maturity-onset diabetes of the young, that are beyond the scope of this text.

From an *epidemiologic* standpoint, diabetes is a severe problem in today's society. Data from the 1982 National Health Interview Survey estimated that there were approximately 5.8 million persons in the civilian noninstitutionalized population of the United States with known diabetes, with the South having the

TABLE 4–40. INSULIN-DEPENDENT DIABETES MELLITUS (TYPE 1): COMMON OCULAR SIGNS AND SYMPTOMS

Fluctuating vision
Binocular vision anomalies (double vision)
Corneal epitheliopathy (recurrent corneal erosion)
Neurologic lid and pupil signs
Accommodative insufficiency
Recurrent infections
Early cataract development
Greater prevalence of glaucoma
Kruckenberg spindle
Optic nerve disease
Retinal vasculopathy

TABLE 4–41. NONINSULIN-DEPENDENT DIABETES MELLITUS (TYPE 2): SYSTEMIC AND OCULAR SIGNS AND SYMPTOMS

Often unaware of disease
Refractive changes
Mild weight loss, fatigue, weakness
Perhaps polyuria, polydipsia, polyphagia
Infection

highest rate. More recent estimates are closer to 14 million affected, with approximately 50 percent of those not yet diagnosed. Other studies estimate that 5 percent of the population has diabetes. There are over 600,000 new cases diagnosed per year, with an estimate that the numbers will double every 15 years. Diabetes is a major national health problem.

Diabetes mellitus is usually *diagnosed* by laboratory tests combined with signs and symptoms. Probably the most common office screening test for diabetes is the fasting blood glucose test. This is performed by asking the patient to fast after 10 PM the night before. The patient then reports to the office early in the morning. A fingerprick is often sufficient to generate a screening fasting glucose level, but is certainly not acceptable as a diagnostic test. Diabetes is suspect in the 100 to 140 mg percent range, and is likely above the 140 mg percent range. This along with a random blood sample, which should not be over 200 mg percent, is often useful in patients who profess to be under control but in whom the clinician finds such signs as ketone breath or severe retinopathy that call the degree of control into question. Never assume that your patients are under good control. If a suspect or abnormal screening level (FBS) is present or if you suspect hypoglycemia, an oral glucose tolerance test (OGTT) should be ordered. The OGTT is an uncomfortable test and should not be ordered in a cavalier fashion, but certainly is diagnostic.

Another useful test to ascertain compliance over a prolonged period is glycated hemoglobin, which is expressed in percentages. Glycated (glycosylated) hemoglobin is a measure of the most abundant component of hemoglobin in normal red blood cells. Hemoglobin A_1C is a variation of the glycated hemoglobin test, and can be elevated as a much as three times in diabetes. The test is particularly sensitive to the degree of glucose control over the preceding 2 to 3 months. Unfortunately different labs use different tests, and the practitioner must rely on the "normal ranges" from the reference laboratories. It can be said that elevated glycated hemoglobin (usually above 11 percent) is definitely a risk factor for the development of preproliferative and proliferative retinopathy as well as a risk factor for cardiovascular disease. The cor-

relation with increased incidence of proliferative retinopathy is the result of the fact that when hemoglobin has an increased glycosylation level, it has a corresponding decrease in the ability to carry oxygen. Screening for traces of protein (microalbuminuria) in the urine has also become an important test, as this is a sensitive indicator of kidney function. Ocular status often reflects the status of the kidneys.

Another important consideration in patients with diabetes is the level of blood lipids. Often lipid levels are elevated in diabetic patients because of the need to catabolize lipid for energy. Should triglyceride, cholesterol, and phospholipids be elevated, retinal vascular complications may occur. Fasting lipid levels may be ordered in patients with diabetes at intervals to ensure the health of the vascular system. Proper management of patients with diabetes includes routine blood work. Never assume proper control of the patient with diabetes.

Proper *management* of types 1 (IDDM) and 2 (NIDDM) diabetes includes a combination of diet modification by a nutritionist, education by a nurse educator, proper timing and proper levels if insulin injection is necessary, control of hepatic glucose production, increasing peripheral uptake and oxidation of glucose by potentiating insulin action, and careful follow-up of the patient, assessing for the complications of diabetes to ensure timely therapeutic intervention. The care of the diabetic is the quintessential example of the need for a multidisciplinary approach to health care. Many health care practitioners must be involved in the care to manage the multitudes of end-organ complications. Optimal care must include communication among the professionals providing care to the patient with diabetes.

> You and I may be experts with our ophthalmoscopes, but let's face it, our friendly retinal specialist, ophthalmologist, and optometrist in all probability are more adept.
> —Marvin Levin, MD,
>   *Diabetes Spectrum* 1991;4:118

> There are four team members that I call the "first team" who should be involved in every case. The patient, the diabetes nurse educator, the dietitian, and . . . the primary care physician, diabetologist, or endocrinologist. . . . The second team is composed of the ophthalmologist, optometrist (especially interested in diabetes and an expert in fundus examination), and the dentist, who should see the patient at least yearly.
> —Marvin Levin, MD,
>   *Clinical Diabetes* Nov/Dec 1989; 94–95

Emergency situations associated with diabetes mellitus include ketoacidosis and hyperosmolar coma. Characteristics of ketoacidosis include (1) lack of insulin, with blood glucose in the 300 to 600 mg percent range, (2) vomiting, (3) abdominal pain from

TABLE 4–42. RISK FACTORS FOR DEVELOPMENT OF DIABETES

91% higher in blacks than whites
61% higher in Hispanics than whites
43% higher in other ethnic groups than whites
Type II 40% higher in native Americans than whites
Type II higher with obesity and family history

TABLE 4–44. RISK FACTORS FOR DEVELOPMENT OF MACULAR EDEMA

Higher levels of glycosylated hemoglobin
Longer duration of diabetes
More severe retinopathy at baseline examination

sodium and potassium loss, (4) labored breathing, and (5) dehydration. Characteristics of hyperosmolar coma include (1) lack of insulin and electrolyte imbalance in an older diabetic with acute illness, (2) severe dehydration, (3) mild ketone elevation, (4) shock, (5) tachycardia, (6) hyperventilation, and (7) possible seizures.

Diabetic Retinopathy: Epidemiology

The American Diabetes Association states that diabetic eye disease is the number-one cause of new blindness in people between ages 20 and 74 in this country, and each year over 5800 Americans lose their sight because of diabetes. Diabetic ocular changes are responsible for 10 percent of the blind population of the United States (Aiello et al, 1981; Harris et al, 1987). Statistics of incidence of diabetic retinopathy in the diabetic population are clouded by definitions. It can be said, however, that the development of diabetic retinopathy increases in incidence with age, and is related to degree of control of the systemic process, according to Diabetes Control and Complications Trial (DCCT) findings. About 5 percent of patients with diabetes have vision-threatening disorders categorized as follows: (1) 200,000 with proliferative diabetic retinopathy (PDR); (2) 200,000 with macular edema; and (3) 200,000 with PDR plus macular edema (Cavallerano, 1991).

The risk of developing diabetic retinopathy with a diagnosis of diabetes prior to age 30 is as follows: (1) 97 percent of patients have some degree of retinopathy after 15 years, (2) 40 percent have worsening of retinopathy, and (3) the incidence of PDR increases with duration of the disease. Type 1 patients have possible ocular manifestations after 5 years but 60 percent

develop some diabetic retinopathy after 10 years, and after 15 to 20 years, 25 to 50 percent progress to sight-threatening PDR (Klein et al, 1984a). With a diagnosis of diabetes after age 30, the risk of developing diabetic retinopathy is as follows: (1) 78 percent of patients have some degree of retinopathy after 15 years, (2) 25 to 34 percent have worsening of retinopathy, (3) the incidence of PDR increases with the duration of the disease, and (4) the risk increases with the use of insulin (Klein et al, 1984b). Type 2 patients have about a 20 percent occurrence of diabetic retinopathy at the time of diagnosis of diabetes, whereas after about 4 years 4 percent develop PDR and after 15 years about 20 percent develop PDR. Risk factors for the development of diabetes and of general complications are shown in Tables 4–42 and 4–43, while specific risk factors for the development of macular edema and severity of retinopathy are illustrated in Tables 4–44 and 4–45.

Probably the greatest risk of vision loss associated with diabetes stems from the fact that patients do not get routine eye examinations. In 1979, Stross and Harlan found that a full 18 months after publication only 28 percent of family practitioners and 46 percent of internists were aware of the positive results reported in the Diabetic Retinopathy Studies concerning the intervention in diabetic retinopathy by photocoagulation. In 1984 it was estimated that 26 percent of type 1 and 36 percent of type 2 diabetics had never had an eye examination. The characteristics of those patients were that they lived in rural America, were elderly, had diabetes for a relatively short period of time, had fewer years of formal education, and were receiving care from a general or family practitioner (Witkin and Klein, 1984). A 1991 study found that about 75 percent of all diabetic patients were cared for by primary care physicians rather than physicians specializing in dia-

TABLE 4–43. RISK FACTORS FOR DEVELOPMENT OF COMPLICATIONS OF DIABETES

Duration of disease
Hypertension—risk of hypertension higher in blacks
Pregnancy
Elevated glycated hemoglobin levels
Proteinuria
Cataract surgery if diabetic retinopathy prior to surgery
Level of control

TABLE 4–45. RISK FACTORS FOR SEVERITY OF DIABETIC RETINOPATHY

Higher levels of glycosylated hemoglobin
Proteinuria
Elevated systolic blood pressure

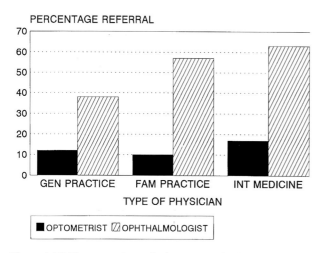

Figure 4–75. The percentage of primary care physicians managing patients with diabetes who routinely refer for eye examinations to rule out diabetic retinopathy. Gen, general; Fam, family; Int, internal. *(Diabetes Care 1991;23:156–158.)*

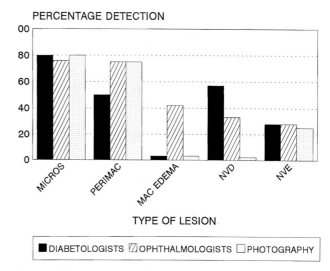

Figure 4–76. Comparison of detecting various forms of diabetic retinopathy by ophthalmologists, diabetologists, and photography. Micros, microaneurysms; Perimac, perimacular; Mac, macular; NVD, neovascularization disc; NVE, neovascularization elsewhere. *(Diabetes Care 1991;14:26–33.)*

betes. Figure 4–75 illustrates the percentage of these primary care physicians who routinely refer for eye examinations (Jacques et al, 1991). Clearly one of the problems is that the primary care physicians are not effectively asking their patients to get routine eye examinations to help prevent the development of vision-threatening retinopathy. In 1990 it was reported that 32 percent of diabetics had never had an eye examination and were found to be at high risk. Of that 32 percent, 61 percent had diabetic retinopathy, glaucoma, cataract, or other abnormalities (Sprafka et al, 1990). In 1991, a report found that of black and Hispanic patients diagnosed with type 2 diabetes, 57.7 percent of Hispanics and 62.7 percent of blacks had mild diabetic retinopathy at their first eye examination. In addition, 42.9 percent of Hispanics and 37.3 percent of blacks had severe preproliferative or proliferative retinopathy at presentation (Appiah et al, 1991).

Another significant risk factor related to the genesis of diabetic retinopathy is the skill level of the doctor involved in diagnosis and management. In two separate reports, it was shown that primary practitioners providing eye care to diabetic patients had a 27 to 57 percent correct diagnosis rate as related to diabetic retinopathy (Sussman et al, 1982; Kleinstein, 1987). In a 1991 report illustrated in Figure 4–76, it was shown that diabetologists performed reasonably well in the detection of diabetic retinopathy when compared to ophthalmologists (Nathan et al, 1991). Unfortunately, all providers involved in the provision of primary eyecare are open for improvement in diagnostic skills. According to a 1991 study, intervention with well-designed and tested postgraduate education improved the ability of nonophthalmologists to detect preproliferative and proliferative retinopathy

from 40 to 85 percent, and the ability to detect macular edema from 17 to 84.8 percent. Regardless of the discipline, education and experience improve diagnostic abilities (Awh et al, 1991).

Blindness from diabetes peaks in incidence between ages 30 and 50 and is race and sex related. Compared to white males, nonwhite females have a 3.8 times higher risk of blindness, nonwhite males a 1.3 times higher risk, and white females a 1.3 times higher risk. As compared to nondiabetics, diabetics are 25 times more prone to blindness, 17 times more prone to renal disease, 20 times more prone to gangrene, and 2 times more prone to myocardial infarct or stroke.

Examination of the Patient With Diabetes

The examination of the patient with diabetes is complex because of the necessity to cover not only the ocular complications but also the systemic complications and an assessment of the degree of control. A number of factors affect the genesis of diabetic retinopathy, and the primary care practitioner must be cognizant of all of these factors. The following represents the minimal acceptable examination procedure for the patient with diabetes.

Crucial Points in the Examination and Management of the Patient With Diabetes

1. *Establish the type of diabetes,* type 1 versus type 2. Type 1 has more of a tendency to develop severe retinopathy sooner in the life of the disease than type 2, while type 2 has more of a tendency to present with retinopathy at the time of diagnosis.

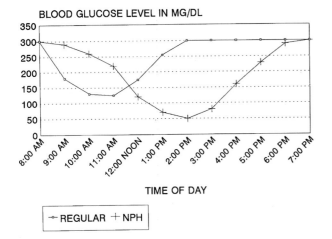

Figure 4–77. Comparison of the action of NPH and regular insulin over the course of the day.

2. *Establish, as best possible, the duration of the diabetes.* Duration of the disease is the most important predictive risk factor for the genesis of diabetic retinopathy.
3. *Establish a family history.* A family history of diabetic retinopathy is a risk factor, and family history of type 2 diabetes is definitely a risk factor for the development of type 2 diabetes in other family members.
4. *Determine the type of control of the diabetes.*
   - Oral (generation) vs. insulin. At this point in time it is believed that even some type 2 patients have been found to benefit from a combination of oral hypoglycemic agents plus insulin, but this is controversial. It is also important to distinguish between first- and second-generation oral hypoglycemic agents, as second-generation agents may create refractive shifts even while controlling blood glucose.
   - Type of insulin and dosage levels. Human insulin has been reported to create less of an immunological reaction than porcine insulin; thus

the patient usually feels better and purportedly has fewer complications. It has also been shown that patients on human insulin have fewer ocular complications. The two basic types of insulin are regular, which is a quick release; and NPH, which is timed release. The slow release go by many different names, including Lente and Super Lente. There are also varieties of insulin that are premixed with different proportions of regular and NPH. The patient on the pump has a fairly constant infusion of regular insulin to control the fluctuations in blood glucose.
   - Determine if split dosages. Regular insulin is a quick-release form causing a rather rapid yet short-lived response, while NPH is more of a timed-release variety. A combination of the two given in split dosages over the day has a tendency to smooth the blood glucose curve, which is thought to minimize complications and make the patient feel more comfortable. Figure 4–77 compares the action of NPH and regular insulin.
5. *Ask if the patient's vision fluctuates.* Fluctuating vision indicates relatively poor control or hyperinsulinemia.
6. *Ask if the patient performs self-monitoring of blood glucose (SMBG).* A positive response to this question usually indicates the level of sophistication of the education of the patient regarding the disease. Often a well-educated patient performs monitoring two to four times a day. Because of the potential side effect of subtle color vision compromise in the diabetic patient, it is wise to test color vision with a D-15 and to advise the patient to perform SBGM with an instrument to avoid the color confusion potential.
7. *Ask for the name and address of the diabetic physician and when he or she was last seen.* A significant part of the care of the patient with diabetes is effective communication between health care providers.

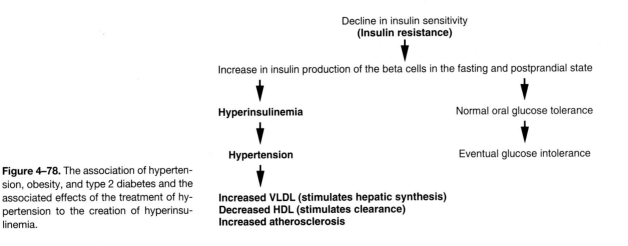

Figure 4–78. The association of hypertension, obesity, and type 2 diabetes and the associated effects of the treatment of hypertension to the creation of hyperinsulinemia.

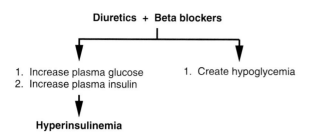

Diuretics + Beta blockers

1. Increase plasma glucose
2. Increase plasma insulin

1. Create hypoglycemia

Hyperinsulinemia

Figure 4–79. The associated effects of the treatment of hypertension to the creation of hyperinsulinemia.

8. *Ask about other medications being used,* especially antihypertensive agents and corticosteroids. Corticosteroids decrease the body's ability to properly metabolize glucose, resulting in altered blood glucose, usually poor control. Certain antihypertensives, especially beta blockers, are thought to actually create a situation of hyperinsulinemia, precipitating cardiovascular complications. Figures 4–78 through 4–80 are a representation of the current concerns regarding beta blocker usage in the patient with diabetes.

9. *Check blood glucose levels (glycated hemoglobin) and blood pressure.* Glycated hemoglobin (Hgb A₁C) is a measure of the level of glucose control over about the past 60 days, and glycated protein level (ROTAG) is a measure of the level of glucose control over about the past week. Measurement of blood pressure is crucial in all patients with diabetes, as hypertension is a strong risk factor for the development of diabetic retinopathy, kidney and heart disease, and many other complications of diabetes.

10. *Consider performing or ordering fasting lipid levels.* Many patients with diabetes also have elevated lipid levels, which increase the risk of associated coronary artery disease.

11. *Evaluate the cornea for epithelial basement membrane dystrophy, keratoconjunctivitis sicca, and any other potential abnormalities.*

12. *Perform tonometry and then dilate the pupils.* There is a significant risk for primary open-angle glaucoma and neovascular glaucoma in the patient with diabetes. Although only a screening test, tonometry may uncover an occasional patient with glaucoma. Far more important in the detection of glaucoma is examination of the pupillary frill of the iris for neovascularization and the optic nerve heads for asymmetry and excavation. Dilation of the pupils is crucial, as it is thought that up to 50 percent of diabetic retinopathy may be overlooked without dilation. Dilation is best accomplished in the diabetic with a combination of ½ or 1% Mydriacyl combined with 2½% phenylephrine. As with all patients, some degree of caution must be exercised with the use of phenylephrine, because of potential associated cardiovascular risks. Figures 4–81 and 4–82 compare dilation in the patient with diabetes with and without the addition of phenylephrine.

13. *Evaluate the anterior segment and crystalline lens for early cataract development and neovascularization at the pupillary frill.*

14. *Evaluate the fundus with multiple examination techniques.*
    • Direct ophthalmoscopy may detect dot-blot hemorrhages, neovascularization of the disc, hard exudates, and intraretinal microvascular

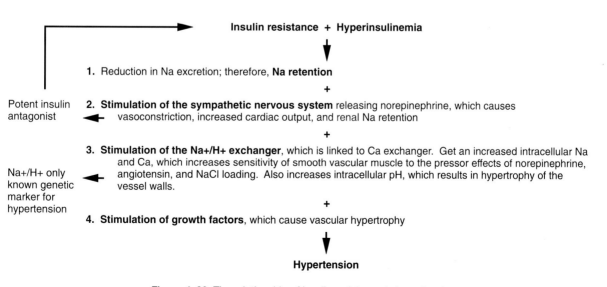

Insulin resistance + Hyperinsulinemia

1. Reduction in Na excretion; therefore, **Na retention**

+

Potent insulin antagonist

2. **Stimulation of the sympathetic nervous system** releasing norepinephrine, which causes vasoconstriction, increased cardiac output, and renal Na retention

+

Na+/H+ only known genetic marker for hypertension

3. **Stimulation of the Na+/H+ exchanger,** which is linked to Ca exchanger. Get an increased intracellular Na and Ca, which increases sensitivity of smooth vascular muscle to the pressor effects of norepinephrine, angiotensin, and NaCl loading. Also increases intracellular pH, which results in hypertrophy of the vessel walls.

+

4. **Stimulation of growth factors,** which cause vascular hypertrophy

Hypertension

Figure 4–80. The relationship of insulin resistance to hypertension.

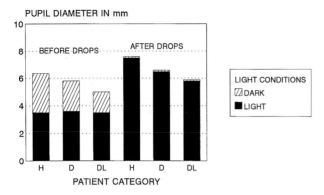

Figure 4–81. Comparison of the pupil size in healthy eyes, eyes with diabetic retinopathy, and eyes that have been treated by laser after the instillation of 0.5% tropicamide. H, healthy; D, diabetic; DL, diabetic laser. *(Br J Ophthalmol 1985;69:425–427.)*

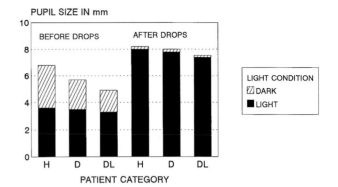

Figure 4–82. Comparison of the pupil size in healthy eyes, eyes with diabetic retinopathy, and eyes that have been treated by laser after the instillation of 0.5% tropicamide plus 10% phenylephrine. H, healthy; D, diabetic; DL, diabetic laser. *(Br J Ophthalmol 1985; 69:425–427.)*

abnormalities, but may miss other diabetic retinopathy features.

- Binocular indirect ophthalmoscopy may detect hard exudate patterns, cotton-wool spots, neovascularization elsewhere, vitreous hemorrhage, and traction retinal detachment but may miss other diabetic retinopathy features.
- A Volk 78 or contact fundus lens evaluation is necessary to detect macular edema and other subtle macular changes as well as the excavations and elevations of the optic nerve head associated with glaucoma, ischemic optic neuropathy, and diabetic papillopathy.
- Fluorescein angiography is the definitive diagnostic test when there is any doubt about the status of the retina, especially when there is concern about macular edema, capillary nonperfusion, and/or subtle neovascularization.

15. *Apply the standards of care for the management of diabetic retinopathy.*
16. *Explain the situation to the patient.* Patient education is the most crucial aspect of the care of the patient with diabetes. Record in the chart that you have educated the patient. Make the patient aware of the benefits of the American Diabetes Association as well as other support groups.
17. *Recommend follow-up according to duration of the diabetes, type of diabetes, general systemic status, status of retina, level of glycated Hgb, and other factors listed in Table 4–46.*
18. *Send a letter to the patient's physician regarding the status of the eyes and the recommended follow-up period.*

■ ■ ■ ■ ■ ■
Clinical Notes Regarding Modification of Management Plans

1. Always communicate your findings to the primary care physician
2. Management should be tempered by your assessment of the patient's general level of control of systemic diabetes.
   - Are random blood glucose levels below 200 mg/dL in office?
   - Are glycated hemoglobin or fructosamine levels within normal range?
   - Is hypertension under control?
   - Is the patient taking medication that might impact negatively on diabetes control?
   - Is there microalbuminuria (proteinuria)?
   - Is the patient performing self-monitoring of blood glucose (SMBG)?
   - Is the patient on the proper oral hypoglycemic agent or the proper insulin regimen?
   - Remember that the longer the patient has had diabetes, the more likely the presence of diabetic retinopathy and the more likely it will progress.

Diabetic Retinopathy: Genesis

The genesis of diabetic retinopathy is certainly controversial, but seems to be secondary to changes in the capillary basement membrane or capillary walls leading to focal development of microaneurysms, vascular loops, and dilated capillaries allowing for the development of leakage. This is combined with sticky

TABLE 4–46. GENERAL GUIDELINES FOR MANAGEMENT OF DIABETIC RETINOPATHY

Category	Characteristics	Management
Normal or minimal nonproliferative diabetic retinopathy	Rare microaneurysms	5–10% progress in 1 year. Document and follow up in 1 year
Mild nonproliferative diabetic retinopathy without macular edema	Microaneurysms, occasional dot-blot hemorrhages or hard exudates away from macula	16% of type 1 progress to proliferation in 4 years. Document and follow up in 6–12 months depending on extent of lesions
Moderate nonproliferative diabetic retinopathy or transitional diabetic retinopathy. **Early hypoxia.**	Hemorrhages and/or microaneurysms in 4 fields, or cotton-wool spots, venous beading, or IRMA	12–27% risk of progression to PDR within 1 year and 33% risk in 5 years. Document and follow up in 3–6 months. Consider retinal consultation with IRMA or 3 or more signs
Severe nonproliferative diabetic retinopathy or preproliferative diabetic retinopathy. **Hypoxia.**	Cotton-wool spots, venous beading, and IRMA in at least 2 fields, large hemorrhages present, or IRMA present	52% risk of progression to proliferation in 1 year and 60% risk in 5 years. If mild, follow in 3 months. If severe or 3 or more signs, get a retinal consultation. Get a retinal consultation with IRMA
Clinically significant macular edema	Retinal thickening within ½ DD of fovea, hard exudates within ½ DD of fovea, retinal thickening at least 1 DD within 1 DD of fovea	Retinal consultation. ETDRS finds intervention of benefit
Proliferative diabetic retinopathy	Neovascularization of the disc, neovascularization elsewhere, fibrotic proliferation	75% risk of progression to high risk in 5 years. Retinal consultation. DRS finds intervention of benefit
High-risk proliferative diabetic retinopathy	Neovascularization of the disc greater than ¼ to ⅓ DD, neovascularization of the disc less than ¼ DD with accompanying preretinal or vitreous hemorrhage, neovascularization elsewhere with accompanying preretinal or vitreous hemorrhage	Retinal consultation. 25–40% risk of visual loss over 2 years
Vitreous hemorrhage	Retrovitreous or intravitreous hemorrhage	Retinal consultation. DRVS finds early vitrectomy improves visual outcome
Traction retinal detachment	Retinal detachment associated with fibrotic proliferation	Retinal consultation
Neovascularization of iris	Any new vessel growth starting at the iris sphincter and growing toward the angle	Retinal consultation, as this is indicative of severe ocular hypoxia. Possible development of neovascular glaucoma.

ETDRS = Early Treatment Diabetic Retinopathy Study; DRVS = Diabetic Retinopathy Vitrectomy Study.

blood, resulting in nonperfusion in the capillary bed. This nonperfusion results in hypoxia. The combination of hypoxia and altered vascular wall structure (selective loss of intramural pericytes) unfolds into diabetic retinopathy. The vascular dilatation is thought to be the result of hyperglycemia and tissue hypoxia. There is also considerable discussion regarding the direct effects of insulin on retinal vascular structure causing an increase in the likelihood of the development of retinopathy. A great deal of research is now being done in the area of the conversion of glucose to sorbitol by aldose reductase because of the implication that accumulation of sorbitol is a possible trigger in the genesis of diabetic retinopathy. Unfortunately the work in the area of aldose reductase inhibitors has not produced any strong evidence to support widespread implementation into the care of the patient with diabetes. Figure 4–83 summarizes some of the current theory regarding the genesis of diabetic mi-

crovasculopathy. Unfortunately, the answer to the problem is still evading the health care community.

Once the basic microvasculopathy is established, a number of retinal vascular changes can occur. Figures 4–84 to 4–86 illustrate potential retinal vascular changes associated with diabetes. It should be noted that large-vessel disease (atherosclerosis) also increases in patients with diabetes. Patients with diabetes have twice the risk of stroke, five times the risk of myocardial infarction, and eight times the risk of peripheral vasculopathy. In addition, other systemic diseases such as systolic hypertension have an effect on the precipitation of diabetic retinal changes.

Diabetic retinopathy is one of the more serious complications of diabetes, as most persons fear the loss of vision above all of their senses. Vision is lost in diabetes by (1) leaking microaneurysms and small intraretinal vessels creating edema in the macular area and (2) relative retinal hypoxia precipitating the

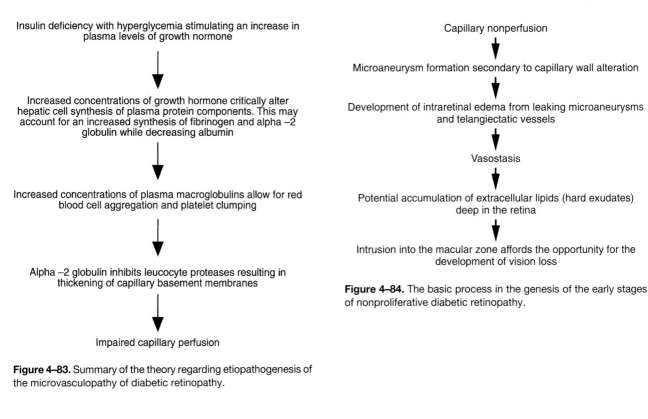

Insulin deficiency with hyperglycemia stimulating an increase in plasma levels of growth normone

↓

Increased concentrations of growth hormone critically alter hepatic cell synthesis of plasma protein components. This may account for an increased synthesis of fibrinogen and alpha −2 globulin while decreasing albumin

↓

Increased concentrations of plasma macroglobulins allow for red blood cell aggregation and platelet clumping

↓

Alpha −2 globulin inhibits leucocyte proteases resulting in thickening of capillary basement membranes

↓

Impaired capillary perfusion

Figure 4–83. Summary of the theory regarding etiopathogenesis of the microvasculopathy of diabetic retinopathy.

Capillary nonperfusion

↓

Microaneurysm formation secondary to capillary wall alteration

↓

Development of intraretinal edema from leaking microaneurysms and telangiectatic vessels

↓

Vasostasis

↓

Potential accumulation of extracellular lipids (hard exudates) deep in the retina

↓

Intrusion into the macular zone affords the opportunity for the development of vision loss

Figure 4–84. The basic process in the genesis of the early stages of nonproliferative diabetic retinopathy.

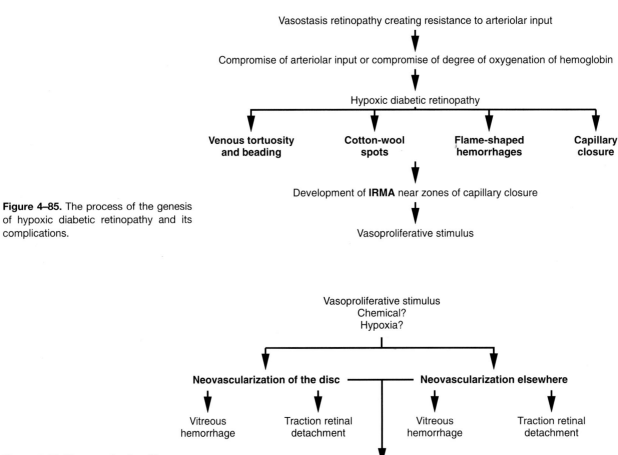

Vasostasis retinopathy creating resistance to arteriolar input

↓

Compromise of arteriolar input or compromise of degree of oxygenation of hemoglobin

↓

Hypoxic diabetic retinopathy

Venous tortuosity and beading   **Cotton-wool spots**   **Flame-shaped hemorrhages**   **Capillary closure**

↓

Development of **IRMA** near zones of capillary closure

↓

Vasoproliferative stimulus

Figure 4–85. The process of the genesis of hypoxic diabetic retinopathy and its complications.

Vasoproliferative stimulus
Chemical?
Hypoxia?

Neovascularization of the disc —————— **Neovascularization elsewhere**

Vitreous hemorrhage   Traction retinal detachment   Vitreous hemorrhage   Traction retinal detachment

Figure 4–86. The genesis of proliferative diabetic retinopathy.

Application of photocoagulation to create regression of neovascularization

development of neovascular nets that may rupture, creating vitreous hemorrhage or developing fibrotic glial tissue that may result in retinal detachment. The edema in the macular area can be secondary to either focal leakage or a generalized or diffuse leakage caused by an overall breakdown of the inner blood-retinal barrier. The general categories of diabetic retinopathy are illustrated in Table 4–46 and should serve as general guidelines for the management of the patient. The recommendations often refer to standard photos developed for reference by the Airlie House Classification System. All of these guidelines must be modified according to new discoveries in the management techniques. Current classification systems have evolved from the Early Treatment Diabetic Retinopathy Study Group (ETDRS), and are often referred to as nonproliferative diabetic retinopathy and proliferative diabetic retinopathy with a subcategory of diabetic macular edema. Nonproliferative retinopathy consists of the components of microaneurysms, hard exudates, dot-blot and flame-shaped hemorrhages, cotton-wool spots, intraretinal microvascular abnormalities, capillary and arteriolar occlusion, and venous caliber abnormalities such as beading and tortuosity. Proliferative retinopathy encompasses neovascularization of the disc and elsewhere, fibrotic proliferation, and vitreous hemorrhage. In the macular area, the classification is broken down into macular edema, hard exudates, and capillary nonperfusion.

Rather than strict categorization, I feel that the practitioner should concentrate on what the retinopathy signs mean and how they serve as a sign for possible vision compromise. Retinal edema is characterized by retinal swelling, hard exudates, microaneurysms, and the presence of dot-blot hemorrhages. Should these signs start to appear within 500 μm from the macula, a fluorescein angiogram should be performed to ascertain the advisability of interventive photocoagulation. The appearance of superficial retinal vascular changes such as flame hemorrhages, preretinal hemorrhages, cotton-wool spots, capillary and arteriolar occlusion, intraretinal microvascular abnormalities (IRMA), and venous caliber changes indicate hypoxia with the increased risk for the development of proliferative changes. Any signs of proliferative changes put the patient in imminent danger.

Nonproliferative Diabetic Retinopathy

Broad statements about background (nonproliferative) diabetic retinopathy (BDR) being relatively benign can be very misleading. Certain components of nonproliferative diabetic retinopathy can have a negative impact on vision when the changes are located in the macular area. The retinal vasculopathy components commonly attributed to nonproliferative diabetic retinopathy are microaneurysms, dot-blot (deep) retinal hemorrhages, flame hemorrhages, cotton-wool spots, IRMA, capillary and arteriolar occlusion, venous caliber changes, and hard exudate formation. The specifics of each of these components are discussed in detail in the section on the clinicopathologic basis of retinal vasculopathy.

Microaneurysms are balloon-like structures along weakened capillary walls. These microaneurysms usually are not visible by ophthalmoscopy but become readily apparent with fluorescein angiography. Microaneurysms leak into the retina, creating edema. Should this edema spread into the macula, visual acuity may become compromised. If there is demonstrable leakage into the macular area, fluorescein angiography is indicated to determine the advisability of photocoagulative intervention. Should the microaneurysms become hyalinized, they will be visible because of the white sheath. If there is evidence of microaneurysmal formation away from the macular area, it is safe to follow this patient in 1 year. Always instruct diabetic patients to use some method of monocular home monitoring of vision. It is important to question degree of control of the diabetes whenever there are all signs of diabetic retinopathy.

Dot-blot or deep retinal hemorrhages represent ruptures in weakened capillary walls. Once the hemorrhage occurs, the condition is static, but hemorrhages indicate the presence of deep intraretinal edema. A dot-blot hemorrhage in the macular area indicates edema encroaching into the foveal avascular zone (FAZ) and an immediate threat to vision. Dot-blot hemorrhages are not treatable, because they resolve of their own accord. Dot-blot hemorrhages do, however, offer a sign of diabetic microvasculopathy and intraretinal edema. If dot-blot hemorrhages are not in the macular area, they may be followed in 12 months using some method of home monitoring. However, if dot-blot hemorrhages are present in the macular area, fluorescein angiography is indicated to determine the advisability of photocoagulative intervention. A preponderance of widespread dot-blot hemorrhages indicates the need for investigation for either an evolving CRVO or ocular ischemia. In general, the rules listed in Table 4–46 may be followed in regard to dot-blot hemorrhaging, remembering that the more extensive the hemorrhaging, the more likely the progression of the diabetic retinopathy, because this usually reflects an increase in the general retinal hypoxia.

Hard exudates represent areas of lipid deposits that are a sign of chronic retinal edema secondary to leaking microaneurysms or a choroidal neovascular net. The exudates in and of themselves are benign but indicate long-standing edema. Most often, the exudates will circle the area of leakage, and if they are around the macula, are known collectively as circinate maculopathy. The hard exudates indicate the boundary of the intraretinal edema and often remain for a time after resolution of the edema. They are the ring around an area of nonperfused retinal microvasculopathy. Because exudates are a sign of long-standing edema, their presence around the macular area or in the foveal avascular zone (FAZ) indicates relatively poor prognosis for return of good vision, because the macular retinal tissue has been compromised for a prolonged period. If the hard exudates are remote to the macular region, it is safe to follow the patient in 6 to 12 months after establishing a system of monitor-

ing the monocular vision at home. Should diabetic maculopathy—clinically significant macular edema with hard exudates in the macula, encroaching to within 500 μm of the macula or surrounding the macula—be present, fluorescein angiography is indicated to assess the desirability of photocoagulative intervention. Prognosis for treatment in diabetic maculopathy is shown in Table 4–47. The advent of grid photocoagulation has improved the prognosis for cases of diabetic maculopathy that were previously thought unmanageable. When in doubt, a competent retinal specialist should be consulted. **See color plates 26, 27, and 31.** Unfortunately, the downside to photocoagulation is the potential for compromise of the reti-

Pearls

Nonproliferative Diabetic Retinopathy

Category	Characteristics	Management
Normal or minimal nonproliferative diabetic retinopathy	Rare microaneurysms	5 to 10 percent progress in 1 year. Document and follow up in 1 year
Mild nonproliferative diabetic retinopathy without macular edema	Microaneurysms, occasional dot-blot hemorrhages, or hard exudates away from the macula	16 percent of type 1 progress to proliferation in 4 years. Document and follow up in 6 to 12 months, depending on the extent of the lesions
Moderate nonproliferative diabetic retinopathy or transitional. **Early hypoxia.**	Hemorrhages and/or microaneurysms in 4 fields or cotton-wool spots, venous beading, or IRMA	12 to 27 percent risk of progression to PDR within 1 year and 33 percent risk in 5 years. Document and follow up in 3 to 6 months. Consider retinal consultation with IRMA or 3 or more signs
Severe nonproliferative diabetic retinopathy or preproliferative. **Hypoxia.**	Cotton-wool spots, venous beading, and IRMA in at least 2 fields, and large hemorrhages present in fields	52 percent risk of progression to proliferation in 1 year and 60 percent risk in 5 years. If mild, follow in 3 months. If severe or 3 or more signs, get a retinal consultation. Get a retinal consultation with IRMA
Clinically significant macular edema	Retinal thickening within ½ disc diameter (DD) of the fovea (center of macula), hard exudates within ½ DD of fovea, retinal thickening at least 1 DD within 1 DD of fovea	Retinal consultation, ETDRS proves benefit of intervention

Δ Make sure that nonretinal signs of diabetes are absent
Δ Carefully evaluate for glaucoma and corneal problems
Δ Evaluate blood pressure
Δ Consider a fasting lipid profile
Δ In office, evaluate status of random blood glucose—should be under 200 mg%
Δ Definitely order a glycated hemoglobin level test if not performed within 3 months for a type 1 or 6 months for a type 2 diabetic patient
Δ Communicate your findings to the primary care physician to assure quality comanagement
Δ Schedule follow-up visits according to retinal status and other contributing factors

TABLE 4–47. PROGNOSIS IN DIABETIC MACULOPATHY

Poor Prognosis	Good Prognosis
Hard exudates in fovea	Exudates away from a foveal avascular zone
Poor initial acuity	
Long-term maculopathy	Good initial acuity
Diffuse nonidentifiable leakage	Short-term maculopathy
	Focal identifiable leakage
Break in perifoveal capillary net	Healthy perifoveal capillary net

nal pigment epithelium-Bruch's membrane barrier, allowing for enlargement of the resulting scotoma and/or development of choroidal neovascular membranes. This complication is a reality and should be watched for within 8 weeks postoperatively even on the subtle application of burns associated with grid photocoagulative procedures.

Recognition of the signs of hypoxic diabetic retinopathy within the framework of nonproliferative retinopathy is absolutely crucial in the management of the patient with diabetes. All of the retinal signs of hypoxia are indicators of the immediate precursor to the vasoproliferative stimulus that potentiates retinal neovascularization. The retinal signs of hypoxia include cotton-wool spots, IRMA, venous tortuosity and beading, arteriolar abnormalities such as flame-shaped hemorrhages, and areas of capillary nonperfusion. The specifics of each of these components other than capillary closure are discussed in detail in the section on the clinicopathologic basis of retinal vasculopathy. Cotton-wool spots are the result of microinfarcts of arterioles in the nerve fiber layer. The

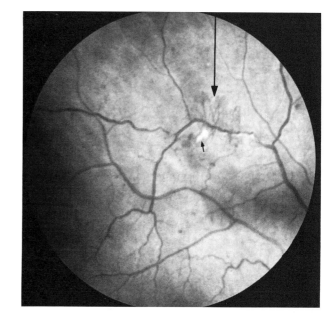

Figure 4–88. The long arrow points to a zone of IRMA, and the small arrow points to a cotton-wool spot.

cotton-like presentation is the result of axoplasmic stasis, with resultant deposition of debris. The cotton-wool spots never occur in the macular area and are usually confined to a distribution pattern within 3 disc diameters of the disc. The spots may cause small scotomas with threshold visual field testing but are essentially benign and nontreatable. Cotton-wool spots serve as an indicator of retinal hypoxia. Eyes with cotton-wool spots should be monitored according to the Early Treatment Diabetic Retinopathy Study (ETDRS) standards at 3- to 4-month intervals. Cotton-wool spots are best detected with the binocular indirect ophthalmoscope because of its increased resolution over other methods of examination.

IRMA (intraretinal microvascular abnormalities; Figs. 4–87 to 4–89) represents an intraretinal shunting system associated with tortuous capillaries in an area of severe capillary nonperfusion. IRMA forms to attempt to drain an area of stasis and is of no immediate threat to vision. IRMA is an indicator of stasis severe enough to create retinal hypoxia, and is thought to be the germination bed of neovascularization. Eyes with IRMA deserve a retinal consultation and should be followed at 3- to 4-month intervals after performance of fluorescein angiography. The presence of IRMA is a relatively ominous sign.

Venous tortuosity and beading (development of strictures within the venous column) is the result of sludging or slowing of venous blood, causing localized areas of venous dilatation. Again, tortuosity is of no threat to vision, but represents stasis to the point that retinal hypoxia exists. Venous tortuosity or beading is a sign that retinal hypoxia is present, and the pa-

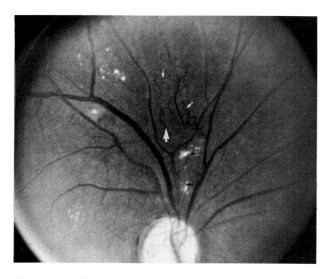

Figure 4–87. The white arrows point to zones of IRMA, and the black arrows point to hard exudates.

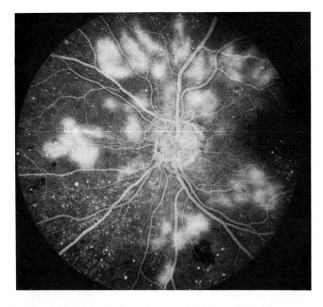

Figure 4–89. Fluorescein angiogram of IRMA evolving into severe neovascularization elsewhere, as evidenced by the leaking hyperfluorescence. Note the glowing microaneurysms spread throughout the posterior pole.

tient should be monitored according to ETDRS guidelines, returning in at least 3 to 4 months.

Arteriolar abnormalities occur as superficial flame-shaped hemorrhages or areas of focal arteriolar narrowing. The flame-shaped hemorrhages are the result of compromised arterioles in the nerve fiber layer. The flames usually present within the area of radial peripapillary distribution. Any arteriolar compromise may result in localized hypoxia. With the presence of flame-shaped hemorrhages, the patient with diabetes should be followed according to ETDRS guidelines, returning in at least 3 to 4 months. **See color plates 26, 28, and 48.**

Areas of capillary closure are evident only on high-resolution fluorescein angiography, appearing as dark spots in the normally lighted-with-fluorescein capillary bed. This area of capillary closure represents an area of localized infarct (multiple) of the capillary bed. This infarct will cause relative hypoxia in the area of capillary distribution. Areas of capillary closure indicate the need for a retinal consultation, with the patient being recalled in 3 to 4 months.

The Diabetic Retinopathy Study (DRS) (1976, 1978, 1979, 1981, 1987) found that approximately 50 percent of eyes with at least three hypoxic signs progress to proliferative diabetic retinopathy within 2 years. Fluorescein angiography is indicated if there are three or more signs of retinal hypoxia. When faced with signs of retinal hypoxia, a consultation with a retinal specialist is not an error but rather an indication that the practitioner is acting conservatively in the best interest of the patient.

■ ■ ■ ■ ■ ■
Clinical Notes: Asymmetrical Diabetic Retinopathy

Any diabetic retinopathy that occurs in an asymmetrical fashion should be considered secondary to unilateral internal carotid or ophthalmic artery stenosis until proven otherwise. Although studies have been controversial in this area, the assumption of asymmetry being secondary to internal carotid stenosis or stenosis within the ophthalmic arterial system is sound. In these cases, always at least palpate the internal carotid area for asymmetrical pulsation, and auscultate for carotid sinus bruits. Should internal carotid stenosis be suspected, consultation requesting at the least a duplex ultrasonography should be arranged. Remember that patients with diabetes have large-vessel disease secondary to the associated hypertension and the effects of hyperinsulinemia on atherosclerosis.

Proliferative Diabetic Retinopathy

Proliferative diabetic retinopathy (PDR) is beyond the realm of primary care. Almost without exception, the patient with PDR should have a consultation with a competent retinal specialist to ascertain the advisability of intervention. PDR was devastating before the development of laser photocoagulation. In the past, patients with PDR had an extremely poor visual prognosis, with radical intervention, such as pituitary ablation, as their only hope. Every component of PDR has the potential to create blindness. The components

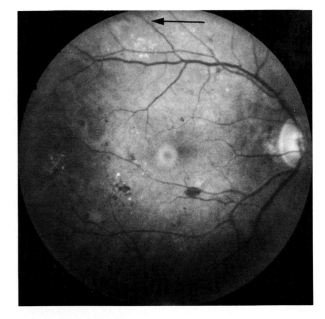

Figure 4–90. Black-and-white photograph of apparent background diabetic retinopathy. The arrow points to a zone that proved to be neovascularization.

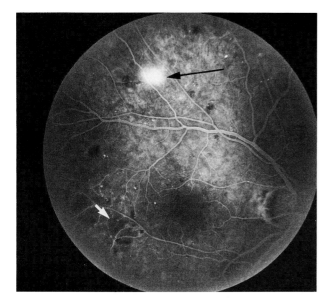

Figure 4–91. Early-stage angiogram of Figure 4–90, demonstrating the neovascularization (*black arrow*) and an area of capillary dropout (*white arrow*).

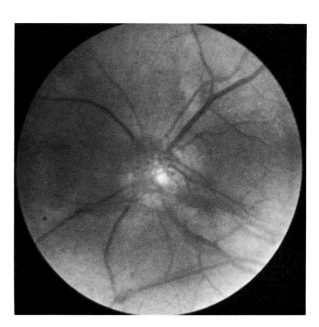

Figure 4–93. Black-and-white photograph demonstrating fragile neovascularization of the disc. Note the haze over the disc created by the leaking neovascularization.

of PDR include neovascularization of the disc, neovascularization elsewhere, fibrotic proliferation accompanying the neovascularization, traction retinal detachment, and vitreous hemorrhages (Figs. 4–90 to 4–96). The specifics of these components are discussed in detail in the section on the clinicopathologic basis of retinal vasculopathy earlier in this chapter. Effective care of the diabetic patient with proper moni-

toring should avert development of PDR in most patients. If, however, the components of PDR are present, laser photocoagulation and vitrectomy offer some hope. There is approximately a 50 percent risk of blindness in an eye with PDR within 5 years after the onset of neovascularization if laser intervention is not applied.

Neovascularization of the disc (NVD) occurs in

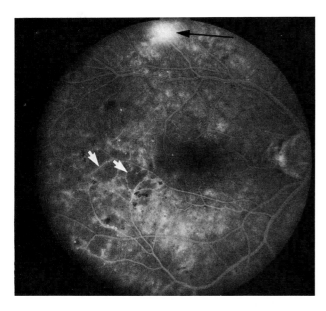

Figure 4–92. Late-stage angiogram of Figure 4–90.

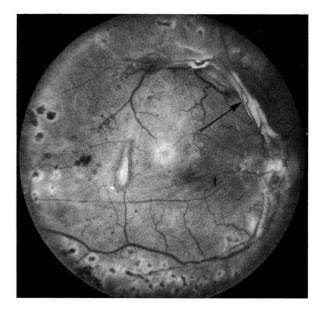

Figure 4–94. An example of proliferative diabetic retinopathy. The long arrow points to fibrotic scaffolding, and the short arrow to the traction created by the proliferation.

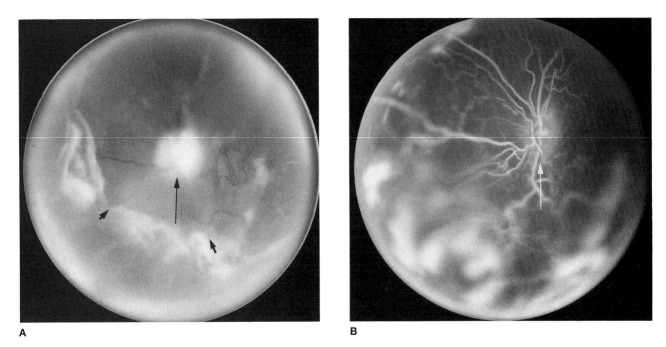

Figure 4–95. A traction retinal detachment associated with proliferative diabetic retinopathy. **A.** The small arrows point to the forward detachment of the retina. **B.** Fluorescein angiograms of the detachment.

approximately 25 percent of the patients who develop PDR as a response to hypoxia in the retinal tissue. NVD and neovascularization elsewhere (NVE) both seem to progress more rapidly in young patients with diabetes than in older patients with diabetes. NVD and NVE both usually appear after a minimum of 15 years of diabetes. NVD initially occurs as a very fine network arising from the disc capillaries, which soon establishes connections with larger retinal veins in the immediate area. This early neovascularization grows slowly but is not restricted by an internal limiting membrane at the disc. All new vessels leak, and the

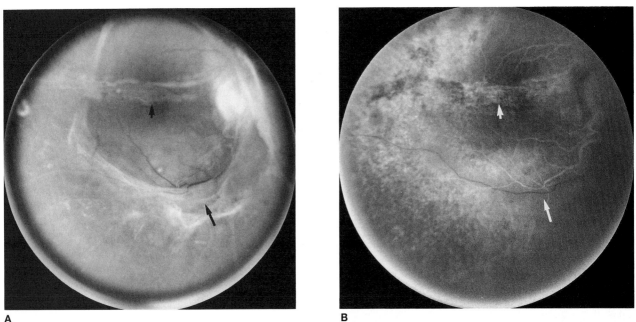

Figure 4–96. This is the fellow eye to that in Figure 4–95, also with a detachment. A band of traction coarses directly through the macula of the photograph (**A**) and the angiogram (**B**).

clinician may notice a hazy appearance to the disc borders and fine vessels of the disc as the result of this leakage. These exposed vessels are subject to trauma and posterior vitreous detachment that may lead to intravitreous or retrovitreous hemorrhage. The haze over the disc is an important ophthalmoscopic diagnostic sign in any diabetic patient.

Should the NVD progress unchecked, a fibrotic scaffolding will become more prominent. The addition of fibrotic scaffolding increases the likelihood of the future development of traction retinal detachment. As the net expands, there is a greater chance of vitreal hemorrhage. The hypoxia may be severe enough at this stage to initiate iris neovascularization, complicating the eye with neovascular glaucoma. At all points in the examination of the patient with diabetes, the practitioner must be cognizant of the possibility of iris neovascularization at the pupillary sphincter area.

Eventually, hypoxia will be severe enough to actually create retinal death, which reduces the hypoxic stimulus. With a reduction of oxygenated blood, the new vessels may regress, leaving the fibrotic scaffolding to do its damage through traction retinal detachment.

NVE takes a similar course to NVD, albeit more insidious. The new vessels are thought to sprout from areas of IRMA in the capillary bed. The new vessels eventually may perforate the internal limiting membrane to proliferate along the retinal surface. These vessels adhere to the vitreal hyaloid membrane and grow rapidly. They may later regress, but the accompanying fibrotic scaffolding remains adherent to the membrane. With vitreous syneresis and collapse, there is potential for both vitreous hemorrhage and retinal detachment. The vitreous detachment in the patient with diabetes is more insidious than in the nondiabetic, creating pockets of detachment. These pockets may create isolated retrovitreous hemorrhage or isolated areas of retinal detachment. NVE may

Pearls

Proliferative Diabetic Retinopathy

Category	Characteristics	Management
Proliferative diabetic retinopathy	Neovascularization of the disc, neovascularization elsewhere, fibrotic proliferation	75 percent risk of progression to high risk in 5 years. Retinal consultation. Diabetic Retinopathy Study Research Group finds intervention of benefit
High-risk proliferative diabetic retinopathy	Neovascularization of the disc greater than ¼ to ⅓ DD, or less than ¼ DD with accompanying preretinal or vitreous hemorrhage, neovascularization elsewhere with accompanying preretinal or vitreous hemorrhage	Retinal consultation. 25 to 40 percent risk of visual loss over 2 years
Vitreous hemorrhage	Retrovitreous or intravitreous hemorrhage	Retinal consultation. Diabetic Retinopathy Vitrectomy Study Research Group finds early vitrectomy improves visual outcome
Traction retinal detachment	Retinal detachment associated with fibrotic proliferation	Retinal consultation
Neovascularization of iris	Any new vessel growth starting at the iris sphincter and growing toward the angle	Retinal consultation, as this is indicative of severe ocular hypoxia. Possible development of neovascular glaucoma

△ Make sure that there are no nonretinal signs of diabetes
△ Carefully evaluate for glaucoma and corneal problems
△ Evaluate blood pressure
△ In office, evaluate status of random blood glucose—should be under 200 mg%
△ Definitely order a glycated hemoglobin level if not performed within 3 months on a type 1 or 6 months on a type 2 diabetic patient
△ Verify that the patient has shown up for the retinal consultation
△ Communicate your findings to the primary care physician to assure quality comanagement
△ Schedule follow-up visits according to retinal status and other contributing factors

regress to the point where no treatment is necessary (15 percent). **See color plates 32, 33, and 49.**

The Diabetic Retinopathy Study Group established the standard of care in the case of NVD and NVE, demonstrating that the risk of severe vision loss—visual acuity at less than 5/200 at two consecutive 4-month follow-up visits—was much greater without photocoagulation than with it.

Although many theories exist about the most effective method of application of panretinal photocoagulation (PRP) and when to photocoagulate, the statistics support the efficacy of photocoagulation in PDR. Photocoagulation actually destroys retina, eliminating the need for oxygen and short-circuiting the vasoproliferative stimulus. Elimination of hypoxia results in regression of new vessel growth. Remember, however, that the fibrotic scaffolding remains. Management of NVD or NVE is fluorescein angiography to assess the potential for photocoagulative intervention. There are complications to PRP or panretinal ablation. The common complications are listed in Table 4–48. A skilled retinal specialist is the consultant of choice to minimize complication rates.

Fibrotic proliferation is the response of retinal glial cells to provide a support scaffold for new vessel growth. The presence of the vitreous is necessary to support this scaffolding. Elimination of the vitreous by vitrectomy effectively prevents future scaffolding for neovascularization. Vitrectomy also cuts and eliminates existing scaffolding. The attachment of the scaffolding between the retina and vitreous face is the point of genesis of a traction retinal detachment when vitreous degeneration occurs. Again, vitrectomy may be used to cut the abnormal adhesions and allow the relief of retinal traction. Fibrotic scaffolding does not directly alter vision, but its presence opens the potential of traction retinal detachment even resulting in retinal tears and rhegmatogenous retinal detachment. The fibrotic scaffolding will remain even with regression of neovascularization. Fibrotic scaffolding re-

sulting in areas of potential retinal traction should be seen by a retinologist to determine if vitrectomy would be of benefit.

Hemorrhage into the vitreous may result in a broad range of reduced acuities. If the hemorrhage is only partial, it may be possible to ascertain the site of the bleeding and intervene with photocoagulation. Should intravitreal blood totally block the view of the retina, the retinologist has the option of waiting to allow blood to clear (6 to 12 months) before performing photocoagulation or vitrectomy, or clearing some of the hemorrhage by pars plana vitrectomy and then performing endophotocoagulation. With further clearing of blood, addition of photocoagulation or vitrectomy may be necessary. Recent studies (Diabetic Retinopathy Vitrectomy Study Group, 1985a, 1985b, 1988), however, indicate that early intervention with vitrectomy actually improves the long-term prognosis. Vitrectomy is not without risk; Table 4–49 lists some of the complications.

Benefits of Photocoagulation and Vitrectomy in Diabetic Retinopathy

Although the general rules put forth have revolved around the suggestion that photocoagulation and vitrectomy will be of benefit in the treatment of diabetic retinopathy, does evidence exist to support the recommendations? Several well-designed and well-controlled studies have been published to support the benefits of intervention. The Diabetic Retinopathy Study Research Group found that panretinal photocoagulation reduced the risk of severe visual loss in diabetic retinopathy by at least 50 percent (Fig. 4–97). The beneficial effects of the photocoagulation were sustained for a minimum of 6 years of follow-up. Sullivan also reported in 1990 that 69 percent of all patients and 82 percent of patients followed for 10 years maintained good vision in the better eye after photocoagulation for the treatment of PDR. The DRS group also found that argon laser was preferred over

---

TABLE 4–48. COMMON COMPLICATIONS ASSOCIATED WITH PANRETINAL PHOTOCOAGULATION

Constriction of visual fields
Mild acuity reduction
Transient cystoid macular edema
Mobility problems, especially at night
Cornea and lens burns
Choroidal neovascularization in scars
Retinal/choroidal detachments
Flattened anterior chamber-angle closure
Transient retinal hemorrhage
Altered pupillary response (parasympathetics)
Decreased accommodative response (parasympathetics)
Pain

TABLE 4–49. POTENTIAL COMPLICATIONS ASSOCIATED WITH VITRECTOMY

Corneal folds
Corneal edema
Iris damage with hemorrhage
Neovascularization of the Iris
Cataract formation
Intraocular hemorrhage
Retinal breaks
Retinal detachment
Fibrinoid syndrome (cornea decomposition + vitreous strands → retinal detachment)
Endophthalmitis

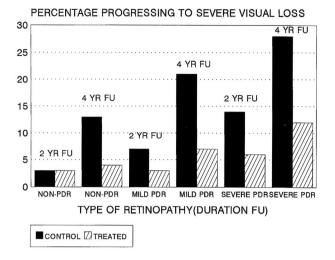

Figure 4–97. Results of the intervention applied to diabetic retinopathy in the Diabetic Retinopathy Studies, pointing to the efficacy of laser treatment in the prevention of progression to severe vision loss. Non-PDR, non-progressive diabetic retinopathy; PDR, progressive diabetic retinopathy; FU, follow up.

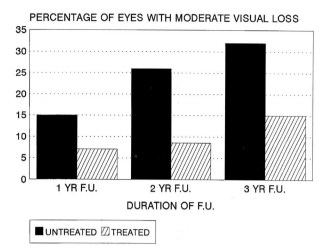

Figure 4–99. Results of focal laser treatment applied to diabetic macular edema with the center of the macula involved in the Early Treatment Diabetic Retinopathy Studies. FU, follow up.

xenon because more harmful side effects occurred with the xenon group. It has also been reported that PRP is often effective in causing a regression of rubeosis iridis associated with diabetes and diabetic retinopathy.

There have also been reports of the benefits of cryotherapy application for diabetic proliferative retinopathy and rubeosis iridis. No prospective, randomized controlled studies exist to support widespread use of this technique.

The Early Treatment Diabetic Retinopathy Study (ETDRS) carried the work of the DRS group a few steps further, finding that panretinal photocoagulation was indicated for eyes only with DRS high risk

characteristics, as a number of the eyes assigned to the study never even progressed to high risk. The ETDRS also found that aspirin treatment was of no benefit in altering the progression of diabetic retinopathy. The ETDRS also addressed the benefits of treating clinically significant macular edema, defined as (1) retinal thickening at or within 500 µm of the macula center (fovea); (2) hard exudates at or within 500 µm of the macula center if associated with thickening of the adjacent retina; or (3) retinal thickening at least 1 disc area in extent, any part of which is within 1 disc diameter of the macula center. The results, summarized in Figures 4–98 to 4–100, indicate the benefits of photocoagulative treatment intervention in macular

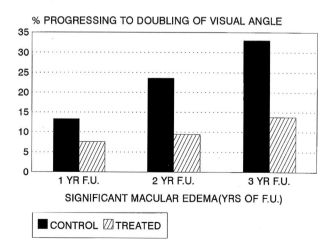

Figure 4–98. Results of the intervention applied to diabetic macular edema with the center of the macula uninvolved in the Early Treatment Diabetic Retinopathy Studies, pointing to the efficacy of laser treatment in minimizing vision loss. FU, follow up.

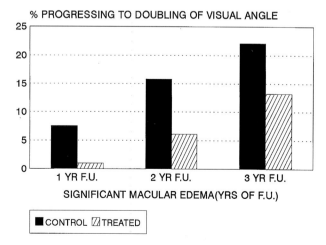

Figure 4–100. Results of the intervention applied to diabetic macular edema with the center of the macula involved in the Early Treatment Diabetic Retinopathy Studies pointing to the efficacy of laser treatment in minimizing vision loss. FU, follow up.

TABLE 4–50. INDICATIONS FOR PHOTOCOAGULATION OF DIABETIC MACULAR EDEMA

Focal retinal thickening including all leaking lesions 500 to 3000 μm from macula center creating macular edema should be treated by focal photocoagulation

Diffuse retinal thickening including all areas 500 to 3000 μm from macula center creating macular edema should be treated with grid photocoagulation

Retinal avascular zones (capillary dropout) including all areas 500 to 3000 μm from macula center associated with macular edema should be treated with grid photocoagulation

edema. The indications for treatment as determined by ETDRS are presented in Table 4–50. All patients should be seen 2 to 4 months following photocoagulative treatment for diabetic macular edema.

The Diabetic Retinopathy Vitrectomy Study Research Group (DRVS) found certain benefits to vitrectomy. Early vitrectomy for vitreous hemorrhage of at least 1 month duration is indicated for bilateral vitreous hemorrhage causing severe bilateral visual loss, unilateral vitreous hemorrhage causing severe visual loss with poor vision in the fellow eye, and in vitreous hemorrhage in type 1 (IDDM) diabetes causing vision to be reduced to less than 20/800. Other indications for vitrectomy include nonclearing of hemorrhage after 3 to 6 months, recent macular traction, combined traction and retinal detachment, and eyes with active proliferative retinopathy with extensive new vessels. Figures 4–101 and 4–102 summarize the positive results of early vitrectomy.

PERCENTAGE WITH V.A. BETTER THAN 20/40

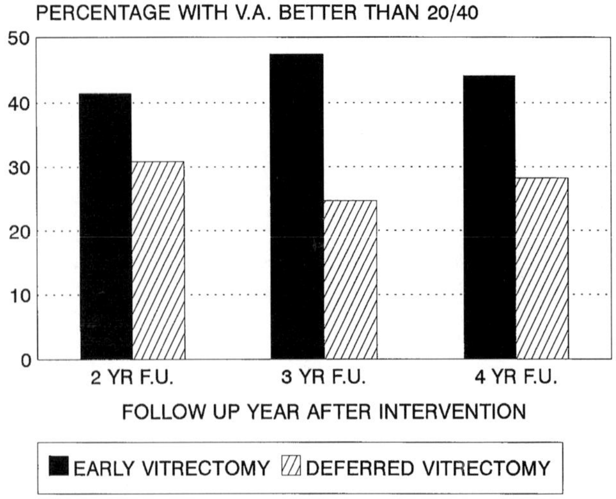

Figure 4–102. Results of early vitrectomy with severe proliferative diabetic retinopathy as reported in the Diabetic Retinopathy Vitrectomy Studies. VA, visual acuity; FU, follow up.

RADIATION RETINOPATHY

Introduction and Description. Radiation therapy is becoming much more common in today's society as we are experiencing significant improvement in morbidity and mortality associated with intervention in cancer treatment. With therapy, however, side effects can and do occur. The more common effects, such as overall ill feeling, hair loss, dietary modifications, and reductions in saliva output, are well known. In addition, keratoconjunctivitis sicca, cataract formation, and radiation retinopathy are possible sequelae to treatment in spite of precautions.

Radiation retinopathy typically presents 3 months to 3 years after x-ray radiation affecting the orbital region. A total dose of 30 to 35 Gy is usually needed to precipitate the retinal changes. The cause is the actual direct damage to the vascular endothelial layer of the ocular structures often precipitating ocular ischemia. The ocular signs simulate diabetic retinopathy and include microaneurysms, telangiectatic vessels, retinal hemorrhages, exudates, cotton-wool spots, macular edema, optic disc edema, capillary nonperfusion, and retinal pigment epithelial destruction. The long term may bring retinal neovascularization, vitreous hemorrhage, rubeosis iridis, and traction retinal detachment. The risk of worsened retinal changes is enhanced with systemic diseases such as hypertension, diabetes, and systemic chemotherapy.

Management. Management of the ocular signs of radiation parallel the management protocol for the ocular signs of diabetic retinopathy. Panretinal photocoagulation is effective in the management of ocular

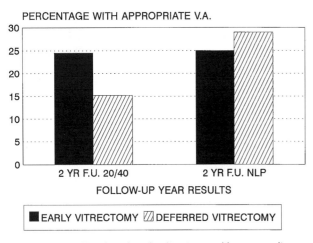

PERCENTAGE WITH APPROPRIATE V.A.

Figure 4–101. Results of early vitrectomy with severe vitreous hemorrhage as reported in the Diabetic Retinopathy Vitrectomy Studies. FU, follow up; NLP, no light perception.

Radiation Retinopathy

Characteristics

Δ Usually occurs 3 months to 3 years after x-ray irradiation near the orbital region (30 to 35 Gy total)

Δ Ocular signs
Microaneurysms and telangiectatic vessels
Hemorrhages, cotton-wool spots, exudates
Capillary nonperfusion and macular edema
Optic disc edema
RPE changes
Retinal neovascularization with vitreous hemorrhages and traction detachment
Iris neovascularization and neovascular glaucoma

Management

Δ Apply the rules for photocoagulation of diabetic retinopathy to the treatment of radiation retinopathy

Δ Follow patients with a history of irradiation near the orbital area every 6 months for 3 years, or more often if there are systemic risk factors

Eales' Disease

Characteristics

Δ Healthy men in their 20s and 30s

Δ If unilateral, most often affects left eye

Δ Bilateral idiopathic presentation

Δ Perivasculitis with occasional anterior uveitis

Δ Vitritis possible

Δ Peripheral neovascularization secondary to areas of nonperfusion

Δ Occasional vitreous hemorrhage may be the presenting sign; it then becomes a diagnosis by exclusion

Management

Δ Rule out tuberculosis with tuberculin test and chest x-ray

Δ Fluorescein angiography if neovascularization suspected

Δ Retinal consultation should be considered if any neovascularization and/or posterior pole telangiectasia coupled with macular edema

Δ Photocoagulation in areas of capillary nonperfusion may benefit peripheral neovascularization

Δ Photocoagulation in areas of telangiectasia may benefit macular edema

---

neovascularization. Photocoagulation application in macular edema is also beneficial in minimizing the risk for vision loss.

Patients with a history of irradiation near the orbit should be followed postirradiation for 3 years every 6 months, or more often if there are associated systemic risk factors such as chemotherapy, diabetes, and hypertension.

EALES' DISEASE (RETINAL PERIPHLEBITIS)

Introduction and Description. The classic form of Eales' disease occurs in otherwise healthy young men in their 20s and 30s. The condition appears as an idiopathic bilateral perivasculitis most often affecting the veins. If unilateral, the left eye is involved most often. There may be an associated anterior uveitis. The cause is obscure, most often being attributed to a nonspecific inflammatory reaction to antigens. There is often a positive association with tuberculoprotein hypersensitivity, with a number of patients having a positive PPD. About 25 percent of patients also have vestibuloauditory problems.

The signs and symptoms vary depending on the severity of the disease. Early in the disease, acuity is usually unaffected, with complaints associated with floaters. In the periphery, there is perivascular sheathing and peripheral retinal capillary nonperfusion that extends into the posterior pole with evolution of the disease. The ensuing peripheral neovascularization may create associated hemorrhages that emanate into the vitreous. Vitritis naturally occurs overlying the inflammatory locus. Retinal capillary telangiectatic formations may occur, creating associated macular edema. Vision eventually may be compromised secondary to vitreous blood, retinal traction, or macular edema. The venous stasis may spread to the posterior pole, resulting in considerable manifestations of retinal edema.

Management. The patient presumed to have Eales' disease should have a complete medical evaluation, including a tuberculin test and chest x-ray, to rule out tuberculosis. The vitreous hemorrhage may be allowed to clear on its own, or vitrectomy may be used. Areas of leakage and neovascularization in the retina should be assessed by fluorescein angiography (Fig. 4–103). Should there be active leakage or neovascularization, photocoagulation to areas of capillary nonperfusion may be attempted. Photocoagulation of paracentral telangiectatic formations may be of benefit in reducing macular edema. Intervention as early as possible will improve the chances of retention of retinal function. A patient suspected of having Eales' disease must have fluorescein angiography to determine if a retinal consultation is necessary.

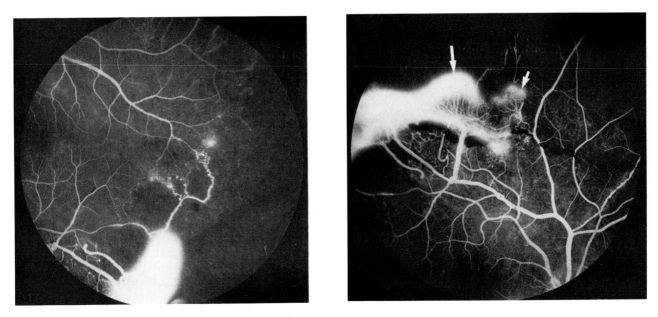

Figure 4–103. Fluorescein angiograms demonstrating neovascularization in a case of Eales' disease.

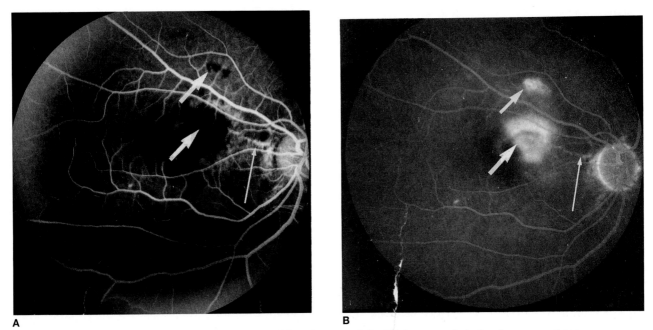

A

B

Figure 4–104. Early-stage (**A**) and late-stage (**B**) angiograms of choroidal neovascularization (*large arrows*) secondary to angioid streaks (*small arrows*) in a case of sickle-cell disease.

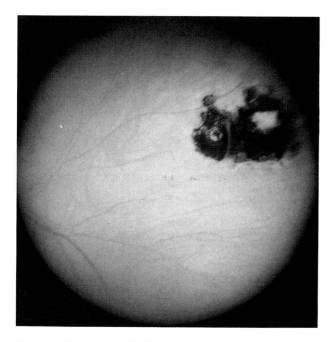

Figure 4–105. A sunburst lesion in the retinal periphery associated with sickle-cell anemic retinopathy.

SICKLE-CELL RETINOPATHY

Introduction and Description. Sickle-cell retinopathy is the result of compromise of normal retinal circulation by abnormal hemoglobin. The result is retinal hypoxia, which then stimulates abnormal vascular growth. The majority of activity occurs preequatorial, with a predilection for the temporal retina. At this location there is inherent vascular narrowing, lending to closure by sickled red blood cells combined with inherently reduced oxygenation in the periphery.

The normal population has only hemoglobin A, whereas sickle-cell patients have an abnormal hemoglobin because of an inherited substitution of amino acid valine for glutamic acid (hemoglobin S) or lysine for glutamic acid (hemoglobin C) in the beta chain. Sickle-cell beta-thalassemia contains a mixture of hemoglobin S, hemoglobin A, hemoglobin A_2, and hemoglobin F. Approximately 10 percent of American blacks have a variety of hemoglobinopathy. About 80 percent of those have the trait (SA), 10 percent have sickle thalassemia (S-thal), 4 percent have sickle cell anemia (SS), and 1 to 2 percent have SC hemoglobinopathy. The SC and S-thal patients have higher hematocrit levels, leading to increased viscosity. This increased viscosity, combined with sickling and hypoxia, creates a higher incidence of proliferative retinopathy than the other hemoglobinopathies. Sick-

led hemoglobin has the potential to have a lower oxygen-carrying ability as well as developing unusual shapes that block vessels. This blockage usually occurs near the arteriole–capillary zone.

Ocular manifestations of sickling hemoglobinopathies have a standard classification system as shown in Table 4–51. The nonproliferative signs of

Pearls

Sickle-Cell Retinopathy

Characteristics

Δ Result of alteration of retinal circulation by sickled hemoglobin coupled with hypoxia in the peripheral retina

Δ Nonproliferative signs
　Salmon patch intraretinal hemorrhages
　Refractile spots representing hemosiderin from old hemorrhages
　Black sunburst lesions, the result of RPE hyperplasia in the zone of old hemorrhages
　Venous tortuosity
　Angioid streaks—watch for choroidal neovascular membranes!

Δ Proliferative signs
　A/V anastomoses at the junction of the vascular postequatorial retina and the avascular preequatorial retina
　Sea fan retinal neovascularization
　Fibrotic scaffolding
　Vitreous hemorrhage
　Traction retinal detachment

Management

Δ Diagnose a nondiagnosed sickle-cell patient with hemoglobin electrophoresis—include good medical and family history

Δ Obtain a medical consultation for potential systemic problems

Δ Routine evaluation of the nonproliferative retinal changes

Δ Retinal consultation for proliferative signs

Δ Careful routine follow-up and communication with primary physician

TABLE 4–51. CLASSIFICATION SYSTEM FOR SICKLING HEMOGLOBINOPATHIES

Stage	Characteristics
I	Peripheral retinal arteriolar occlusions
II	Peripheral retinal arteriolar–venule anastomoses
III	Neovascularization and fibrotic proliferation
IV	Vitreous hemorrhage
V	Retinal detachment

From Goldberg MF. Classification and pathogenesis of proliferative sickle retinopathy. *Am J Ophthalmol.* 1971;71:649–665.

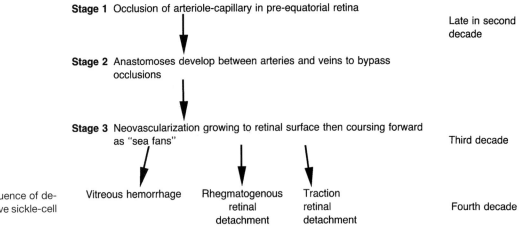

Stage 1 Occlusion of arteriole-capillary in pre-equatorial retina

Late in second
decade

Stage 2 Anastomoses develop between arteries and veins to bypass
occlusions

Stage 3 Neovascularization growing to retinal surface then coursing forward
as "sea fans"

Third decade

Vitreous hemorrhage   Rhegmatogenous   Traction
                          retinal   retinal
                          detachment   detachment

Fourth decade

Figure 4–106. The sequence of development of proliferative sickle-cell retinopathy.

sickling retinopathy are the result of necrosis of the vessel wall, and include (1) salmon patches, which are fresh intraretinal hemorrhages, (2) refractile spots, which are deposits from old resorbed hemorrhage below the internal limiting membrane, (3) black sunburst lesions, which are hemosiderin (from resorbed hemorrhage) deposits associated with retinal pigment epithelial hyperplasia (see figure 4–105), (4) venous tortuosity, and (5) angioid streaks with their potential sequelae (see figure 4–104). With the exception of the complication of choroidal neovascularization associated with angioid streaks, the nonproliferative changes serve only as signs of ocular involvement. Dark without pressure in the posterior pole is at times associated with sickle-cell retinopathy, and should prompt careful patient questioning with the performance of a Sickledex test.

The proliferative retinopathy is the result of arteriolar occlusion that results in arteriolar–venule anastamoses at the junction of the nonvascularized pre-equatorial retina and the vascularized postequatorial retina. The most susceptible zone of the retina is the temporal periphery, because it is most distal from the oxygenated blood source. Neovascularization forms as the result of the hypoxia in the area and is often described as a sea fan. The ensuing fibrotic scaffolding may then contract, creating retinal breaks, vitreous hemorrhage, and traction retinal detachment. Often the neovascularization will spontaneously regress, leaving a characteristic whitish tuft. Figure 4–106 illustrates the sequence of development of proliferative retinopathy.

Management. The undiagnosed patient presenting with sickling hemoglobinopathy must have a Sickledex test plus hemoglobin electrophoresis (patients with hemoglobin C and with the sickle-cell trait may have a negative Sickledex test). The patient should also have a consultation to ascertain the systemic status.

Other than the possible complication of the choroidal neovascular net in angioid streaks, the nonproliferative signs of sickling hemoglobinopathies have no indication for treatment. The proliferative changes, including sight-threatening retinal neovascularization and vitreous hemorrhage, may benefit from photocoagulation and/or vitrectomy. Both sector scatter and circumferential scatter demonstrate regression, while the feeder vessel technique has demonstrated equivocal results. Cryotherapy appears to have a high complication rate and it is recommended only when opacities prevent accurate visualization. Unfortunately, no significant studies substantiate the benefit of photocoagulation. Nevertheless, the proliferative sickle-cell hemoglobinopathies necessitate a retinal consultation if active and threatening vision.

The complication of vitreous hemorrhage is often allowed to clear on its own. Should a retinal tear occur, it is usually at the base of the lesion, and often creates a rhegmatogenous retinal detachment. Surgical intervention, often with scleral buckling, is necessary. The risk of anterior segment necrosis secondary to buckling is very high (70 percent) in patients with sickle-cell retinopathy as compared to under 5 percent in non-sickle-cell patients. A skilled surgeon is of utmost importance for these patients.

Patients with nonproliferative and proliferative sickling retinopathies should be scheduled for routine follow-up based on the severity of their presentation.

RETINOPATHY OF PREMATURITY (RETROLENTAL FIBROPLASIA)

Introduction and Description. Retinopathy of prematurity (ROP) has once again surfaced as a severe problem as the result of improved technology in neonatology. The incidence of ROP has actually in-

TABLE 4–52. ZONES OF RETINA USED IN CLASSIFICATION OF RETINOPATHY OF PREMATURITY

Zone	Characteristics
1	Innermost zone with radius defined as twice distance from disc to fovea
2	Surrounding zone 1 with radius defined as distance from zone 1 to nasal ora serrata
3	Remaining temporal crescent from zone 2 to ora serrata

creased to the epidemic rates that were registered in the 1943 to 1953 era. ROP is associated with prematurity (under 36 weeks gestation), low birthweight (under 4 lbs 6 oz, but worsening with lower weight), xanthine administration, maternal bleeding, the bright lights of the neonatal units, and supplemental oxygen therapy. As discussed previously, retinal vascularization to the oral region is just barely complete at full gestation in the human. The last area of the retina to be vascularized is the temporal periphery. If birth occurs before full gestation, this peripheral retinal region is susceptible to altered vasculopathy because of incomplete maturation. Retinopathy of prematurity has three distinctive stages: (1) vaso-obliterative, (2) proliferative, and (3) cicatricial.

The classification system for ROP involves zones of the retina, the extent of involvement, and the severity. The zones are listed in Table 4–52. The extent of the disease involvement is described in clock hours. The stages of the disease are outlined in Table 4–53.

The vaso-obliterative phase is related to the rise in available oxygen when the premature infant is placed in oxygen-rich incubation. The excessive oxygen stunts the normal maturation of vessels (vaso-obliteration). Once the infant is returned to room air, there is a sudden deficiency in oxygen, creating a demand that cannot be met by the infant's existing vessels. Vaso-

proliferation then ensues to satisfy the demand. As one would expect, this activity occurs most frequently in the temporal periphery, appearing first as endothelial nodules in the inner retina, followed by proliferation of intraretinal capillaries. This neovascularization breaks through the internal limiting membrane to proliferate on the retinal surface, and may then spread into the vitreous in the form of hemorrhage, fibrotic proliferation, and retinal traction. Traction can cause retinal detachment as well as mild forms of retinal dragging that may result in heterotopic macula. The extent of proliferation is determined by several factors, including the elapsed time of the oxygen therapy. Spontaneous recovery from vasoproliferative ROP occurs in a very high percentage of patients, resulting in mild temporal periphery changes that are typically static.

The cicatricial phase is considered the regressive phase and is identified by pigment irregularities, vit-

TABLE 4–53. STAGES OF SEVERITY OF RETINOPATHY OF PREMATURITY

Stage	Characteristics
1	Development of distinct demarcation line between avascular and vascular retina
2	Demarcation line becomes more distinct and forms elevated ridge
3	Fibrovascular proliferation develops and extends posterior to ridge in vitreous
4	Partial retinal detachments develop that a. Involve fovea b. Do not involve fovea
5	Total retinal detachment
Plus disease	Engorgement of veins and tortuous arteries in posterior pole are poor prognostic sign

Pearls

Retinopathy of Prematurity

Characteristics

Δ Risk factors
  Prematurity under 36 weeks gestation
  Low birthweight—under 4 lbs 6 oz
  Xanthine administration
  Maternal bleeding
  Supplemental oxygen therapy
Δ Classified by
  Zone of involvement (1 to 3)
  Clock hours of involvement
  Stages of severity
Δ Vaso-obliterative stage due to high oxygen
Δ Vasoproliferative stage secondary to return to room air, manifesting as neovascularization, fibrotic scaffolding, hemorrhage, and retinal detachment
Δ Cicatricial stage characterized by dragged retina, retinal folds, pale optic nerve, and retrolental mass

Management

Δ Attempts at prevention
Δ Examination of suspect neonates and follow-up according to risk factors
  Initial examination for all at risk
  Frequent follow-up for all under 2 lbs 12 oz
  Repeat examination at 12 to 14 weeks for others
Δ Retinology consultation at first signs of vasoproliferation or complications
Δ Possible prophylactic cryotherapy according to Cryotherapy for Retinopathy of Prematurity Cooperative Group guidelines
Δ Watch for development of glaucoma

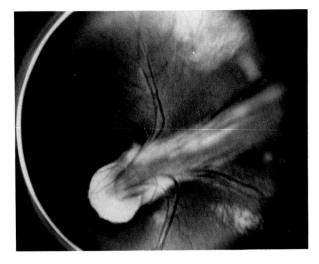

Figure 4–107. The dragged disc characteristic of severe stages of retinopathy of prematurity.

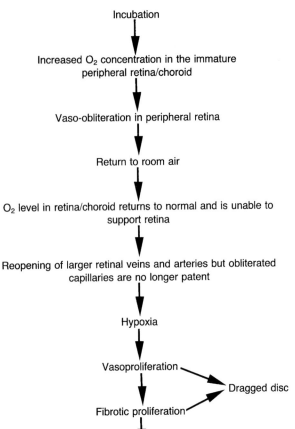

Incubation

↓

Increased O₂ concentration in the immature peripheral retina/choroid

↓

Vaso-obliteration in peripheral retina

↓

Return to room air

↓

O₂ level in retina/choroid returns to normal and is unable to support retina

↓

Reopening of larger retinal veins and arteries but obliterated capillaries are no longer patent

↓

Hypoxia

↓

Vasoproliferation

↓

Fibrotic proliferation → Dragged disc

↓

Cicatricial stage

Figure 4–108. Flowchart demonstrating the development of retinopathy of prematurity.

reoretinal membranes, pale optic nerve head with temporally dragged vessels, retinal folds, and a retrolental mass in the pupillary area (Fig. 4–107). The development of ROP is summarized in Figure 4–108. Most of the time, the retinal vasculopathy is bilateral, but the author has observed unilateral cases.

Management. The importance of recognition and management of ROP is apparent when considering the severe visually debilitating results of progression. Recognition and diagnostic difficulties are compounded by the difficulty of examining the peripheral retina of the infant. Maximal dilation (0.5 percent cyclopentolate + 0.5 percent tropicamide + 2.5 percent phenylephrine), in addition to mild anesthesia, is preferable for complete examination. For all patients under 2 lbs 12 oz, a complete examination should be performed every 2 weeks until age 14 weeks, followed every 1 to 2 months at first and later about every 6 to 12 months. For other patients at risk, if there are no initial signs of ROP, a repeat examination should be performed at week 12 to 14, but risk for development after this is minimal. Should an active phase—a vasoproliferative component—be diagnosed, a retinal consultation is indicated for possible photocoagulative or cryopexy intervention. Photocoagulation has proven to be of some benefit in the management of some of the neovascular components of ROP. Vitrectomy in skilled hands may also be beneficial. Should the patient have cicatricial components of ROP and such potential complications as retinoschisis and retinal detachment, the individual complications must be managed by proper surgical protocol. It is also important to watch for other complications such as glaucoma.

The best method of management of retinopathy of prematurity is prevention. Although strides constantly are being made in monitoring of blood gases and improved neonatologic techniques, some cases are unavoidable. Recent work has indicated that prophylactic cryopexy of low-birthweight infants may delay or eliminate the development of ROP. The Cryotherapy for Retinopathy of Prematurity Cooperative Group recommends that cryotherapy should be given to one eye of a patient with stage 3+ ROP in zone 1 or 2 involving at least 5 contiguous clock hours or at least 8 cumulative clock hours. The group added that cryotherapy should be considered for both eyes whenever stage 3+ involves zone 1 of both eyes. The increased success in neonatology also results in more potential candidates for ROP. Research in this area is aggressive, but recent setbacks indicate that retinopathy of prematurity is a difficult problem in eye care.

BEHÇET'S DISEASE

Introduction and Description. Behçet's disease is a systemic occlusive vasculitis thought to be an immune complex disease. It is characterized by recurrent iridocyclitis, mucous membrane ulcers of the mouth and genitals, and central nervous system and joint disorders (acute polyarthritis). Behçet's disease affects young (18 to 40 years) adults (male/female 2:1) and is more common in Japan (20 to 30 percent of iridocyclitis) and the Mediterranean area. The systemic findings include genital ulcers, oral ulcers, cutaneous manifestations such as erythema nodosum and subcutaneous thrombophlebitis, epididymitis, and gastrointestinal lesions. Ocular findings include anterior and posterior uveitis with sterile hypopyon as the most prevalent ocular feature, but vaso-occlusive manifestations may occur as peripheral retinal vasculitis (26 percent of patients) in the form of hemorrhages and infarction. Late-stage complications include rubeosis iridis, retinal neovascularization, glaucoma, cataract, retinal detachment, and optic atrophy.

In the retina, the small peripheral veins are affected most often. With this, there is retinal edema, exudates deep in the retina, sheathing, and large vessel occlusion. This is a necrotizing vasculitis, and as such is irreversible. The ophthalmoscopic view is often hampered by the almost omnipresent cells of the accompanying uveitis.

Management. Management includes topical and periocular steroids to control the anterior and posterior uveitis. Recalcitrant signs and symptoms may be alleviated in consultation with a collagen vascular specialist with trials of systemic steroids and immunosuppressive agents such as those being used in collagen vascular disorders. There has been little information in the literature regarding the success of photocoagulation in the effective treatment of retinal neovascularization associated with the disorder, but the appearance necessitates a retinal consultation. Vision-threatening occlusive vasculitis also requires a retinal consultation.

Follow-up of the ocular condition depends on the retinal status, but should be performed at least every 6 months. The disorder is systemic and must be managed in concert with other health care providers.

Pearls

Behçet's Disease

Characteristics

△ Systemic occlusive vasculitis thought to be an immune complex disorder

△ Affects young adults (18 to 40), most often in Japan and Mediterranean area

△ Systemic characteristics
  Genital ulcers
  Oral ulcers
  Cutaneous manifestations
  Epididymitis
  Central nervous system involvement
  Gastrointestinal lesions

△ Ocular characteristics
  Recurrent anterior and posterior uveitis
  Sterile hypopyon
  Necrotizing retinal vasculitis (peripheral)
  Late-stage sequelae including rubeosis iridis, glaucoma, retinal neovascularization, cataract, retinal detachment, optic atrophy

Management

△ Topical and periocular steroids for uveitis

△ Possible systemic steroids and/or immunosuppressive agents

△ Retinal consultation for
  Ocular photocoagulation for neovascular developments
  Necrotizing vasculitis

△ Systemic consultation for associated disorders with collagen vascular specialist

△ Follow-up dictated by extent of ocular involvement, but in 6 months at a minimum

---

ACUTE RETINAL NECROSIS SYNDROME

Introduction and Description. Acute retinal necrosis syndrome (ARNS) is a severe occlusive vasculitis that primarily involves the arteries of the retina and choroid, preferentially affecting the peripheral retina. In the majority of untreated cases, the result is a delayed occurrence of rhegmatogenous retinal detachment. The strongest evidence implicates herpes-family viruses as the precipitating factor in the process. ARNS typically affects patients between 20 and 60 years of age, with peaks at ages 20 and 50 years. Herpes simplex virus (HSV) infections usually become manifest in the younger patients, whereas varicella zoster virus (VZV) infections are more closely related to the appearance of ARNS in the older population. There appears to be no racial predilection, but males are affected slightly more often than females. There is bilateral involvement in 33 percent of patients, but often there is a delay of several weeks before involvement of the second eye. There is thought to be an immunogenetic predisposition to the development of ARNS based on HLA-DQw7 antigen findings.

Clinical symptoms at the presentation of ARNS include mild to moderate ocular or periorbital pain, foreign body sensation, and a red eye. Pain on motion may occur because of concurrent optic neuritis and myositis. Severe pain often typical of acute anterior uveitis is rare. Visual complaints vary but include hazy vision, floaters, and the perception of side vision problems. Central vision loss may occur late associated with optic neuritis or retinal detachment.

Clinical signs include mild to moderate conjunctival injection, episcleritis, chemosis, lid edema, subconjunctival hemorrhage, and mild proptosis. Should the patient be immunocompromised, other viral infective signs may be present. Mild to moderate anterior granulomatous uveitis is typical with the possibility of hypopyon. A paradox in this disease is the fact that the intraocular pressure is often elevated in the ARNS form of anterior uveitis. The classic triad of signs in the posterior segment include retinal and choroidal vasculitis, retinal necrosis, and vitritis. The retinal vasculitis primarily affects the arteries, manifesting as narrowing and sheathing of the larger vessels. Venous inflammation (phlebitis) is unusual. Small retinal hemorrhages may occur following the course of the vascular involvement.

The retinal necrosis appears as confluent areas of retinal whitening that may present as small or larger zones and obscure underlying choroidal detail. The necrosis usually develops concurrent with or soon after the vasculitis. The area between the necrosis and normal retina is well circumscribed and may develop as pseudopods. The peripheral retina is usually involved first, with a spread toward the posterior pole in a geographic pattern.

Vitreous cells are a consistent feature of ARNS and their absence suggests another disease. In chronic ARNS the vitreous actually may opacify, with severe vitreous fibrosis and traction as a late complication.

Pearls

Acute Retinal Necrosis Syndrome (ARNS)

Characteristics

Δ Acute occlusive vasculitis involving arteries of the retina and choroid, initially involving the peripheral areas

Δ Herpes-family viruses implicated, with age ranges of 20 to 60 years and the thought of immunogenetic predisposition
  HSV in younger patients
  VSV in older patients

Δ Bilateral involvement in 33 percent, but may delay several weeks

Δ Symptoms include mild to moderate ocular pain, foreign body sensation, red eye, pain on movement, hazy vision, floaters, peripheral vision problems, late central loss

Δ Signs include
  Anterior
    Mild to moderate conjunctival injection, episcleritis, chemosis and lid edema, subconjunctival hemorrhage, possible mild proptosis, anterior granulomatous uveitis, elevated intraocular pressure
  Posterior
    Retinal and choroidal vasculitis, retinal necrosis, vitritis, optic neuritis, exudative retinal detachment, neovascularization, vitreous hemorrhage, macular edema, vitreous traction, vitreous opacification, retinal tears at junction of normal and abnormal retina, rhegmatogenous retinal detachment

Δ Retinal process is self-limiting in 6 to 12 weeks

Management

Δ Retinal consultation

Δ Diagnostic vitrectomy if signs and symptoms are equivocal

Δ Diagnostic tests if using acyclovir
  Complete blood count
  Creatinine
  Blood urea nitrogen
  Liver function tests

Δ Diagnostic tests if using systemic corticosteroids
  Tuberculin test
  Chest x-ray

Δ Other possible diagnostic tests
  HIV titer
  Acute and Convalescent titers to HSV1, HSV2, VZV, CMV
  RPR
  FTA-ABS
  Angiotensin-converting enzyme
  Gallium scan
  Toxo titers
  Lumbar puncture
  CT or MRI

Δ Fluorescein angiography demonstrates early blockage of choroidal fluorescence and characteristic "cut off" of vascular flow

Δ Treat with
  Intravenous acyclovir 1500 mg/m^2 per day in three doses for 5 to 10 days followed by oral acyclovir 400 to 600 mg five times a day for 6 weeks
  Antithrombotic, aspirin 125 to 650 mg once or twice a day
  High dosage (60 to 80 mg per day) of corticosteroids, but this is of questionable efficacy
  Prophylactic photocoagulation posterior to areas of active retinitis
  Surgical reattachment of retina

Other posterior segment signs include optic neuritis, branch vaso-occlusive disease, exudative retinal detachment, retinal and disc neovascularization, vitreous hemorrhage, and macular edema.

The inflammatory process is self-limiting in 6 to 12 weeks, with affected retinal areas demonstrating atrophic retinal pigment epithelium in a scalloped pattern. Complications include the formation of full-thickness retinal holes appearing during the recovery stage of the process. They usually appear in the posterior pole at the junction of the normal and abnormal retina, are large, and are often multiple. The retinal tears accompanied by the vitreous traction lend to the development of both rhegmatogenous retinal detachment and proliferative vitreoretinopathy in up to 75 percent of ARNS patients. The stages of ARNS are summarized in Table 4–54. The long-term visual prognosis for ARNS is improving with intervention, with recent reports indicating that less than 33 percent of patients will lose vision to 20/200 or worse.

Associated systemic findings include herpes zoster skin lesions, cutaneous herpes simplex ulcers, acute varicella infections, aphthous ulcerations, low-grade fever, mild headache, sinus pain, or nuchal rigidity. There is also a reported association with viral encephalitis in immunosuppressed patients.

Management. The diagnosis of ARNS is made on the basis of history and associated physical findings. Diagnostic vitrectomy or endoretinal biopsy may produce positive viral cultures to confirm the diagnosis. Immunofluorescence studies of aqueous humor may also test for VZV and HSV antibody production, but the sensitivity and specificity have yet to be determined. Standard laboratory diagnostic tests will not confirm the diagnosis of ARNS, but are useful in determining systemic immunodeficiency and in monitoring medical therapy for possible complications. For those patients being placed on acyclovir, a complete blood count, creatinine, blood urea nitrogen, and liver function tests should be performed prior to initiation of therapy. If systemic corticosteroids are to be used, a tuberculin test and chest x-ray should be performed to rule out active tuberculosis. HIV titer testing is also imperative in any patient suspected of having ARNS. Although often nonproductive, the suggestion has been made that acute and convalescent titers to HSV1, HSV2, VZV, and CMV be performed. With suspicion of associated diseases, the practitioner may opt to order a rapid plasma reagin (RPR), fluorescent treponemal antibody absorption (FTA-ABS) test, angiotensin-converting enzyme (ACE), gallium scan, Toxo titers, and investigation of the CNS with lumbar puncture, CT, or MRI studies.

Fluorescein angiography demonstrates early blockage of underlying choroidal fluorescence in areas of active retinitis, with a "characteristic" cut-off of the artery and vein flow pattern. Minimal blood flow in the affected areas exists late in the fluorescein. B-scan ultrasonography has value in determining the presence of a retinal detachment when the vitreous is so compromised that a standard view is impossible.

Medical therapy is based on the assumption that the majority of ARNS is due to either HSV or VZV infections. Intravenous acyclovir has in vitro activity against HSV1, HSV2, and VZV without affecting normal cells. The recommended dosage is 1500 mg/meters^2 per day in three doses for 5 to 10 days. Treatment results in regression of the necrosis within 4 days, while progression usually occurs over the first 48 hours. The treatment results in improvement in the retinal and optic nerve signs. Following the intravenous treatment, oral acyclovir is given at 400 to 600 mg five times a day for 6 weeks, because of the fact that the second eye may be involved within 6 weeks of onset of the first eye. In immunosuppressed patients, acyclovir is less effective, necessitating the use of ganciclovir. Ganciclovir is, however, much more toxic than acyclovir. In addition to the antiviral, antithrombotic therapy in the form of aspirin 125 to 650 mg once or twice a day is indicated for the hyperactivity of the platelets in ARNS. High-dosage systemic corticosteroid therapy (60 to 80 mg per day for 1 week followed by tapering) may suppress the intraocular inflammation as well as improve clearing of the vitreous but has questionable efficacy because of the theoretical contraindication with IV and oral antiviral agents.

Surgical therapy of ARNS includes prophylactic confluent laser photocoagulation applied posterior to the areas of active retinitis. The photocoagulation appears to have a positive effect on the incidence of subsequent retinal detachment. Scleral buckling and pars plana vitrectomy also have a place in the management of patients with ARNS in spite of the fact that successful anatomic reattachment of the retina is difficult.

TABLE 4–54. CLINICAL STAGES OF ACUTE RETINAL NECROSIS SYNDROME

Category	Clinical Features
Stage 1	Necrotizing. Areas of peripheral retinitis leading to confluence, optic neuritis, and macular edema
Stage 2	Vitreous opacification and potential traction
Stage 3	Cessation of necrotic activity (6–12 weeks) with secondary atrophic changes in retina including full-thickness holes associated with further vitreous changes
Stage 4	Tears and traction leading to retinal detachment or development of proliferative vitreoretinopathy

FROSTED BRANCH ANGIITIS

Introduction and Description. Frosted branch angiitis (periphlebitis) is a condition classically described as a sudden bilateral loss of vision and thick sheathing of the retinal veins in an otherwise healthy patient. There are, however, cases reported of a unilateral presentation. The sheathing is more prevalent in the veins and presents as thick, confluent, and white. There may be optic disc edema and extensive intraretinal and preretinal hemorrhaging, with edema causing a serous macular detachment. The fluorescein angiograms demonstrate late leakage from the retinal veins without evidence of stasis or occlusion. The anterior chamber is usually unaffected, but there may be cells in the vitreous.

The cause of frosted branch angiitis is elusive, but there has been the suggestion that there is a relationship to the herpes virus family. There may even be a concurrent flu-like condition, but the condition is probably more related to an immune-mediated process. It should be noted that other periphlebitic conditions of the eye may be related to sarcoidosis, syphilis, tuberculosis, multiple sclerosis, HIV, and connective tissue disorders. All of these conditions must be considered when ruling in or ruling out frosted branch angiitis.

Management. A retinal consultation is indicated if there is the suspicion of frosted branch angiitis. If therapy is instituted quickly, the prognosis for the condition is reasonable. Because frosted branch angiitis is thought to be an immune-mediated condition, oral corticosteroid therapy is indicated and does create a resolution of the problem. A loading dose of prednisone at 80 mg/day is recommended, with tapering after resolution of the ophthalmoscopic picture. The resolution often takes 1 to 2 months. It is also important to consider the other causes of retinal periphlebitis and rule out those causes with appropriate laboratory diagnostic testing.

RETINAL VASCULAR TUMORS

Several different tumors arise from the vascular tissues of the retina and optic nerve, some of which may threaten vision. In addition to ocular signs, there may be associated lesions in other systems of the body, including the skin, central nervous system, and visceral tissues. When retinal vascular tumors are associated with remote changes in other systems, the complex is sometimes grouped under the term "phakomatoses" or "systemic hamartomatoses."

Cavernous Hemangioma of the Retina

Introduction and Description. Cavernous hemangioma of the retina is a relatively rare condition that occurs at an average age of 23 years. In the past, however, it was often misdiagnosed as one of the other retinal vascular tumors or abnormalities. The majority of the patients reported in the literature are white. Cavernous hemangioma usually is unilateral, with no preference for laterality. There is increasing evidence in the literature that cavernous hemangioma of the retina is inherited in an autosomal dominant pattern, with highly variable penetrance and expressivity.

Cavernous hemangioma of the retina appears ophthalmoscopically as dark red saccular clusters projecting from the inner retinal layers (Fig. 4–109). There is usually an associated overlying white epiretinal membrane. The saccular clusters rarely demonstrate change over time, but the epiretinal membrane may increase in size and density. Exudation and hemorrhage are extremely rare, which contrasts with Coats' disease (retinal telangiectasia) and capillary hemangioma of the retina. When a cavernous hemangioma occurs on the disc, the ophthalmoscopic appearance is similar.

The patient with a cavernous hemangioma is usually asymptomatic and has good visual acuity if the epiretinal membrane does not tug on the macula. The visual fields may show a scotoma corresponding to the site of the lesion if assessed at threshold. Vision may become compromised if a rare vitreous hemorrhage occurs. There may be an associated extraocular muscle palsy if the central nervous system is the peripheral site of a similar tumor.

Pearls

Frosted Branch Angiitis (Periphlebitis)

Characteristics

△ Sudden bilateral or unilateral loss of vision

△ Thick white venous sheathing, optic disc edema, possible intraretinal and preretinal hemorrhage, serous macular detachment, vitritis, and variable anterior chamber reaction

△ Cause is elusive but tied to herpesvirus family
  Must rule out other causes of phlebitis such as sarcoidosis, syphilis, tuberculosis, multiple sclerosis, HIV, and connective tissue disorders

Management

△ Retinal consultation

△ Rule out all causes of retinal phlebitis

△ Long-term high-dose (80 mg) oral corticosteroids

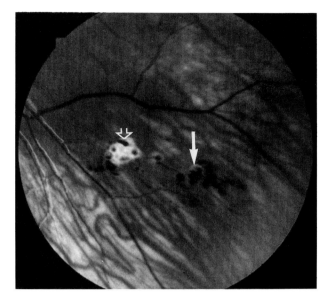

Figure 4–109. Black-and-white photograph of a retinal cavernous hemangioma. The solid arrow points to the saccular dilatations, and the open arrow points to a preretinal membrane.

The most important diagnostic test in all retinal vascular tumors is fluorescein angiography, which produces results that are very characteristic, if not pathognomonic, of cavernous hemangioma of the retina. The epiretinal membrane may produce a mild

autofluorescence. The prearterial (choroidal flush) phase of fluorescein angiography demonstrates hypofluorescence of the area of the lesion, whereas the surrounding retina is normal. The hypofluorescence remains throughout the arterial phase. During the later parts of the venous phase, fluorescein begins to slowly enter the clusters of the hemangioma. The fluorescein pools in the plasma in the superior portion of each vascular space, whereas the blood collects in the inferior portion of the ballooning of the vessel. This plasma–erythrocyte sedimentation pattern is pathognomonic of cavernous hemangioma. There is usually no leakage of dye into the surrounding tissue. The fluorescein angiography findings may be summarized as slowed venous drainage, no arteriovenous shunting, no leakage into or under surrounding retinal tissue, and the classic plasma–erythrocyte sedimentation.

Cavernous hemangiomas of the retina and optic nerve are composed of multiple isolated saccular dilatations of blood vessels that replace the normal tissue of the inner half of the retina and optic nerve head (Fig. 4–110). The saccular dilatations are lined with a continuous layer of nonfenestrated endothelial cells. Electron microscopic studies have shown normal anatomic features for retinal vessels within a cavernous hemangioma. Within the hemangioma, the vessels often abut one another with lumen connected by small orifices. The saccular dilatations are rela-

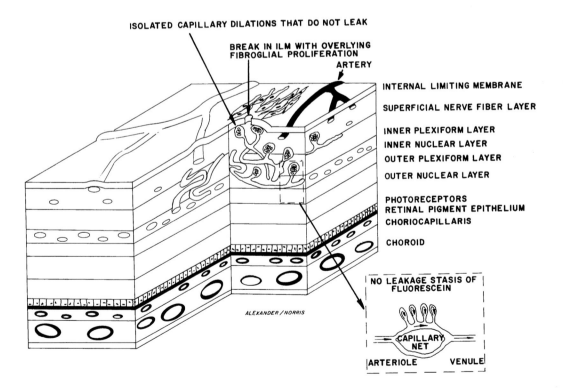

Figure 4–110. Schematic retinal cross section demonstrating the development of a retinal cavernous hemangioma. (*Reprinted with permission from Alexander LJ, Moates KN. Cavernous hemangioma of the retina. J Am Optom Assoc. 1988;59:539–548.*)

Cavernous Hemangioma of the Retina

Pearls

Characteristics

△ Congenital malformation characterized by clusters of vascular abnormalities
△ Usually unilateral, intraretinal, and often covered by a preretinal membrane
△ No demonstrable vision-threatening consequences
△ Possible associated hemangiomas in the central nervous system

Management

△ Ruling out neurologic signs and routine eye examinations
△ A retinal consultation is indicated if the feeling is that the lesion needs to be obliterated

TABLE 4–55. SYSTEMIC ANOMALIES ASSOCIATED WITH CAVERNOUS HEMANGIOMA OF THE RETINA

Neuro-oculocutaneous syndrome
Congenital cardiovascular anomalies
Hypogammaglobulinemia
Cranial nerve palsies
Angioma serpiginosum
Agenesis of the internal carotid system
Blue rubber bleb syndrome

tively independent of the remainder of the retinal vascular system. The endothelial lining is responsible for the fact that leakage is not a factor in a cavernous hemangioma, as contrasted to some of the other vascular tumors with fenestrated vessel walls.

In addition to the saccular dilatations, the internal limiting membrane overlying these tumors is altered. In places, the internal limiting membrane is thin to absent, allowing for communication between the inner retina and the vitreous face. Migration of retinal glial cells up through these focal breaks allows for proliferation of the glial tissue on the surface of the internal limiting membrane. The proliferation and subsequent contraction of these glial cells produce the epiretinal membrane often associated with cavernous hemangioma.

Management. Emphasis should be placed on ruling out associated central nervous system dysfunction and symptoms. The patient should be questioned carefully about cutaneous vascular anomalies. Cutaneous vascular lesions may occur in a variety of ways and may even give an appearance similar to the fundus lesion. The classic skin lesion is a cherry hemangioma. The clinician must always consider the possibility of an associated vascular tumor elsewhere in the body. A number of conditions associated with cavernous hemangioma of the retina has been reported, as shown in Table 4–55.

Probably the most important clinical association is the triad of cavernous hemangioma of the retina, intracranical vascular lesions, and cutaneous angiomas. Pedigree analysis of the neuro-oculocutaneous presentation supports an autosomal dominant inheritance pattern with variable penetrance and ex-

pressivity. A few cases have been presented in which the entire neuro-oculocutaneous syndrome has been transmitted. Any history of seizure, cranial nerve palsies, paresthesias, convulsions, visual field variations, strokes, and neurologic seizure in a patient with a cavernous hemangioma of the retina may be indicative of central nervous system involvement. The clinician should refer all questionable signs and symptoms in patients for computed tomography (CT) or magnetic resonance imaging (MRI). The lesions in the brain are often amendable by surgical intervention.

Angiomatosis Retinae (Retinal Capillary Hemangioma)

Introduction and Description. Angiomatosis retinae (capillary hemangiomas) is a benign retinal angioma that usually occurs within the first few decades of life. The lesion is inherited in an autosomal dominant manner, with incomplete penetrance and variable expressivity. The condition is bilateral in 50 percent of the cases. Capillary hemangioma may appear at the optic nerve head (Fig. 4–111) or within the retina. When the ocular lesion is associated with an intracranial or spinal cord hemangioblastoma, the syndrome is referred to as von Hippel–Lindau disease. Angiomas and cysts may also occur in the liver, kidney, pancreas, ovary, and epididymis. Approximately 25 percent of patients with retinal capillary hemangiomas have von Hippel–Lindau disease. Patients with von Hippel–Lindau disease have an incidence of retinal angiomas greater than 60 percent, a similar incidence of hemangioblastomas, an incidence of medullary hemangioblastomas over 10 percent, spinal and renal hemangioblastomas, renal cell carcinoma, pancreatic cystadenoma, pancreatic islet cell tumor, adrenal pheochromocytoma, liver adenoma, renal cysts, pancreatic cysts, and liver cysts. There is also a coincidence of polycythemia in some cases.

Angiomatosis retinae usually occurs as an ophthalmoscopically observable lesion in the 20- to 40-

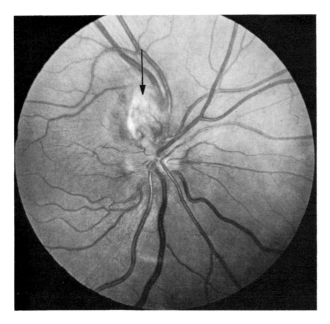

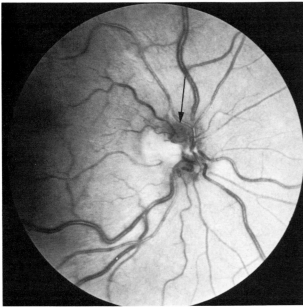

Figure 4–111. Two cases of capillary hemangioma of the optic nerve head.

velop into a large fistular single arteriole and venous channel. As the blood is shunted to the tumor from the surrounding retina, microvasculopathy occurs in the capillary bed. This nonperfused area may then develop intraretinal edema, hemorrhages, and exudation (Fig. 4–112). The intraretinal edema may lead to cystoid maculopathy. If allowed to progress unchecked, the hemangioma decompensates, allowing for intraretinal and subretinal exudation with the potential for retinal detachment. Figure 4–113 summarizes the sequence in the development of angiomatosis retinae. The exudation has a strong propensity for the posterior role, resulting in reduced acuity (Fig. 4–114). Fluorescein angiography will demonstrate the tumor and the leakage from the site. **See color plates 50 and 51.**

Management. Treatment is indicated whenever there is a threat to the macular function by exudation. Because it is most likely that the angioma will progress, it is important to intervene surgically as soon as possible. The exception to this is the case of the optic nerve hemangioma, which is difficult to treat without coincidental destruction of central vision. The earlier the angioma is treated, the better the prognosis. Cryopexy and photocoagulation are both effective methods of treatment when in experienced hands. Photocoagulation is the treatment of choice for angiomas smaller than 2.5 disc diameters spread over multiple treatment sessions to avoid the risk of secondary exudative retinal detachment. Cryotherapy is

year-old patient. The temporal periphery is the most common location of the hemangioma, which originates as a proliferation of endothelial cells between arterioles and venules in the capillary bed. At this stage, the lesion is small, with a red-gray color. As the hemangioma enlarges to occupy the sensory retina, arteriovenous communications develop, with further growth of the capillaries surrounding the hemangioma. The lesion then assumes a pink balloon pattern. The capillary growth exists to supply and drain the tumor. These capillary channels eventually de-

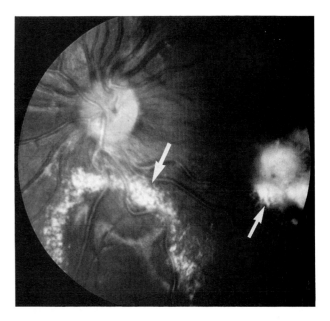

Figure 4–112. The exudative response associated with a retinal capillary hemangioma (*arrows*).

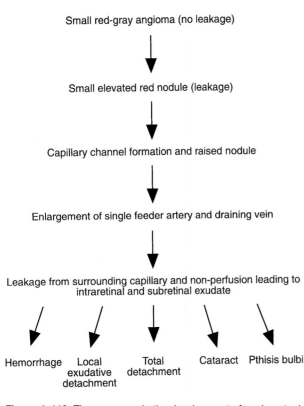

Small red-gray angioma (no leakage)

↓

Small elevated red nodule (leakage)

↓

Capillary channel formation and raised nodule

↓

Enlargement of single feeder artery and draining vein

↓

Leakage from surrounding capillary and non-perfusion leading to intraretinal and subretinal exudate

↙ ↓ ↓ ↘ ↘

Hemorrhage | Local exudative detachment | Total detachment | Cataract | Pthisis bulbi

Figure 4–113. The sequence in the development of angiomatosis retinae. (*Reprinted with permission from Alexander LJ, Moates KN. Cavernous hemangioma of the retina. J Am Optom Assoc. 1988; 59:539–548.*)

Pearls

Angiomatosis Retinae

Characteristics

△ Retinal angioma transmitted as autosomal dominant with incomplete penetrance
△ No sexual predilection
△ Bilateral in 50 percent of cases
△ Approximately 25 percent have coincidental von Hippel–Lindau disease with all of the associated complications
　Hemangioblastomas of the nervous system and renal system
　Other systemic tumors including renal, pancreatic, adrenal, epididymis, and liver
　Cysts in the renal, pancreatic, and liver systems
　Polycythemia
△ Most often in the 20s to 40s in temporal periphery
△ Clinical picture
　Orange-red tumor fed by dilated tortuous vessels
　Associated development of macular exudate
　Potential development of nonrhegmatogenous retinal detachment
　Potential retinal and/or vitreous hemorrhage

Management

△ Genetic counseling
△ Neurologic and/or systemic consultation to rule out the possible association with von Hippel–Lindau disease
△ Retinal consultation for possible photocoagulation should exudation be threatening macular function

used for small peripheral lesions or when the media precludes effective photocoagulation. Larger angiomas are difficult to treat with any modality and sometimes need surgical excision. Genetic counseling is indicated in cases of angiomatosis retinae, as is a neurologic consultation to rule out intracranial and spinal hemangioblastomas and the possibility of pheochromocytomas.

Coats' Disease

Introduction and Description. Retinal telangiectasia is often confused with cavernous hemangioma. Coats' disease is a variety of exudative retinopathy resulting from telangiectasias of the retinal vessels. Leber's miliary aneurysms are similar telangiectatic vessels without the presence of extensive exudation. Coats' disease usually occurs unilaterally in the first

to second decades. It is about four times more common in males than females, and is usually discovered in the first to second decades in spite of the fact that the telangiectasias are actually congenital.

The congenital vascular anomalies are altered over time, leading to leakage, degeneration, and development of hard exudates. It has been proposed that the conversion of benign congenital telangiectasias is stimulated by a growth hormone. Figure 4–115 illustrates the clinicopathology of retinal telangiectasias.

The breakdown in the blood–retinal barrier results in the development of cystic cavities filled with proteinacious fluid and accumulation of lipid-rich fluid within and underneath the retina. The macrophages pick up the lipids and migrate, resulting in intraretinal and subretinal exudation (Fig. 4–116). In addition to exudation creating vision loss,

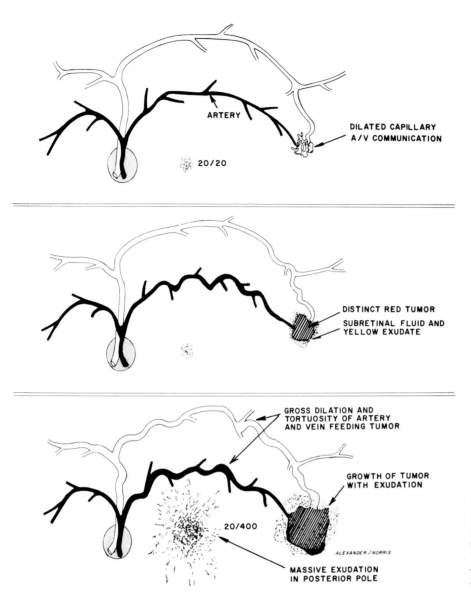

ARTERY

DILATED CAPILLARY
A/V COMMUNICATION

20/20

DISTINCT RED TUMOR
SUBRETINAL FLUID AND
YELLOW EXUDATE

GROSS DILATION AND
TORTUOSITY OF ARTERY
AND VEIN FEEDING TUMOR

GROWTH OF TUMOR
WITH EXUDATION

20/400

MASSIVE EXUDATION
IN POSTERIOR POLE

ALEXANDER / NORRIS

Figure 4–114. Schematic illustrating progression of a retinal capillary hemangioma. (*Reprinted with permission from Alexander LJ, Moates KN. Cavernous hemangioma of the retina. J Am Optom Assoc. 1988;59:539–548.*)

the intraretinal edema may spread to the posterior pole, creating cystoid macular edema. Ischemic foci may develop within the capillary bed near the telangiectasias. Retinal hemorrhage, neovascularization, and subsequent vitreous hemorrhage may occur in these areas of hypoxia. As the exudative process evolves and becomes more chronic, cholesterol crystals accumulate, and tortuous vessels develop in the periphery with the potential toward arteriovenous shunting. Ghost cells characteristic of Coats' disease appear, and are thought to originate from retinal histocytes, retinal pigment epithelial cells, or lipid-laden macrophages.

The clinical findings can be quite variable. With mild changes there are localized areas of retinal telangiectasia with localized areas of exudation and mild retinal hemorrhage. At the other end of the spectrum, larger areas of telangiectasia can present

Pearls

Coats' Disease

Characteristics

△ Occurs unilaterally in 90 percent of patients
△ Most often in males under age 20 years
△ No genetic association
△ No systemic disease association
△ Irregular dilatation of retinal vessels with a wide variation in clinical presentation
△ May progress to intraretinal and subretinal exudate accumulation with a poor visual prognosis

Management

△ A retinal consultation is indicated if there is a threat to vision
△ Patients with normal vision and minimal peripheral exudative changes may be followed every 3 months, watching carefully for intrusion into the macular area or for the threat of detachment

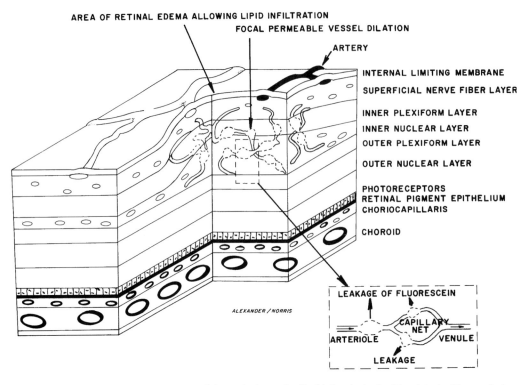

Figure 4–115. Schematic illustrating the clinicopathology of retinal telangiectasia. (*Reprinted with permission from Alexander LJ, Moates KN. Cavernous hemangioma of the retina. J Am Optom Assoc. 1988;59:539–548.*)

with capillary nonperfusion, hemorrhage, massive exudation, retinal edema, and retinal detachment. Table 4–56 outlines the stages of development of Coats' disease, with recommended therapeutic intervention.

Fluorescein angiography in Coats' disease demonstrates the aneurysmal dilations of arteries, veins, and capillaries within the mainstream of the vascular tree, and that arteriovenous collateral channels are present. Variable leakage of fluorescein dominates the picture.

Management. The patient suspected of having Coats' disease should have fluorescein angiography performed to determine if the lesions that are threatening vision are amendable by photocoagulation. The best candidates for photocoagulation include patients with central visual loss due to exudation from focal extramacular telangiectasia, and children, because of the poorer prognosis when the disease presents at an earlier age. The earlier the disease is detected with application of therapy, the better the prognosis. The end result of Coats' disease, if allowed to progress unchecked, is retinal detachment. Table 4–57 compares cavernous hemangioma, retinal telangiectasia, and capillary hemangioma.

Parafoveal and perifoveal retinal telangiectasia may also occur as an isolated entity not associated directly with Coats' disease or Leber's miliary aneurysms. Parafoveal retinal telangiectasia occurs as capillary malformation at the edge of the foveal avascular zone. This condition usually occurs as vision reduction in the third to fifth decades of life, and has a possible relationship to diabetes. Treatment by photocoagulation is controversial, because results are sometimes poor.

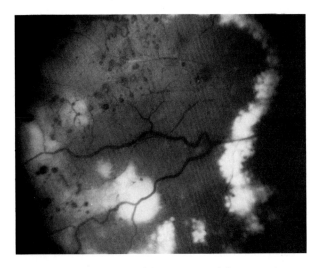

Figure 4–116. An example of the severe exudation occurring secondary to the leakage associated with telangiectasia.

TABLE 4–56. CLINICAL STAGES OF COATS' DISEASE WITH RECOMMENDATIONS REGARDING THERAPEUTIC INTERVENTION

Clinical Stage of Coats' Disease	Recommendations Regarding Therapeutic Intervention After Fluorescein Angiography
I. Retinal vessel telangiectasia (dilated tortuosity, edema, minor exudates)	I. Xenon (children) or argon photocoagulation to areas of telangiectasia A. Thermal necrosis of telangiectasia B. Possible cryopexy
II. Localized intraretinal exudates (obscuration of telangiectasia by exudate)	II. Higher energy photocoagulation or cryopexy
III. Localized (partial) retinal detachment (sensory RD by subsensory exudate)	III. A. Photocoagulation to affected area (often repeated) B. Drainage of subretinal exudate C. Cryopexy
IV. Total retinal detachment (massive exudation and subretinal membrane)	IV. Same as stage III with addition of scleral buckle
V. Uveitis, phthisis bulbi, glaucoma, cataract, massive subretinal membrane	V. Symptomatic relief of pain

TABLE 4–57. COMPARISON OF CAPILLARY HEMANGIOMA, RETINAL TELANGIECTASIA, AND CAVERNOUS HEMANGIOMA

Characteristics	Capillary Hemangioma	Retinal Telangiectasia	Cavernous Hemangioma
Age of onset	1st–2nd decade	1st–2nd decade	1st–2nd decade
Laterality	Bilateral 50%	Unilateral	Unilateral
Sex	No pattern	Male	Female
Genetics	Autosomal dominant with variable penetrance and expressivity	None	Possible autosomal dominance with variable expressivity and penetrance
Progression	Common	Common	Only epiretinal membrane
Ophthalmoscopic appearance	1. Distinct red tumor with large feeder 2. Arteriovenous shunt 3. Massive intraretinal and subretinal exudation 4. Surrounding retina involved	1. No distinct tumor 2. Arteriovenous collaterals 3. Intraretinal and subretinal exudation 4. Surrounding retina involved	1. Dilatations isolated from vascular tree 2. No collaterals 3. No exudation 4. No involvement of surrounding retina 5. Preretinal membrane
Histology	Abnormal blood–retinal barrier	Abnormal blood–retinal barrier	Intact blood–retinal barrier
Fluorescein angiography	Dye leakage	Dye leakage	No dye leakage but classic sedimentation
Complications	Hemorrhage Retinal detachment Glaucoma	Retinal detachment Hemorrhage	Rare hemorrhage
Associated systemic conditions	25% with CNS involvement	Usually no association	Possible Neuro-oculocutaneous syndrome
Treatment	Photocoagulation Cryopexy Scleral buckle Genetic counseling Neurologic consultation	Photocoagulation Cryopexy Scleral buckle	Not indicated Possible Neurologic consultation

Modified from Alexander LJ, Moates KN. Cavernous hemangioma of the retina. *J Am Optom Assoc.* 1988;59:539–548.

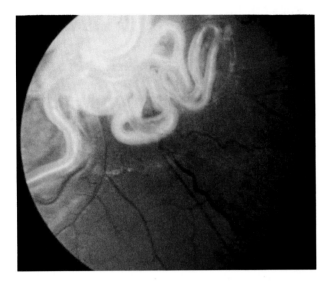

Figure 4–117. An example of a racemose hemangioma emanating from and returning to the optic nerve head. (*Photo courtesy of J. Potter.*)

Racemose Hemangioma

Introduction and Description. Racemose hemangioma (Fig. 4–117) usually occurs unilaterally as extremely dilated, tortuous arteriovenous communications associated with reduced acuities occurring with vein occlusion and/or hemorrhage. The AV malformations are typically classified into three groups: (1) small AV malformations with a capillary network between a normal-caliber artery and vein, (2) direct AV malformation with no capillary network but a direct communication between an artery and vein, and (3) large convoluted communication with no capillary network. There are usually no other ocular anomalies. With fluorescein angiography, it appears as if there is no capillary bed between the arteriovenous communication in the group 2 and 3 variations. Leakage occurs in the larger formations with no apparent associated intervening capillary bed.

Management. Racemose hemangioma does not progress and does not have strong tendencies toward leakage. Photocoagulation and cryopexy are not beneficial in eliminating the lesion. Photocoagulation is, however, of benefit when vein occlusions result in macular edema and/or retinal, disc, or iris neovascularization. There is some concern that racemose hemangioma may be associated with similar aberrant vasculature within the optic nerve and intracranial cavity. The AV malformations that are severe may have in excess of 40 percent association with systemic AV malformations. The Wyburn–Mason syndrome is the phakomatosis consisting of retinal and midbrain arteriovenous malformations. A neurologic consultation is, therefore, recommended in severe cases of racemose hemangioma.

Choroidal Hemangioma

Introduction and Description. Choroidal hemangiomas occur as unilateral lesions either in the localized form with no systemic association or in the diffuse form with the systemic association to Sturge–Weber syndrome. The localized forms occur in adult life and may create a reduction in vision. The diffuse form is usually detected in childhood because of the presentation of Sturge–Weber syndrome, which consists of ipsilateral choroidal, facial, and neurological angiomas.

The choroidal hemangiomas are cavernous vascular spaces within the choroid with overlying retinal pigment epithelial changes and potential retinal changes. In the localized form, there is an orange to red oval to circular choroidal mass in the posterior pole that may extend into the macula. Subretinal fluid, cystoid macular edema, and RPE alterations may present in this form. In the diffuse form, there are larger areas of the fundus with a reddish-orange coloration. During fluorescein angiography there is an early hyperfluorescence of the larger choroidal vessels and a late staining of the tumor because of the seepage. B-scan ultrasonography demonstrates tumor reflectivity. A secondary concern is the complication of

Pearls

Racemose Hemangioma

Characteristics

△ Extremely dilated tortuous arteriovenous communications of varying degrees

   Small AV malformation with a capillary network between a normal caliber artery and vein

   Direct AV malformation with no capillary network but a direct communication between an artery and vein

   Large convoluted communication with no capillary network

△ Reduced acuities may occur from vein occlusion or hemorrhage

Management

△ Retinal consultation if associated retinal venous occlusive disease creating edema or neovascularization

△ The AV malformation cannot be destroyed by photocoagulation or cryopexy

△ Possible intracranial associations in the stage 3 networks, necessitating a neurologic consultation

Pearls

Choroidal Hemangiomas

Characteristics

Δ Localized form presenting in adult life with no systemic association

  Appears as round, orange-red tumor in the posterior pole

  May create subretinal fluid leakage into macula

  Early filling, late leakage on fluorescein angiography

  May have associated secondary glaucoma

Δ Diffuse form is usually associated with Sturge–Weber syndrome, which is choroidal, facial, and neurologic angiomas

Δ Appears as large area of reddish-orange discoloration

Δ Early filling, late leakage on fluorescein angiography

Δ May have associated secondary glaucoma

Management

Δ Photocoagulation to areas of subretinal fluid threatening macular function

Δ In diffuse variety consider systemic manifestations of Sturge–Weber syndrome and assure coverage of these possibilities

Δ Recheck both varieties on a regular basis, and inform patient of self-monitoring to minimize risk to macular function

Δ Follow both varieties carefully for the potential development of secondary glaucoma

glaucoma associated with the mechanical elevation of the episcleral pressure.

Management. In the localized form, intervention is unnecessary unless there is leakage creating a serous retinal detachment threatening macular function. If there is leakage, argon green or yellow dye photocoagulation may be considered as long as the total obliteration of the tumor is not attempted. The photocoagulation is used solely to assist in the obliteration of the subretinal fluid accumulation. In the diffuse form, it is incumbent on the practitioner to determine if there are associated threatening systemic manifestations of Sturge–Weber syndrome. In addition, especially for the diffuse variation, there must be constant vigilance for the development of secondary glaucoma.

In addition, it is important to follow both varieties on a regular basis to assure that there is not intrusion of subretinal fluid into the macular area. The patient should be on some sort of home monitoring system to assure prompt detection of retinopathy threatening macular function.

REFERENCES

Elschnig Spots

Casser Locke L. Ocular manifestations of hypertension. *Optom Clin.* 1992;2:47–76.

Photocoagulation

Acheson RW, et al. Intraocular argon laser photocoagulation. *Eye.* 1987;1:97–105.

Bloom SM, Brucker AJ. *Laser Surgery of the Posterior Segment.* Philadelphia: Lippincott; 1991.

Brancato R, et al. Clinical applications of the tunable dye laser. *Lasers Ophthalmol.* 1986;1:115–118.

Charles S. Endophotocoagulation. *Retina.* 1981;1:117–120.

Glaser BM, et al. Retinal pigment epithelial cells release an inhibitor of neovascularization. *Arch Ophthalmol.* 1985;103:1870–1875.

L'Esperance FA. Clinical applications of the organic dye laser. *Ophthalmology.* 1985;92:1592–1600.

Machemer R. The importance of fluid absorption, traction, intraocular currents, and chorioretinal scars in the therapy of rhegmatogenous retinal detachments: XLI Edward Jackson memorial lecture. *Am J Ophthalmol.* 1984;98:681–693.

Marshall J. Lasers in ophthalmology: The basic principles. *Eye.* 1988;2:S98–S112.

Singerman IJ, Kalski RS. Tunable dye laser photocoagulation for choroidal neovascularization complicating age-related macular degeneration. *Retina.* 1989;9:247–248.

Yannuzzi LA, Shakin JL. Krypton red laser photocoagulation of the ocular fundus. *Retina.* 1982;2:1–14.

Retinal Macroaneurysms

Abdel-Khalek MN, Richardson J. Retinal macroaneurysm: Natural history and guidelines for treatment. *Br J Ophthalmol.* 1986;70:2–11.

Asdourian GK. Vascular anomalies of the retina. *Perspect Ophthalmol.* 1979;3:111–119.

Joondeph BC, et al. Retinal macroaneurysms treated with the yellow dye laser. *Retina.* 1989;9:187–192.

Lavin MJ, et al. Retinal arterial macroaneurysms: A retrospective study of 40 patients. *Br J Ophthalmol.* 1987;71:817–825.

Lewis RA, et al. Acquired arterial macroaneurysms of the retina. *Br J Ophthalmol.* 1976;60:21–30.

Magargal LE. Venous macroaneurysms following branch retinal vein obstruction. *Ann Ophthalmol.* 1980;12:685–688.

Mainster MA, Whitacre MM. Dye yellow photocoagulation of retinal arterial macroaneurysms. *Am J Ophthalmol.* 1988;105:97–98.

Palestine AG, et al. Macroaneurysms of the retinal arteries. *Am J Ophthalmol.* 1982;93:164–171.

Rabb MF, et al. Retinal arterial macroaneurysms. *Surv Ophthalmol.* 1988;33:73–96.

Schulman J, et al. Large capillary aneurysms secondary to retinal venous obstruction. *Br J Ophthalmol.* 1981;65:36–41.

Idiopathic Juxtafoveal Telangiectasia

Chopdar A. Retinal telangiectasis in adults: Fluorescein angiographic findings and treatment by argon laser. *Br J Ophthalmol.* 1978;62:243–250.

Gass JDM. *Stereoscopic Atlas of Macular Diseases: Diagnosis and Treatment.* 3rd ed. St Louis: Mosby; 1987.

Hutton WI, et al. Focal parafoveal retinal telangiectasis. *Arch Ophthalmol.* 1978;96:1362–1367.

Lipemia Retinalis

Alexander LJ. Ocular signs and symptoms of altered blood lipids. *J Am Optom Assoc.* 1983;54:123–126.

Retinal Emboli

Alexander LJ. Variations in physician response to consultation requests for Hollenhorst plaques: A pilot study. *J Am Optom Assoc.* 1992;63:326–332.

Appen RE, et al. Central retinal artery occlusion. *Am J Ophthalmol.* 1975;79:374–381.

Becker WL, Burde RM. Carotid artery disease. A therapeutic enigma. *Arch Ophthalmol.* 1988;106:34–39.

Berguer R. Idiopathic ischemic syndromes of the retina and optic nerve and their carotid origin. *J Vasc Surg.* 1985;2:649–653.

Bruno A, et al. Retinal infarction during sleep and wakefulness. *Stroke.* 1990;21:1494–1496.

Bruno A, et al. Concomitants of asymptomatic retinal cholesterol emboli. *Stroke.* 1992;23:900–902.

Bunt TJ. The clinical significance of the asymptomatic Hollenhorst plaque. *J Vasc Surg.* 1986;4:559–562.

Chawluk JB, et al. Atherosclerotic carotid artery disease in patients with retinal ischemic syndromes. *Neurology.* 1988;38:858–863.

Coleman K, et al. Electroretinography, retinal ischemia and carotid artery disease. *Eur J Vasc Surg.* 1990;4:569–573.

Ehrenfeld WK, et al. Embolization and transient blindness from carotid atheroma. *Arch Surg.* 1966;93:787–794.

Fisher CM. Observations of fundus oculi in transient monocular blindness. *Neurology.* 1959;9:333–347.

Flory CM. Arterial occlusion produced by emboli from eroded aortic atheromatous plaques. *Am J Pathol.* 1945;21:549–565.

Hollenhorst RW. Significance of bright plaques in the retinal arterioles. *JAMA.* 1961;178:23–29.

Hollenhorst RW, et al. Experimental embolization of the retinal arterioles. *Trans Am Ophthalmol Soc.* 1962;60: 316–333.

Javitt JC, et al. Detecting and treating retinopathy in patients with type I diabetes mellitus. A health policy model. *Ophthalmology.* 1990;97:483–495.

Jorgensen R, et al. Monocular ischemia: The influence of carotid atherosclerosis versus primary ocular disease on prognosis. *Surgery.* 1988;104:507–511.

Kirshner RL, et al. Ocular manifestations of carotid artery atheroma. *J Vasc Surg.* 1985;2:850–853.

Pfaffenbach DD, Hollenhorst RW. Morbidity and survivorship of patients with embolic cholesterol crystals in the ocular fundus. *Am J Ophthalmol.* 1973;75:66–72.

Roper WL, et al. Effectiveness in health care. An initiative to evaluate and improve medical practice. *N Engl J Med.* 1988;319:1197–1202.

Savino PJ, et al. Retinal stroke. Is the patient at risk? *Arch Ophthalmol.* 1977;95:1185–1189.

Schwarcz TH, et al. Hollenhorst plaques: Retinal manifesta- tions and the role of carotid endarterectomy. *J Vasc Surg.* 1990;11:635–641.

Trobe JD. Carotid endarterectomy. Who needs it? *Ophthalmology.* 1987;94:725–730.

Preretinal Membrane Formation

Alexander LJ. Pre-retinal membrane formation. *J Am Optom Assoc.* 1980;51:567–572.

Pesin SR, et al. Vitrectomy for premacular fibroplasia. *Ophthalmology.* 1991;98:1109–1114.

Branch Retinal Vein Occlusion

Alexander LJ. Implications of retinal vaso-occlusive disease. *S J Optom.* 1986;4:20–34.

Alexander LJ. Retinal vein occlusion. A literature update. *J Am Optom Assoc.* 1986;57:557–560.

Blankenship GW, Okun E. Retinal tributary vein occlusion: History and management by photocoagulation. *Arch Ophthalmol.* 1973;889:363–368.

Branch Vein Occlusion Study Group. Argon laser scatter photocoagulation for prevention of neovascularization and vitreous hemorrhage in branch vein occlusion: A randomized clinical trial. *Arch Ophthalmol.* 1986;104:34–41.

Branch Vein Occlusion Study Group. Argon laser photocoagulation for macular edema in branch vein occlusion. *Am J Ophthalmol.* 1985;99:218–219.

Branch Vein Occlusion Study Group. Argon laser photocoagulation for macular edema in branch vein occlusion. *Am J Ophthalmol.* 1984;98:271–282.

Brown GC, et al. Neovascular glaucoma. Etiologic considerations. *Ophthalmology.* 1984;91:315–320.

Frucht J, et al. Intraocular pressure in retinal vein occlusion. *Br J Ophthalmol.* 1984;68:26–28.

Grunwald JE. Effect of topical timolol on the human retinal circulation. *Invest Ophthalmol Vis Sci.* 1986;27:1713–1719.

Gutman FA. Discussion of macular branch vein occlusion. *Ophthalmology.* 1980;87:98–104.

Gutman FA, et al. Photocoagulation in retinal branch vein occlusion. *Ann Ophthalmol.* 1981;13:1359–1363.

Gutman FA, Zegarra H. Macular edema secondary to occlusion of the retinal veins. *Surv Ophthalmol.* 1984;18: 462–470.

Hayreh SS, et al. Ocular hypotony following retinal vein occlusion. *Arch Ophthalmol.* 1978;96:827–833.

Jaffe L, et al. Macular branch vein occlusion. *Ophthalmology.* 1980;87:91–97.

Jalkh AE, et al. Chronic macular edema in retinal branch vein occlusion: Role of laser photocoagulation. *Ann Ophthalmol.* 1984;16:526.

Johnston RL, et al. Risk factors of branch retinal vein occlusion. *Arch Ophthalmol.* 1985;103:1831–1832.

Kado M, Trempe CL. Role of the vitreous in branch retinal vein occlusion. *Am J Ophthalmol.* 1988;105:20–24.

McGrath MA, et al. Systemic factors contributory to retinal vein occlusion. *Arch Intern Med.* 1978;138:216–220.

Orth DM, Patz A. Retinal branch vein occlusion. *Surv Ophthalmol.* 1978;22:357–376.

Osterloh MD, Charles S. Surgical decompression of branch retinal vein occlusions. *Arch Ophthalmol.* 1988;106: 1469–1471.

Roseman RL, Olk RJ. Krypton red laser photocoagulation for branch retinal vein occlusion. *Ophthalmology.* 1987;94: 1120–1125.

Shilling JS, Jones CA. Retinal branch vein occlusion: A study of argon laser photocoagulation in the treatment of macular edema. *Br J Ophthalmol.* 1984;68:196–198.

Central Retinal Vein Occlusion

Alexander LJ. Implications of retinal vaso-occlusive disease. *S J Optom.* 1986;4:20–34.

Brown GC, et al. Neovascular glaucoma. Etiologic considerations. *Ophthalmology.* 1984;91:315–320.

Brown GC, et al. Central retinal vein obstruction and carotid artery disease. *Ophthalmology.* 1984;91:1627–1633.

Brunette I, Boghen D. Central retinal vein occlusion complicating spontaneous carotid cavernous fistula. Case report. *Arch Ophthalmol.* 1987;105:464–465.

Carter JE. Panretinal photocoagulation for progressive ocular neovascularization secondary to occlusion of the common carotid artery. *Ann Ophthalmol.* 1984;16:572–576.

Dodson PM, et al. Retinal vein occlusion and the prevalence of lipoprotein abnormalities. *Br J Ophthalmol.* 1982;66: 161–164.

Gonder JR, et al. Central retinal vein obstruction associated with mitral valve prolapse. *Can J Ophthalmol.* 1983;18: 220–222.

Grunwald JE. Effect of topical timolol on the human retinal circulation. *Invest Ophthalmol Vis Sci.* 1986;27:1713–1719.

Gutman FA. Evaluation of a patient with central retinal vein occlusion. *Ophthalmology.* 1983;90:481–483.

Gutman FA, Zeyarra H. Macular edema secondary to occlusion of the retinal veins. *Surv Ophthalmol.* 1984;28 (suppl):462–470.

Hanson LL, et al. A randomized prospective study on treatment of central retinal vein occlusion by isovolemic hemodilution and photocoagulation. *Br J Ophthalmol.* 1985;69:108–116.

Hayreh SS. Classification of central retinal vein occlusion. *Ophthalmology.* 1983;90:458–474.

Hayreh SS, et al. Ocular neovascularization with retinal occlusion, III. Incidence of ocular neovascularization with retinal vascular occlusion. *Ophthalmology.* 1983;90: 488–506.

Klein MI, Finkelstein D. Macular grid photocoagulation for macular edema in central retinal vein occlusion. *Arch Ophthalmol.* 1989;107:1297–1302.

Kohner EM, et al. The management of central retinal vein occlusion. *Ophthalmology.* 1983;90:484–487.

Laatikainen I, et al. Panretinal photocoagulation in central retinal vein occlusion: A randomized controlled clinical study. *Br J Ophthalmol.* 1977;61:741–753.

Magargal LE, et al. Efficacy of panretinal photocoagulation in preventing neovascular glaucoma following ischemic central retinal vein obstruction. *Ophthalmology.* 1982;89: 780–784.

Magargal LE, et al. Neovascular glaucoma following central retinal vein obstruction. *Ophthalmology.* 1981;88: 1095–1101.

May DR, et al. Xenon arc panretinal photocoagulation for central retinal vein occlusion: A randomised prospective study. *Br J Ophthalmol.* 1979;63:725–734.

Mason G. Iris neovascular tufts. *Ann Ophthalmol.* 1980;12: 420–422.

McGrath MA, et al. Systemic factors contributory to retinal vein occlusion. *Arch Intern Med.* 1978;138:216–220.

Minturn J, Brown GC. Progression of nonischemic central retinal vein obstruction to the ischemic variant. *Ophthalmology.* 1986;93:1158–1162.

Roberts SP, Haefs TMP. Central retinal vein occlusion in a middle-aged adult with HIV infection. *Optom Vis Sci.* 1992;69:567–569.

Smith RJ. Rubeotic glaucoma. *Br J Ophthalmol.* 1981;65: 606–609.

Zegarra H, et al. The natural course of central retinal vein occlusion. *Ophthalmology.* 1979;86:1931–1942.

Hemicentral Retinal Vein Occlusion

Alexander LJ. Retinal vein occlusion. A literature update. *J Am Optom Assoc.* 1986;57:557–560.

Brown GC, et al. Neovascular glaucoma. Etiologic considerations. *Ophthalmology.* 1984;91:315–320.

Chopdar A. Dual trunk central retinal vein incidence in clinical practice. *Arch Ophthalmol.* 1984;102:85–87.

Hayreh SS, Hayreh MS. Hemi-central retinal vein occlusion. Pathogeneses, clinical features, and natural history. *Arch Ophthalmol.* 1980;98:1600–1609.

Sanborn GE, Magargal LE. Characteristics of the hemispheric retinal vein occlusion. *Ophthalmology.* 1984;91: 1616–1626.

Zegarra H, et al. Partial occlusion of the central retinal vein. *Am J Ophthalmol.* 1983;96:330–357.

Branch Retinal Arterial Occlusions and Central Retinal Arterial Occlusions

Alexander LJ. Diseases of the retina. In: Bartlett JD, Jaanus SD, eds. *Clinical Ocular Pharmacology.* Boston: Butterworths; 1989.

Alexander LJ. Implications of retinal vaso-occlusive disease. *S J Optom.* 1986;4:20–34.

Hypertensive Retinopathy

Casser Locke L. Ocular manifestations of hypertension. *Optom Clin.* 1992;2:47–76.

Schwartz GL. Diagnosis, pathogenesis, and management of essential hypertension. *Optom Clin.* 1992;2:31–46.

Cerebrovascular Disease and the Eye

Alexander LJ. National health care issues: Stroke. *J Am Optom Assoc.* 1992;63:361–364.

Ocular Ischemic Syndrome

Brown GC. Macular edema in association with severe carotid artery obstruction. *Am J Ophthalmol.* 1986;102: 442–448.

Brown GC, et al. Arterial obstruction and ocular neovascularization. *Ophthalmology.* 1982;89:139–146.

Campo RV, Reeser FH. Retinal telangiectasia secondary to bilateral carotid artery occlusion. *Arch Ophthalmol.* 1983; 101:1211–1213.

Coppeto JR, et al. Neovascular glaucoma and carotid artery obstructive disease. *Am J Ophthalmol.* 1985;99:567–570.

Duker JS, Belmont JB. Ocular ischemic syndrome secondary to carotid artery dissection. *Am J Ophthalmol.* 1988;106: 750–752.

Eggleston TF, et al. Photocoagulation for ocular ischemia associated with carotid artery occlusion. *Ann Ophthalmol.* 1980;12:84–87.

Johnston ME, et al. Successful treatment of the ocular ischemic syndrome with panretinal photocoagulation and cerebrovascular surgery. *Can J Ophthalmol.* 1988;23: 114–119.

Kahn M, et al. Ocular features of carotid occlusive disease. *Retina.* 1986;6:239–252.

Kearns TP. Ophthalmology and the carotid artery. *Am J Ophthalmol.* 1979;88:714–722.

Knox DL. Ischemic ocular inflammation. *Am J Ophthalmol.* 1965;60:995–1002.

Young LHY, Appen RE. Ischemic oculopathy: A manifestation of carotid artery disease. *Arch Neurol.* 1981;38: 358–361.

Diabetes and Diabetic Retinopathy

Aaberg TM, Abrams GW. Changing indications and techniques for vitrectomy in management of complications of diabetic retinopathy. *Ophthalmology.* 1987;94:775–779.

Aiello LM, et al. Diabetic retinopathy in Joslin clinic patients with adult onset diabetes. *Ophthalmology.* 1981;88: 619–623.

Appiah AP, et al. Delayed diagnosis of diabetic retinopathy in black and Hispanic patients with diabetes mellitus. *Ann Ophthal.* 1991;23:156–158.

Awh CC, et al. Improved detection and referral of patients with diabetic retinopathy by primary care physicians. *Arch Int Med.* 1991;151:1405–1408.

Aylward GW, et al. Extensive argon laser photocoagulation in the treatment of proliferative diabetic retinopathy. *Br J Ophthalmol.* 1989;73:197–201.

Benedett R, et al. Transconjunctival anterior retinal cryotherapy for proliferative diabetic retinopathy. *Ophthalmology.* 1987;94:612–619.

Benson WE, et al. Chorioretinal and subretinal proliferations: Complications of photocoagulation. *Ophthalmology.* 1979;86:283–289.

Blankenship G. A clinical comparison of central and peripheral argon laser panretinal photocoagulation for proliferative diabetic retinopathy. *Ophthalmology.* 1988; 95:170–177.

Bresnick GH. Diabetic macular edema: A review. *Ophthalmology.* 1986;93:989–997.

Brouhard BH. Antihypertensive therapy for patients with diabetes mellitus. *Diabetes Care.* 1992;15:918–921.

Cavallerano J. Diabetic retinopathy: The new imperative. *Rev Optom.* 1991;7:50–59.

Cignarelli M, et al. High systolic blood pressure increases the prevalence and severity of retinopathy in NIDDM patients. *Diabetes Care.* 1992;15:1002–1008.

Diabetes Control and Complications Trial Research Group. Are continuing studies of metabolic control and microvascular complications in insulin-dependent diabetes mellitus justified? *N Eng J Med.* 1988;318:246–250.

Diabetes Control and Complications Trial Research Group. Color photography vs. fluorescein angiography in the detection of diabetic retinopathy in the Diabetes Control and Complications Trial. *Arch Ophthalmol.* 1987a;105: 1344–1351.

Diabetes Control and Complications Trial Research Group. Diabetes Control and Complications Trial (DCCT) results of feasibility study. *Diabetes Care.* 1987b;10:1–19.

Diabetes Control and Complications Trial Research Group. The Diabetes Control and Complications Trial (DCCT) design and methodologic considerations for the feasibility phase. *Diabetes.* 1986;35:530–545.

Diabetic Retinopathy Study Research Group. Four risk factors for severe visual loss in diabetic retinopathy: The third report from the Diabetic Retinopathy Study. *Arch Ophthalmol.* 1979;97:654–655.

Diabetic Retinopathy Study Research Group. Indications for photocoagulation treatment of diabetic retinopathy. Diabetic Retinopathy Study report no. 14. *Int Ophthalmol Clin.* 1987;27:239–253.

Diabetic Retinopathy Study Research Group. Photocoagulation treatment of proliferative diabetic retinopathy: Clinical applications of Diabetic Retinopathy Study (DRS) findings. DRS report no. 8. *Ophthalmology.* 1981b;88: 583–600.

Diabetic Retinopathy Study Research Group. Photocoagulation treatment of proliferative diabetic retinopathy: The second report of Diabetic Retinopathy Study findings. *Ophthalmology.* 1978;85:82–106.

Diabetic Retinopathy Study Research Group. Preliminary report on effects of photocoagulation therapy. *Am J Ophthalmol.* 1976;81:383–396.

Diabetic Retinopathy Study Research Group. Report 6: Design, methods, and baseline results. *Invest Ophthalmol Vis Sci.* 1981a;21:149–209.

Diabetic Retinopathy Vitrectomy Study Research Group. Early vitrectomy for severe proliferative diabetic retinopathy in eyes with useful vision: Results of a randomized trial—Diabetic Retinopathy Vitrectomy Study report 3. *Ophthalmology.* 1988;95:1307–1320.

Diabetic Retinopathy Vitrectomy Study Research Group. Early vitrectomy for severe vitreous hemorrhage in diabetic retinopathy: Two-year results of a randomized trial: Diabetic Retinopathy Vitrectomy Study report 2. *Arch Ophthalmol.* 1985a;103:1644–1652.

Diabetic Retinopathy Vitrectomy Study Research Group. Two-year course of visual acuity in severe proliferative diabetic retinopathy with conservative management. *Ophthalmology.* 1985b;92:492–502.

Early Treatment Diabetic Retinopathy Study Group. Photocoagulation for diabetic macular edema: Early Treatment Diabetic Retinopathy Study report number 4. *Int Ophthalmol Clin.* 1987b;27:265–272.

Early Treatment Diabetic Retinopathy Study Group. Treatment techniques and clinical guidelines for photocoagulation of diabetic macular edema: Early Treatment Diabetic Retinopathy Study report number 2. *Ophthalmology.* 1987a;94:761–774.

Early Treatment Diabetic Retinopathy Study Group. Techniques for scatter and local photocoagulation: Early Treatment Diabetic Retinopathy Study report number 3. *Int Ophthalmol Clin.* 1987;27:254–264.

Early Treatment Diabetic Retinopathy Study Group. Photocoagulation for diabetic macular edema: Early Treatment Diabetic Retinopathy Study report number 1. *Arch Ophthalmol.* 1985;103:1796–1806.

Ferris FL, et al. Macular edema in diabetic retinopathy study patients: Diabetic Retinopathy Study report number 12. *Ophthalmology.* 1987;94:754–760.

Harris MI, et al. Prevalence of diabetes and impaired glucose tolerance and plasma glucose levels in U.S. population aged 20-74 yr. *Diabetes.* 1987;36:523–534.

Hubar MJ, et al. Mydriatic drugs for diabetic patients. *Br J Ophthalmol.* 1985;69:425–427.

Jacobson DR, et al. The treatment of angle neovascularization with panretinal photocoagulation. *Ophthalmology.* 1979;86:1270–1275.

Jacques CHM, et al. Reported practice behaviors for medical care of patients with diabetes mellitus by primary-care physicians in Pennsylvania. *Diabetes Care.* 1991;14:712–717.

Kaufman SC, et al. Factors associated with visual outcome after photocoagulation for diabetic retinopathy: Diabetic Retinopathy Study Report number 13. *Invest Ophthalmol Vis Sci.* 1989;30:23–28.

Klein R, et al. The Wisconsin Epidemiologic Study of Diabetic Retinopathy, II. Prevalence and risk of diabetic retinopathy when age at diagnosis is less than 30 years. *Arch Ophthalmol.* 1984a;102:520–526.

Klein R, et al. The Wisconsin Epidemiologic Study of Diabetic Retinopathy, III. Prevalence and risk of diabetic retinopathy when age at diagnosis is 30 or more years. *Arch Ophthalmol.* 1984b;102:527–532.

Klein R, et al. The Wisconsin Epidemiologic Study of Diabetic Retinopathy, IV. Diabetic macular edema. *Ophthalmology.* 1984c;91:1464–1474.

Klein R, et al. Glycosylated hemoglobin predicts the incidence and progression of diabetic retinopathy. *JAMA.* 1988;260:2864–2871.

Klein R, et al. The Wisconsin Epidemiologic Study of Diabetic Retinopathy, IX. Four-year incidence and progression of diabetic retinopathy when age at diagnosis is less than 30 years. *Arch Ophthalmol.* 1989a;107:237–243.

Klein R, et al. The Wisconsin Epidemiologic Study of Diabetic Retinopathy, X. Four-year incidence and progression of diabetic retinopathy when age at diagnosis is 30 years or more. *Arch Ophthalmol.* 1989b;107:244–249.

Klein R, et al. The Wisconsin Epidemiologic Study of Diabetic Retinopathy, XI. The incidence of macular edema. *Ophthalmology.* 1989;96:1501–1510.

Kleinstein RN, et al. Detection of diabetic retinopathy by optometrists. *J Am Optom Assoc.* 1987;11:879–882.

Kroc Collaborative Study Group. Blood glucose control and the evolution of diabetic retinopathy and albuminuria. *N Engl J Med.* 1985;311:365–372.

Kroc Collaborative Study Group. Diabetic retinopathy after two years of intensified insulin treatment: Follow-up of the Kroc Collaborative Study. *JAMA.* 1988;260:37–41.

McDonald HR, Schatz H. Grid photocoagulation for diffuse macular edema. *Retina.* 1985;5:65–72.

Nathan DM, et al. Role of diabetologist in evaluating diabetic retinopathy. *Diabetes Care.* 1991;14:26–33.

Olk RJ. Modified grid argon (blue-green) laser photocoagulation for diffuse diabetic macular edema. *Ophthalmology.* 1986;93:938–950.

Pavan PR, et al. Diabetic rubeosis and panretinal photocoagulation: A prospective, controlled, masked trial using fluorescein angiography. *Arch Ophthalmol.* 1983;101:882–884.

Phelps RL, et al. Changes in diabetic retinopathy during pregnancy: Correlations with regulation of hyperglycemia. *Arch Ophthalmol.* 1986;104:1806–1810.

Ross WH, Gottner MJ. Peripheral retinal cryopexy for subtotal vitreous hemorrhage. *Am J Ophthalmol.* 1988;105:377–382.

Singerman LJ, et al. Krypton laser for proliferative diabetic retinopathy: The Krypton Argon Regression of Neovascularization Study. *J Diabet Complications.* 1988;2:189–196.

Sprafka JM, et al. Prevalence of undiagnosed eye disease in high-risk diabetic individuals. *Arch Int Med.* 1990;150:857–861.

Stross JK, Harlan WR. The dissemination of new medical information. *JAMA.* 1979;241:2622–2624.

Sunness JS. The pregnant woman's eye. *Surv Ophthalmol.* 1988;32:219–238.

Sullivan P, et al. Long-term outcome after photocoagulation for proliferative diabetic retinopathy. *Diabetic Med.* 1990;7:788–794.

Sussman EJ, et al. Diagnosis of diabetic eye disease. *JAMA.* 1982;247:3231–3234.

Vernon SA, Cheng H. Panretinal cryotherapy in neovascular disease. *Br J Ophthalmol.* 1988;72:401–405.

Warram JH, et al. Excess mortality associated with diuretic therapy in diabetes mellitus. *Arch Int Med.* 1991;151:1350–1356.

Witkin SR, Klein R. Ophthalmologic care for persons with diabetes. *JAMA.* 1984;251:2534–2537.

Radiation Retinopathy

Axer-Siegel R, et al. Radiation retinopathy treated with the krypton red laser. *Ann Ophthalmol.* 1989;21:272–276.

Brown GC, et al. Radiation retinopathy. *Ophthalmology.* 1982;89:1494–1501.

Chee PHY. Radiation retinopathy. *Am J Ophthalmol.* 1968;66:860–865.

Kinyoun JL, et al. Photocoagulation treatment of radiation retinopathy. *Am J Ophthalmol.* 1988;105:470–478.

Eales' Disease

Eliot AJ. 30-year observation of patients with Eales' disease. *Am J Ophthlamol.* 1975;80:404–408.

Gass JDM. *Steroscopic Atlas of Macular Diseases: Diagnosis and Treatment.* 3rd ed. St. Louis: Mosby; 1987.

Magargal LE, et al. Treatment of Eales' disease with scatter laser photocoagulation. *Ann Ophthalmol.* 1989;21:300–302.

Renie WA, et al. The evaluation of patients with Eales' disease. *Retina.* 1983;3:243–248.

Spitznas M, et al. Treatment of Eales' disease with photocoagulation. *Arch Klin Exp Ophthalmol.* 1975;194:193–198.

Zeki SM, Dutton GN. Photocoagulation of raised new vessels by long-duration low-energy argon laser photocoagulation: A preliminary study. *Br J Ophthalmol.* 1988;72:837–840.

Sickle Cell Retinopathy

Condon PI, et al. A randomized clinical trial of feeder vessel photocoagulation of proliferative sickle cell retinopathy, II. Update and analysis of risk factors. *Ophthalmology.* 1984;91:1496–1498.

Condon PI, Serjeant GR. Behaviour of untreated proliferative sickle retinopathy. *Br J Ophthalmol.* 1980;64:404–411.

Goldberg MF. Retinal neovascularization in sickle retinopathies. *Trans Am Acad Ophthalmol Otolaryngol.* 1977; 83:409–431.

Goldberg MF. Classification and pathogenesis of proliferative sickle retinopathy. *Am J Ophthalmol.* 1971;71:649–665.

Hanscom TA. Indirect treatment of peripheral retinal neovascularization. *Am J Ophthalmol.* 1982;93:88–91.

Jampol LM, et al. An update on vitrectomy surgery and retinal detachment repair in sickle cell disease. *Arch Ophthalmol.* 1982;100:591–593.

Jampol LM, Goldbaum MH. Peripheral proliferative retinopathies. *Surv Ophthalmol.* 1980;25:1–14.

Kimmel AS, et al. Peripheral circumferential retinal scatter photocoagulation for treatment of proliferative sickle retinopathy: An update. *Ophthalmology.* 1986;93: 1429–1434.

Nagpal KC, et al. Angioid streaks and sickle hemoglobinopathies. *Br J Ophthalmol.* 1976;60:31–34.

Rednam KRV, et al. Scatter retinal photocoagulation for proliferative sickle cell retinopathy. *Am J Ophthalmol.* 1982; 93:594–599.

Retinopathy of Prematurity

Barr CC, et al. Angioma-like mass in a patient with retrolental fibroplasia. *Am J Ophthalmol.* 1980;89:647–650.

Cryotherapy for Retinopathy of Prematurity Cooperative Group. Multicenter trial of cryotherapy for retinopathy of prematurity: Three month outcome. *Arch Ophthalmol.* 1990;108:195–204.

Cryotherapy for Retinopathy of Prematurity Cooperative Group. Multicenter trial of cryotherapy for retinopathy of prematurity: Preliminary results. *Arch Ophthalmol.* 1988; 106:471–479.

Flynn JT, et al. Retinopathy of prematurity. Diagnosis, severity and natural history. *Ophthalmology.* 1987;94: 620–629.

Majima A, et al. Clinical observation of photocoagulation on retinopathy of prematurity. *Jpn J Clin Ophthalmol.* 1976;30: 93–97.

Nagata M. Treatment of acute proliferative retrolental fibroplasia with xenon-arc photocoagulation: its indications and limitations. *Jpn J Ophthalmol.* 1977;21:436–459.

Veith J, Scharre JE. Retinopathy of prematurity—review of the pathophysiology and classification. *J Am Optom Assoc.* 1992;63:496–499.

Behçet's Disease

Godfrey WA, et al. The use of chlorambucil in intractable idiopathic uveitis. *Am J Ophthalmol.* 1974;78:415–428.

Graham EM, et al. Neovascularization associated with posterior uveitis. *Br J Ophthalmol.* 1987;71:826–833.

Michelson JB, Chisari FV. Behçet's disease. *Surv Ophthalmol.* 1982;26:190–203.

Acute Retinal Necrosis Syndrome

Cartwright MJ. Acute retinal necrosis: An unusual presentation. *Ann Ophthalmol.* 1991;23:452–453.

Culbertson WW, et al. Chickenpox-associated acute retinal necrosis syndrome. *Ophthalmology.* 1991;98:1641–1646.

Duker JS, Blumenkranz MS. Diagnosis and management of the acute retinal necrosis (ARN) syndrome. *Surv Ophthalmol.* 1991;35:327–343.

Matsuo T, et al. Factors associated with poor visual outcome in acute retinal necrosis. *Br J Ophthalmol.* 1991;75:450–454.

Pepose JS, et al. Herpesvirus antibody levels in the etiologic diagnosis of the acute retinal necrosis syndrome. *Am J Ophthalmol.* 1992;113:248–256.

Rummelt V, et al. Detection of varicella zoster virus DNA and viral antigen in the late stage of bilateral acute retinal necrosis syndrome. *Arch Ophthalmol.* 1992;110:1132–1136.

Frosted Branch Angiitis

Kleiner RC, et al. Acute frosted retinal periphlebitis. *Am J Ophthalmol.* 1988;106:27–34.

Sugin AL, et al. Unilateral frosted branch angiitis. *Am J Ophthalmol.* 1991;111:682–685.

Cavernous Hemangioma of the Retina

Alexander LJ, Moates KN. Cavernous hemangioma of the retina. *J Am Optom Assoc.* 1988;59:539–548.

Asdourian GK. Vascular anomalies of the retina. *Perspect Ophthalmol.* 1979;3:111–119.

Messmer E, et al. Nine cases of cavernous hemangioma of the retina. *Am J Ophthalmol.* 1983;95:383–390.

Angiomatosis Retinae

Alexander LJ, Moates KN. Cavernous hemangioma of the retina. *J Am Optom Assoc.* 1988;59:539–548.

Augsburger JJ, et al. Classification and management of hereditary retinal angiomas. *Int Ophthalmol.* 1981;4: 93–106.

Gass JDM, Braunstein R. Sessile and exophytic capillary angioma of the juxtapapillary retina and optic nerve head. *Arch Ophthalmol.* 1980;98:1790–1797.

Hardwig P, Robertson DM. Von Hippel–Lindau disease: A familial, often lethal, multi-system phakomatosis. *Ophthalmology.* 1984;91:263–270.

Kremer I, et al. Juxtapapillary exophytic retinal capillary hemangioma treated by yellow krypton (568 nm) laser photocoagulation. *Ophthalmic Surg.* 1988;19:743–747.

Lane CM, et al. Laser treatment of retinal angiomatosis. *Eye.* 1989;3:33–38.

Peyman GA, et al. Treatment of large von Hippel tumors by eye wall resection. *Ophthalmology.* 1983;90:840–847.

Whitson JT, et al. Von Hippel–Lindau disease: Case report of a patient with spontaneous regression of a retinal angioma. *Retina.* 1986;6:253–259.

Coats' Disease

Annesley WH, et al. Fifteen-year review of treated cases of retinal angiomatosis. *Trans Am Acad Ophthalmol Otolaryngol.* 1977;83:446–453.

Asdourian GK. Vascular anomalies of the retina. *Perspect Ophthalmol.* 1979;3:111–119.

Ridley ME, et al. Coats' disease: Evaluation of management. *Ophthalmology.* 1982;89:1381–1387.

Silodor SW, et al. Natural history and management of advanced Coats' disease. *Ophthalmic Surg.* 1988;19:89–93.

Tarkkanen A, Laatikainen L. Coats' disease: Clinical, angiographic, histopathological findings and clinical management. *Br J Ophthalmol.* 1981;67:766–776.

Racemose Hemangioma

Alexander LJ, Moates KN. Cavernous hemangioma of the retina. *J Am Optom Assoc.* 1988;59:539–548.

Asdourian GK. Vascular anomalies of the retina. *Perspect Ophthalmol.* 1979;3:111–119.

Mansour AM, et al. Ocular complications of arteriovenous communications of the retina. *Arch Ophthalmol.* 1989;107:232–236.

Mansour AM, et al. Arteriovenous anastomoses of the retina. *Ophthalmology.* 1987;94:35–40.

Choroidal Hemangiomas

Anand R, et al. Circumscribed choroidal hemangiomas. *Arch Ophthalmol.* 1989;107:1338–1342.

Augsburger JJ, et al. Circumscribed choroidal hemangiomas: Long-term visual prognosis. *Retina.* 1981;1:56–61.

Jarrett JH, et al. Clinical experience with presumed hemangioma of the choroid: Radioactive phosphorus uptake studies as an aid in differential diagnosis. *Trans Am Acad Ophthalmol Otolaryngol.* 1976;81:862–870.

Lindsey PS, et al. Bilateral choroidal hemangiomas and facial nevus flammeus. *Retina.* 1981;1:88–95.

Sanborn GE, et al. Treatment of circumscribed choroidal hemangiomas. *Ophthalmology.* 1982;89:1374–1380.

Witschel H, Front RL. Hemangioma of the choroid. *Surv Ophthalmol.* 1976;20:415–431.

Chapter Five ■ ■ ■ ■ ■ ■

Exudative and Nonexudative Macular Disorders

The clinician is well aware of the importance of maintaining the integrity of the macular area of the retina. The concentration of photoreceptors in this area requires an exquisite vascular supply for proper function. This complex and active vascular supply makes the macular area particularly susceptible to compromise, often in the form of edema or leakage from various sources. Often this compromise can be predicted, and with proper and timely intervention, severe loss of vision can be averted, at least over a limited period of time. Prevalence of the various reported macular disorders is on the rise because of the relationship of macular disease to age, the increasing age of the world population, and our improved ability to differentially diagnose. To understand diagnosis and management of macular disease, the clinician must first have a working knowledge of the clinicopathology of the macular region of the retina.

RETINAL ANATOMY RELEVANT TO THE MACULOPATHIES

Gross Anatomy

The central posterior portion of the eye is clinically known as the posterior pole. The area is usually considered to be demarcated by the major vascular arcades (Fig. 5–1). The macula is about 1.5 mm centered around the 0.35–mm fovea. The macular region is brownish yellow as compared to the remainder of the

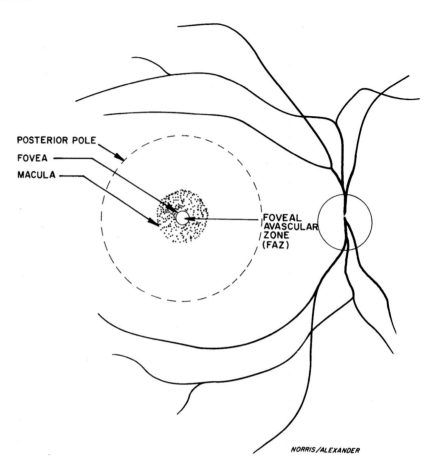

Figure 5–1. A schematic representation of the clinical posterior retina.

NORRIS/ALEXANDER

retina. The yellow coloration is due to xanthophyll pigment and is more apparent in darkly pigmented individuals. This yellow pigment combined with high-density retinal pigment epithelium (RPE) creates blockage of background choroidal fluorescence in all phases. Unfortunately, the yellow xanthophyll pigment also has a tendency to attract and concentrate blue light, which may be a factor in the genesis of some of the age-related maculopathies. The xanthophyll also attracts and concentrates the blue wavelengths incorporated into some of the lasers used to treat the retina. The area devoid of retinal capillaries surrounding the fovea is known as the foveal avascular zone, and is 0.5 to 0.6 mm in diameter. This portion of the retina receives nutrition from the choriocapillaris.

Sensory Retina

The sensory retina is comprised of nine specific layers. From the vitreous toward the RPE the retina consists of the (1) internal limiting membrane, (2) nerve fiber layer, (3) ganglion cell layer, (4) inner plexiform layer, (5) inner nuclear layer, (6) outer plexiform layer, (7) outer nuclear layer, (8) external limiting membrane,

and (9) rod and cone inner and outer portions. For this clinical discussion, these nine layers will be referred to as the sensory retina. The retinal pigment epithelium binds loosely to the sensory retina; then Bruch's membrane binds more firmly to the RPE. The differences in the adherence of the sensory retina to the RPE and the RPE to Bruch's membrane make it easier to detach the sensory retina from the RPE than to detach the RPE from Bruch's membrane. Underneath Bruch's membrane is the swamplike choroid/choriocapillaris. Bruch's membrane, when intact, forms a fluid barrier to prevent the flow from the choroid/choriocapillaris to under the RPE and sensory retina. The collagenous sclera envelopes the entire package, forming a barrier very resistant to escape of fluids.

The retinal structure is markedly different in the macular zone. In the central fovea the only retinal layer present is the photoreceptor layer. The majority of cells in this area are cones. As the fovea unfolds up the clivus, the retina accumulates additional layers from the outer retina inward. Very near the fovea, the outer plexiform layer forms the thickened Henle's layer. This variation of structure in the macular zone lends to the characteristic patterns that develop in many disease processes, such as cystoid macular edema.

Retinal Pigment Epithelium (RPE)

The retinal pigment epithelium (RPE) is a uniform single layer of cells that is situated between the sensory retina and Bruch's membrane. The cells of the RPE are cuboidal, usually heavily pigmented (melanin granules in cytoplasm), and hexagonal in shape. The cells have a reasonably tight junction to one another. The RPE functions to hold structures together, provides a barrier to the swamplike choroid, processes metabolites, and absorbs light.

Bruch's Membrane

Bruch's membrane functions with the RPE to provide a barrier and supportive system to the retina. The interaction of the RPE and Bruch's membrane is crucial in the pathologic process of a number of retinal and choroidal diseases. Bruch's membrane is considered to consist of five layers: (1) basement membrane of the RPE, (2) inner collagenous zone, (3) elastic layer, (4) outer collagenous zone, and (5) basement membrane of the choriocapillaris.

Choroid/Choriocapillaris

The choriocapillaris layer is the capillary complex adjacent to Bruch's membrane. The short posterior ciliary arteries, recurrent branches of the long ciliary arteries, and branches of the anterior ciliary arteries provide the arterial blood supply to this area. This area drains into the vortex veins. The vessels in the choriocapillaris are fenestrated, allowing for a free exchange of fluids with surrounding tissues. The choriocapillaris is the densest beneath the macula. The density at the macula allows for the necessarily high hemodynamic activity and creates the potential for the genesis of vision compromise associated with edema and leakage especially related to the vascular system.

The choroidal stroma lies external to the choriocapillaris. The choroid is comprised of blood vessels, nerves, immune cells, fibroblasts, collagenous supportive tissue, and melanocytes. The larger choroidal vessels seen by ophthalmoscopy are usually veins. The presence of immunologic cells in the choroid speaks to the relationship of choroidal disease to some of the systemic immunologic diseases such as histoplasmosis. The suprachoroid lies between the choroid and the sclera. The choroid is responsible for the nutritional (vascular) supply to the RPE and the outer one third of the sensory retina.

Sclera

The entire ocular structure is surrounded by the predominantly acellular sclera, which functions to maintain the shape and integrity of the intraocular contents. The sclera does not actively participate in ocular metabolism.

THE ISSUE OF DRUSEN

The issue of retinal drusen is complex at best. The term "drusen" means many different things to different people, and it must be realized that it does refer to many different retinal/RPE/Bruch's alterations. The drusen may take on multiple clinical presentation, and the only for-sure thing about drusen is that if you see them in one eye, you should see a mirror image in the fellow eye. If you do not, you may be seeing something other than drusen.

Retinal drusen have been classically described in the following manner according to appearance:

1. Hard drusen, which appear as small, well-defined yellow deposits deep in the retina. Often the overlying RPE appears depigmented. Hard drusen are thought to consist of hyaline material in the inner and outer collagenous layers of Bruch's membrane.
2. Soft drusen, which are larger and more fluffy than hard drusen, and consist of material between the basement membrane of the RPE and the inner collagenous layer of Bruch's membrane. These soft drusen are typically present in over 25 percent of patients over the age of 70 years.
3. Basilar laminar drusen, which are present in young patients and appear as multiple, fine yellow spots. The basilar drusen are thought to be hyaline thickening of the basement membrane of the RPE.
4. Calcific drusen, which are long-standing drusen that have aged and calcified, often appearing as cholesterol glistening deposits.
5. Mixed-variety drusen.

Although neither the true pathogenesis nor the total implications of drusen are entirely understood, it is known that drusen do represent an altered state of the metabolically healthy retinal complex. If multiple extramacular drusen are present, there is an over 80 percent chance of macular degenerative abnormalities as compared to only a 2 percent chance in the population without drusen.

Drusen have been described as hyaline deposits lying underneath the RPE. Drusen are associated with retinal pathology, Bruch's membrane disease, choriocapillaris and choroidal disease, retinal pigment epithelial disease, systemic diseases such as diabetes, and space-occupying lesions of the choroid such as benign choroidal melanomas.

The RPE/Bruch's membrane complex is the area of activity in the genesis of drusen. The RPE is derived from the neuroectoderm and acts to maintain the health of the outer retinal layers. The RPE forms an outer blood–retina barrier, is integral in vitamin A metabolism, works in the transport of metabolites between the choriocapillaris/choroid complex and the retina, manufactures extracellular mucopolysaccharides, functions to eliminate damaged and discarded photoreceptor outer segments, and also works to envelop and negate the effects of developing choroidal neovascular nets. There is a strong juncture between RPE cells known as the zonula occludens that prevents significant fluid seepage between the choriocapillaris and the retina. The metabolism of the RPE is intimately related to the health of the choriocapillaris. It is also important to note that the RPE is tightly adherent to Bruch's membrane and very loosely adherent to the overlying retina.

When RPE cells are not functioning properly, they elaborate an extracellular material such as collagen and basement membrane material, which is deposited or "spit out" onto Bruch's membrane. The resulting excrescences are called drusen and are composed of mucopolysaccharides and lipids. The triggering mechanism is unknown but is thought to be related directly to choriocapillaris disease.

When considering drusen in the macular area, the health of the choriocapillaris has an intimate relationship. The choriocapillaris supply to the macular area is derived primarily from arterioles coming from the short posterior ciliary arteries. These arterioles terminate in small compartments. In the eyes of patients with age-related macular disease (ARM), there is a

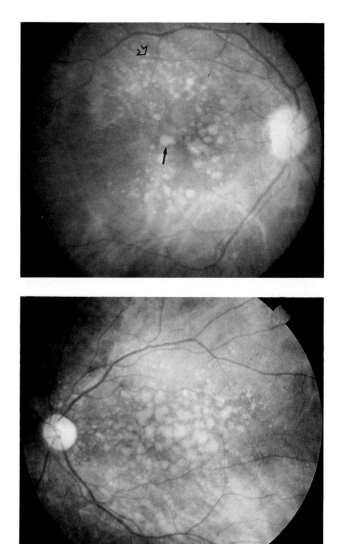

Figure 5–3. The paired photographs represent an example of the confluence of soft drusen in the macular area.

narrowing of the capillary lumen, foci of atrophy of the capillaries, and a loss of cellularity of the capillaries. This situation may create a condition of "zone hypoxia" such as that which occurs overlying a benign choroidal melanoma (choroidal nevus). This zone hypoxia results in a "sick" RPE area that creates the deposition of drusen. The concept of local or zone hypoxia is supported by the occurrence of drusen with systemic vascular diseases such as cardiovascular disease, hypertension, and diabetes.

Drusen may then progress to further changes that can affect the health and architectural integrity of the overlying retina. The drusen are, however, observable in well over 70 percent of the population over the age of 50 years, but do not negatively affect all of those eyes. As the deposition of the drusen increases with age, the RPE cells undergo further thinning and loss

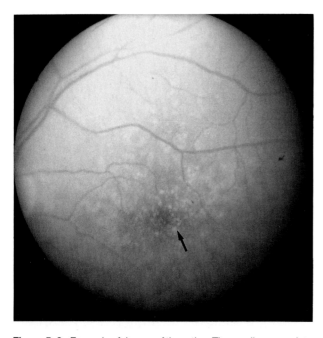

Figure 5–2. Example of drusen of the retina. The small arrow points to the very small hard drusen present in the macular area.

of function. In addition, there are fibrovascular changes within the drusen. There can be a variable color presentation that is associated with lipofuscin accumulation. These zones of drusen may progress on toward calcification (Figs. 5–2 and 5–3) and the development of rifts in Bruch's. The final aging change that occurs related to drusen is the accumulation of granular deposits near the drusen lying between the RPE and Bruch's. These areas of deposition seem to be the actual sites of ingress of choroidal neovascularization. It is well recognized that small, discrete drusen are less likely to be associated with choroidal neovascularization than larger soft "drusen." What in fact may be occurring is the deposition of drusen in the classical sense with nearby granular deposits in a larger area giving the appearance of soft, confluent drusen. These soft, confluent drusen may be localized zones of RPE detachment.

Drusen, then, are signs of RPE abnormalities that are not necessarily an assurance that atrophy of the overlying retina will occur or that choroidal neovascularization will occur, leading to exudative maculopathy. The only absolute is that the appearance of large, soft, fuzzy-white "drusen" indicates a compromised RPE that may lead to the development of dry or wet maculopathy. These fuzzy-white drusen may be referred to as choroidal infiltrates to distinguish them from the less threatening atrophic dry drusen.

One last point to be made is that the risk of choroidal neovascularization and exudative maculopathy decreases as RPE atrophy progresses. Further

progression of RPE atrophy indicates poor choroidal vascular perfusion. If the choroidal vessels are dying, it is impossible to support new vessel growth. Therefore, when significant RPE loss occurs or if drusen calcify with cholestrin crystal deposition, the possibility of growth of neovascularization is reduced. **See color plates 53 to 55.** Further discussion of this topic is included in "Biochemical/Vitamin/Light Damage Associated With Macular Degeneration" later in the chapter.

THE ISSUE OF CHOROIDAL NEOVASCULARIZATION AND RPE DETACHMENT

Once an alteration of Bruch's membrane occurs, there is the possibility of choroidal neovascular growth and infiltration under the RPE, sensory retina, or both. Figures 5–4 to 5–6 show the progression of the ocular changes toward the development of choroidal neovascularization. Figures 5–7 to 5–11 depict variations on the development of choroidal neovascular membranes and RPE detachments. There is also the possibility that seepage through the alterations may occur, creating a localized RPE detachment. The primary area of concern within the retina is the macular zone, as the hemodynamic activity is very high in this area, and small changes in oxygenated blood flow can create dramatic changes in function and structure.

Detachment of the RPE without choroidal neo-

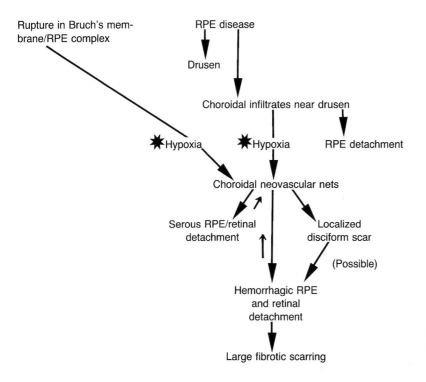

Figure 5–4. A flowchart demonstrating the stages in the evolution of choroidal neovascular nets.

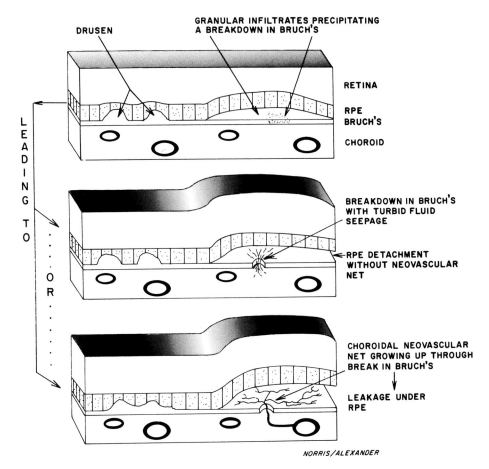

Figure 5–5. This figure illustrates alterations of Bruch's membrane in the form of drusen and granular infiltration. The granular infiltration allows for choroidal neovascular net development.

NORRIS/ALEXANDER

vascularization can occur. This usually occurs associated with other signs of RPE dysfunction such as drusen. In over 90 percent of cases of RPE detachment, an associated sensory detachment occurs as well. RPE detachments in patients under the age of 55 have an associated excellent visual prognosis and rarely lead to choroidal neovascularization. In patients over the age of 55, RPE detachment is a poor prognostic sign. The associated visual loss may be the result of atrophy, choroidal neovascularization, or a retinal pigment epithelial tear. If there is turbidity (haziness) of the accompanying fluid or if there is hemorrhage, the prognosis is up to 90 percent likelihood of 20/200 or less as compared to a prognosis of 20/200 in only up to 33 percent of patients with only a serous detachment.

Up to 30 percent of patients with RPE detachments over age 55 years will develop choroidal neovascularization; RPE tears develop in about 10 percent. The diagnosis of the RPE detachment requires a combination of stereoscopic observation and fluorescein angiography. When the detachment occurs without hemorrhage, the appearance is a dome with turbid intralesional fluid that may have accompanying hard exudate deposition. On fluorescein angiog-

raphy, the lesion glows early and evenly and remains stained late into the process. The presence of an RPE detachment does not necessarily guarantee the presence of a choroidal neovascular net. It is possible to have spontaneous RPE detachment remission or progression toward further retinal destruction. Choroidal neovascularization can occur in many ocular disease processes. A number of these are listed in Table 5–1.

Choroidal neovascularization is often classified by type according to the location in the macula, as follows.

1. A subfoveal neovascular membrane extends underneath the center of the foveal avascular zone.
2. A juxtafoveal neovascular membrane extends to within 1 to 199 microns from the center of the foveal avascular zone.
3. An extrafoveal neovascular membrane extends no closer than 200 microns from the center of the foveal avascular zone.

There are several routes of retinal destruction associated with choroidal neovascularization. All routes of destruction start with the growth of a neovascular net up through an area of compromise in the RPE/Bruch's complex. This neovascular net initially

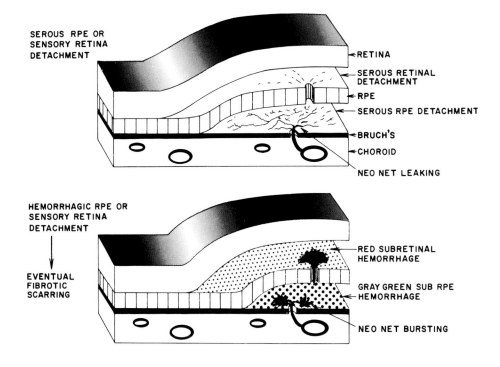

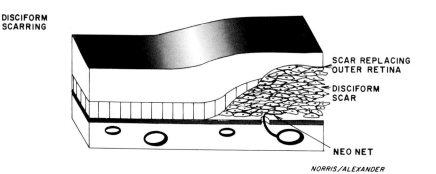

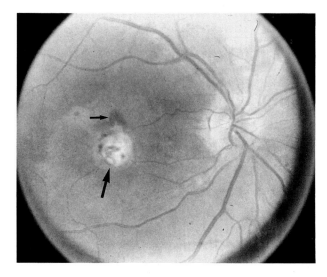

Figure 5–6. The possible consequences of the development of choroidal neovascularization.

NORRIS/ALEXANDER

TABLE 5–1. CONDITIONS ASSOCIATED WITH CHOROIDAL NEOVASCULAR DEVELOPMENT

Wet age-related maculopathy
Presumed ocular histoplasmosis
Inflammatory chorioretinal diseases
Postphotocoagulative scarring
Angioid streaks
Degenerative myopia
Choroidal rupture
Dominant drusen
Vitelliform dystrophy
Optic nerve head drusen—even at a very young age
Benign choroidal melanoma
Rubella retinopathy
Harada's disease
APMPPE
Osseous choroidoma
Geographical helicoid peripapillary choroidopathy
Retinal hamartomas
Cryosurgery
Behçet's disease
Chronic uveitis
Idiopathic

Figure 5–7. This photograph illustrates a "golf-ball" disciform sear (*large arrow*) and subretinal hemorrhage (*small arrow*) secondary to a choroidal neovascular net.

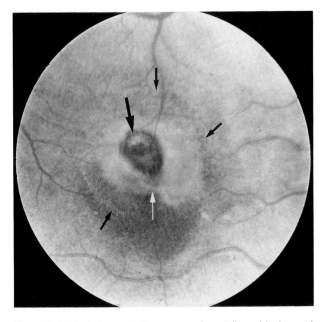

Figure 5–8. A photograph of a neovascular net (*large black arrow*) creating a sensory retinal elevation, the limits of which are indicated by the small black arrows. The white arrow indicates the notch in the sensory elevation at the fovea that occurs because of the anatomic resistance in this area.

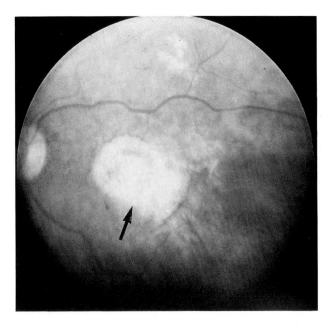

Figure 5–10. Example of a large disciform scar (*arrow*) associated with wet ARM.

appears as a gray-green area. The appearance occurs as the result of fibrosis accompanying the new vessels. As the fibrosis progresses, the color becomes yellowish. With the development of the net there is RPE hyperplasia and leakage, causing RPE, sensory retinal elevation, or both. This elevation creates metamorphopsia, vision reduction, or both. The fluid accumulation associated with the sensory retinal detachment is to be contrasted with that of idiopathic central serous choroidopathy (ICSC). The fluid in ICSC is

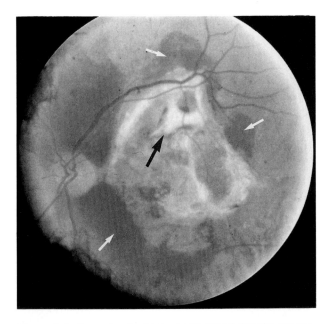

Figure 5–9. Example of a hemorrhagic retinal detachment secondary to a ruptured neovascular net. The small white arrows point to residual hemorrhage, while the large black arrow points to scarring.

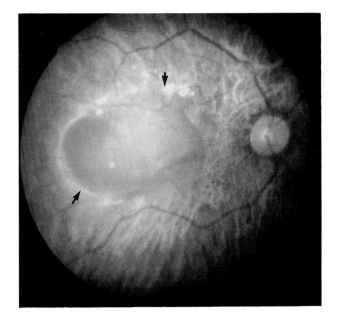

Figure 5–11. Example of the development of a retinal pigment epithelial detachment (non-rhegmatogenous retinal detachment). The small arrows point to the hard exudates (Coats' response) surrounding the detachment.

usually clear, and that associated with choroidal neovascularization creating a sensory retinal detachment is often turbid due to protein extravasation. The RPE detachment associated with choroidal neovascularization is often indistinguishable from a leak-induced RPE detachment until fluorescein angiography is performed. In all cases of choroidal neovascularization, fluorescein angiography will demonstrate an early-onset, hot-spot-spoked wheel that spreads to include the entire area of leakage.

The neovascular net may regress if enveloped by RPE, or it may progress to hemorrhage or disciform scarring. The envelopment is evidenced clinically by a pigmentary hyperplasia occurring in the zone of the neovascular net. When the net hemorrhages, blood first accumulates between Bruch's and the retinal pigment epithelium. The hemorrhage at this phase is gray-green. Should the hemorrhage spread through the RPE into the subretinal space, it will assume a reddish coloration. This type of hemorrhage has also been known to break through into the vitreous cavity. In all stages, subretinal and intraretinal exudate is possible and is classically known as Coat's response. In fact, hard exudate formation in the absence of ophthalmoscopically visible retinal vascular disease is a very strong indicator of choroidal neovascular disease or conditions such as retinal macroaneurysms or retinal vascular tumors.

During the involutional stage, the hemorrhage can organize with accompanying fibrotic scarring, resulting in severe, widespread retinal destruction and a resultant extensive central scotoma.

TABLE 5–2. CLINICAL FINDINGS COMMON TO CHOROIDAL NEOVASCULAR MEMBRANES

Ophthalmoscopic Findings

Subretinal or subretinal pigment epithelial blood
Retinal, subretinal, or subretinal pigment epithelial exudates
Subretinal fluid accumulation
Subretinal pigment ring
Retinal pigment epithelial detachment
Subretinal plaque
Disciform scar
Macular edema
Folds extending from the scar or subretinal activity

Angiographic Findings

Lacy neovascularization early in the fluorescein process
Diffuse subretinal leakage late in the fluorescein process
Diffuse leakage with some blockage of fluorescence secondary to hemorrhage or exudate
Retinal pigment epithelial detachment flume throughout the fluorescein process
Irregular filling or blockage of background choroidal fluorescence
Tortuous vessels due to retinal folding seen early in the fluorescein process
Cystoid petalliform filling

The neovascular net may also pursue a more insidious course of development. The net may grow, being somewhat retarded by disciform scarring and RPE hyperplasia. The development of the disciform scar complex will initially limit the totality of retinal destruction and limit the size of the central scotoma. This scar may, however, reactivate, leading to a more destructive hemorrhagic scar. **See color plates 56 through 71.** Table 5–2 summarizes the typical clinical appearances of choroidal neovascular membranes.

BIOCHEMICAL/VITAMIN/LIGHT DAMAGE ASSOCIATED WITH MACULAR DEGENERATION

As a major cause of blindness and visual disability, age-related macular degeneration afflicts millions of Americans. The problem is becoming more apparent because of the increased numbers of elderly patients within our society. Age-related macular degeneration is characterized by two forms, dry and wet, with both involving alteration of the retina, RPE, Bruch's membrane, and choroidal complex. The deterioration is most severe in the outer layers of the macular zone of the retina. Several theories exist regarding the specific pathogenic factors involved in the involutionary changes, all being the consequences of vascular insufficiency and deposition of abnormal materials within the ocular tissues. Drusen are considered to be the hallmark of macular degeneration, with the soft variety being strongly suggestive of the development of neovascular membranes. The true composition of the drusen is controversial, but is known to vary throughout the eye. All variations of drusen indicate a breakdown of the RPE/Bruch's membrane complex.

Lipofuscin accumulation also increases within the RPE with age. This lipofuscin accumulation is thought to be related to photo-oxidative mechanisms. The deposition of lipofuscin is secondary to "stressed" RPE as well as an accumulation of shed components of the photoreceptor outer segments. This combination has been implicated as a possible factor in macular degeneration. The lipofuscin deposition is accelerated with dietary deficiencies of antioxidants such as vitamin A.

The risk factors for age-related macular degeneration include (1) increasing age (peak ages at 75 to 85 years), (2) positive family history, (3) weakness of hand grip, (4) hyperopia, (5) light-colored irides and hair, (6) suggestions that whites are more affected than blacks, (7) association of solar radiation with retinal damage and (8) smoking.

Solar radiation is thought to be a major contributing factor in macular degeneration. Laboratory studies support the conclusion that damage to the retina from visible radiation is localized in the RPE and rod and cone layer and is most evident in the macular area. The high-energy short-wavelength end of the spectrum (blue light hazard) is much more hazardous than the longer wavelengths of light. Refer to Figure 5–12 to understand the effect of blue light on the retina. Photochemical damage created by high energy is thought to be additive, as the biological system may be unable to control the damage and repair the system, especially as the patient ages. The most dramatic evidence of this irreversible photochemical damage is solar retinopathy. The melanin within the RPE has a tendency to afford protection by actually absorbing some of the energy. On the other hand, the lipofuscin in the RPE is an aggregation of damaged molecules that absorb more energy and re-emit this energy into the photoreceptors to create even more damage. With age, melanin concentration decreases while lipofuscin concentration increases, setting the stage for further photo-oxidative damage.

The retina is protected from most ultraviolet radiation (UVR) by the facial anatomy; the cornea, which absorbs 100 percent of UV-C (290 to 100 nm); and the crystalline lens, which absorbs UV-B (320 to 290 nm). As the crystalline lens ages, the absorption increases, to include most radiation of 370 nm and below. Unfortunately, a lot of blue-end light is allowed penetration to the retina. The UVR effect on the retina should, therefore, be more prevalent in unprotected aphakic patients. The National Health and Nutrition Examination Survey (NHANES) suggests that light-induced damage does create an increase of age-related macular degeneration in aphakic eyes. The initial findings of the population-based Chesapeake Bay watermen found no association with UV-A or UV-B and

macular degeneration. However, a reanalysis of the data establishing the relationship of exposure to blue and visible light to age-related macular degeneration revealed differing conclusions. Increasing duration of exposure to blue and visible light demonstrated an associated increase in more severe grades of age-related macular degeneration. The conclusion was drawn that there was a strong association between exposure to blue and visible light over the prior 20 years, suggesting that early life exposure is not as significant as exposure later in life. This is probably related to the decreased ability of the retina to repair solar damage as the patient ages. When evaluating the action spectrum shown in Figure 5–12 it becomes apparent that wavelengths shorter than 430 nm should be filtered out to minimize the risks of the development of age-related macular degeneration and cataracts.

In addition to physical structural changes, photodynamic effects can produce chains of events altering oxygen to a superoxide-free radical, which can then initiate a chain of lipid peroxidation. This chain can then alter cell membranes or can create abnormal molecular aggregates. The reaction then leads to further formation of lipofuscin within the RPE, creating more degradation. The process is very dynamic within the retina, as the oxygen flow in the RPE/photoreceptor complex is higher than at any site in the body. The oxidation process puts the rod and cone outer segments at particularly high risk.

There are molecular mechanisms within the retina that can exert damage control in the photodynamic process. The enzyme superoxide dismutase (photoreceptor outer segments) scavenges the superoxide radical, converting it to harmless H_2O_2 and O_2. Glutathione peroxidase (retina and RPE) protects against the formation of lipid hydroperoxides and hydrogen. It is believed that glutathione peroxidase requires selenium for function, and that riboflavin is important in reducing oxidized glutathione. Catalase is linked to rod outer segment degradation phagocytosis and prevention of lipid peroxidation in the RPE. The catalase activity is highest in the RPE and decreases with age and macular degeneration. Iron, zinc, and copper are essential cations in the formation of all of these enzymes.

Vitamins C and E are antioxidants that quench singlet oxygen and terminate chain reactions. Vitamin E deficiency in laboratory animals actually induces increases in RPE lipofuscin deposition rates. Aging, however, results in increases in vitamin E levels in the retina and RPE, as does light adaptation. This "naturally occurring phenomenon" may then be serving as a protective function within the retina. Vitamin E deficiency has been implicated in degenerative diseases including age-related macular degeneration and phototoxic degeneration of photoreceptor cells. The the-

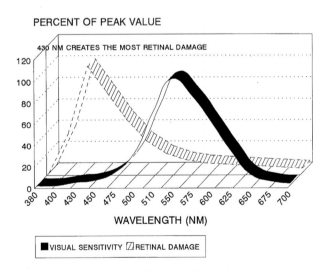

Figure 5–12. Comparison of the visual sensitivity peak spectrum and the peak spectrum for damage to the retina. (*Reproduced with permission from Alexander LJ. Ocular vitamin therapy. A review and assessment. Optom Clin. 1992;2:1–34.*)

ory is that peroxidation of unsaturated fatty acids in phospholipids, which produce toxic intermediates, results in cellular damage in the absence of sufficient vitamin E. The rod outer segments and the RPE are particularly sensitive to the peroxidation activity, and both of these layers have the highest concentration of vitamin E. These tissues are usually last to give up their concentrations of vitamin E during dietary deprivation. One study (Katz and Eldred, 1989) challenges the antioxidative activity of vitamin E in cyclic light exposure, finding that Vitamin E deficiency did not enhance the photo-oxidative effects. This study concludes that photosensitized autoxidation is unlikely to play a significant role in light-mediated damage to the retina.

In laboratory animals, if there is a dietary deprivation of vitamin E and the retina is irradiated, there is a notable increase in the amount of hydroperoxide formed in the retina. It has also been shown that dietary supplementation of vitamin C raises the level of ascorbate in the retina and RPE, thereby reducing the quantity of hydroperoxides formed, which minimizes the overall cellular damage. There is also evidence suggesting that beta-carotene (vitamin A) reduces radiation damage to the retina in primates.

A 1988 study by Newsome and co-workers brought vitamin therapy for age-related macular degeneration into the spotlight. In a clinical study, this group investigated the effects of oral zinc administration on the visual acuity outcome in 151 subjects with drusen or macular degeneration. The "treated" group received 100 mg of oral zinc sulfate twice a day with meals. Although some eyes in the zinc-treated group lost vision, the treated group had significantly less visual loss than the placebo group after 12 to 24 months of follow-up (Figs. 5–13 and 5–14). It was carefully noted in the study that "because of the pilot nature of

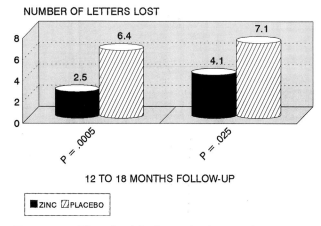

Figure 5–14. Effect of oral zinc in macular degeneration as gauged by visual loss with time. (*Reproduced with permission from Alexander LJ. Ocular vitamin therapy. A review and assessment. Optom Clin. 1992;2:1–34.*)

the study and the possible toxic effects and complications of oral zinc, . . . that . . . widespread use of zinc in macular degeneration is not now warranted." Newsome and associates also cautioned about the effects of zinc on copper depletion with the possible consequence of anemia.

In a non-refereed symposium report in the April, 1991, *Ocular Surgery News*, Pomerance and associates discuss the effect of antioxidants on visual acuity and contrast sensitivity in patients with macular degeneration. The data are summarized in Figure 5–15, showing vision and contrast sensitivity improvement in different initial visual acuity groups after 6 months of treatment. The study was performed on 192 patients with age-related macular degeneration. The patients were placed on ICAPS Plus, a nutritional supplement, at 2 tablets a day if they were under 132 pounds and 4 tablets a day if over 132 pounds. The authors main-

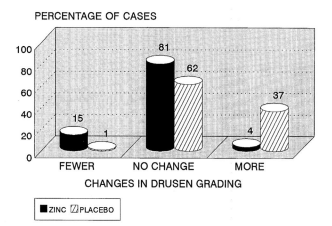

Figure 5–13. Effect of oral zinc in macular degeneration changes associated with grading of drusen. (*Reproduced with permission from Alexander LJ. Ocular vitamin therapy. A review and assessment. Optom Clin. 1992;2:1–34.*)

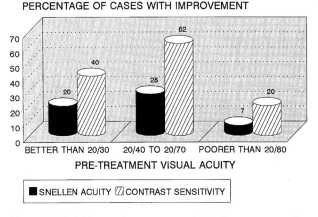

Figure 5–15. Vision and contrast sensitivity improvement after 6-month treatment with ICAPS Plus (192 patients with ARM). (*Reproduced with permission from Alexander LJ. Ocular vitamin therapy. A review and assessment. Optom Clin. 1992;2:1–34.*)

tain that contrast sensitivity is an excellent means of assessing progress because of the tolerance of the consequences of outside effects such as patient reliability and attention span. The study found that 63.5 percent of all the patients treated reported better-quality vision even if they did not demonstrate acuity or contrast sensitivity improvement. Keep in mind, however, that this study is not in a refereed journal. In the same symposium report, Mamalis and co-workers reported the results shown in Figure 5–16. His group addressed the effect of compliance of the use of ICAPS Plus on the resultant visual acuity. Their conclusion was that good compliance resulted in less vision loss than poor compliance. Again, however, the study does not appear in a refereed journal. Faulkner, in the same symposium report, makes the point that the results from vitamin supplementation in age-related macular degeneration are not to be expected immediately. He says to tell the patients not to expect anything for a year, because his anecdotal experience is that improvement is not attained until 9 to 12 months into therapy. This symposium also suggests that the vitamin supplementation may be of benefit in other macular conditions such as cystoid macular edema. Other unpublished studies also support the efficacy of oral vitamin and mineral supplementation for the patient with macular degeneration.

Currently there are well-controlled clinical trials being designed and conducted (Age-related Eye Disease Study) that may once and for all answer the question regarding the benefits of vitamin supplementation as it relates to age-related macular degeneration. Further studies should also address the claims that interferon-alpha$_{2a}$ injected every other day for 6 to 8 weeks may have a positive effect on retarding macular degeneration.

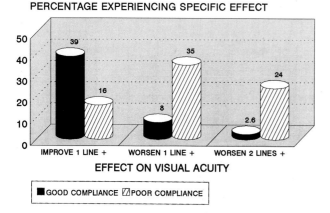

PERCENTAGE EXPERIENCING SPECIFIC EFFECT

Figure 5–16. Effect of compliance on visual change in patients with macular degeneration receiving ICAPS Plus vitamin supplement. (*Reproduced with permission from Alexander LJ. Ocular vitamin therapy. A review and assessment. Optom Clin. 1992; 2:1–34.*)

Current commercially available ocular vitamin supplements contain the beta-carotene form of vitamin A, ascorbic acid (vitamin C), vitamin E, zinc, and copper. The most significant controversy as to which is the best surrounds the form of zinc contained in each product. It is contended that the bioavailability of zinc oxide is not as great as other water-soluble forms of the element. Prasad (1978) contends that zinc acetate achieves a higher blood plasma level than zinc oxide in a shorter interval of time. He also states that zinc aminoate and zinc acetate were almost identical in action. This finding is, however, controversial. The zinc oxide form is not water soluble and purportedly maintains its concentration longer. All forms of zinc have the strong potential to aggravate the gastrointestinal system. If you were to choose to recommend an over-the-counter multivitamin, to achieve the same therapeutic level for beta-carotene, zinc, and copper as one of the ocular vitamins, a potential overdose could occur with vitamins A and D, which each have a significant toxicity.

The latest word regarding management of patients with macular degeneration is to (1) recommend a healthy diet that includes more fruits and vegetables and less fat, (2) caution patients about potential risks of taking megadoses of vitamins and minerals, and (3) tell those patients already taking supplements for eye disease that supplementation has not yet been proven to be helpful and that more definitive research is now under way. Any supplemental vitamin therapy must be approached with caution. Early results from a large multicenter case-controlled study show high carotenoid intake may actually reduce the risk of ARM by 70 percent, and that high serum levels of vitamins C and E also created a 20 to 40 percent risk reduction. These early findings also suggest that selenium and zinc supplementation do not create a significant positive effect.

Some studies support the use of antioxidant supplementation to control the development of cataracts and are based on the same principles as those governing the development of retinal disease.

AGE-RELATED MACULAR DEGENERATION

Age-related macular degeneration (ARM) is the number one cause of legal blindness in the United States in persons over 65 years of age. Age-related macular degeneration is present in about 10 percent of the population over age 52, and in up to 33 percent of persons over the age of 75 years. The Framingham Eye Study reports rates of up to 7 percent of the aged population. There are two distinctive forms of ARM, with variations within these categories. The more common form of ARM is dry ARM, or geographic RPE atrophy. This is present in about 15 percent of eyes by the age of 80 years. Of the patients with ARM who are not legally blind, about 90 percent have dry ARM. The less common form of ARM is wet ARM. Wet ARM can be of several forms: (1) choroidal neovascularization, (2) exudative degeneration, (3) hemorrhagic degeneration leading to fibrotic scarring, or (4) disciform macular degeneration. Of the patients who are legally blind from ARM, about 90 percent have the wet variety. Wet age-related maculopathy is more common in whites than blacks, and is probably related to the increased presence of melanin in the retinas of blacks. Although etiology and predisposing factors are uncertain, some reports suggest a familial tendency in the development of ARM. One interesting finding is that the more lightly pigmented the iris is in a patient, the more likely the patient is to develop ARM at an earlier age. This is consistent with the reduced protective levels of melanin pigment in the retina.

The distinction between wet and dry ARM is crucial, as the severe vision loss of wet ARM may be delayed or prevented by timely photocoagulative intervention. The more benign dry ARM will now be differentiated from the potentially vision-threatening wet ARM.

Dry (Nonexudative) ARM

Introduction and Description. The discussion of dry ARM is a direct extension of the previous section on RPE/Bruch's membrane abnormalities. Patients with macular drusen are at an increased risk of developing ARM both dry and wet. An increase in the

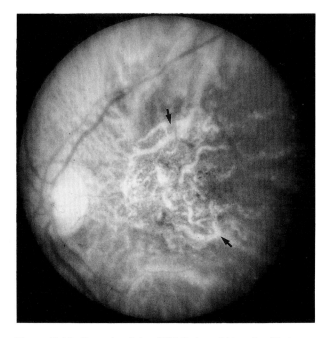

Figure 5–18. Example of dry ARM that could be classified as a geographic variety. The small arrows delineate the boundaries of the atrophy.

incidence of drusen and of dry ARM occurs in patients over 60 years of age.

From an ophthalmoscopic view, there is initially an observable alteration of the RPE in dry ARM (Figs. 5–17 and 5–18). This alteration is usually bilateral and eventually somewhat symmetrical. There are areas of depigmentation, areas of granular clumping of RPE, and areas of RPE hyperplasia, all reflecting a basic disease process of the RPE. Patterns of presentation are unpredictable. With time these areas of RPE change may coalesce into geographic patterns.

Geographic atrophy is a gradually progressive loss of the combination of the RPE and the choriocapillaris in a very specific pattern. Secondarily, there is loss of photoreceptor function. These areas typically develop after coalescence of drusen, but may also occur in a state of "burned-out" retinal pigment epithelial detachments. Geographic atrophy appears as well-circumscribed areas that may appear in a multiple pattern or may appear as a single compromised area. These changes usually present close to the macular area by definition and vary in size from 200 to over 5000 microns. The atrophy may be present unilaterally, but is bilateral in up to 55 percent of eyes. Choroidal neovascularization will usually not occur within the atrophic zone as nonviable choriocapillaris will not support the growth, but in up to 20 percent of the eyes may develop at the margin of the atrophy. Visual prognosis is variable.

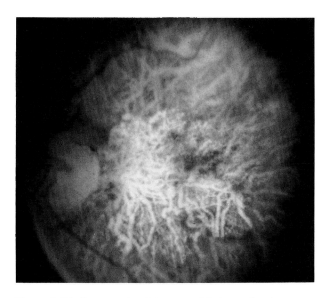

Figure 5–17. An example of dry age-related macular degeneration. Note the choriocapillaris and choroidal atrophy as well as the loss of RPE.

Dry (Nonexudative) ARM

Characteristics

△ Usually over age 60 years
△ Presentation of drusen is variable
△ Granular disorganization of the RPE in macular area in the form of RPE hyperplasia and/or RPE degeneration
△ Degeneration of outer retinal layers
△ Geographical atrophy that may be multiple or singular
   Usually near the macula
   200 to 5000 microns in size
   Bilateral in 55 percent of cases
   May develop choroidal neovascularization at edge in 20 percent of cases
△ Variable bilateral loss of central vision, color vision compromise
△ Rare severe loss of central vision

Management

△ Patient education and home monitoring of vision
△ Maximize visual correction, consider low-vision devices, utilize proper lighting, consider psychological counseling if deemed necessary
△ Consider vitamin supplementation, consider blocking blue hazard light
△ Follow patient at 3- to 12-month intervals
△ Fluorescein angiography and retinology consultation if threat of "wet" ARM

From a clinicopathologic standpoint, in all forms of dry or nonexudative ARM it appears that there is initially a change noted in the RPE cells that may be the result of isolated poor vascular supply from the choriocapillaris. The RPE cells eventually undergo complete degeneration resulting in photoreceptor loss. This degeneration creates a situation where the inner nuclear layer actually comes in contact with Bruch's membrane. The outer retinal layers then degenerate. In the past it was thought that the underlying choriocapillaris was also lost, but recent work implies that it is kept intact. **See color plates 54 and 55.**

Dry ARM creates a variable degree of loss of central vision that usually becomes bilateral but may have variable acuity in both eyes. Because of loss of cone function, color vision may also be compromised. It is well known that "wet forms" of degeneration may coexist with the dry forms, and therefore other symptoms such as metamorphopsia may present.

Management. Visual acuity is rarely reduced to legal blindness in dry ARM. The primary goal in management of the patient with dry ARM is education and maximizing usable vision. The patient must be educated regarding the potential of progression of dry to wet ARM. These individuals must be on some form of home monitoring and must be followed at routine intervals (every 3 to 12 months). Should signs of "soft drusen" or other exudative signs develop (hard exudates or intraretinal hemorrhages), fluorescein angiography must be performed. At this time it is difficult to accurately predict which, if any, of the patients with dry ARM will convert to wet ARM. The suggestion has been made that as drusen calcify and RPE disappears, the risk of progression to wet ARM in that area is virtually nonexistent but neovascularization may develop in the adjacent retinal areas. My conservative approach is to assume the worst, to cover for the possibility, and to be ecstatic when nothing occurs. Supplemental vitamin therapy as well as blocking undesirable "blue-hazard" light may also be of benefit to the patient.

To maximize usable vision, the doctor must provide the best prescription, low-vision devices, advice on proper lighting, and patient education regarding eccentric viewing. The elderly patient facing the compromise of vision may also benefit from psychological counseling regarding the problem.

Wet (Exudative) ARM

Introduction and Description. It has long been regarded as true that drusen are the visible precursors of wet ARM even though the neovascular growth actually occurs away from visible drusen in areas of RPE/Bruch's breakdown. If a patient has bilateral macular drusen, it appears that about 10 percent develop exudative maculopathy over a 4.3-year period. Table 5–3 summarizes the risk factors for the development of exudative macular degeneration. There is suspicion that extramacular drusen and macular degeneration have similar pathogenic mechanisms.

As suggested previously, wet ARM may assume four patterns: (1) choroidal neovascularization, (2) ex-

TABLE 5–3. RISK FACTORS FOR DEVELOPMENT OF WET ARM

Risk Factors	Risk
Bilateral drusen only	2 to 4% of eyes will develop exudative macular degeneration
Fellow eye has exudative macular degeneration	10% of fellow eyes per year will develop exudative macular degeneration
Confluence of drusen	55% in the unilateral exudative group
Focal RPE hyperpigmentation	43% in the unilateral exudative group
Increased age over 75 years	45% in the unilateral exudative group

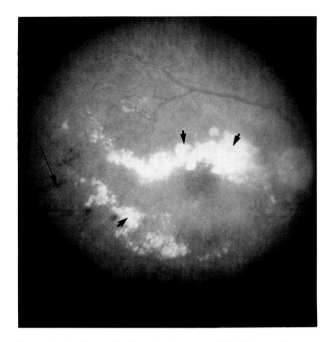

Figure 5–19. Example of a variation of wet ARM. The small arrows point to massive exudation (Coats' response), whereas the longer arrow points to intraretinal hemorrhage associated with the condition.

udative degeneration, (3) hemorrhagic degeneration, and/or (4) disciform degeneration (Figs. 5–19 to 5–21).

Choroidal neovascularization occurs as the result of disruption in the RPE/Bruch's barrier. New vessels from the choriocapillaris grow up through the disruption in Bruch's in response to a hypoxic stimulus. The neovascularization may then (1) leak, creating an RPE detachment or a sensory retinal detachment, (2)

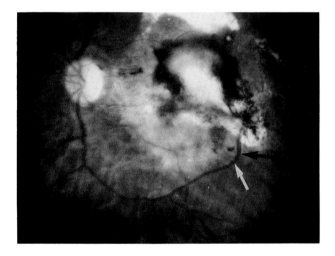

Figure 5–20. Example of a retinal vascular tumor that simulates the same picture as wet exudative macular degeneration. A tell tale differentiating sign is the feeder vessel entering the lesion (*arrows*) as well as the usual early age onset of the lesion.

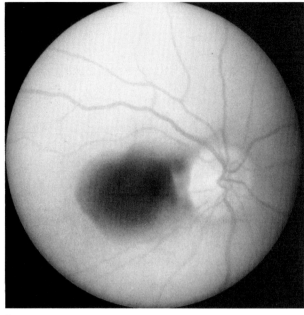

A

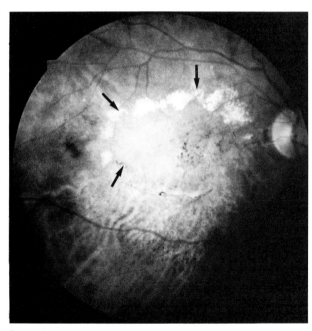

B

Figure 5–21. Examples of variations of wet ARM. **A.** A large subretinal hemorrhage resulting from a choroidal neovascular net near the disc margin. **B.** Hard exudates (Coats' response) surrounding an area of sensory retinal elevation created by a leaking choroidal neovascular net. Note the RPE clumping and loss of choroidal detail.

hemorrhage, creating a sub–RPE or subretinal hemorrhage, or (3) form a disciform scar. Whichever option is pursued, the results are visually devastating. **See color plate 71.**

Another process of vision loss associated with RPE disease and wet ARM is RPE tear, which can be

Wet (Exudative) ARM

Characteristics

∆ With bilateral macular drusen, 10 percent of patients develop exudative maculopathy over a 4.3-year period

∆ In aged patients with drusen/choroidal infiltrates as precursors

∆ May present as:
    Choroidal neovascularization—gray-green net
    Exudative degeneration—hard exudates
    Hemorrhagic degeneration
    Disciform degeneration

∆ Retinal pigment epithelial tear
    Appears as crescent-shaped RPE defect
    Rolled edge may progress, creating vision loss

∆ Reduced vision, altered color vision, or meta morphopsia

Management

∆ Consider benefits of blocking blue-hazard light

∆ Consider potential benefits of vitamin/antioxidant therapy

∆ Elderly patients with metamorphopsia or reduced vision should be suspected of neovascular nets and should have fluorescein angiography within 72 hours

∆ If one eye has a disciform scar, assume the other eye will develop vision loss, and monitor appropriately

∆ If there is suspicion of development of a net, ask for a retinal consultation
    Hard exudates in the absence of demonstrable retinal vascular disease
    Macular hemorrhages in the absence of demonstrable retinal vascular disease

∆ Watch soft choroidal infiltrates carefully, or ask for a retinal consultation
    Coalescence of soft drusen or choroidal infiltrates is suspicious

∆ If the choroidal net is treatable, it must be performed in a timely fashion and by an experienced retinal specialist
    Krypton red or dye yellow laser for juxtafoveal neovascular nets
    Argon laser for extrafoveal neovascular nets

∆ Scarification may be managed by vitreoretinal procedures to minimize the secondary scotoma

∆ Postoperative management:
    Color photodocumentation with comparison to preoperative drawing to assess success
    Reapplication of laser if inadequate
    Follow with fluorescein angiography in 1, 3, and 6 months because of strong possibility of recurrence
    Repeat exams thereafter every 3 to 6 months
    Employ self-monitoring

visually devastating if it extends into the foveal area. RPE tears occur in ARM as the result of lipofuscin accumulation in the RPE with progression to drusen development. The tears occur when traction from isolated RPE detachments, neovascular nets, or traction induced by photocoagulation leads to excessive force on the RPE, allowing for a rift to develop. The RPE tear appears as a crescent-shaped RPE defect whose outer arc demarcates the edge of the tear and whose inner arc is always toward the center of the detachment with the rolled edge of the RPE. The fluorescein angiogram demonstrates the tear with a crescent of early hyperfluorescence and an adjacent area of hypofluorescence.

Often the only complaint of a patient with evolving wet ARM is reduced vision, distorted vision, or color distortion. Unfortunately a lot of patients come into the office after irreversible damage has already occurred. When this is the case, the best option is to guard against involvement of the fellow eye. **See color plates 67 and 68.**

Management. Untreated, prognosis for usable vision in wet ARM is poor. Functional vision, such as reading large print, currency discrimination, and color recognition, is known to be significantly better with better Snellen acuity. It is best to attempt some sort of intervention within reasonable guidelines, rather than to tempt fate by relying on natural progression. The argument for protection with blocking short-wavelength blue and the use of vitamin supplementation is very compelling when the side effects of vitamin therapy as well as the limitations are carefully considered. The goal is maintenance of the best possible vision.

Primary care practitioners must recognize the early signs of the evolution of wet ARM. All elderly patients with macular drusen should be placed on home monitoring systems to be used daily, and should be followed at least at yearly intervals. All elderly patients with unexplained vision reduction or distortion should be suspected of having choroidal neovascularization, RPE detachments, or RPE tears until proven otherwise. The appearance of soft drusen—really choroidal infiltrates or RPE detachments—should heighten the practitioner's suspicion. All hard exudates (Coats' response) or hemorrhages in the macular area in the absence of documented retinal vascular disease should alert the practitioner to the possibility of choroidal neovascular nets. All gray-green areas in the macular area should be assumed to be choroidal neovascular nets until disproven by fluorescein angiography. Any unusual appearance in the macular area in an elderly patient that cannot be explained should have a fluorescein angiography evaluation. Should the evolution of the choroidal neovascular membrane progress to hemorrhage or disciform scarring, laser intervention will be of little value. Recent work has, however, demonstrated that surgical excision of scarification may be of value in the improvement of long term visual function.

Should a patient be suspected of having a choroidal neovascular membrane or other signs of wet ARM, a fluorescein angiogram should be performed within 72 hours. Delay in the instances of treatable lesions can be devastating. Up to 73 percent of untreated extrafoveal lesions can become subfoveal within 1 year. Choroidal neovascular membranes can be expected to grow up to 5 to 10 microns per day once the process has started. Improper treatment can also be devastating. Inadequately treated choroidal neovascularization is a major cause of treatment failure and of regrowth. The retinal specialist treating the membrane will typically perform a preoperative drawing and discuss the procedure of intervention with the patient and the family members.

It has been shown that expertly placed laser photocoagulation applied in a timely manner reduces the risk of severe vision loss for patients with extrafoveal wet ARM degeneration. About 5 percent of choroidal neovascular membranes are treatable with argon photocoagulation according to the original Macular Photocoagulation Study, which confined treatment to angiographically defined areas of neovascularization at least 200 microns from the center of the fovea. Eyes with poorly defined or subfoveal choroidal neovascularization have even a poorer visual prognosis. The elapsed time of choroidal neovascular development is crucial. It has been estimated that at least 75 percent of patients with wet ARM degeneration secondary to choroidal neovascularization pass through a potentially treatable stage. At the same time it has been suggested that only 20 percent of patients with symptoms secondary to choroidal neovascularization will be treatable after 8 weeks, and only 15 percent after 4 months. Up to 80 percent of patients with visual symptoms for less than 2 weeks and over 50 percent with symptoms less than 4 weeks will be treatable. There is a small window for success; therefore, early detection and rapid intervention are crucial. It should be noted that once the eye is treated, proper follow-up is mandatory, as the recurrence rate is as high as 25 percent, and 12 percent of fellow eyes develop wet ARM.

Photocoagulative intervention is indicated in well-defined choroidal neovascular membranes with no overlying retinal pigment epithelial detachment. Krypton laser photocoagulation is recommended for juxtafoveal choroidal neovascular membranes in nonhypertensive patients with ARM, and argon laser has

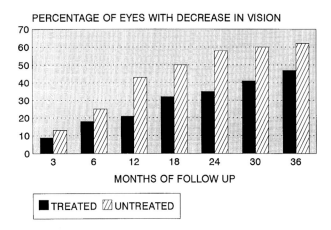

PERCENTAGE OF EYES WITH DECREASE IN VISION

MONTHS OF FOLLOW UP

■ TREATED ▨ UNTREATED

Figure 5–22. Percentage of eyes with a decrease in visual acuity associated with ARM, with and without interventive treatment. (*Arch Ophthalmol.* 1986;104:694–701.)

been shown to be beneficial for extrafoveal choroidal neovascular nets. In choroidal neovascular membranes with overlying retinal pigment epithelial detachments, photocoagulation may be beneficial in the preservation of vision. Figure 5–22 demonstrates the risk of decreased vision in macular degeneration with and without laser intervention.

The operative procedure consists of the use of retrobulbar anesthesia if the membrane is close to the fovea or if there is anticipated excessive eye movements. The type of laser (argon, krypton, dye) used is at the discretion of the retinal specialist. Green argon is the most popular wavelength currently used, but is not as beneficial in juxtafoveal membranes because of the absorption of the wavelength by the xanthophyll pigment with spread of heat to associated structures. Dye yellow (577 nm) photocoagulation can be used in juxtafoveal membranes because of minimal absorption by the xanthophyll pigment, and may be of benefit in treating red neovascular nets as the yellow is absorbed by hemoglobin. The absorption by hemoglobin makes dye yellow unacceptable in cases of neovascular membranes associated with subretinal hemorrhage. The theory behind use of the krypton or dye red photocoagulation is that it allows treatment closer to the fovea than argon because of krypton's (red) specificity for choroidal layers. Krypton is especially useful in cases where neovascular membranes are associated with melanin pigmentation, where overlying hemorrhage does not absorb red krypton, and in the juxtafoveal nets. Studies of patients with choroidal neovascularization within the foveal avascular zone treated with krypton laser demonstrated that improvement of stabilization may occur. In addition to these findings, there is a strong argument that the resultant scar created by the krypton laser will create a smaller scotoma than if the neovascular net had progressed naturally. The smaller scar and resultant scotoma create improved functional vision for the patient. There appear to be no major differences in outcome between argon and krypton if criteria are followed carefully in the hands of a skilled retinal surgeon. Photocoagulation of RPE detachments by argon and krypton laser has also demonstrated some encouraging results. The photocoagulation can actually collapse the detachment, and good results may be achieved if the detachment is away from the fovea.

Current retinal vitreal procedures include surgical excision and removal of disciform and fibrotic scars associated with wet ARM. The objectives of the procedure are not restoration of vision but rather a minification of the size of the scotoma secondary to the scarification. Surgical intervention includes vitrectomy, diathermy, retinotomy, peeling of a subretinal scar, drainage of subretinal fluid, endophotocoagulation, and retinal tacks.

In all, early recognition and expeditious consultation with a highly competent retinal specialist is indicated, as the visual prognosis for the forms of wet ARM untreated is very grim. Improper treatment is almost as dangerous as no treatment because of the potential of the future development of recurrent neovascular nets.

Postoperative management must include photodocumentation. There should be color photodocumentation immediately after surgery and then at least 48 hours after application of the laser treatment. Assessment of pretreatment drawings compared to posttreatment drawings is important in addressing the success of the procedure. Should the treatment be inadequate, reapplication of laser is indicated. Platelet inhibitors, heavy lifting, and potential trauma should be avoided until documentation is secure regarding regression of the choroidal neovascularization because of the strong possibility of secondary hemorrhage. The patient should be followed with fluorescein angiography at 1, 3, and 6 weeks after treatment because of the strong possibility of recurrence. Repeat examinations should occur every 3 to 6 months depending on the patient's status, with fluorescein angiography performed should any suspicion of reneovascularization develop. The patient should also be maintained on home Amsler grid or other methods of self-monitoring. Recurrences occur and are a major problem. Most choroidal neovascular membranes recur within 1 year of treatment and are not amendable by retreatment. The majority of recurrences are at the foveal side of the treated scar due to the increased hemodynamic activity in the foveal area. Risk of recurrence is associated with cigarette smoking, females, and a younger age. Recurrences occur in up to 60 percent of treated eyes. Figure 5–23 gives a sense of the rate of recurrence of neovascularization in ARM.

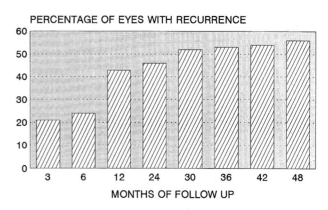

Figure 5–23. Cumulative percentage of eyes with recurrent choroidal neovascular membranes associated with photocoagulation for ARM. (*Arch Ophthalmol.* 1986;104:503–512.)

CHOROIDAL NEOVASCULARIZATION RELATED TO CHORIORETINAL SCARRING

The initiating factor in the development of choroidal neovascularization is a combination of the disruption in the RPE/Bruch's membrane barrier coupled with the occurrence of hypoxia. Certainly degenerative changes such as ARM can create the situation for the development of alterations in the barrier. There is also the possibility that physical damage to the eye can create the possibility for a disruption in the membranes, leading to neovascular development. There are many possibilities for this disruption, including trauma, postuveitic scarring, postcryopexy scarring, postphotocoagulation scarring, and neovascularization arising from a drainage site after scleral buckling procedures.

Choroidal Ruptures

Introduction and Description. Choroidal ruptures (Figs. 5–24 and 5–25) in the posterior pole are fairly common complications of contusion injuries to the eye. The ruptures may be singular or multiple, and are typically the result of contrecoup shock waves generated in blunt trauma. The ruptures are usually crescentric in nature with the concavity toward the disc. Depending on the severity of the blow, there may be hemorrhages of the following types: intrachoroidal, subretinal pigment epithelium, subretinal, intraretinal, and vitreous. The hemorrhages often obscure the underlying rupture immediately after the injury. As the hemorrhage resorbs and the retinal and choroidal edema disappear, a scar forms with migration and hyperplasia of the overlying RPE. Despite the damage, the overlying retina and retinal vessels often remain intact.

Vision loss or visual field defects vary considerably, depending on the severity, particular area in-

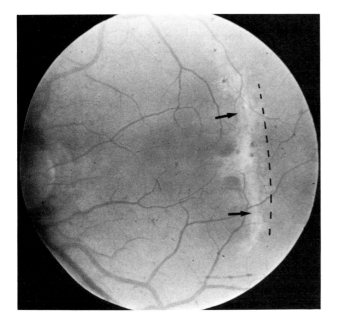

Figure 5–24. Example of a choroidal rupture (*arrows*). The contour is indicated by the dotted line and follows the contour of the disc.

Choroidal Ruptures

Characteristics

Δ Result of blunt trauma with contrecoup shock waves

Δ Appearance is crescentic or curvilinear following contours of the disc

Δ An active rupture usually has an associated bleed, which obscures the choroidal rupture

Δ As the hemorrhage resorbs, scarification ensues

Δ Vision and visual field loss is variable

Δ Possibility of development of choroidal neovascularization in zone of the scar up to 5 years later

Management

Δ Patient education and yearly monitoring

Δ Home monitoring of vision

Δ Protective eyewear

Δ Photocoagulation of developing choroidal neovascular nets may be necessary if an immediate threat to vision, but there is a distinct possibility of spontaneous involution of the choroidal membrane

volved, and extent of retinal edema. The visual field defect may be larger than that expected because of inherent damage to the nerve-fiber layer. There is no particularly effective management for the acute phase of choroidal rupture.

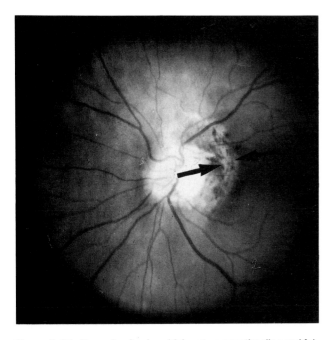

Figure 5–25. Example of a choroidal rupture near the disc and following the contour of the disc. Note the associated RPE hyperplasia.

One of the concerns regarding choroidal rupture is the possibility of delayed onset of complications. It is possible that choroidal neovascularization can occur within the scar up to 5 years after the original trauma. This choroidal neovascularization has the potential toward leakage, hemorrhage, or disciform scarring. Photocoagulation of the developing neovascular net may create variable results, as the RPE/Bruch's membrane barrier is already very fragile from the trauma. In addition, there are reports that spontaneous involution of the choroidal neovascular net is possible.

Management. The management of the patient with choroidal rupture in the posterior pole consists of patient education, monitoring on a yearly interval, home monitoring of vision, and provision of protective eyewear in eye hazard situations. Photocoagulation of the neovascular net is only to be performed if there is an immediate threat to vision as spontaneous involution of the nets appear to occur. **See color plate 72.**

Postphotocoagulative and Postcryopexy Scarring and Other Surgical/Trauma-induced Neovascular Development

Introduction and Description. Photocoagulation and cryopexy have provided the ophthalmic surgeon with effective tools to combat blindness. Unfortunately, the scar created by these processes represents a destruction of tissue that may support choroidal neovascular growth when a situation of hypoxia oc-

Postphotocoagulative and Postcryopexy Scarring and Other Surgical/Trauma-induced Neovascular Development

Characteristics

△ Choroidal neovascularization may develop in photocoagulation or cryopexy scars—it may be delayed by 6 years

△ Occurs in photocoagulation treated Eales disease, sickle-cell proliferative retinopathy, sarcoid retinopathy, proliferative diabetic retinopathy, idiopathic central serous choroidopathy, choroidal hemangioma, choroidal melanoma, choroidal neovascularization, and focal/grid photocoagulation for diabetic macular edema

△ Surgical trauma and intraocular foreign bodies that affect the choroid may also induce choroidal neovascular development

△ All may develop after a considerably delayed time frame

Management

△ Prevention by proper photocoagulation and cryopexy. If the net occurs, it appears that the best results occur with no intervention

△ Intervention may actually convert a choroidal net to a choriovitreal net with enhanced threat to vision

△ Routine follow-up examinations

curs. The first reported cases of choroidal neovascular net development within photocoagulative scars were in association with Eales' disease. Other reports have associated choroidal neovascular net development secondary with heavy photocoagulative intervention in sickle-cell proliferative retinopathy, sarcoidosis, proliferative diabetic retinopathy, idiopathic central serous choroidopathy, choroidal hemangioma, choroidal melanoma, choroidal neovascularization, and focal treatment for diabetic macular edema. There are even reports of secondary choroidal neovascular development in cases of grid photocoagulation for diabetic macular edema. In the past, over 60 percent of photocoagulated proliferative retinopathy has been shown to develop neovascular nets in the scars. It has also been shown that there may be up to a 6–year delay in the development of nets within the scars. **See color plate 73.**

New approaches to photocoagulation have been undertaken to minimize the likelihood of the choroidal neovascularization. The type of photocoagulative procedure that is most likely to create a situation conducive to neovascular growth is a combination of small spot size, short exposure durations, high peak power, and retreatment.

Surgical trauma such as drainage of subretinal fluid and peeling of an epiretinal membrane may also result in the genesis of choroidal neovascular development. External trauma such as metallic intraocular foreign bodies associated with choroidal injury may also serve as the initiating factor in the development of choroidal neovascular membranes. All trauma-induced nets may present after a delay between the trauma and the development of the net.

Management. Once a neovascular net develops within a scar, it is recommended that no treatment be applied unless there is active, symptomatic vitreous hemorrhage. There may be evidence for the treatment of photocoagulation-induced extrafoveal macular neovascularization, although definitive proof does not currently exist. It appears that outcome is better with no intervention, and that treatment may actually convert the choroidal neovascularization to a choriovitreal neovascularization, which is a much more significant threat to vision.

DEGENERATIVE OR PATHOLOGIC MYOPIA

Introduction and Description. Degenerative or pathologic myopia differs significantly from the more prevalent refractive myopias in that there is a true alteration of structure of the globe that is progressive and often leads to blindness. The condition also differs from the congenital forms of posterior staphylomas, which typically do not progress but do offer some threat to the development of retinal tears and detachments. True degenerative myopia has a prevalence of only about 2 percent in the United States and seems to have an ethnic predilection for Chinese, Japanese, Arabians, and Jews. Although low in prevalence, pathologic myopia is the seventh leading cause of blindness in the United States. Ocular and systemic diseases associated with pathologic myopia are listed in Table 5–4.

The clinician cannot rely on refractive error as the

TABLE 5–4. OCULAR AND SYSTEMIC CONDITIONS ASSOCIATED WITH PATHOLOGIC MYOPIA

Fetal alcohol syndrome	Low birthweight
	Infantile glaucoma
Ocular albinism	Hereditary vitreoretinal dystrophies
Pigmentary retinal dystrophy	Retinopathy of prematurity
	Ehlers–Danlos syndrome
Down syndrome	Marfan's syndrome

sole predictor of pathologic myopia, as many highly myopic patients will never progress toward pathologic alteration of ocular structure. The diagnosis of degenerative myopia is based primarily on ophthalmoscopically observable signs.

Myopia has been categorized into three easily clinically definable conditions. Stationary myopia typically develops during periods of rapid body growth and rarely exceeds 6 to 9 diopters. Although there is an increased incidence of retinal detachment in these individuals, the pathologic changes found in degenerative myopia are usually absent in the stationary myopias. Late myopia begins after bodily growth ceases and is often associated with work conditions. This differentiation can best be characterized by the myopia a first-year law student develops associated with an inordinate amount of reading. Degenerative myopia typically develops in youth and progresses through stages as the patient ages. Some individuals are, however, born with staphylomas of the globe that are usually associated with the later stages of development of degenerative myopia. Whether congenital or developmental, the ocular structure changes associated with pathologic myopia often lead to vision-threatening complications.

Pathologic myopia presents in two stages that are age dependent, the developmental and degenerative stages. Ocular alterations during the developmental stage are the direct result of axial length changes, whereas the degenerative phase is secondary to vascular changes.

With pathologic myopia, the primary alteration is a posterior elongation of the eyeball. This bulging is often age related and as such can be divided into stages. The earliest stages present between birth to the age of 30 years. About 30 percent of patients with pathologic myopia have onset at birth, whereas about 60 percent of patients present from the ages of 6 to 12 years. Approximately 10 percent of patients with pathologic myopia present early changes after the age of 12 years.

The elongation of the eyeball in the posterior segment occurs as a result of progressive thinning of the sclera, resulting in a bulge or ectasia. This thinning seems to be the result of meridional collagen-bundle thinning and deformity. The posterior staphylomas (Fig. 5–26) are a poor visual prognostic sign, with over 50 percent of eyes with staphylomas over the age of 60 years being considered legally blind. Some feel that there is a genetic factor involved that initiates abnormal RPE changes leading to scleral degeneration. Ophthalmoscopically, this appears as thinning of the retinal pigment epithelium. The thinning of the RPE and choroid is also present histologically.

The elongation of the globe continues with age, resulting in chorioretinal changes manifesting as patches of choriocapillaris and choroidal atrophy. These patches may coalesce, creating a very dramatic picture. As the choriocapillaris and choroidal complex breaks down, rifts may develop in Bruch's membrane that appear as jagged lines known as lacquer cracks. Lacquer cracks are present in 4 percent of eyes with

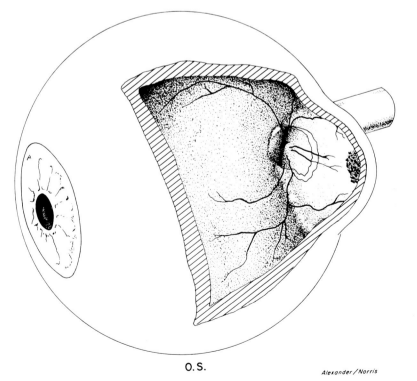

O. S.

Alexander/Norris

Figure 5–26. A schematic illustrating a posterior staphyloma in a left eye in the macular area. The bulging pulls on the edge of the nerve head, creating a temporal scleral crescent and straightening or "dragging" of the vessels exiting the disc.

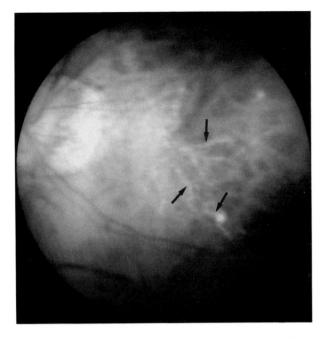

Figure 5–27. Example of lacquer cracks (*small arrows*) associated with degenerative myopia.

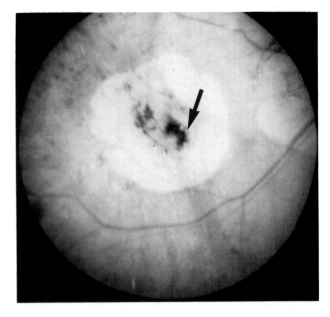

Figure 5–28. Example of a Fuch's spot in degenerative myopia with the classical association of RPE hyperplasia indicated by the large arrow. The RPE hyperplasia is a reaction to the development of an underlying choroidal neovascular net.

axial lengths of at least 26.5 mm. These cracks are known to be mobile from one visit to the next, and certainly open an avenue for the genesis of choroidal hemorrhages. Lacquer cracks are seen most often in young men (Fig. 5–27). These lacquer cracks, or breaks, in Bruch's membrane also open the channel for the development of choroidal neovascular nets. Lacquer cracks are present in 82 percent of eyes with choroidal neovascularization and in 97 percent of eyes with subretinal hemorrhage without associated choroidal neovascularization. These nets usually develop with overlying RPE hyperplasia and are classically known as Fuchs' spots. The onset of Fuchs' spot is typically in the fourth to sixth decade and may be preceded by sensory retinal elevations. Fuchs' spot is similar to the choroidal neovascular net associated with other varieties of exudative maculopathies, but has more of a tendency toward hyperplasia of the RPE (Fig. 5–28). Fuchs' spot may hemorrhage or develop into a disciform scar. Five to ten percent of eyes with degenerative myopia develop a Fuchs' spot. Unfortunately, as with other choroidal neovascular nets, there is a predilection for the macular area.

In addition to the extensive choroidal atrophy of the posterior pole (Fig. 5–29) there are peripheral retinal changes that predispose to retinal detachment. Because of the continual stretching of the retina and tugging at the vitreoretinal interface, several retinal changes may develop. These changes include white without pressure, lattice degeneration, atrophic and operculated retinal holes, chorioretinal cobblestone degeneration, retinal breaks, and retinal detachment.

The risks of detachment rise significantly with an increase in the extent of myopia.

Structural changes also occur at the optic nerve head, but are of no direct threat to vision. With ectasia in the macular area, there is a pulling away of the choroid and RPE from the edge of the optic nerve head. This results in the classical scleral crescent (Fig. 5–30). Because of this physical tugging, the vessels em-

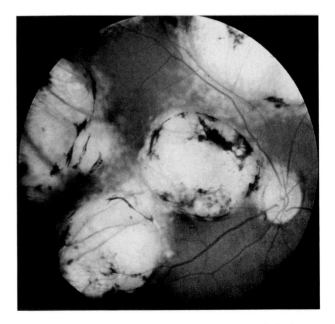

Figure 5–29. Areas of gross choroidal atrophy in pathologic myopia.

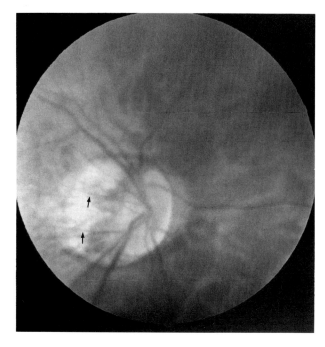

Figure 5–30. Scleral crescent in a highly myopic eye. The arrows point to straightened disc vessels.

anating from the disc that run temporally are also stretched. The disc may also appear tilted toward the ectatic area, with the nasal aspect of the nerve head slightly elevated, known as supertraction. If a posterior staphyloma encircles the disc, the lamina is displaced anteriorly, and the optic nerve head is elevated above the retina.

Anterior chamber alterations are often present in patients with high myopia secondary to posterior staphylomas. These alterations are iris remnants and increased iris processes. These alterations may lead toward an increased incidence of primary open-angle glaucoma in the patient with pathologic myopia.

Pathologic myopia is a continuing spectrum of change. Initially, the clinician must be concerned about optimizing the refraction. As the degeneration progresses, the retinal changes increase the threat of neovascular nets and retinal detachment. The overall incidence of open-angle glaucoma is also significantly higher, and its detection is complicated by the gross refractive errors and the physically altered disc appearance. The inevitability of some vision compromise is omnipresent.

Management. The patient with pathologic myopia must be monitored constantly, especially as he or she ages. With age the incidence of Fuchs' spot, vitreous liquefaction and traction, peripheral retinal degenerative changes, and glaucoma all increase. With the threat of glaucoma, fields must be performed with a contact lens prescription often in the form of a disposable lens with an over-refraction and a lot of attention to detail. Intervention must be provided at the

first sign of destructive peripheral retinal disease or glaucoma. Intervention with laser application to Fuchs' spots provides only equivocal results; in fact, the laser may actually worsen the condition. A high percentage of the choroidal neovascular membranes actually stabilize in the form of an atrophic scar or regress without intervention. All patients with Fuchs' spots should, however, have fluorescein angiography performed. A retinal consultation is advised when a Fuchs' spot develops.

Because of the inherent alteration of the retinal and choroidal infrastructure, the patient should be cautioned regarding trauma and should be advised to

Pearls

Degenerative Myopia

Characteristics

△ Not associated with either stationary myopia or congenital staphylomas

△ Typically begins in youth and progresses through stages with aging

△ Developmental stage

Posterior elongation of the globe evidenced by thinning of the RPE and choroid

Development of scleral crescent and vessel straightening secondary to the physical bulging

Peripheral vitreoretinal degenerations such as lattice are also possible

Disc tilting and supertraction as the result of progressive ectasia

△ Degenerative stage

Patches of choriocapillaris/choroidal atrophy may develop

Lacquer cracks present in 82 percent of eyes with choroidal neovascularization, and in 97 percent of eyes with subretinal hemorrhages without choroidal neovascularization

Choroidal neovascularization—Fuchs' spot—in the fourth to sixth decade

△ Increased incidence of primary open–angle glaucoma secondary to anterior chamber alterations

Management

△ Provision of best possible prescription in protective eyewear

△ Caution regarding trauma and eye hazard

△ Routine monitoring for development of peripheral vitreoretinal disease

△ Routine monitoring for development of neovascular nets

△ Retinal consultation if a Fuchs' spot develops or if peripheral retinal disease becomes a threat

△ Laser intervention may actually worsen condition as a high percentage of choroidal neovascularization actually involutes on its own

△ Follow up at least yearly

use protective eyewear in eye hazard situations. The patient should be examined at least on a yearly basis.

ANGIOID STREAKS

Introduction and Description. Angioid streaks (Figs. 5–31 and 5–32) are an anatomic phenomenon secondary to pathologic changes in the RPE, Bruch's membrane, and the choroid/choriocapillaris. There seems to be a higher prevalence of angioid streaks in whites with an increase in appearance with age. It should also be noted that the incidence of buried drusen of the optic nerve head is 20 to 50 times greater than in the healthy population. The majority of patients have pseudoxanthoma elasticum or Grönblad–Strandberg syndrome (80 to 90 percent of affected patients have streaks), whereas some patients have Paget's disease (8 to 15 percent of affected patients have streaks), Ehlers–Danlos syndrome, or sickle-cell disease (1 to 2 percent of affected patients have streaks). Conversely, it is estimated that about 50 percent of patients with angioid streaks have either psuedoxanthoma elasticum, Paget's disease, or sickle-cell hemoglobinopathy. Other associations with angioid streaks are listed in Table 5–5. There are, however, some patients with no systemic association whatsoever. The strong association with elastic tissue diseases indicates that angioid streaks will probably present in a bilateral but often asymmetrical manner.

Angioid streaks are a manifestation of breaks in thickened and calcified Bruch's membrane. There is

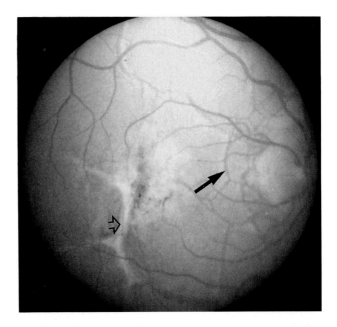

Figure 5–32. Example of a variation of the presentation of angioid streaks. The large black arrow points to the angioid streaks, while the small open arrow points to a scar associated with the underlying compromise of the RPE/Bruch's membrane barrier. Note how the scar simulates the choroidal rupture in Figure 5–25.

then a loss or migration of pigment granules in the RPE. When full-thickness breaks occur in Bruch's membrane, there is a disruption of the choriocapillaris, atrophy of the RPE, and loss of overlying photoreceptor cells. The cracks in Bruch's membrane result in leakage or, coupled with hypoxia, in development of choroidal neovascular nets. The nets may then develop into disciform scars or hemorrhage, creating a classical exudative maculopathy. The development of choroidal membranes does not usually occur until the 40s or 50s.

The ophthalmoscopic signs of angioid streaks develop in a characteristic pattern, but all seem to have

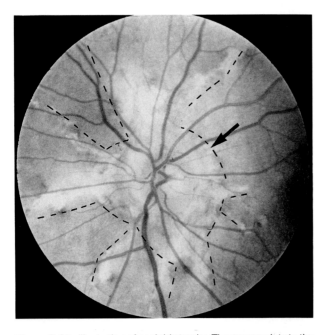

Figure 5–31. Illustration of angioid streaks. The arrow points to the "hub" around the disc, while the dotted lines follow the contour of the streaks emanating from the "hub."

TABLE 5–5. SYSTEMIC ASSOCIATIONS WITH OCULAR ANGIOID STREAKS

Pseudoxanthoma elasticum
Paget's disease
Sickling hemoglobinopathies
Ehlers–Danlos syndrome
Diabetes mellitus
Hemochromatosis
Acquired hemolytic anemia
Hypercalcinosis
Hyperphosphosphatemia
Lead poisoning
Neurofibromatosis
Sturge-Weber syndrome
Tuberous sclerosis
Acromegaly
Familial polyposis—CHRPE as well

individuality in their clinical appearance. There also appears to be no particular predictability to the rate of progression. **See color plate 74.** An area of circumpapillary degeneration appears as the hub for the outward radiation of spokes of irregularly placed, jagged lines. The lines often vary in color from gray, red-gray, red-brown, to red, depending on the overall ocular pigmentation. In black patients the lines may be enhanced by extensive RPE migration and proliferation. A mottled fundus appearance (peau d'orange) temporal to the macula may present with or actually precede the development of the streaks, and probably represents an alteration of the RPE overlying the streaks. This mottled appearance may extend to the temporal equator. The author has observed this mottled appearance throughout the entire retina with the exception of the macula.

In some cases poorly defined red-brown spots occur in pairs on either side of the light-colored area along the margins of the streaks. These spots are usually less than ½ disc diameter (DD) in size. Another characteristic that may be seen is peripheral focal chorioretinal lesions that are salmon in color and resemble histo spots. When these spots occur along with the peripapillary atrophy and macular lesions, presumed ocular histoplasmosis may be suspected. Two other fundus characteristics, disc drusen and short, vertical lines concentric to the disc margins, may also be present with angioid streaks.

Often signs and symptoms are not present initially with angioid streaks. The patient may enter the office for a routine eye examination, and the streaks may be found on routine binocular indirect ophthalmoscopy. Unfortunately, the patient may present at the first sign of vision loss either to a moderate degree, associated with macular degeneration, or to a more severe degree, associated with disciform maculopathy.

Management. Visual compromise can occur in angioid streaks secondary to progression and extension of the cracks in Bruch's membrane into the macular area. A very high percentage of patients develops some form of (dry) macular degeneration, creating some vision loss, whereas others develop choroidal neovascular nets (14 percent), leading to severe vision loss. There seems to be an association of vision loss to trauma even though this may be difficult to elicit in a case history. Studies vary regarding the presence of neovascular membranes, as does the success rate for treating the membrane with photocoagulation. Although choroidal neovascularization is a treatable lesion, one must remember that photocoagulation will only further break down an already weakened Bruch's membrane, enhancing future development of neovascular nets. If indications and methods are well chosen and there is no alternative, photocoagulation in the hands of a skilled retinal surgeon is indicated to

Pearls

Angioid Streaks

Characteristics

△ Occur in pseudoxanthoma elasticum (80 to 90 percent), Paget's disease (8 to 15 percent), Ehlers–Danlos syndrome, sickle-cell disease (1 to 2 percent), or associated with no identifiable systemic disease

△ Approximately 50 percent have associated systemic disease

△ Usually bilateral but may be asymmetrical

△ Result of breaks in thickened and calcified Bruch's membrane

△ Area of circumpapillary degeneration serves as the hub for outward radiation of spokes or breaks in Bruch's membrane

△ Possible peau d'orange appearance temporal to macula, which is the result of changes in the overlying RPE

△ May have peripheral focal chorioretinal lesions

△ May develop macula degeneration and/or choroidal neovascular nets (14 percent)

△ Loss of central vision in 70 percent of angioid streaks associated with pseudoxanthoma elasticum and 20 to 50 times the incidence of associated buried drusen in these patients

Management

△ Watch for development of neovascular nets and use fluorescein angiography to confirm

△ Schedule retinal consultation when indicated

△ Rule out associated and at times life-threatening systemic diseases
  Pseudoxanthoma elasticum
  Paget's disease
  Sickling hemoglobinopathies

△ Recommend safety lenses and advise about trauma

△ Schedule for routine examinations at least yearly

abort the development of the net. Prophylactic photocoagulation is definitely not indicated.

In addition to being watchful for the development of neovascular nets with routine examination and home monitoring of vision, it is important to rule out the possibility of associated systemic disease. Pseudoxanthoma elasticum presents in the second to fourth decade of life as changes in the skin of the neck, axillae, inguinal areas, and periumbilical zone. These changes appear as thickened, grooved, inelastic areas that may have associated plaque formation. Pseudoxanthoma elasticum is the result of a defect in elastin biosynthesis. The disease is usually autosomal recessive, but a rarer autosomal dominant form may present; a pedigree may assist in the differential diagnosis. The autosomal dominant form usually has the skin lesions but not the cardiovascular complications. In addition, the cardiovascular system may suffer occlusions in the form of premature atherosclerosis, angina, myocardial infarctions, valvular heart disease, and peripheral vascular calcifications, which may lead to gastrointestinal and intracerebral hemorrhaging. Up to 70 percent of patients with pseudoxanthoma and angioid streaks develop loss of central vision. Add the association of buried drusen of the optic nerve head with the resultant peripheral field loss and the patient with pseudoxanthoma elasticum is at great risk for severe vision problems over the age of 50 years.

Paget's disease is the result of abnormal bone formation leading to thickened and weakened bone. Paget's disease presents with bone pain, osteoarthritis, and neurologic problems. Thickened bone in the skull of the patient with Paget's disease may reduce the size of the optic foramen and the orbit, resulting in muscle palsies and optic nerve dysfunction. Increased intraocular pressure may also occur secondarily to the compressed episcleral venous channels. Ehlers–Danlos syndrome and sickle-cell disease must also be ruled out. The systemic implications of all of these conditions must be addressed.

The patient should also be prescribed polycarbonate lenses because of the fragility of the system and be advised against potentially traumatic situations, such as contact sports or occupations at high risk of trauma. The patient should also be on some type of home monitoring and should be examined at least every year. Should there be any sign of choroidal neovascular development or serous leakage, it is advisable to perform a fluorescein angiography and ask for a retinal consultation.

IDIOPATHIC CENTRAL SEROUS CHORIORETINOPATHY (ICSC)

Introduction and Description. Idiopathic central serous chorioretinopathy (ICSC) is an enigma in that there are transient episodes of serous retinal or pigment epithelial detachments in the macular area of the posterior pole of eyes of young to middle-aged patients, with none of the common predisposing conditions, such as drusen (Figs. 5–33 and 5–34). ICSC is usually unilateral but the underlying RPE disease is often bilateral and progressive. The average age in years of onset of ICSC is the mid-30s, with a range from the late 20s to the late 50s. ICSC affects males more than females by a 10 to 1 ratio and whites more than nonwhites. If the patient presents with a serous retinal detachment over the age of 55 years, the primary diagnosis should not be ICSC; fluorescein angiography should be used to rule out an age-related choroidal neovascular membrane. Other causes of choroidal neovascular membranes in younger patients, such as presumed ocular histoplasmosis, must be considered as well.

The initial problem in ICSC seems to originate at the level of the RPE. The RPE cells are typically strongly adherent to one another and to Bruch's membrane. They are only loosely adherent to the overlying sensory retina. This tight bond prevents leakage from the spongy choroidal layer from seeping up under the sensory retina. Should the RPE be compromised by poor circulation, the cells may break down, allowing the seepage to occur, which creates a sensory retinal detachment. Further breakdown of the RPE bonds may allow a separation from the underlying Bruch's membrane. This precipitates an RPE detachment. **See color plates 75 and 76.** ICSC usually consists of a small RPE detachment within a larger localized serous sensory detachment. If leakage is excessive, the localized detachment can spread, leading to an extensive bullous retinal detachment.

Type A personality patients (competitive, aggressive, hostile) seem to be more prone to the development of ICSC. The breakdown of the RPE in ICSC has been hypothesized to occur secondary to vasomotor instability or sympathetic nervous excitation. The vascular excitability may create a localized breakdown in choriocapillaris blood supply to the RPE. The propensity of ICSC for the macula speaks to the high hemodynamic activity at the macula. Because of the compromise of the RPE, the practitioner will often find pigmentary migration and hyperplasia associated with ICSC as well as some microcystic changes.

The ophthalmoscopic view of the active condition is variable. Binocular indirect ophthalmoscopy gives the best overall view of the dome of elevated retina. The change is subtle, and the clinician must rely on color variation and reflections from the internal limiting membrane. There may be a loss of foveal reflex. The details of the dome are best observed under high magnification with a Hruby or Volk lens. The dome can also be transilluminated to enhance the view. Should the detachment be long standing, the dome may present with yellow precipitates. The appearance of the precipitates indicates a poorer prognosis for visual recovery, as these deposits are a sign of longevity of the lesion.

Evidence of past bouts of ICSC present as RPE disturbances or cystlike areas in the macula. In most cases of ICSC, the clinician can observe a one third DD or less area of RPE detachment beneath the detached retina. This area is usually yellow and is referred to as a lemon-drop nodule. This nodule may transilluminate as a golden glowing area. Infrequently this nodule may be larger, sometimes up to 1 DD, and may even lie outside the area of retinal detachment.

In all cases of ICSC, fluorescein angiography of-

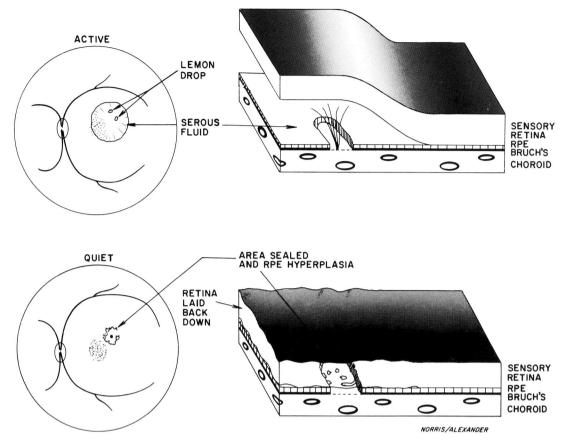

Figure 5–33. A schematic illustrating both active and quiet stages of ICSC.

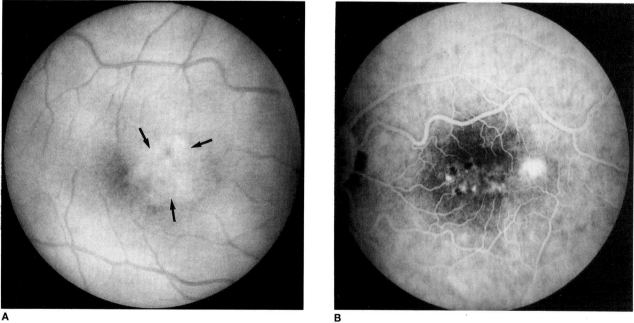

Figure 5–34. Examples of macular changes associated with ICSC. **A.** Illustrates the RPE changes (bounded by the *small arrows*). **B.** Demonstrates the picture of the leakage with fluorescein angiography.

Idiopathic Central Serous Chorioretinopathy (ICSC)

Characteristics

△ ICSC occurs in young to middle-aged patients and is associated with anxiety or stress

△ Usually unilateral but reflects bilateral RPE disease

△ Affects males 10:1 over females and is associated with Type A personalities

△ Dome of elevated retina is associated with loss of foveal reflex resulting from a small RPE detachment within a larger sensory retinal detachment

△ If long standing, there are yellow precipitates in the area

△ The area of swelling shows RPE disturbance and may have a lemon-drop nodule within

△ With cessation of activity may notice RPE hyperplasia

△ Fluorescein angiography is diagnostic, especially when concerned about the possibility of a choroidal neovascular membrane

△ Metamorphopsia, delayed photostress recovery, and vision loss are symptoms; the clinician may also notice a hyperopic shift in the refraction

△ Percentage recovery of vision is high 1 to 6 months after bout

△ Recurrence rate is 20 to 30 percent

△ May be associated RPE decompensation or the sick retinal pigment epithelial syndrome

Management

△ Rule out other causes of serous retinal detachments

△ Reassurance

△ Indications for photocoagulation
  Patient intolerant of symptoms
  Accumulation of turbid subretinal fluids
  Severe recurrence
  Long-standing cases (4 months) outside of foveal avascular zone
  Cases developing CME
  Concordance of choroidal neovascular membranes
  Serous macular detachment

△ Possible photocoagulation
  Direct photocoagulation decreases the duration of serous elevation but does not improve visual outcome
  Indirect photocoagulation may increase recurrence rates
  Direct photocoagulation may improve outcome in RPE decompensation threatening vision
  Photocoagulation is of benefit in situations of secondary development of choroidal membranes

△ Vitamin supplementation?

△ Psychological counseling?

△ Home monitoring of vision

△ Yearly routine eye examinations

---

fers the definitive diagnosis, in most cases showing a focal punctate stain that grows in size and holds its fluorescence into the late stages. Ultimately, the stain diffuses into the area of the sensory retinal detachment. Fluorescein angiography will demonstrate no leakage in cases where the RPE has resealed itself.

ICSC typically presents as a sudden onset of unilateral distortion (metamorphopsia) or slight loss of central vision. The patient may also complain of a haze over vision or a slight color perception problem. Contrast sensitivity will be altered, as well as macular photostress recovery time. There may be a unilateral hyperopic shift, but this is a weak diagnostic sign. General health is usually good, with no particular association with systemic disease. There is, however, often an association with anxiety or stress. Past bouts of ICSC may present as areas of RPE migration and hyperplasia.

Management. ICSC carries a relatively good prognosis with no intervention whatsoever. A very high percentage of patients recover vision to a 20/40 level within 1 to 6 months after the onset of symptoms. Up to 60 percent recover vision to the 20/20 level. When associated with the stress of pregnancy, the symptoms typically resolve by the third trimester.

There is always some residual metamorphopsia, but it is rarely noticed by the patient. The major problem associated with ICSC is recurrence. Up to 20 to 30 percent of patients have recurrences that may progress to reduced vision associated with RPE atrophy. It is, however, very rare to have permanent vision loss below 20/40. The fellow eye may develop ICSC even after a considerable time delay, but this occurrence is also very rare. An exudative retinal detachment may occur as well as RPE decompensation after multiple attacks. The RPE decompensation, also known as the "sick retinal pigment epithelium syndrome," may lead to the formation of localized RPE changes known as an RPE gutter or may lead to generalized loss of function that may support the development of choroidal neovascular membranes.

Localized photocoagulation affords the only proven mode of therapeutic intervention, and should be considered only after a 3- to 4-month waiting period to allow for the possibility of spontaneous resolution. It is believed that under certain circumstances photocoagulation may be effective in sealing the site of RPE damage and leakage. As there is a very strong tendency for excellent spontaneous recovery, *photocoagulation must be applied only after strong consideration.* Indications for photocoagulation are as follows.

1. A patient who is intolerant of symptoms and is willing to take a risk.
2. Accumulation of turbid subretinal fluid.
3. Severe bouts of recurrence with a direct threat to vision.
4. Long-standing cases where photocoagulation is not a direct threat to macular function (as with a leakage point outside of the foveal avascular zone).
5. Cases where there is a defect in the fellow eye from recurrent bouts of ICSC.
6. Cases with anatomic changes in the macula such as cystoid macular edema.
7. The occurrence of secondary choroidal neovascular membranes.
8. Serous detachment of the macula.

The photocoagulation technique of direct application at the site of angiographic leakage decreases the duration of serous detachment of the macula but does not appreciably improve the final visual acuity nor does it appreciably affect recurrence rates. Direct krypton appears to have less of a recurrence rate than direct argon. Indirect photocoagulation away from the site of the leakage does not positively affect outcome; in fact it has a tendency to increase the rates of recurrence, and appears to be far inferior to the direct management. Treatment of exudative retinal detachment with argon or krypton appears to effectively precipitate the resolution of the detachment.

Photocoagulative intervention in cases of RPE decompensation with leakage compromising vision improves or stabilizes vision when compared to untreated eyes. It is important to recognize that there is no cookbook for photocoagulative intervention in ICSC. A delay of up to 4 months prior to treatment is important because of the distinct possibility of spontaneous resolution. Treatment should be avoided within ½ DD of the foveal center.

There appears to be no known medical therapy for ICSC, and the obvious technique of stress reduction has no validation. Patients should be made aware of their condition and should monitor their vision, as choroidal neovascular membrane development is always a possibility. It is also sound to schedule the patient for yearly routine examinations. There have been some indications that vitamin/mineral supplementation may be of benefit, but there is no proof.

CYSTOID MACULAR EDEMA (CME)

Introduction and Description. Cystoid macular edema (CME) may be secondary to many ocular conditions. These include retinal vaso-occlusive disease, postcataract surgery (Irvine-Gass syndrome), idiopathic central serous chorioretinopathy, pars planitis, severe carotid or ophthalmic artery disease, retinitis pigmentosa, progressive pigmentary degeneration, YAG laser posterior capsulotomy, relaxing corneal incision, retinal surgery, radiation retinopathy, ocular inflammatory conditions, and ocular tumors. The macular area is very sensitive to fluid accumulation, and as such even remote lesions such as angiomatosis retina can precipitate cystoid macular edema. CME can be vascularly mediated, RPE mediated, or idiopathic. The clinician must also rule out toxic substances, such as all forms of epinephrine, or propine use in treatment of primary open-angle glaucoma, as their use may be related to the accumulation of edema in the macular area.

When CME occurs secondary to cataract extraction (Irvine–Gass syndrome), there is usually a delay in onset of the edema. The peak occurrence is usually at about the sixth postoperative week. By using fluorescein studies it has been shown that up to 50 percent of postsurgical aphakic eyes develop CME, but only an extremely small percentage of these are symptomatic. There seems to be no race, age, or sexual predilection for CME. There does seem to be an in-

Pearls

Cystoid Macular Edema (CME)

Characteristics

△ Occurs secondary to many ocular or systemic conditions

△ Strong association with cataract surgery with vitreous displacement

△ Usually loss of foveal reflex, as the elevation is subtle

△ Fluorescein angiography gives definitive diagnosis—petalliform appearance in the macula

△ Reduced vision, metamorphopsia, and prolonged photostress recovery may occur along with the signs and symptoms of the precipitating conditions

△ A dominantly inherited form occurs with initial loss of vision starting in the 30s and progressing insidiously over the following years

Management

△ High percentage of spontaneous recovery

△ Controversy as to the benefit of prostaglandin inhibitors or corticosteroids both in inhibition and in treatment

△ Possible grid photocoagulation intervention

△ Possible benefit to intervention with pars plana vitrectomy

△ Retinology consultation is indicated

△ Provision of best refractive correction and routine yearly examinations

crease in the percentage occurrence of CME associated with vitreous prolapse with vitreal adherence to anterior chamber structures (the vitreous wick syndrome). This relationship lends support to the theory that the etiopathogenesis of CME is related to vitreous fiber adhesions to the macula, predisposing this area to the development of edema with displacement of the vitreous.

CME usually is secondary to fluid seeping into the unusual arrangement of fibers in Henle's layer, where the internal limiting membrane is the thinnest. The etiology of fluid accumulation is sometimes obscure.

The ophthalmoscopic picture is rarely dramatic. Often all that is evident is loss of foveal reflex, which is not particularly useful in older patients, who inherently have a loss of foveal reflex. When CME is suspected, fluorescein angiography is the definitive diagnostic test; the radiating cystoid spaces of CME present a glow simulating the petals of a flower. If the CME is chronic, the cystoid spaces may coalesce, facilitating the development of a lamellar or through-and-through macular hole.

The patient with CME may complain of variable reduction in vision; this is often the presentation postoperatively in the cataract patient who has had better visual acuity at previous postoperative visits. This reduction would be most obvious with contrast sensitivity. Slight metamorphopsia may be evident on Amsler grid, and a prolonged photostress recovery time will occur. As CME is associated with many other ocular conditions, numerous other unrelated signs and symptoms may be present.

Management. Prognosis for untreated Irvine–Gass syndrome is very good, as about 50 percent of eyes recover normal vision in about 6 months. Twenty percent of these patients will, however, have the condition for up to 5 years.

Several studies support use of prostaglandin inhibitors for the treatment of aphakic and pseudophakic CME. Topical indomethacin (1 percent) drops given four times a day for 1 to 4 months as treatment or prophylaxis against CME has been effective. The prostaglandin inhibitor coupled with 1 percent topical steroids may also be of some value. The question still exists as to whether intervention or prophylactic treatment is indicated, as such a small percentage of angiographically proven CME ever creates any visual problem at all. When CME is secondary to another ocular or systemic condition, the associated conditions must always be managed.

If CME stands alone as the primary condition, the intervention question becomes even more clouded. Oral inhibitors of prostaglandins, oral corticosteroids, and topical steroids all have variable efficacy and unpredictable side effects. Periocular corticosteroid injections are likewise unpredictable. Pars plana vitrectomy may be considered if vitreoretinal traction is present. Pars plana vitrectomy has also been shown to benefit CME that is unresponsive to corticosteroids. Grid photocoagulation has also produced some positive results.

■ ■ ■ ■ ■ ■

Clinical Note: Dominantly Inherited Cystoid Macular Edema

There are also reports of dominantly inherited cystoid macular edema. This form of macular dystrophy has its onset at approximately age 30 years, with an insidious progression to moderate to severe vision loss over the following decades. The dominant pathologic changes in this form of macular edema are in the inner nuclear layer, appearing as large retinal cysts, atrophy, disorganization of the inner nuclear layer, preretinal membranes, and degeneration of Müller cells.

MACULAR HOLES

Introduction and Description. The etiology of macular hole formation is somewhat confusing. Trauma with subsequent cystoid macular edema was originally considered the primary causative factor. It is now considered that any condition that precipitates cystoid macular edema may be implicated in facilitating the genesis of the macular hole. There is also some thought that macular hole formation may be related to the tugging at the macular area secondary to posterior vitreous detachment. The latest work implies that the macular hole actually occurs secondary to traction pulling the photoreceptors apart in the macular area. It is important to note that vitreous cortex can remain at the fovea after a total posterior vitreous detachment. Idiopathic macular holes usually occur in patients over 60 years of age. The incidence of bilaterality varies from 6 to 22 percent and affects women more frequently than men.

Stages of macular hole development have been proposed. Stage 1 (the macular cyst) is considered the point at which focal contraction of the prefoveal vitreous cortex elevates the retina, creating a tractional detachment or an impending hole. There is no evidence of vitreous detachment at stage 1, but mild reduction in visual acuity and metamorphopsia. Stage 2 is the result of further contraction causing a tear typically at one edge of the fovea. Over several months the tear enlarges to the fully developed hole, or stage 3.

Macular Holes

Characteristics

△ May be idiopathic associated with age, or may be related to degenerative or pathologic myopia

△ Idiopathic in patients over age 60 years and more frequent in females

△ Bilateral in 6 to 22 percent of patients

△ Macular pseudoholes are the result of contraction of epiretinal membranes around the tightly adherent foveal area

    Elliptical with the longest axis vertical

    Presence of epiretinal membrane

    Probable zonal tortuous vessels due to tugging

    No yellow dot, no PVD, no cuff of subretinal fluid

△ Stage 1 (macular cyst)

    Focal contraction of prefoveal vitreous with retinal elevation and loss of foveal pit

    Yellow spot forms in pit and may enlarge to a ring

    No evidence of PVD at this stage

    Mild reduction in vision and metamorphopsia

    May have spontaneous loss of traction and aborting of development of the hole with a plug of condensed vitreous over fovea (PVD)

    May have mild rip of inner layer of retina resulting in lamellar hole with mild reduction of vision, presence of PVD, and a round, oval, or petal-shaped color variation over the fovea

    50 percent progression to stage 3

△ Stage 2

    Result of further traction on stage 1 with a rip developing in the edge of the hole

    Stronger likelihood of progression (70 percent) to stage 3

△ Stage 3 (through-and-through macular hole)

    Circular to oval depression in avascular area of macular

    One-fourth to one-third DD reddish area surrounded by gray edema

    Yellow deposits at base known as pathologic drusen

    Severely reduced acuity and a central scotoma

Management

△ Differentiate stages and rule out a pseudohole

△ 50 percent chance of stage 1 developing into a true hole

△ If macular hole in one eye and PVD in other, little chance of fellow eye developing hole

△ If macular hole in one eye and no PVD in other, 28 to 44 percent chance of fellow eye developing hole

△ RPE disturbances in fellow eye to macular hole are an 80 percent risk factor

△ Retinal thinning in fellow eye to macular hole is a risk factor

△ Vitrectomy is of tremendous benefit in helping to abort the development of a macular hole from stage 1; obtain a retina/vitreous consultation

△ Vitrectomy may be of some value in improving outcome in stages 2 and 3; obtain a retina/vitreous consultation in stage 2 and in a fresh stage 3

△ Possibility of retinal detachment is remote in idiopathic holes related to aging

△ Macular holes associated with pathologic myopia have a high incidence of retinal detachment

    The higher the myopia, the greater the risk

    Chorioretinal degeneration is a risk

    Posterior staphylomas are a risk

△ Recommend safety lenses and educate the patient to avoid trauma, especially in high myopia

△ Recommend home monitoring and follow according to risk factors

During stage 1, traction and loss of the foveal depression, the xanthophyll pigment concentrated at the base of the fovea becomes more apparent as a yellow spot, which enlarges to a ring as the traction continues. The yellow spot may be a similar presentation as the yellow nodule in the middle of an ICSC lesion. In approximately 50 percent of patients the process is aborted at stage 1, resulting in a relaxation of the retina and a return of vision. At this aborted stage, a plug of condensed vitreous may present in front of the fovea. The other clinical presentation at this aborted stage is the inner lamellar hole created by stripping away of inner retinal tissue. The inner lamellar hole has evidence of a vitreous detachment, the presence of a foveal depression, and a round, oval, or petal-shaped depression in the macular area. If progression occurs, the retina is pulled apart in this area, resulting in significant vision loss.

The important aspect of macular hole management is the differentiation of the stages of the macular holes and the differentiation from macular pseudoholes (Figs. 5–35 to 5–37), so that intervention with vitrectomy and/or photocoagulation may be presented if it is a viable option. Careful biomicroscopic examination with appropriate fundus lenses is crucial to differentiating the stages of macular hole evolution. It has been suggested that green laser source, a narrow beam, and maximal brightness enhance the ability to properly view the macular architecture. The use of digitized imagery with the optic nerve head scopes now being developed may assist in the differential diagnosis.

Macular pseudoholes may be the result of the contraction of epiretinal membranes with a baring of the tightly bound foveal area. The contrast of the whitish epiretinal membrane with the foveal color and the sharply circumscribed borders may create the illusion of a macular hole. Pseudoholes are usually el-

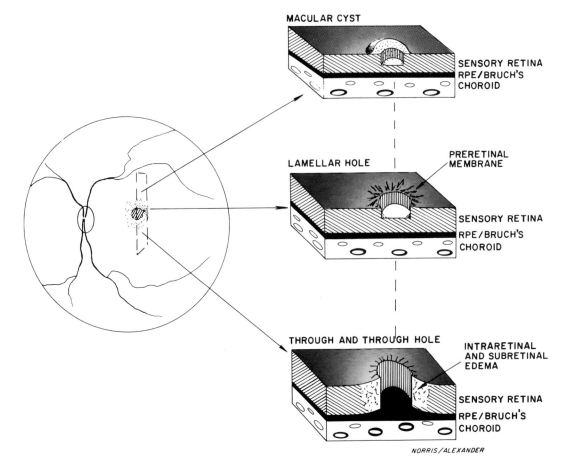

Figure 5–35. A schematic illustrating the differences between macular cysts, lamellar macular holes, and through-and-through macular holes.

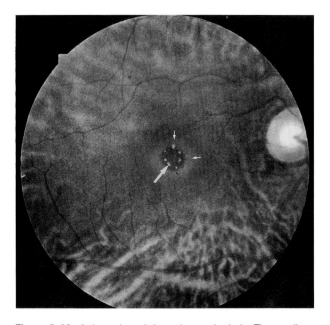

Figure 5–36. A through-and-through macular hole. The small arrows point to the surrounding retinal "edema," while the large arrow points to the yellow deposits in the base of the hole.

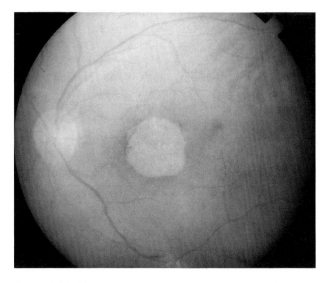

Figure 5–37. Example of a macular coloboma that had been improperly diagnosed as a macular hole.

liptical, with the vertical axis longer, and have the absence of features typically associated with macular holes, such as a foveolar detachment in an impending situation, yellow dot in the center of the fovea, cuff of subretinal fluid, yellow deposits at the base of the hole, and overlying operculum of detached vitreous. The pseudohole also has an associated preretinal membrane with characteristics such as locally tortuous vasculature made even more apparent by fluorescein angiography or red-free photographs. Visual acuity is also usually better in the eye with the pseudohole as compared to the true macular hole, but the membrane can actually reduce vision as well.

A macular hole is a circular to oval depression in the avascular area of the macula. The color variation from the surrounding edematous retina makes identification with the binocular indirect ophthalmoscope quite obvious. Macular cysts are often the result of coalescence of macular cystoid areas into a larger cavity and are the equivalent of stage 1 macular holes.

Macular holes are usually divided into two distinct entities, lamellar holes and full-thickness holes. Although this distinction may be inappropriate, it is still considered in the clinical definition by many clinicians. The lamellar hole is the result of the rupture of the thin, inner retinal layer of a macular cyst. There is a slight reddish coloration of the hole. This makes the lamellar hole a partial-thickness macular excavation usually with some maintenance of visual acuity.

A full-thickness macular hole is an excavation that is either entirely devoid of retinal tissue or has a nondistinguishable outer retinal layer. The classic full-thickness hole is one-fourth to one-third DD in size, appearing as a reddish area often surrounded by grayish retinal elevation and appearing like a doughnut. There are yellowish deposits in the base of the hole that may be migratory. Macular cysts and lamellar holes do not have the dramatic color of a through-and-through hole, but visual acuity and stereoscopic observation are necessary to validate the diagnosis. Retinal glial membranes may also grow onto the surface of the retina surrounding a lamellar or through-and-through macular hole.

In the early arteriovenous phase of fluorescein angiography, a through-and-through hole will demonstrate hyperfluorescence, while a lamellar hole or cyst will hypofluoresce. In the late stages, cysts may hyperfluoresce like true holes. **See color plates 77 and 78.**

Patients with lamellar holes and macular cysts will present with slightly reduced acuity and metamorphopsia in addition to the classic ophthalmoscopic picture. The true macular hole will create significantly reduced visual acuity, a central scotoma, and the potential for the effects of a retinal detachment.

Management. If a patient presents with a stage 1 macular hole (macular cyst), there is considerable controversy as to whether this will develop into a full-thickness hole. This question will only be resolved by a high-population carefully controlled study. Hole development is thought to be associated with a posterior vitreous detachment (PVD). The identification of a PVD is a pretty good indicator of stability. Approximately 70 percent of stage 2 holes progress to stage 3 without intervention.

If a patient has a true macular hole in one eye, there are predictors of hole formation in the fellow eye. If PVD is present in the fellow eye, there is little to no risk of development of a true macular hole. If a PVD is not present, 28 to 44 percent of fellow eyes have been reported to develop macular holes. Patients with pigment epithelial defects in the macula of the fellow eye to a macular hole showed an 80 percent risk of developing a macular hole. The pigment epithelial defects indicate a basic disease problem in the retinal structure, allowing for retinal thinning. Posterior vitreous detachment, RPE defects, disturbances in the macula, and retinal thinning at the macula all represent risk factors for the development of macular holes in fellow eyes.

Understanding that the vitreoretinal adhesion may be a risk factor for the precipitation of a macular hole lays the foundation for understanding the potential benefits of interventive vitrectomy. Studies documenting vitrectomy performed in stage 1 holes demonstrate that development of through-and-through macular holes is aborted. Although stage 2 holes do not show an improvement in visual acuity with vitrectomy, they do show stability of acuity. This can apparently be achieved with attention to the core vitreous and without manipulation of the prefoveal cortical vitreous in stage 1, but may not be as beneficial in stage 2. There are even suggestions that vitrectomy may collapse full-thickness macular holes, resulting in improved visual acuity although there may be associated RPE changes with the procedures that could harbinger future chorioretinal problems.

Secondary retinal detachment of the retina caused by liquefied vitreous seeping under the retina through the hole occurs at a very low rate associated with idiopathic holes related to aging. When detachment does occur, there is a fairly good success rate with reattachment. There has even been the recommendation that cyanoacrylate tissue adhesive retinopexy may improve the outcome of patients with retinal detachments secondary to macular holes. The glue is literally placed at the macular hole. Prophylactic photocoagulation is indicated in myopic eyes over 6D because of the high incidence of secondary detachment. The higher the myopia and the more associated chorioretinal degeneration, the more likely it is that retinal detachment will occur associated with retinal holes. The presence of a posterior staphyloma in pathologic myopia is also a grim prognostic indicator, and the presence of the posterior vitreous detachment in the patient with pathologic myopia is apparently not protective, as it is in the idiopathic age-related hole. It is believed that the macular hole and the associated retinal detachment evolve from different mechanisms in pathologic myopia and in the idiopathic condition associated with aging. Argon photocoagulation may be of benefit in minimizing the surrounding shallow retinal elevation and may stabilize visual acuity.

The key feature for management of the patient with an impending macular hole or a through-and-through hole is the recognition of the stage of the development of the hole. At all stages, there are reports of improvement with vitrectomy intervention. It must be remembered, however, that fewer than 50 percent of impending holes (stage 1) will ever progress to stage 3. At the same time the practitioner must realize that vitrectomy intervention may result in totally aborting the progression of all stage 1 holes and some stage 2 holes. Stage 1 and 2 holes deserve a retina/vitreous consultation to ascertain whether surgery would be of benefit. Stage 3 holes may also collapse, resulting in a slight improvement in acuity. The clinician has the responsibility of explaining the condition to the patient, mentioning the risk factors for involvement of the fellow eye, discussing the risk factors of vitrectomy intervention, providing polycarbonate lenses for protection, advising against avoidable trauma, and reevaluating at frequent intervals.

The use of transforming growth factor-B2 (TGF-B2) has been recommended for the treatment of macular holes. The use of this method is based on the ability of TGF-B2 to induce chorioretinal adhesion around retinal tears. This would flatten the edges of the macular hole, assisting in the resolution of the subclinical retinal detachment surrounding the hole. The use of this treatment appeared to improve or stabilize holes, but zeal must be tempered by the fact that a core vitrectomy was performed prior to the application and the vitrectomy could be the cure rather than the TGF-B2 (Glaser et al, 1992).

■ ■ ■ ■ ■ ■
Clinical Note: Solar Retinopathy

Solar retinopathy, eclipse burn, and foveomacular retinitis all refer to a condition resulting from direct sungazing, for whatever the reason. Several hours after the sungazing, the vision drops to the 20/30 to 20/100 range, with patient complaints of a small scotoma, chromatic changes in vision, metamorphopsia, and photophobia. As one would expect, the condition is usually bilateral but asymmetrical.

The end results of solar maculopathy may simulate a true macular hole, as a small yellow foveal lesion develops and about 2 weeks after the event, a small oval-shaped red depression appears in the foveal area. Fluorescein angiography may demonstrate an early hyperfluorescence, but is often entirely normal. Vision may return to the 20/20 to 20/40 range over 3 to 6 months, but the patient may still sense the small scotoma. There should certainly be no progression of vision loss. The small size and variable visual acuity of 20/25 to 20/80 often assist in the differential diagnosis.

Foveomacular retinitis is considered by some to be a separate entity from solar maculopathy. Foveomacular retinitis has been reported to present as macular edema followed by a macular cyst surrounded by a one-half to 1 disc diameter gray area. This lesion may then progress to further macular degeneration, resulting in an irregular macular hole and acuity between 20/25 and 5/200.

INFLAMMATORY MACULOPATHIES

Presumed Ocular Histoplasmosis Syndrome (POHS)

Introduction and Description. Presumed ocular histoplasmosis syndrome (POHS) is a fungal disease endemic in many river valleys of the world. Histoplasmin sensitivity is particularly prevalent in the United States in individuals who have lived in or visited the Ohio–Mississippi River Valley. It is believed that the ocular syndrome is the result of bloodborne *Histoplasma capsulatum* organisms reaching choroidal circulation during a bout of systemic dissemination. The hypothesis of the disease origin is that the fungus is inhaled early in life and the macular lesions reactivate 10 to 30 years later in life within the choriocapillaris and grow through prior breaks in Bruch's membrane. Systemic histoplasmosis has a wide variety of presentations, from a flulike illness to a disseminated disease in the young, aged, and immunosuppressed. It must be remembered that acquired immunodeficiency syndrome (AIDS) has the potential to create reactivation of POHS. Signs of disseminated disease and ocular manifestations do not usually coexist.

Patients typically present with POHS between ages 20 and 50, with rare occurrences outside this range. Macular involvement associated with POHS usually occurs more frequently in patients over the age of 30 years. POHS only rarely occurs in blacks (six times as frequent in whites than blacks), and when it does occur, macular involvement is less than 20 per-

Presumed Ocular Histoplasmosis Syndrome

Characteristics

△ Associated with persons who were born in or visited the Ohio–Mississippi River Valley

△ Six times more frequent in whites than blacks, and blacks have 20 percent the macular involvement of whites

△ Usually presents between 20 and 50 years of age, with macular involvement over 30 years of age

△ Macular involvement may lag the initial infection by up to 30 years

△ Bilateral macular involvement more common in men than women

△ Circumpapillary choroidal scarring, peripheral atrophic histoplasmosis spots, and exudative maculopathy secondary to choroidal neovascular membranes

   May also have linear streaks of chorioretinal atrophy in the retinal periphery

△ Progression of macular lesions
   Stage 1 is the development of a yellow fluffy focus of active choroiditis near the macula
   Stage 2 is the development of a pigment ring or nodule in the macular area with an overlying sensory serous detachment
   Stages 3 through 5 are the exudative stages of development, with severe reduction in vision

△ Absence of vitritis and anterior uveitis

△ Patient is asymptomatic until macular involvement, which shows as vision reduction and/or metamorphopsia

△ If one eye has a disciform scar secondary to POHS, the fellow eye has a 30 percent chance of development within 6 to 7 years after the first with the presence of histoplasmosis lesions in the macula

Management

△ Educate patient regarding the condition and the possibilities for loss of vision

△ Routine follow–up and home monitoring of vision, especially if there are histoplasmosis lesions near the macula

△ Fluorescein angiography and retinal consultation at first sign of active macular involvement

△ Medical intervention with steroids and antifungals are of no proven value

△ Juxtafoveal neovascular membranes are treatable by krypton laser photocoagulation

△ Extrafoveal neovascular membranes are treatable by argon laser photocoagulation

cent of that in whites. POHS has no sexual predilection. Involvement in both maculae occurs more frequently in men than women. It is also important to note that the macular form of the disease may not occur until up to 30 years after the disseminated form appears. It is also of note that the macular form is often precipitated by stress.

POHS is characterized by a triad of circumpapillary choroidal scarring, peripheral atrophic histo (choroidal) spots, and macular compromise secondary to choroidal neovascularization. There is neither the anterior uveitis nor the vitritis that often accompany other intraocular inflammatory processes.

The lesions surrounding the optic nerve head resemble the histoplasmosis spots spread throughout the periphery. The diffuse choroidal inflammation results in choroidal degenerative changes and RPE hyperplasia. This ring of scarring can be up to 0.5 DD in width. It is important not to confuse circumpapillary chorioretinal scarring with circumpapillary chorioretinal atrophy associated with aging. Up to 10 percent of POHS patients develop hemorrhage secondary to choroidal neovascularization in the circumpapillary area. Those who do hemorrhage have a poor prognosis for vision. The changes surrounding the optic nerve head are at the level of the choroid and RPE, which eventually compromises the overlying retina.

The choroidal granulomatous lesions can also occur spread throughout the retina. The majority of atrophic histoplasmosis spots, which are yellow-white and usually less than 1 mm in diameter, occur posterior to the equator and may number up to 70. In addition, linear streaks of chorioretinal atrophy may occur in the peripheral retina. **See color plates 79 through 82.** Bilaterality is the rule (over 60 percent). It is assumed that the *Histoplasma capsulatum* or its byproducts reach the choroidal circulation, creating a granulomatous inflammatory mass that may create breaks in Bruch's membrane on the way to scarring. The active peripheral choroiditis is usually so mild that it is not clinically observable. The lesion typically heals in a few weeks. If these lesions are outside the major temporal vascular supply, the eye will not suffer any associated visual loss. The breaks in Bruch's membrane in peripheral scars rarely lead to neovascularization or serous retinopathy. The peripheral scars are usually 0.2 to 0.7 DD in size and may present with or without RPE hyperplasia.

Macular lesions of POHS seem to progress through specific stages of development (Figs. 5–38 to 5–42). Although the basic pathogenesis is similar to wet ARM, there are usually no drusen as precursors. In stage 1 of POHS maculopathy, a yellowish focus of active choroiditis occurs near the macular area. This may also be considered a choroidal infiltration, as the activity is characterized by fuzzy white borders. These

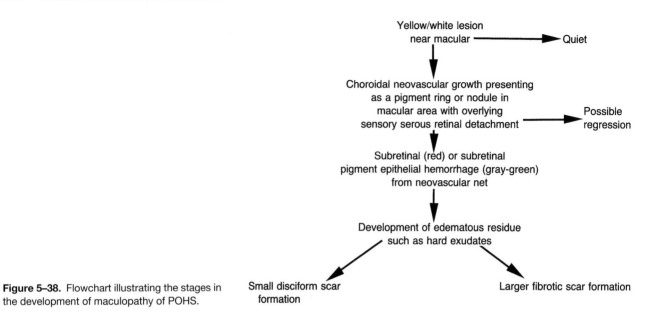

Figure 5–38. Flowchart illustrating the stages in the development of maculopathy of POHS.

infiltrates are less than 1 DD in size and may remain in a holding pattern indefinitely; but the majority will progress toward the development of exudative macular disease. The clinicopathology of this stage is characterized by a small choroidal granulomatous mass that extends through Bruch's membrane to the RPE. There is no leakage during fluorescein angiography at this stage.

Stage 2 is characterized by a pigment ring or pigment nodule in the macular area with an overlying

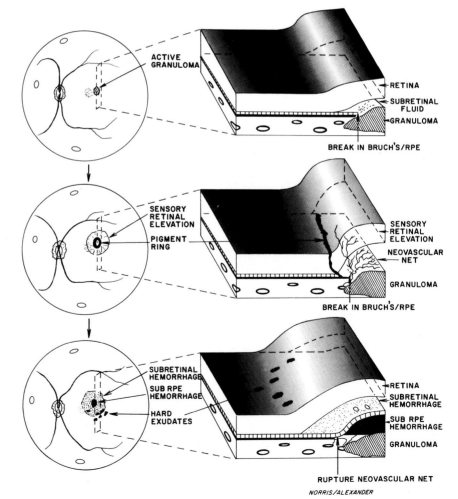

Figure 5–39. A schematic illustrating the stages in the development of macular lesions in POHS.

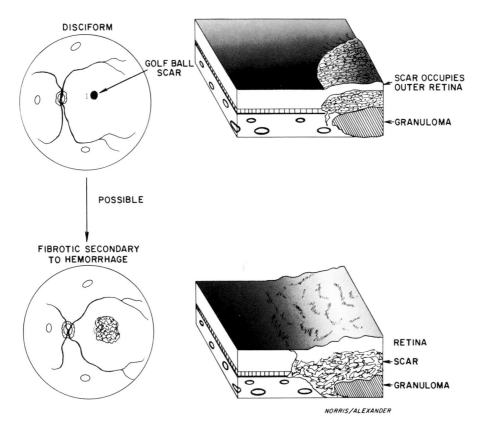

Figure 5–40. A schematic illustrating the development of two types of macular scarring in POHS.

sensory retinal serous detachment. These changes occur because of the choroidal neovascular growth through the compromised Bruch's membrane and the reactive RPE hyperplasia in the area of the lesion. The RPE actually attempts to envelop the growing net and

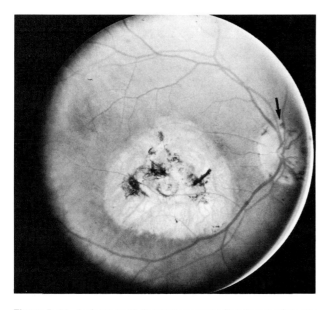

Figure 5–41. A photograph illustrating a large fibrotic macular scar and circumpapillary choroiditis (*arrow*) in POHS.

retard its growth. The growing, leaking neovascular net only adds to the development of serous sensory retinal elevation. This stage will be obvious in all stages of fluorescein angiography. This stage may also stop and regress, leaving only a small scotoma.

Stage 3 of POHS consists of hemorrhages emanating from the neovascular net of stage 2. If the hemorrhage occurs under the RPE, it is gray-green, and if it dissects through to the subsensory retinal space, it will appear red. At this stage, lipid exudates may accumulate around the area of serous elevation. The lipid exudate accumulation is considered by some to indicate longevity of the lesion, and is often referred to as stage 4.

Stage 5 is considered to be the end stage of the development of maculopathy. This stage usually indicates maculopathy of 2 years or more duration. This is the stage of scarring that is seen as a white, elevated lesion, indicating a chronic disciform detachment of the sensory retina with microcystic degeneration. The lesions vary in size up to 1 DD. If hemorrhage has occurred, the scar may be fibrotic and may have less distinct characteristics. The fibrotic scarring usually occupies more territory than the disciform scar, creating a larger scotoma.

Choroidal neovascular membranes may develop in any patient with a history of ocular histoplasmosis,

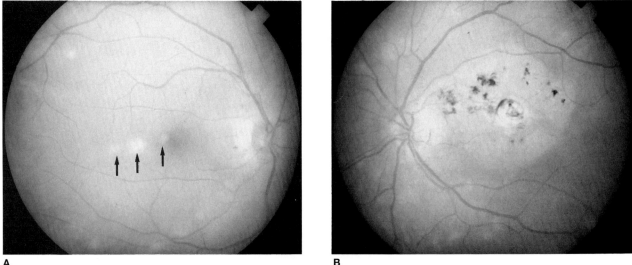

A   **B**

Figure 5–42. Example of a variation on the presentation of POHS. In (**A**), the small arrows point to reactivation granulomas, while (**B**) illustrates the fellow eye with significant macular scarring, peripheral histoplasmosis spots, and circumpapillary choroiditis.

and the development carries a grave visual prognosis. If one eye has an existing disciform scar, there is about a 30 percent chance of the fellow eye developing a neovascular membrane, especially with the presence of macular or perimacular histoplasmosis spots.

The patient with POHS is usually asymptomatic until the macula or circumpapillary area is involved. At that point, vision reduction and metamorphopsia are variable, depending on the proximity of the lesion to the macula. Symptoms of flashing lights, waviness, and field loss may occur with active circumpapillary choroidopathy. Laboratory diagnostic tests are of no value in the differential diagnosis of POHS.

Management. Once choroidal neovascularization begins near the macular area, the prognosis for good vision is poor. Resultant vision of less than 20/200 occurs in over 60 percent of untreated cases. Bilateral loss of vision occurs in 20 to 30 percent of patients, with a mean onset of the second eye 6 to 7 years after the first. Involvement of the second eye usually results in better acuity than the first.

The key to successful management of POHS is the early detection of stages 1 and 2 macular involvement. In general, the peripheral lesions and the circumpapillary chorioretinal lesions are of no threat to vision. All patients with POHS should be on routine followup and home Amsler grid monitoring, especially during the high-risk years of ages 30 to 50. Once the macular vision is threatened, fluorescein angiography is indicated.

Two modes of therapy are used for the prevention of severe vision loss secondary to POHS. Steroids,

both oral and depot injection, are used often to quiet the inflammatory reaction of the disease process. The use of steroids may also be of benefit in the management of recurrences of macular POHS. There is, however, no firm evidence of the benefit of steroids or antifungal agents in the treatment of POHS. Controlled studies have yet to confirm the benefit of any medical management of the ocular disease process.

Numerous studies have demonstrated the benefit of photocoagulative intervention for patients with POHS who are developing neovascular nets outside the foveal areas. Patients who meet certain criteria have a significant reduction in the potential for severe loss of vision over untreated eyes when photocoagulation is properly applied. At the first sign of macular

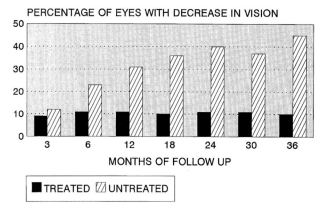

Figure 5–43. Percentage of eyes with a 6-line decrease in visual acuity in POHS treated with argon laser versus those not treated with argon laser. (*Arch Ophthalmol.* 1986;104:694–701.)

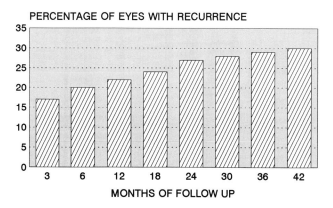

PERCENTAGE OF EYES WITH RECURRENCE

Figure 5–44. Cumulative percentage of eyes developing recurrence of a choroidal neovascular membrane associated with argon photocoagulation for POHS. (*Arch Ophthalmol.* 1986;104:503–517.)

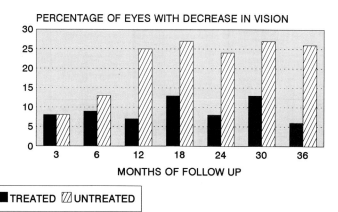

PERCENTAGE OF EYES WITH DECREASE IN VISION

■ TREATED ▨ UNTREATED

Figure 5–45. Percentage of eyes with a 6-line decrease in visual acuity in POHS treated with krypton laser versus those not treated with krypton laser. (*Arch Ophthalmol.* 1987;105:1499–1507.)

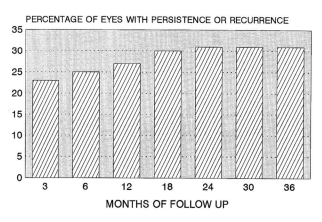

PERCENTAGE OF EYES WITH PERSISTENCE OR RECURRENCE

Figure 5–46. Cumulative percentage of eyes with persistent or recurrent choroidal neovascularization after krypton photocoagulation for POHS. (*Arch Ophthalmol.* 1989;109:344–352.)

involvement, fluorescein angiography is indicated in addition to a consultation with a retinal specialist. Juxtafoveal choroidal neovascular membranes with no overlying RPE detachment benefit from krypton red photocoagulation. Extrafoveal choroidal neovascular membranes benefit from intervention with argon photocoagulation. As with other conditions, prophylactic photocoagulation of inactive histoplasmosis spots is not of benefit, and may actually precipitate the development of choroidal neovascular membranes.

Figures 5–43 to 5–46 demonstrate the positive benefits of photocoagulative intervention and the rate of recurrence of choroidal neovascular membranes in eyes with POHS that were treated with photocoagulation. It should be noted that in the argon laser study that 30 percent of treated eyes did experience recurrence of the neovascular membrane. In the krypton study, there were 23 percent of eyes demonstrating persistence of the neovascular membrane posttreatment, with recurrence in 8 percent of the eyes; but 60 percent of these eyes were eligible for retreatment. Recurrence usually occurred on the foveal side of the treatment scar much the same as the situation with the treatment of age-related maculopathy. In either case, argon or krypton, recurrence was associated with the development of severe vision loss.

Ocular Toxoplasmosis

Introduction and Description. *Toxoplasma gondii* is an obligate intracellular protozoan parasite that produces either a congenital or acquired retinochoroiditis as well as neurologic manifestations. Toxoplasmosis (Figs. 5–47 to 5–50) is one of the more likely causes of posterior uveitis in the United States. Reactivation of both ocular and cerebral toxoplasmosis is also a common occurrence associated with human immunovirus infection. In most cases of activation, compromise of the patient's immune status is the basis for reactivation that creates the inflammatory response. It is estimated that at least 50 percent of the human population would show serologic evidence of exposure to toxoplasmosis.

Fewer than 1 percent of patients with documented acquired toxoplasmosis with lymph node involvement (adenopathy demonstrable in 90 percent) develop retinitis, but over 80 percent of patients with congenitally acquired toxoplasmosis develop retinitis at some time. Congenital toxoplasmosis is an omnipresent threat, with 60 to 70 percent of females at risk during the childbearing years. Congenital infection occurs because of primary maternal infection during pregnancy. It is important to realize that toxoplasmosis can only be transmitted to the fetus during maternal parasitemia. The most common route of maternal infection is exposure to cat feces, as the cat is the natural host for the parasite. The second child of an

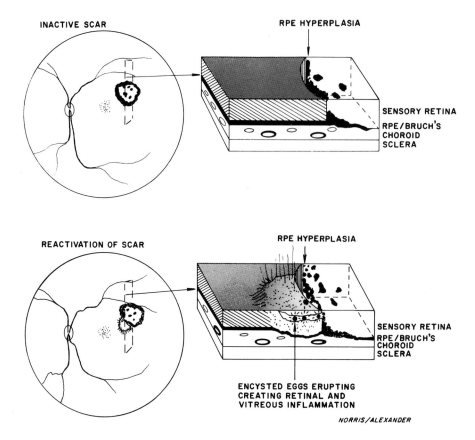

Figure 5–47. A schematic illustrating both an inactive toxoplasmosis scar and a reactivated toxoplasmosis scar.

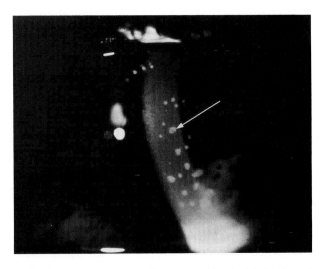

Figure 5–48. The greasy mutton-fat keratitic precipitates (*arrow*) seen in granulomatous anterior uveitis often associated with active ocular toxoplasmosis.

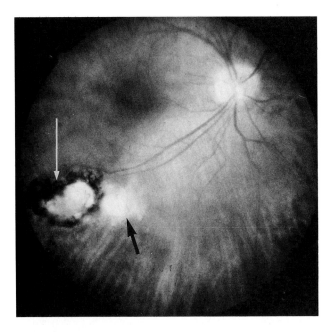

Figure 5–49. The white arrow points to the pigmented toxoplasmosis scar, while the black arrow points to the "headlight in the fog" area of reactivation.

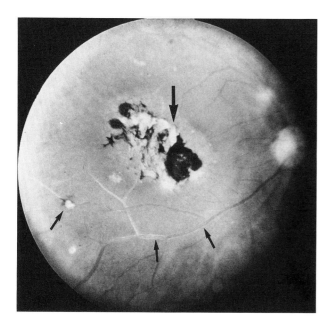

Figure 5–50. The large arrow in this photograph points to an inactive macular toxoplasmosis scar, while the small arrows point to areas of active vasculitis secondary to toxoplasmosis.

exposed mother stands no chance of transplacental infection. The rate of fetal infection increases throughout pregnancy, and the incidence of congenital infection is 0.01 percent of live births.

The *Toxoplasma gondii* parasite may exist in three forms. In the host, the cat, the parasite is in the intestine as a sporozoite contained in oocysts. In the intermediate host the parasite may exist as a tachyzoite, which is the proliferative form; or as a bradyzoite, which is an encysted form. The toxoplasmic protozoa enters the eye of the human via the circulatory system, but then locates within the nerve fiber layer, setting up the potential for the development of an acute necrotizing retinochoroiditis. Once the organism is within the nerve fiber layer, it may actively invade cells, which burst and allow for infection of nearby cells. If the host's resistance is high, the cells may encyst the still-viable organisms. The organisms may remain viable within the cysts for over 25 years. The cysts often encircle old toxoplasmic focal scars. The bradyzoite may exist asymptomatically for several years in the inner retina, but with immunocompromise may multiply, liberating tachyzoites into adjacent tissue. The ocular inflammation caused by the infestation and hypersensitivity reaction manifests as the "headlights in the fog." Eventually, the host immunity will suppress the tachyzoites, causing them to become retransformed to bradyzoites, resulting in a calming of the inflammatory response.

A granulomatous anterior uveitis usually accompanies a reactivation of congenital toxoplasmosis. The anterior uveitis is an extension forward of the posterior inflammation that is believed to be a manifestation of hypersensitivity. The organism has never been recovered from the anterior chamber. **See color plates 83 and 84.**

When inactive, a toxoplasmosis scar is often indistinguishable from other chorioretinal scars. When active, the lesion usually appears as a white lesion next to a pigmented scar, will vary in size from 1/10 to 5 DD, and will have overlying vitreous cells. These cells will cast a haze on the underlying retinal structure. The active lesion may also appear with no apparent accompanying pigmented scar. The lesions may also be multiple and may have an accompanying optic-nerve head locus. Active toxoplasmosis may also manifest as an isolated elevated choroidal nodule. In the case of isolation of the toxoplasmosis lesion in the choroid, it is likely that there will be no associated vitritis or anterior chamber reaction.

There may be an accompanying posterior vitreous detachment, retinal arteritis, occlusive vasculitis, optic neuritis (papillitis), granulomatous anterior uveitis, or macular edema. The arteritis may be so severe as to obscure all other retinal signs, especially in very large inflammatory foci.

It is also well established that reactivation of congenital toxoplasmosis can manifest itself neurologically. The neurologic lesions are a very common complication of human immunovirus infection, while ocular complications are relatively rare.

The patient with active toxoplasmic retinitis may present with blurred vision or floaters secondary to the vitritis, vision or visual field loss secondary to optic nerve inflammation or retinal inflammation near the macula, or a red eye secondary to the anterior uveitis. All granulomatous anterior uveitis should be investigated by a dilated fundus examination to rule out toxoplasmic retinitis.

In the congenital form, the neonatal presentation of toxoplasmosis can be varied, but the classical severe case has the triad of convulsions, cerebral calcifications, and chorioretinitis.

Management. Recurrent attacks of congenital toxoplasmic retinitis can occur between ages 5 and 60 years, with the first attack often occurring in the 20s. The duration of each attack averages 4 months but can be much shorter, with most patients having no more than three attacks. Retinal scarring occurs with each attack. The scarring can compromise vision if it occurs near the macula or within the optic nerve.

Retinal tears near scars open the channel for retinal detachment. Choroidal neovascularization provides a threat for disciform macular disease. The brain and eye share a common vascular system, allowing for neurologic involvement, including convulsions and intracranial calcifications.

Ocular Toxoplasmosis

Characteristics

Δ One of the more likely causes of granulomatous posterior uveitis in the United States

Δ Congenital toxoplasmosis is most common, resulting from primary maternal infection during pregnancy due to exposure to cat feces or ingestion of undercooked meat

Δ The organism is transferred to the fetus via the circulatory system

Δ The organism lodges in nerve fiber layer initially as tachyzoite or proliferative form that may encyst as a bradyzoite awaiting immunocompromise and reactivation

Δ Organisms may remain viable as bradyzoites surrounding old scars for up to 25 years

Δ First active attack of congenital reactivation often in 20s

Δ Active toxoplasmosis presents as anterior granulomatous uveitis, focal white fuzzy retinitis, and overlying vitritis

Δ May have focus of inflammation in nerve head

Δ May have focus of inflammation limited to the choroid with no associated vitritis or anterior uveitis

Δ Patient complains of hazy vision, floaters, field loss, or a red eye (granulomatous anterior uveitis) with reactivation

Management

Δ Attempt to educate the community regarding expectant mother avoidance of cat litter and undercooked meat

Δ Educate patient regarding inactive scars and follow at routine intervals

Δ An active attack usually is self-limiting, lasting up to 4 months

Δ Active lesions/laboratory tests
 Serum antitoxoplasma antibody at 1:1 dilution
 FTA-ABS
 PPD with anergy panel
 Chest x-ray
 Toxocara ELISA
 HIV test if patient at high risk

Δ Active lesions indications for treatment
 Lesions near or threatening the optic nerve
 Lesions severe enough to cause vitreous traction with potential for retinal detachment
 Active lesions near the macula

Δ Active lesions/treatment
 Sulfadiazine 2 to 4 g po load then 1 g po qid. for 4 to 6 weeks
 Pyrimethamine at meals 75 mg po load for 2 days, then 25 mg po daily for 4 to 6 weeks, checking at least weekly for platelet levels and CBC. MUST ALTER IF PLATELETS DROP BELOW 100,000
 Folic acid at 5 mg po three times a week for 4 to 6 weeks to prevent bone marrow depression
 Clindamycin (possible) at 300 mg po tid. to qid. for 4 to 6 weeks, but discontinue if more than four bowel movements per day. Tetracycline is an alternative
 Prednisone at 40 to 60 mg po for 4 to 6 weeks but never alone without antimicrobials

Δ Manage anterior uveitis
 Mydriatics/cycloplegics
 Topical corticosteroids with high penetrability

Δ Watch for retinal tears near scars

Δ Photocoagulation is contraindicated

Δ Cryopexy may be of benefit

Δ Vitrectomy may be of benefit in nonresolving vitreous opacification

The proper diagnosis must be made, as virtually all active toxoplasmic retinitis should be treated if threatening vision. Several laboratory tests may be used to assist in the diagnosis, including the Sabin–Feldman methylene blue dye test (SFDT). The SFDT is, however, of limited value in congenital toxoplasmosis, as the mother's antibodies cross the placenta whether or not the infection is transmitted. The complement fixation test measures antibodies of comparatively short duration and therefore has value in children who have been infected during the first 6 years of life. Serum antitoxoplasma antibody titer (1:1 dilution) is of value because the IgM antibody will not pass the placental barrier, therefore indicating infection by the toxoplasmic organism. To rule out other causes of granulomatous disease, it is also important to order FTA-ABS, PPD with anergy panel, a chest x-ray, a toxocara ELISA, and an appropriate HIV test if the case is atypical or if you feel the patient is at high risk. The reader may refer to Chapter 2 for a further discussion of the workup for the patient with granulomatous anterior uveitis.

Toxoplasmic retinitis must be treated when there is a threat to macular function because of the associated necrosis of retinal tissue. Interestingly enough, there are no controlled studies establishing the efficacy of medical intervention in active ocular toxoplasmosis. Indications for treatment include (1) lesions near or threatening the optic nerve or peripapillary bundle, (2) lesions severe enough to cause vitreous traction or retinal detachment, and (3) active lesions near the macula. In fact, there are only rare instances when aggressive therapy should not be instituted for the above-cited situations, one of those being pregnancy.

Systemic therapy consists of the synergistic employment of triple sulfonamides with pyrimethamine and oral corticosteroids to suppress the inflammatory reaction. Steroids should never be used in the absence of antimicrobials. The therapy is not without risk, as the antitoxoplasmic agent (pyrimethamine) may alter white blood cell and platelet production. Other agents, such as chlortetracycline, clindamycin, and spiramycin, may also be used. Clindamycin carries the risk of pseudomembranous colitis. The standard treatment protocol calls for (1) sulfadiazine 2 to 4 g po load, then 1 g po qid. for 4 to 6 weeks; (2) pyrimethamine (at meals) 75 mg po load for 2 days, then 25 mg po daily for 4 to 6 weeks; (3) folic acid with pyrimethamine to prevent bone marrow depression at 5 mg po three times a week for 4 to 6 weeks; (4) possibly Clindamycin (tetracycline at 2 g load po followed by 250 mg po qid. is an alternative for persons over 12 years and nonpregnant females) at 300 mg po tid. to qid. for 4 to 6 weeks but discontinue with more than four bowel movements per day; and possibly (5) prednisone at 40 to 60 mg po for 4 to 6 weeks. The accompanying anterior uveitis should be managed by mydriatic/cycloplegic agents combined with topical steroids with high ocular penetrability (Pred forte 1% qid. or Flarex qid.). If the patient is on pyrimethamine, a platelet count and CBC must be performed at least weekly, and if the platelet count falls below 100,000, the dosage must be reduced and the folic acid dosage must be increased. Follow-up should be in 3 to 7 days depending on the severity of the lesion.

Surgical treatment of the active lesions has value only when all medical modalities have been exhausted. Photocoagulation is not recommended for the treatment of ocular toxoplasmosis. Cryopexy offers more opportunity for eradication of the lesion because of the organism's sensitivity to cold. Vitrectomy may be of benefit for severe nonresolvable vitreous opacification creating a compromise of vision.

Ocular Parasititis

Introduction and Description. Migration of parasitic larvae to the eye is an important cause of blindness in many parts of the world. The most common of these parasites in the United States is the nematode larvae of *Toxocara canis*. This parasite infects dogs and other canids and is transferred to humans by fecal material (Fig. 5–51). *Cysticercus cellulosae* is the larval form of the pork tapeworm that may also infect the ocular area. Many other parasites, including giardiasis and onchocerciasis, have been implicated in eye infections.

Human intraocular infestation by all worms may cause a diffuse subacute neuroretinitis. This condition is characterized by a unilateral decrease in vision in young adults, with an accompanying vitritis, papillitis, and recurrent patches of grayish outer RPE lesions. With time, optic atrophy and diffuse RPE changes may occur. The various nematodes have been reported to remain viable in the subretinal area for up to 3 years.

Human infestation by the Toxocara larvae manifests as ocular larval migrans and visceral larval migrans. Table 5–6 summarizes the differences between ocular and visceral forms. The infestation usually presents between the ages of 2 and 40 years, but most commonly in ages 7 or 8 years old; it is most commonly diagnosed in the south central and southeastern regions of the United States. The infestation is usually associated with ingestion of the eggs of the parasite and is often associated with eating dirt (geophagia) or contact with puppies. The ingested eggs may remain viable for years and develop into viable larvae at any point in time. These larvae then enter the lymph and blood systems to form foci of granulomas throughout the host's body.

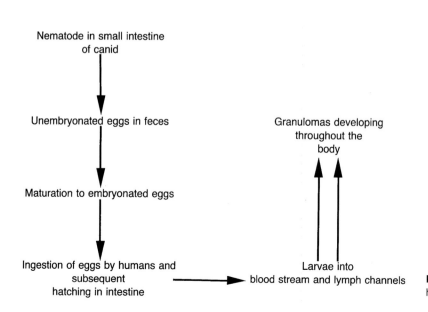

Figure 5–51. Flowchart illustrating the route of human infestation by the Toxocara organism.

TABLE 5–6. CHARACTERISTICS OF OCULAR AND VISCERAL TOXOCARA INFESTATION

Characteristics	Ocular Form	Visceral Form
Age at onset	6 to 7 years	2 years
Ocular findings	Posterior pole and/or peripheral retinal granuloma, anterior uveitis	
White count	Normal	Elevated
Eosinophil count	Normal	Elevated
Enzyme-linked immuno-assay	Low (<1:512)	High (<1:16)
Visceral signs	Absent	Present

The ocular manifestations of Toxocara as well as other nematodes (Figs. 5–52 and 5–53) may present as peripheral focal lesions, posterior pole focal lesions, or diffuse vitreous involvement with associated retinal detachment in addition to the diffuse unilateral subacute neuroretinitis. These lesions may be the result of a nematode that has been present in the subretinal space for 4 years or more. Anterior uveitis, hypopyon, and vascular occlusion secondary to neuroretinitis have also been reported. Virtually any condition associated with an inflammatory response may present.

The choroid may be involved with extension into the retina and vitreous, or the retina may be the focus of infestation. The nematode may be present both within or below the retina. The retinal lesion is typically round, raised, white, and about 1 DD in size. **See color plate 85.** There is often an associated reactive RPE hyperplasia and fibrotic bands radiating from the lesion.

The visceral form of Toxocara is associated with a cough, chest pain, intermittent fever, loss of appetite, and at times, right upper abdominal pain. In children, eruptions and nodules may present over the trunk and lower extremities.

Ocular Toxocara may present with a mild iritis, but is often discovered when a child is examined because of decreased vision, leukocoria, strabismus, or all three. It is rare to have any systemic manifestations associated with the primary ocular condition.

The clinical diagnosis is based on the ELISA test for Toxocara, which gives a diagnostic sensitivity of 78 percent with a specificity of 92 percent. Diagnostic B-scan ultrasonography may also be of assistance for differentiating the white raised lesion from other causes for a similar appearance.

Onchocerciasis (river blindness) is a very common cause of blindness in underdeveloped nations. The cause is the bite of the blackfly, which transfers the parasite and usually goes unnoticed. The worm then develops after a latent interval of 1 to 2 years. The infective larvae mature into adult worms, which release microfilariae. The adult worms form skin nodules often associated with the joints. The nodules are more common around the pelvic area in the individuals infected in Africa, but occur around the head and shoulders in those infected in Central America.

The earliest sign of ocular involvement in onchocerciasis is the result of the invasion by the microfilariae. They may be seen in the anterior chamber of the eye, especially if the patient sits with the head between the knees for a few minutes prior to examination. The microfilariae appear as small white, wiggling worms in the anterior chamber. The microfilariae may be accompanied by inflammatory infiltration in the cornea and a sclerosing keratopathy may develop with time. Eventually the entire cornea may become opacified. The retina may demonstrate RPE migration, atrophy, or hyperplasia, or more commonly a granular atrophy of the RPE. Areas of active inflammation may appear as retinal edema with leakage on fluorescein angiography. The macula is often spared until the end stage of the disease process.

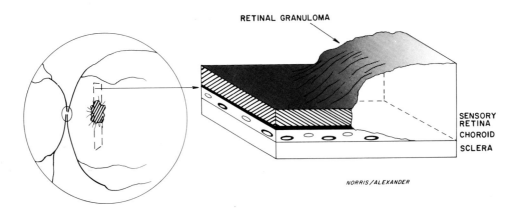

Figure 5–52. A schematic illustrating a granuloma created by the Toxocara organism.

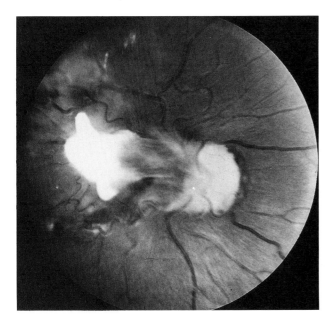

Figure 5–53. A photograph of a retinal granuloma created by Toxocara. (*Photo courtesy of R. Coshatt.*)

Management. Initially it is necessary to differentiate the condition from other potentially more serious causes of leukocoria in youth. Table 5–7 provides the major causes of leukocoria in youth.

Should the inflammatory process invade the posterior pole and the granuloma become established, hopes for recovery of vision are poor. If the larva is active and seen away from the capillary free zone, several modes of therapy may be attempted. Steroid therapy by mouth may act to suppress the inflammatory response but has not been proven in clinical studies. Thiabendazole, photocoagulation applied directly to the live nematode, and cryopexy have all been attempted with variable success. Clearly the most effective measure against ocular parasititis is prevention. The public must be educated regarding the impact of geophagia (eating of dirt by children and some adults) and the consumption of all undercooked meat. Should one eye have reduced vision associated with the condition, the best correction in the form of

TABLE 5–7. PRIMARY CAUSES OF LEUKOCORIA IN YOUTH

Retinopathy of prematurity
Congenital cataract
Persistent hyperplastic primary vitreous
Retinoblastoma
Toxocariasis
Coats' disease
Trauma
Retinochoroidal coloboma
Retinal detachment

Pearls

Ocular Parasititis

Characteristics

Δ May manifest from infestation by many different kinds of worms

Δ Most common form in the United States is Toxocara, most frequently in ages 7 to 8 years

Δ Toxocara is the result of children or adults eating dirt (geophagia) and of eating undercooked meat

Δ There is both a visceral and ocular form

Δ Diffuse subacute neuroretinitis may manifest with any ocular worm infestation
  Unilateral decrease in vision
  Young adults
  May have vitritis, papillitis, recurrent patches of grayish RPE lesions
  May result in optic atrophy and diffuse RPE changes

Δ Ocular form presents as a round, raised, white lesion in the posterior pole that is about 1 DD in size

Δ Ocular form may remain viable in the subretinal area for up to 3 years

Δ Ocular form may have anterior uveitis and vitritis

Δ A cause of decreased vision, leukocoria, and strabismus in children

Δ ELISA for toxocara to confirm diagnosis

Management

Δ Rule out other causes of leukocoria

Δ Prevention and education by cautioning against geophagia and the eating of undercooked meat

Δ Retinal consultation if active, as photocoagulation of the worm may be of benefit

Δ Best possible correction if established and protection of fellow eye

Δ Routine yearly eye examinations

safety glasses is in order. Routine yearly examinations are necessary in all cases.

OCULAR MANIFESTATIONS OF SARCOIDOSIS

Introduction and Description. Sarcoidosis is a systemic disease of noncaseating granulomas suspected to be an antigenic reaction of the reticuloendothelial system. The disease is granulomatous with a multifaceted presentation. Age of onset is usually between 20 to 60 years, with approximately 27 to 50 percent (average, 40 percent) of patients having ocular involvement. Blacks are afflicted more often than whites, and females more than males (Fig. 5–54).

Ocular involvement includes affectation of the lacrimal gland (enlarged and keratoconjunctivitis sicca) in about 7 percent of patients. Granulomatous

Ocular Manifestations of Sarcoidosis

Characteristics

Δ Sarcoidosis is a systemic disease of noncaseating granulomas suspected to be antigenic in origin

Δ Granulomatous disease with age of onset at 20 to 60 years, with 27 to 50 percent of patients having some ocular involvement

Δ More prevalent in blacks and females

Δ Ocular signs include:
   Lacrimal gland affectation and keratoconjunctivitis sicca
   Granulomatous anterior uveitis
   Busacca and Koeppe nodules on the iris
   Equatorial periphlebitis
   String of pearls vitreous opacities
   Various vascular complications
   Optic nerve head edema and granulomas
   Equatorial choroidal granulomas
   Multiple other ocular signs

Δ Vision compromise may occur from tissue destruction and/or choroidal neovascular nets

Δ Systemic signs include:
   Hilar adenopathy on chest x-ray
   Facial nerve palsies
   Erythema nodosum
   Arthritis
   Hepatomegaly
   Spleenomegaly
   Lymphadenopathy

Management

Δ Diagnosis of systemic sarcoidosis
   Primary
      Chest x-ray
      Serum ACE
      PPD with anergy panel
   Secondary
      Limited gallium scan of head, neck, and chest
      Serum lysozymes
      Serum protein electrophoresis
      Biopsy

Δ A disease to be managed by many disciplines, watching for remissions and exacerbations

Δ Control the anterior uveitis with cycloplegia/mydriasis and penetrating topical steroids
   May need to back up with periocular injections of steroids

Δ If vision-threatening sarcoid retinopathy or optic disc edema occurs, systemic pharmaceutical management in the form of oral steroids at 60 to 80 mg of prednisone is indicated. If control is not achieved, other agents such as immunosuppressants may be necessary.

Δ If choroidal, peripheral, or disc neovascularization occurs, fluorescein angiography and a retinal consultation are indicated

Δ If no threats to vision, re-examine in 6 months

Δ If on steroids, reexamine in 2 to 7 days, and then follow closely for IOP while titering dosage

Δ Communicate with other physicians throughout the care of the patient

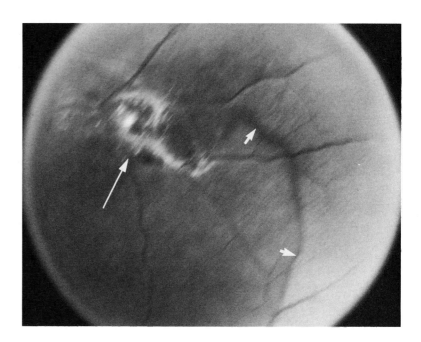

Figure 5–54. Example of the associated ocular signs of sarcoidosis.

anterior uveitis is often the most prevalent ocular manifestation, often with Busacca nodules on the iris surface and Koeppe nodules at the pupillary margin. Up to 37 percent of patients manifest retinal involvement in the form of string of pearls vitreous opacities, periphlebitis with candle-wax drippings, retinal vein occlusions, retinal hemorrhages, chorioretinitis, macular edema, optic disc edema, and optic nerve head granulomas (Fig. 5–55). Periphlebitis in equatorial retinal veins is the most common retinal sign. The periphlebitis appears as creamy white perivascular exudations. It is believed that the sarcoid granulomas actually compress the vascular lumens, precipitating the ocular signs. Focal choroidal granulomas appearing similar to choroidal masses may occur elsewhere in the retina. Whitish fluffy infiltrates may also occur in the vitreous over the choroidal nodules. Optic disc edema or choroidal neovascular membranes, as well as peripheral retinal neovascularization or disc neovascularization, may also be part of the picture of sarcoid ophthalmopathy. The author has also seen a preganglionic Horner's syndrome secondary to an apical lung granuloma. Conjunctival granulomas, extraocular muscle palsies, proptosis, and macular edema may also occur with sarcoidosis.

Systemic signs include hilar adenopathy on chest x-ray, facial nerve palsies (Bell's), erythema nodosum (tender nodules beneath the skin in the anterior tibial area), arthritis, lymphadenopathy, hepatomegaly, spleenomegaly, CNS alterations, and many other signs and symptoms. Sarcoidosis is the epitome of the multisystem systemic disease. As such, a multidisciplinary approach with excellent communication between the health care providers is essential.

Diagnosis of sarcoidosis may be made by laboratory techniques. The chest x-ray is the anchor of the diagnostic process. Chest radiographs will pick up lung changes. Elevation of serum angiotensin-converting enzyme (ACE) occurring in patients with the manifestations of sarcoid is strongly suggestive of the disease. It is important to recognize that the ACE may also be elevated in tuberculosis, diabetes, leprosy, and histoplasmosis, and may not even be elevated in active sarcoidosis. The PPD with an anergy panel will help to distinguish sarcoidosis (anergy in 50 percent) from tuberculosis (usually 10 mm or more). Limited gallium scans of the head, neck, and chest will show increased uptake and may be of use in diagnosing patients suspected of having sarcoidosis but not proven by more noninvasive tests. Serum lysozymes may be elevated, and serum protein electrophoresis may demonstrate hypergammaglobulinemia in active cases. Kveim biopsy used to be the standard, but is now rarely available; biopsy of nodules in the skin, lymph node, or conjunctiva may be diagnostic.

Sarcoidosis is a disease of remissions and exacerbations. The remissions occur more frequently in the first 3 years, ultimately leading to chronicity. Visual signs and symptoms recur and must be managed to prevent long-term tissue damage. Blurred vision, discomfort, redness, and photophobia accompany the anterior uveitis. Long-term vision loss may occur with the choroidal granulomas and neovascularization.

Management. The most important aspect of management of the patient with sarcoidosis is the recognition that it is a multisystem disease and needs to be coordinated by an internist or pulmonary specialist with exquisite communication among the specialists.

A final visual acuity of at least 20/30 can be expected if ocular inflammation is properly controlled and if choroidal and retinal neovascularization is held at bay. If vision-threatening sarcoid retinopathy occurs, oral and/or topical steroid therapy is indicated. Initially, if vision is threatened, the patient is treated with 60 to 80 mg per day of steroids. Concomitant use of an H_2 antihistaminic is often necessary with oral corticosteroid use to minimize gastrointestinal distress. If unresponsive to steroids, chlorambucil as well as other immunosuppressive agents may be tried as well as phenylbutazone, oxyphenbutazone, and chloroquine. The accompanying anterior uveitis must also be managed appropriately with cycloplegic/mydriatics and deeply penetrating topical steroids such as 1% Pred forte q 1 to 6 hours depending on the degree of inflammation. If the uveitis does not respond

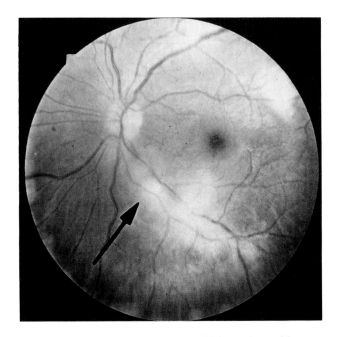

Figure 5–55. The arrow points to a choroidal granuloma of the posterior pole. It is larger and more posterior than sarcoid lesions. Diagnosis by blood tests determined this to be a toxoplasmosis lesion.

TABLE 5–8. COMPARISON OF INFLAMMATORY LESIONS OF THE POSTERIOR POLE (MACULA)

	Toxoplasmosis	Histoplasmosis	Toxocariasis	Sarcoid Ophthalmopathy
Typical age range	All ages; average 25 years	20–50 years	6–30 years	20–40 years (blacks)
Layer of primary affectation	Retina	Choroid	Retina/choroid	Retina/choroid
Anterior uveitis	Yes	No	Yes	Yes
Vitritis	Yes	No	Yes	Yes
Exudative maculopathy	Rare	Yes	Rare	No
Characteristics appearance	White area 0.2–15 DD, hazy white when active	Pigment ring at macula ↓ Exudative macula, atrophic histo spots, circumpapillary scarring	1 DD granuloma (white) raised	Yellow 0.25 DD nodules near vessels

to topical application of steroids, periocular steroids may be necessary. Should choroidal, peripheral, or disc neovascularization occur, fluorescein angiography is indicated as well as a retinal consultation for possible photocoagulative intervention.

Regardless of the mode of management, the patient must be followed routinely. If there is no threat to vision and if the patient is under reasonable systemic control, the follow-up examination may be in 6 months. If the patient has been placed on any type of steroid for the ocular manifestations, they must be followed within 2 to 7 days and the steroids adjusted gradually according to the treatment response. As the patient is being followed, intraocular pressure must be routinely monitored as well. As the disease is chronic, the long-term use of steroids may precipitate posterior subcapsular cataract formation. Very often the patient has an associated keratoconjunctivitis sicca that must be managed with nonpreserved tears and ointments as well as a strong consideration of silicone punctal implants and plugs because of the chronicity of the systemic disease.

Sarcoidosis is a multisystem disease, and as such one must never ignore its potential systemic morbidity. Sarcoidosis must be managed by the entire health care team.

Table 5–8 lists the characteristics of inflammatory lesions of the posterior pole.

HUMAN IMMUNOVIRUS AND THE EYE

Introduction and Description. The initial case of acquired immunodeficiency syndrome (AIDS) was diagnosed in 1981. In the United States alone as of December 1987, the Centers for Disease Control (CDC) had on file over 47,000 reports of adult or adolescent cases of AIDS. Over 57 percent of the reported cases had died. As of November 1991, there were 202,843 persons diagnosed with AIDS in the United States. It is estimated that there are over 1.5 million persons infected with the human immunovirus (HIV) in the United States, with over 10 million persons infected worldwide. Of these totals in the adult and adolescent category, approximately 70 percent have been the result of homosexual and bisexual intercourse, about 20 percent of intravenous (IV) drug use, approximately 4 percent of heterosexual intercourse, 3 percent of blood and blood product transfusions, and the remainder undetermined. The heterosexual percentages, however, appear to be on the rise in spite of previous beliefs that the transfer in this manner was unlikely.

The CDC defines a case of AIDS as an illness characterized by (1) the presence of one or more opportunistic diseases (Table 5–9) that are at least moderately indicative of immunodeficiency, (2) absence of all known underlying causes of immunodeficiency, and (3) absence of all other possible causes of reduced resistance ordinarily associated with the opportunistic diseases.

The recognized cause of AIDS is a retrovirus of the human T–cell lymphotropic class (HTLV–III). The virus has also been called the lymphadenopathy–associated virus (LAV), and is referred to as HTLV–III/LAV by the CDC or, more recently, as human immunovirus (HIV). When the virus enters the host cell, the HIV virus genetic information is incorporated into the host cell DNA. The HIV virus primarily infects T-helper cells, which are crucial to normal immunologic function. Alteration of these cells results in immunocompromise characteristic of AIDS. The cell may remain quiescent for many years, but activation results in viral proliferation within the infected cell, with release of the mature virus into the system. It is believed that all HIV-positive individuals will develop AIDS. Approximately 25 percent of infected individuals have the lymphadenopathy syn-

Human Immunovirus and the Eye

△ Over 10 million persons infected with HIV world-wide

△ Recognized cause is the HIV retrovirus, primarily infecting T-helper cells, resulting in immuno-compromise

△ Transmission by
Sexual contact with exchange of bodily fluids
Infusion of blood or blood products
Passage from infected mother to child

Characteristics

△ Immunosuppression allowing for destruction by opportunistic infections

△ Ocular or neuro-ocular manifestations in

1 percent at HIV positive
40 percent in AIDS-related complex (ARC)
67 percent in AIDS

△ Ocular manifestations include

Cotton-wool spots (67 percent)
Retinal hemorrhages (40 percent)
Ischemic macular edema
Cytomegalovirus retinopathy (15 to 46 percent of AIDS)
Acute retinal necrosis syndrome (ARNS)
Toxoplasmosic retinopathy (toxoplasmosis is more common as a neurologic manifestation)
Histoplasmosic retinopathy
Kaposi's sarcomas (18 percent with conjunctival lesions)
Papilledema
Opportunistic disseminated choroiditis

△ Neurologic manifestations (40 percent of AIDS patients) include

Cerebral toxoplasmosis (5 to 10 percent)
Primary CNS lymphoma
Metastatic systemic lymphoma
Cranial nerve palsies
AIDS dementia complex (ADC)
Acute septic meningitis
Vacuolar myelopathy
Sensory neuropathy, polyneuropathy, demyelinizing neuropathy
Neurosyphilis
Cerebral infarction
Visual field loss

△ Diagnosis by Western blot test and by specialized testing for the opportunistic infections

Management

△ Education

△ Prevention

△ Specific medication for opportunistic infections

△ Antiviral therapy such as ganciclovir, foscarnet, zidovudine

TABLE 5–9. CONDITIONS SUGGESTIVE OF UNDERLYING IMMUNODEFICIENCY

Conditions	Symptoms/Signs
Protozoal and Helminthic Infections	
Cryptosporidosis	Diarrhea for over 1 month
Pneumocystis carinii	Pneumonia
Strongyloidosis	Disseminated infection
Toxoplasmosis	Cerebral infection, retinitis
Fungal Infections	
Candidiasis	Esophagitis
Cryptococcosis	Central nervous system or other infection
Viral Infections	
Herpes zoster	Vessicular eruptions/pain
Cytomegalovirus	Infection, retinitis
Herpes simplex	Persistent (1 month) mucocutaneous lesions
Bacterial Infections	
Mycobacterium avium–intracellulare	Disseminated infection
Mycobacterium tuberculosis, kansasii	Disseminated infection
Cancer	
Kaposi's sarcoma	Reddish/blue skin lesions
Lymphoma/diffuse lymphoma	
Hodgkin's disease	
Miscellaneous	
Histoplasmosis	Ocular reactivation

drome, which is characterized by fever, fatigue, night sweats, malaise, weight loss, thrush, or diarrhea. About 25 percent of HIV-positive individuals will develop AIDS within 7 years, and 50 percent will develop the syndrome within 11 years. Patients with AIDS can be expected to live about 3 years.

Transmission of the HIV is by anal or vaginal intercourse, infusion of blood or blood products, or transplacental passage from infected mother to child.

Individuals with AIDS will probably have at least one ocular or neuro–ocular manifestation at some point during the disease process, especially as the disease progresses from the HIV-positive stage (1 percent), to the AIDS complex (up to 40 percent), to the AIDS syndrome (up to 67 percent). HIV retinopathy consists of several components, and often resembles some form of diabetic or hypertensive retinopathy. The retinal vascular changes are thought to occur as the result of the HIV infection of the retina and the retinal vascular endothelial architecture combined with increased blood viscosity from the elevated fibrinogen levels. Cotton-wool spots occur in about 67 percent of patients and last 4 to 6 weeks. Flame, white centered, or dot-blot hemorrhages are seen in up to 40 percent of patients. Ischemic macular edema is seen in up to 6 percent of patients with AIDS. Most of the manifestations of HIV retinopathy are relatively benign. There are reports, however, of central retinal vein occlusion in patients with HIV infection.

The true vision-threatening changes associated with AIDS are the result of cytomegalovirus (CMV) retinopathy, occurring in 15 to 46 percent of patients with AIDS; and less frequently, toxoplasmosis and histoplasmosis. CMV retinopathy is the most common severe ocular manifestation of AIDS, affecting up to 45 percent of patients. Most adults (50 to 80 percent) in the United States have been exposed to CMV, but the immunosuppressive system subdues the virus. Almost all HIV-positive homosexual males have CMV antibodies and more than 50 percent demonstrate the virus in their urine or semen. When the patient is immunocompromised and the virus is allowed to proliferate, CMV causes a necrotizing retinopathy, creating full-thickness retinal destruction (Fig. 5–56). The symptoms of the onset of the disease depend on the location of the retinopathy and may include floaters, variable loss of vision, and altered visual fields. The early stage of CMV retinopathy consists of white, granular lesions near major vessel arcades near the disc, which have a tendency to coalesce. The destruction spreads outward in a brushfire fashion as white retinal necrosis accompanied by hemorrhages engulfing the entire retina within 6 months. The leading edge is most involved, leaving behind chorioretinal atrophy and granularity. There may also be forms of vasculitis accompanying the development of the full-blown disease. There may be a minimal vitritis. Optic neuritis and retinal detachment (one third of

treated patients may develop) may also be associated with CMV retinopathy. The retinal detachment is similar to that caused by ARNS. The end stage results in retinal destruction and optic atrophy. Because of the severity of CMV retinopathy, patients who are HIV-positive should have dilated fundus examinations every 3 to 6 months, and patients with AIDS should have dilated fundus examinations at least every 3 months.

Frosted branch angiitis may also be associated with CMV retinopathy. Frosted branch angiitis manifests as profound sheathing of retinal vessels. The perivascular infiltration is usually very thick and white, affecting both veins and arteries near veins. Fluorescein angiography demonstrates leakage from both arteries and veins. Frosted branch angiitis is usually not directly associated with any particular disease process and presents most frequently in young patients.

Another possible ocular complication in AIDS is the acute retinal necrosis syndrome (ARNS), which is frequently complicated by retinal detachment. ARNS is described elsewhere and is typically treated with intravenous acyclovir.

Although toxoplasmosis can reactivate within the eye in AIDS, it is a far more common neurologic complication. Toxoplasmosis is, in fact, the most common neurologic complication of AIDS, occurring in 5 to 10 percent of patients. It is the most frequent presenting syndrome leading to the diagnosis of AIDS. Patients present with a subacute alteration in cognition and consciousness, headache, ataxia, incontinence, hemisensory deficit, cranial nerve paresis, aphasia, anisocoria, pain, hemianopsia, diplopia, and photophobia. Ocular toxoplasmosis in AIDS patients is usually associated with central nervous system involvement and presents in a manner similar to ARNS with multifocal bilateral necrotizing retinochoroiditis. In the case of toxoplasmosis, the expected vitritis and anterior granulomatous uveitis are common, which contrasts with CMV retinopathy. All other opportunistic infections may affect the eye, including syphilis (neurosyphilis is reported to be very prevalent in AIDS patients), presumed ocular histoplasmosis, bilateral multifocal retinitis, primary ocular malignant lymphoma, and choroiditis. Cryptococcal meningitis occurs in about 5 percent of AIDS patients, presenting as a subacute illness with headache, alteration of cognition and consciousness, nuchal rigidity, fever, nausea with vomiting, and at times focal seizures.

The choroiditis associated with AIDS may be secondary to *Pneumocystis carinii*, mycobacteria, and Candida. *Pneumocystis carinii* pneumonia is the most common infection in patients with AIDS, and disseminated choroiditis is often the first sign of the spread of Pneumocystis infection. The choroiditis is

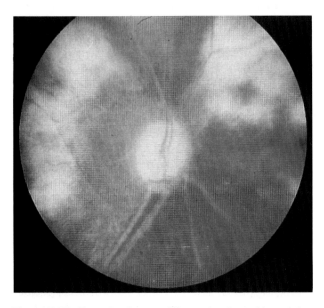

Figure 5–56. Example of some of the ocular signs of human immunovirus.

insidious in its progress, with small, yellow-white irregular choroidal infiltrates with no associated inflammation. The lesions are usually confined to the postequatorial zone. The lesions are not a threat to vision and do not need treatment. The systemic condition does, however, require treatment. The choroiditis connected with mycobacteria is usually characterized by granulomatous disease, often affecting the anterior segment as well. Candidial infection in AIDS patients presents as fluffy yellowish retinochoroidal lesions that may spread into the vitreous cavity, creating a mild vitritis. Treatment involves use of systemic anticandidial therapy and perhaps eventual vitrectomy.

Kaposi's sarcoma may present in the ocular area, often as reddish-purple tumors near the medial canthus or inferior cul-de-sac. Kaposi's sarcomas occur in 24 percent of AIDS victims, with 18 percent of those also having the conjunctival lesions. Other HIV-associated neoplasia include primary central nervous system lymphoma and metastatic lymphoma. The primary CNS lymphoma presents with alterations in cognition or consciousness, hemiparesis, aphasia, seizures, and cranial neuropathies simulating cerebral toxoplasmosis. Systemic metastatic lymphoma manifests as cranial neuropathy and headache.

Neuro-ocular disorders such as cranial nerve palsies and neurologic disorders may occur in AIDS. At least 40 percent of patients with AIDS show neurologic symptoms. Approximately 10 to 20 percent of patients have neurologic problems as their initial manifestation of AIDS. In the AIDS complex, the prevalence of neurologic symptoms is approximately 35 to 40 percent. It is proposed that the virus either enters the neurologic system tied to lymphocytes and monocytes through a break in the blood–brain barrier or, similar to the retina, as a direct infection of the endothelial cells. The neurologic disorders may vary from mild cognitive impairment to acute septic meningitis. The most common presentation (up to 90 percent of AIDS patients) is dementia, characterized by variable impairment of cognitive, motor, and behavioral function. The dementia is referred to as the AIDS demential complex (ADC), and eventually becomes so severe as to alter activities of daily living. In advanced stages, global cognitive dysfunction develops, leading to loss of motor function. In ADC, the cerebrospinal fluid shows an increase in IgG and total proteins. CT shows cortical atrophy and the more sensitive MRI, leucoencephalopathy.

Vacuolization of the white matter of the spinal cord (vacuolar myelopathy) is a result of direct viral invasion of the spinal cord. This is responsible for the myelopathy presenting in the AIDS patient. There is a progressive paraparesis with spasticity, ataxia, and urinary incontinence. Vacuolar myelopathy is present in about 50 percent of patients with ADC. Cerebral granulomatous angiitis, another neurologic complication, is a rare presentation in AIDS patients, creating multiple infarcts in the brain.

Sensory neuropathy, polyneuropathy, and inflammatory demyelinating neuropathy may occur associated with AIDS. The demyelinating neuropathy usually occurs prior to the development of full-blown AIDS and can simulate Guillaine–Barré syndrome. Significant pain can be associated with any of the forms of peripheral neuropathy. Herpes zoster is another possible presentation in the patient with HIV.

Cerebral infarction is a complication of HIV infection, reported to occur in 12 percent of patients and reported to increase the risk of stroke by up to 100 times.

Papilledema and visual field loss may present secondary to intracranial infection, cerebral infarction, or intracranial tumors. Pupillary abnormalities may also occur associated with the underlying neurologic compromise.

Laboratory diagnosis of HIV is made by the Western blot test. The Western blot is used to specify the fluorescent antinuclear antibody test to detect the HIV and to monitor the AIDS patient's immune system. Multiple other laboratory tests are necessary to diagnose the disorders associated with AIDS.

Management. Currently, prognosis for AIDS and its related ocular complications is grim. Many drugs are under investigation and may create a brief state of quiescence in the systemic or ocular manifestations, but there is a high recurrence rate at cessation of treatment.

CMV retinopathy is treatable by administration of antiviral therapy. Intravenous (necessitating an indwelling catheter) ganciclovir and foscarnet are used to manage the disease and function as virostatic agents. As virostatic agents, they must be used for the life of the patient to control the infectious process. Zidovudine has also been shown to control CMV infection. Myelosuppression is a potential consequence of both zidovudine and ganciclovir; concurrent use is therefore ill-advised. Foscarnet creates renal toxicity and can therefore be used concurrently with zidovudine. Other new agents such as didanosine are on the horizon to control the CMV retinopathy.

Reactivation within 6 months with intravenous antiviral agents varies between 18 and 50 percent of eyes. If there is a resistance to ganciclovir, the reactivation occurs within 3 months. Foscarnet is indicated in ganciclovir resistant situations. As a last resort, intravitreal injections and implantation of ganciclovir may offer some relief to patients.

All opportunistic infections must be managed according to current therapeutic protocol and must often be used concurrently with the antiviral therapy.

TABLE 5–10. RECOMMENDATIONS TO PREVENT THE TRANSFER OF HUMAN IMMUNOVIRUS

General

1. Exercise special care regarding sexual contacts.
2. Wear goggles when there is potential for infected fluids to be splashed into the eyes.
3. Wear masks when examining patients suspected of having airborne opportunistic organisms.
4. Dispose of all needles and syringes in "contaminant" containers.

Ocular

1. Glove when there is potential contact with bodily secretions or blood.
2. Wash hands after each patient contact.
3. Disinfect tonometer tips and all other instruments that make contact with the eye.
   Note: HTLV-III/LAV may be inactivated by
      5- to 10-minute exposure to 3% hydrogen peroxide.
      1:10 dilution of household bleach, or
      70% ethanol or isopropyl alcohol.
4. Disinfect rigid gas-permeable and PMMA contact lenses with hydrogen peroxide.
5. Disinfect soft contact lenses with heat or hydrogen peroxide disinfection systems.

The best management modality for AIDS is prevention. Table 5–10 summarizes current recommendations for prevention of, or prophylaxis against, HIV infection.

NONHEREDITARY RETINAL PIGMENT EPITHELIOPATHIES

Acute Posterior Multifocal Placoid Pigment Epitheliopathy (APMPPE)

Introduction and Description. Acute posterior multifocal placoid pigment epitheliopathy (APMPPE) has been considered a relatively benign bilateral process that usually affects young adults (typically between the ages of 20 and 40 years), although the disease has been reported up to age 66 years. There appears to be no sexual predilection. The disease appears to affect the RPE and is thought to be secondary to some underlying vascular problem of the choroid or choriocapillaris. Another theory is the possibility that there is a direct inflammatory process of the RPE secondary to an infectious or toxic agent, but the vascular theory enjoys more support. There is a strong association with recent bouts of systemic viral disease, and this can be elicited in up to one third of patients. HLA testing reveals a higher positivity to HLA-B7 and HLA-DR2 in affected patients than controls, suggesting an autoimmune aspect to the process. Table 5–11 summarizes conditions reported to be associated with APMPPE.

TABLE 5–11. CONDITIONS REPORTED TO BE ASSOCIATED WITH ACUTE POSTERIOR MULTIFOCAL PLACOID PIGMENT EPITHELIOPATHY (APMPPE)

Viral respiratory infection	Fever and malaise
Headaches	Myalgias
Arthralgias	Lymphadenopathy
Mycobacterial infection	Prior streptococcal pharyngitis
Prior mononucleosis	Thyroiditis
Tinnitus	Vertigo
Acute nephritis	Erythema nodosum
Sarcoidosis	Hepatomegaly
Regional enteritis	Meningoencephalitis
Cerebral vasculitis (death)	Subclinical neuropathy
Transient hearing loss	Family history of tuberculosis
HLA-B7 and HLA-DR2 positivity	

There are also reports of the association of APMPPE with prior treatment with penicillin, ampicillin, tetanus toxoid, tetracycline, triamcinolone, methylprednisolone, sulfamethoxazole, trimethoprim, thyroid replacement, tranquilizers, dextroamphetamine, prochlorperazine, sulfonamides, and swine flu vaccine.

The sudden appearance of dirty yellow-white (creamy) multiple placoid lesions in the posterior pole, followed by the same in the fellow eye, is characteristic of APMPPE. The lesions occur deep in the retina, and there may be associated retinal or optic nerve disease (Fig. 5–57). New additional lesions may appear for up to 3 weeks from the initial onset. Additional ocular findings reported with APMPPE are

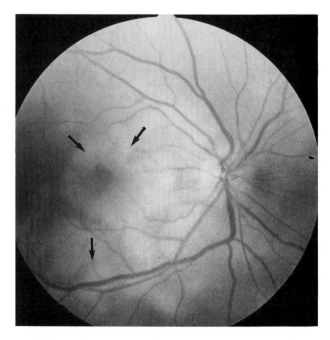

Figure 5–57. Example of the RPE changes in the posterior pole associated with APMPPE. The arrows point to "placoid" areas of RPE alteration.

TABLE 5–12. OCULAR FINDINGS REPORTED TO BE ASSOCIATED WITH ACUTE POSTERIOR MULTIFOCAL PLACOID PIGMENT EPITHELIOPATHY (APMPPE)

Decreased central vision	Paracentral and central scotomas
Metamorphopsia	
Photopsia	Photophobia
Anterior uveitis	Subconjunctival hemorrhage
Papillitis	Episcleritis
Retinal hemorrhages	Optic disc edema
Retinal vasculitis	Dilated tortuous retinal veins
Altered color visio	Retinal detachment
Abnormal EOG	Abnormal ERG

listed in Table 5–12.

Fluorescein angiography exhibits a characteristic pattern that strongly implicates the RPE as the layer of primary affectation. In the early phases of FA there is a blockage of background choroidal fluorescence by the altered RPE. The late stage of FA demonstrates an accumulation of dye in the diseased RPE. Old lesions hyperfluorescence on FA. There is some possibility that the RPE disturbance could be secondary to focal disease of the underlying choriocapillaris. The fundus lesions resolve rapidly over 2 to 4 weeks, leaving evidence of mottled RPE. Should the rare recurrence occur, there may be the appearance of new lesions or enlargement of previously existing lesions.

See color plate 86. APMPPE presents as a rapid loss of vision eventually affecting both eyes. Scotomas will present corresponding to the locations of the lesions. As mentioned previously, there may be a relationship to a recent nondescript illness.

Laboratory testing is usually nonproductive in the diagnosis of underlying conditions associated with APMPPE. HLA class I and class II antigen analysis may reveal positivity to HLA-B7 and HLA-DR2. Anterior uveitis or cells in the vitreous are present in approximately 50 percent of affected patients.

Management. APMPPE is a process that demonstrates rapid resolution of the fundus lesions over 2 to 4 weeks. Remnants of vision compromise or field defects may persist for up to 6 months. There has been a reported low incidence of recurrence, and the large majority of patients recover to an acuity level between 20/20 and 20/30. Recovery to 20/40 or better is expected in 80 percent of cases. There is no reason to intervene therapeutically. Recent reports, however, point to the possibility of recurrence even after delays of up to 7 years. Apparently, the recurrences may present near the old lesions or at totally remote sites. These recurrences have occurred in patients placed on steroid, antimicrobial, and antitubercular therapy.

There is the possibility of long-term development of choroidal neovascularization secondary to

Acute Posterior Multifocal Placoid Pigment Epitheliopathy (APMPPE)

Characteristics

△ Bilateral condition (some unilateral reports) in young adults usually aged 20 to 40 years

△ Strong association with recent bouts of systemic viral disease, but many associated conditions reported including drug sensitivities

△ Reported linkage to HLA-B7 and HLA-DR2 suggesting an immunogenetic predisposition to the condition

△ Yellow-white multiple placoid lesions in posterior pole, with new lesions appearing for up to 3 weeks after the initial onset

△ Fluorescein angiography shows early hypofluorescence and late hyperfluorescence indicative of RPE disease

△ Visual acuity reduction and scotomas are quick to develop

△ Fundus lesions resolve over 2 to 4 weeks, but vision reduction or scotomas may persist 6 months

△ Possibility of anterior uveitis or cells in the vitreous in about 50 percent of patients

Management

△ Up to 80 percent recover vision to 20/40 or better untreated

△ Proper diagnosis is important as there are many differentials; fluorescein angiography is often crucial

△ Manage anterior uveitis with cycloplegia/mydriasis and topical steroids

△ Patient education

△ Watch for long–term development of choroidal neovascular nets

△ Other complications include
  Central serous retinal detachment
  Choroidal vasculitis
  Central retinal vein occlusion
  Hemorrhagic maculopathy
  Optic neuropathy
  Meningoencephalopathy
  Cerebral vasculitis and death

△ After quiescence, follow-up should be every 3 months for at least 1 year with self-monitoring of vision

△ Watch for the possibility of recurrence as more reports are reaching the literature

the altered metabolic state of the RPE. There are also some suggestions that APMPPE is a part of a continuum resulting in extensive chorioretinal disease. Poor recovery and reports of associated deaths bring question to how benign the condition actually is. Complications of APMPPE include central serous retinal detachment, choroidal vasculitis as fluffy whitish deposits deep in the retina, central retinal vein occlusion, hemorrhagic maculopathy secondary to the choroidal neovascular development, optic neuropathy, meningoencephalopathy, and cerebral vasculitis.

Should an accompanying anterior uveitis be present and symptomatic, it must be treated with cycloplegic and adjunctive topical steroid therapy.

In the management plan it is important to differentially diagnose APMPPE from conditions that may simulate the disease. Patient counseling regarding outcome associated with a fluorescein angiography are important. After resolution of the active attack, follow-up at a minimum of every 3 months for the first year with self-monitoring of vision is important.

Geographic Helicoid Peripapillary Choroidopathy (GHPC)

Introduction and Description. Geographic helicoid peripapillary choroidopathy (GHPC) is also known as serpiginous choroidopathy, macular geographic helicoid choroidopathy, and geographic choroiditis. It is a bilateral (may be asymmetrical in presentation) idiopathic disease of the choriocapillaris and RPE. There is the characteristic of recurrence to differentiate GHPC from APMPPE. The involvement of the second eye may be after a time delay and may be asymmetrical. GHPC shows no apparent sexual preference but has been reported more often in whites than blacks. There is also a report of a possible hereditary aspect to the condition. The age range for onset is 30 to 70 years of age, with the average 45 to 50 years of age. Associated ocular findings are rare but may include

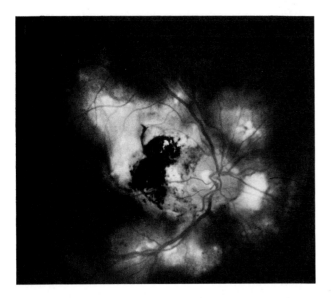

Figure 5–58. A photograph illustrating the destruction of geographical helicoid peripapillary choroidopathy. (*Diagnosis by F. LaRussa.*)

Geographic Helicoid Peripapillary Choroidopathy (GHPC)

Characteristics

Δ Bilateral, idiopathic, recurrent choriocapillaris/RPE disease with asymmetrical presentation

Δ Involvement of the second eye may be after a time delay

Δ Average age of onset 45 to 50 years

Δ Acute phase presents as propellerlike pseudopods extending out from optic nerve head

Δ Creamy lesions develop at the edges of the pseudopods and persist for several weeks (RPE disease)

Δ When the pseudopods creep into the macula, vision is lost, and scotomas occur at sites of pseudopods

Δ Fluorescein angiography shows early hypofluorescence of central scar and hypofluorescence early in active creamy lesions

Δ Variations may occur primarily involving the macula and may have pseudopods extending toward the disc

Δ There is the suggestion of some type of hereditary pattern

Management

Δ Disease characterized by recurrences (even over a 10-year period) and there is controversy regarding efficacy of steroid intervention

Δ Patient education and routine follow–up at least every six months with home monitoring of vision

Δ Choroidal neovascular nets can develop. Should this occur, order fluorescein angiography. Laser intervention has variable results

Δ Provision of best possible correction and low-vision rehabilitation if necessary

serous sensory retinal detachment, anterior uveitis, vitritis, and choroidal neovascular nets. There are no apparent related systemic diseases. Severe visual loss can occur if the macular area is affected. The exact cause of the disease has not been determined.

GHPC is a chronic, recurrent, progressive disease that usually involves the circumpapillary RPE, choriocapillaris, and choroid (Fig. 5–58). In the acute phase, pseudopods extend out from the optic nerve head in a propellerlike fashion (centrifugal). The pseudopods represent subretinal scarring. The scarring may be noncontinuous with "skip zones." During activity, gray or cream lesions will develop at the advancing edge of the scar at the level of the RPE. The active lesion usually persists only several weeks. Should the pseudopods "crawl" into the macular area, vision will be compromised.

There is a variant of the "classical" GHPC in which the lesions start away from the disc and extend inward toward the disc (centripetal). Another variation may present in the macula without any peripapillary activity. The disease is characterized by remissions and exacerbations. During the stage of inactivity, the ophthalmoscopic picture is that of extensive irregular scars and occasional choroidal neovascularization. The choroidal neovascularization usually occurs at the edge of the inactive chorioretinal scar and may create more extensive disciform scarring. The loss of overlying RPE often results in easy visualization of the large choroidal vessels around the optic nerve head. Optic disc neovascularization has also been reported associated with GHPC.

The fluorescein pattern is characteristic in GHPC. Early in the angiogram, the central part of the inactive lesion hypofluoresces and is surrounded by hyperfluorescence. This is characteristic of active RPE diseases such as APMPPE. During the later phase the fluorescein seeps into the scar, creating spotty fluorescence. The active lesion is hypofluorescent and demonstrates variable fluorescence late in the angiogram. The fluorescein pattern strongly implicates the choriocapillaris as the initial site of the disease. There is a theory that progressive tearing and retraction of the RPE or Bruch's membrane around the optic disc may be involved in the etiopathogenesis of the disease. The fellow eye, although usually involved, may present nothing more than mild circumpapillary changes that are certainly capable of progression.

In the active phase the patient may report the sudden onset of reduced vision or a paracentral scotoma if the pseudopods have encroached on the macular area. There is usually no accompanying pain, photophobia, or lacrimation. Recurrence is the rule. Patients may report symptoms early if they have been placed on a home monitoring system.

Management. GHPC is characterized by multiple recurrences with development of new scars and extensions of old scars. Active development has been documented as occurring over a 10-year period. During the active lesion, vision drops. In some cases there does seem to be some improvement in acuity with quiescene of the lesions. The time to recovery seems to vary between 2 and 22 months. Some of the patients may, however, have an irreversible drop in visual acuity. Final visual acuity seems to be unpredictable, but GHPC does not inevitably result in severe visual loss.

The issue of management seems to be controversial, as some practitioners advocate aggressive systemic and/or local steroid intervention when the lesions become active, while others point out that no clinical trails are available to support efficacy. The patient nonetheless should be placed on a home vision monitoring system and should report reactivation. Should choroidal neovascularization occur in the scarred areas, fluorescein angiography should be performed to determine if laser photocoagulation would be of benefit. The results of interventive laser photocoagulation are variable in the literature.

One important aspect of management involves patient education and provision of the best possible visual correction. In the later stages of the disease, low-vision rehabilitation may be necessary. Follow-up of the patient should be at least every 6 months but sooner if self-monitoring of vision indicates resumption of activity of the lesions.

Recurrent Multifocal Choroiditis (RMC)

Introduction and Description. Recurrent multifocal choroiditis (RMC) is a clinical entity affecting young (14 to 34 years of age, one reported over 34 years of age), mildly myopic, female patients. The condition has also been referred to as multifocal choroiditis and panuveitis (MCP), progressive subretinal fibrosis, punctate inner choroidopathy, chorioretinopathy with anterior uveitis, and multifocal choroiditis with

---

Pearls

Recurrent Multifocal Choroiditis (RMC)

Characteristics

△ Referred to as pseudo-presumed ocular histoplasmosis syndrome

△ Affects young (14 to 34 years) myopic females

△ Small, multiple, yellow-white lesions (in posterior pole) that become gray and fuzzy during activity

△ During activity there may be vitritis, anterior uveitis, optic disc edema, loss of vision, photopsia, and scotomas associated with acute idiopathic blind spot enlargement syndrome

△ Fluorescein angiography shows early hyperfluorescence of active lesions

△ Recurrences often are next to older lesions but may be anywhere

△ With continued scarring there is a threat for choroidal neovascularizaton or progressive subretinal fibrotic scarring (30 to 40 percent of patients)

△ Association with Epstein–Barr virus

Management

△ Education and home monitoring of vision

△ Systemic steroid therapy may be of value when reactivation occurs after weighing the potential systemic side effects

△ Watch for choroidal neovascularization—poor prognosis even with laser intervention

△ Routine examinations every 6 months with instructions to return if reactivation is noted

disciform macular degeneration. The disease is reported to simulate POHS in its clinical appearance even to the point of having circumpapillary choroiditis, atrophic peripheral scars, macular choroidal neovascularization, and even peripheral linear streaks. The condition may be unilateral or bilateral, is idiopathic, and recurrences are common. One eye may follow the other in development of the lesions. There appears to be no particular relationship to systemic diseases except to the Epstein–Barr virus, and laboratory diagnosis appears to be of no value. There have also been reports of the association of the condition with syphilis, tuberculosis, and sarcoidosis. It has been postulated that the condition presents as a result of alterations in the host immune system. Because of the positive response to corticosteroid therapy, the lesions are thought to be inflammatory (Fig. 5–59).

Ophthalmoscopic findings include small, multifocal, round yellow-white lesions that may have a surround of pigment proliferation. During activity these areas become gray and fuzzy and may be accompanied by vitritis, anterior uveitis, cystoid macular edema, and optic disc edema. There also appears to be the relationship to the acute idiopathic blind spot enlargement syndrome. These lesions of the RPE and choriocapillaris are usually confined to the clinical posterior pole but may encroach on the macular area. With fluorescein angiography, the lesions hyperfluoresce early and remain fuzzy throughout the duration of an angiogram. Recurrences often occur next to older lesions.

Because of the compromise to the RPE/Bruch's membrane zone, there is a significant threat for the development of choroidal neovascularization or progressive subretinal fibrotic scarring (reports of 30 to 40 percent). A variable percentage of patients may develop cystoid macular edema. Recurrences may occur in previously unaffected retinal areas.

The condition may be found on routine eye examination if the lesions have not affected the macular area. When macular function is compromised, visual acuity is rapidly reduced, and metamorphopsia occurs. Isolated scotomas may be demonstrated on visual field testing.

Management. As RMC is a newly described condition, there is considerable variation in the reports on prognosis. Both choroidal neovascularization and subretinal fibrosis carry a poor prognosis, and intervention must occur should either of these complications arise. Acute fundus lesions do respond positively to systemic steroids, but again the response is variable. It appears that laser treatment of the choroidal neovascular nets does not afford excellent results in all cases.

All patients suspected of having RMC must have all other causes of choroiditis ruled out. In addition, the patients should be on some form of home monitoring system. Should activity occur, it is imperative that systemic corticosteroid therapy be instituted immediately at least on a trial basis after the potential side effects have been weighed. Follow-up should be at least every 6 months unless recurrences present.

■ ■ ■ ■ ■ ■

Clinical Note: Punctate Inner Choroidopathy (PIC)

Punctate inner choroidopathy (PIC) is characterized by the appearance of tiny grayish or yellowish punctate lesions scattered randomly throughout the posterior pole between the inner choroid and RPE. The lesions may appear in a linear or cluster configuration. PIC is considered to be a variation of multifocal choroiditis. The condition is more prevalent in myopic women with a dramatic reduction in visual function. There is neither accompanying vitritis nor anterior uveitis. There is often an associated serous retinal detachment due to leakage through the compromised RPE. Choroidal neovascularization is another complication occurring in areas of chorioretinal scarring.

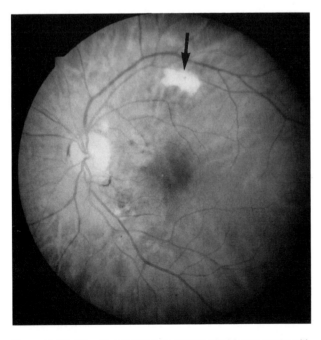

Figure 5–59. Fibrotic scar (*arrow*) associated with recurrent multifocal choroidopathy.

Multiple Evanescent White Dot Syndrome (MEWDS)

Introduction and Description. Multiple evanescent white dot syndrome (MEWDS) is a variant of posterior uveitis that involves the RPE, eventually affecting the overlying photoreceptors. It occurs primarily in

Multiple Evanescent White Dot Syndrome (MEWDS)

Characteristics

Δ Occurs primarily in young females (17 to 38 years of age)

Δ Possible relationship to prior "flulike illness"

Δ Unilateral transient disease appearing as multiple creamy white dots in clinical posterior pole but sparing the fovea

Δ Granularity to affected macula appearing as small white to light orange specks with staining in FA

Δ There may be cells in the vitreous

Δ Patients present because of acute unilateral vision decrease (20/50 to 20/20) and perhaps photopsia

Δ Often an enlarged blind spot, paracentral scotomas, and abnormal electroretinogram during activity

Δ Reported linkage to optic disc edema

Management

Δ Proper diagnosis and patient education are crucial

Δ Vision typically recovers to 20/20 to 20/30 in 1 to 16 weeks

Δ Recurrence and choroidal neovascularization appear to be rare

Δ Routine follow-up eye examinations

young (ages 17 to 38 years) females. This acute onset unilateral transient disease appears to have no particular association with systemic abnormalities, but some patients report a prior "flulike" illness. There appears to be no racial predilection.

Ophthalmoscopically, MEWDS appears as a unilateral presentation of several small, discrete, creamy white dots concentrated in the clinical posterior pole but typically sparing the fovea. The dots appear to be at the RPE level, with their activity causing transient interference in the photoreceptor function. There is a granularity to the macula in the affected eye that appears as tiny white to light orange specks. Cells occur in the vitreous, and fluorescein staining presents in the macula in most cases. There is hyperfluorescence of the disc, with fluorescein angiography in some cases and occasional venous sheathing. There also seems to be a reported relationship to the acute idiopathic blind spot enlargement syndrome, and there is a report linking MEWDS to optic disc edema.

Fluorescein angiography performed during the active stage shows early hyperfluorescence of the lesions with late-stage patchy staining. Electroretinogram testing reveals both a decreased a-wave and ERP amplitude in the active phase, implying impaired photoreceptor function.

As the active stage of MEWDS subsides, the white dots and macular granularity tend to fade. Subtle RPE window defects will always be the sequelae of the process.

The patient with MEWDS usually presents because of acute unilateral reduction in visual acuity and photopsia. Acuity during activity varies between 20/50 (6/12) to 20/200 (6/60). There is often an enlarged blind spot and paracentral scotomas.

Management. Prognosis for MEWDS is excellent. Vision typically recovers to the 20/20 to 20/30 level within 1 to 16 weeks. There is one report of recurrence and one report of the secondary complication of choroidal neovascularization. The responsibility of the clinician is to rule out all other causes of acute unilateral vision loss and to follow the patient for reactivity. It appears that MEWDS, recurrent multifocal choroiditis, and acute idiopathic blind spot enlargement syndrome may have a common etiologic source.

■ ■ ■ ■ ■ ■

Clinical Note: Acute Retinal Pigment Epitheliitis—Krill's Disease

Acute retinal pigment epitheliitis may also cause an acute reduction in acuity in young and middle-aged patients. This condition may be bilateral. The lesions in acute retinal epitheliitis are gray colored (hyperpigmented), presenting as one to four discrete clusters with an irregular halo of white. These clusters are about ¼ DD. Spontaneous resolution of vision from the 20/100 level occurs in 6 to 12 weeks without therapeutic intervention. RPE abnormalities remain after the active phase of the disease has subsided.

Birdshot Retinochoroidopathy

Introduction and Description. Birdshot (vitiliginous) retinochoroidopathy occurs in white middle-aged adults (40 to 60 years) and is most frequently bilateral. There appears to be no sexual predilection. The condition is characterized by multiple, discrete, depigmented or creamy spots about ⅓ to ½ DD in size in the midperiphery to the posterior pole. The lesions appear deep and are often arranged near large choroidal vessels. The depigmented areas do not change much over time. During early fluorescein angiography, these lesions at the level of the RPE hypofluoresce, accumulating some dye in the later phases. Vascular leakage, often in the larger veins, is also a characteristic during fluorescein angiography. Patients have chronic vitritis, retinal vasculitis, optic disc edema, and, ultimately, cystoid macular edema. The primary

Birdshot Retinochoroidopathy

Characteristics

△ Bilateral occurrence in white middle-aged adults

△ Multiple creamy spots in midperiphery to posterior pole

△ Early hypofluorescence with late accumulation of dye and vascular leakage in larger veins

△ Chronic vitritis, retinal vasculitis, cystoid macular edema in 50 percent of cases

△ May develop epiretinal membranes, retinal neovascularization, choroidal neovascularization, and optic atrophy

△ Autoimmune disease with strong relationship to HLA-A29 positivity, atopy, and prior viral infections

Management

△ Benefits are derived from oral and local steroid therapy

△ Possible benefit from immunosuppressive therapy as well as vitrectomy

△ Retinal consultation for laser intervention for choroidal neovascular membranes and retinal neovascularization

△ Provide best possible correction, consider low-vision rehabilitation when necessary, and schedule routine follow-up visits

cause of loss of vision is the macular edema (50 percent of cases), which occurs in a manner similar to that associated with pars planitis. Anterior uveitis is usually not a characteristic. Birdshot is similar to pars planitis without the snowbanks at the ora. The disease is chronic and protracted and may be associated with epiretinal membranes, retinal neovascularization, choroidal neovascularization, and optic atrophy. Birdshot retinochoroidopathy is thought to be an autoimmune disease and is strongly related to HLA-A29 allele. Eighty to 95 percent of patients with birdshot retinochoroidopathy are HLA-A29 positive. HLA-A29 positivity also appears to be related to more posterior pole involvement and a higher incidence of optic disc edema. There is also a relationship of the condition to atopy, elevated serum IgE levels, and viral infection.

Management. Birdshot retinochoroidopathy may benefit from local and/or systemic steroid therapy. It appears that the best resolution occurs with doses of steroids greater than 10 mg/day. Immunosuppressive therapy as well as vitrectomy also appear to be beneficial to the visual outcome. The choroidal neovascularization that may develop appears to respond well to laser intervention assuming reasonable criteria are met. Peripheral neovascularization, neovascu-

larization in the posterior pole, and disc neovascularization all respond reasonably to properly applied photocoagulative intervention.

Birdshot retinochoroidopathy requires a retinal consultation in the active phase. In the quiescent phase the primary care practitioner must be constantly watching for complications and must provide the best vision correction. Low-vision rehabilitation may be necessary late in the disease process. Routine follow-up is necessary.

Table 5–13 lists the characteristics of some of the retinal pigment epitheliopathies.

OCULAR MANIFESTATIONS OF LYME DISEASE

Introduction and Description. Lyme disease is a condition occurring primarily in the summer months associated with a spirochete (*Borrelia burgdorferi*) passed by Ixodes ticks commonly found on white-tailed deer but also present on other animals including domestic animals and birds. If the tick is infected with the spirochete, it may pass it during the bite for the feeding process. There are several endemic regions within the United States including the upper Midwest, the Northeast, and the West. Unfortunately the tick is very small and difficult to detect.

The disease typically progresses through specific stages. In stage 1, the dermatologic stage, there is a flat erythematous bull's-eye skin lesion that enlarges in all directions and that presents 3 to 32 days after the bite. The patient may also have flulike symptoms during this stage. Stage 1 may be intermittent and transient, usually resolving on its own.

Within a few days to months, stage 2 may present. Stage 2 is characterized by meningitis, cranial neuritis, encephalitis, peripheral radiculoneuropathy, and cardiac involvement. Stage 3 has characteristic rheumatologic symptoms that may present months to years after the initial infection. Rheumatoid arthritis occurs in approximately 60 percent of untreated patients.

The ocular manifestations are not inevitable but may be the presenting signs, and as such must be recognized so that the patient can receive interventive systemic therapy. Mild transient conjunctivitis may present in stage 1 of the disease associated with the flulike symptoms. Bilateral interstitial keratopathy in the visual axis with the possibility of delayed onset stromal opacities may occur, as well as acute anterior uveitis. Stage 2 may present with cranial palsies including the sixth and seventh nerves. During this stage there may be headaches, pain on ocular gaze, and photophobia. The optic nerve head may be involved, manifesting optic disc edema (optic neuritis) with associated macular edema up to 2 years after

TABLE 5–13. RETINAL PIGMENT EPITHELIOPATHIES

	Acute Posterior Multifocal Placoid Pigment Epitheliopathy	Geographic Helicoid Peripapillary Choroidopathy	Recurrent Multifocal Choroiditis	Multiple Evanescent White-Dot Syndrome	Acute Retinal Pigment Epitheliitis	Birdshot Retinochoroidopathy	Pigmented Paravenous Retinochoroidal Atrophy
Average age of onset (years)	20–40	45–50	13–34	17–38	Young to middle age	40–60	4–70
Sex	—	—	Females	Females	—	—	Usually males
Active lesion acuity	Rapid reduction	Sudden scotoma or vision loss if pseudopods in macula	Sudden scotoma or vision loss if near macula	Sudden unilateral vision loss to 20/50–20/200	Sudden loss to 20/100	No loss until cystoid macular edema	Asymptomatic
Final visual acuity	20/20–20/30 over 6 months	Variable from good to severe vision loss	Variable from good to severe vision loss	20/20–20/30 within 16 weeks	Good VA within 12 weeks	Variable	Rare progression to severe loss of vision
Clinical appearance	Creamy multiple placoid lesions in posterior pole; anterior uveitis and vitritis in 50%	Pseudopod subretinal scarring extending out from the disc in a propellerlike pattern; gray lesions develop at scars during activity; choroidal neo may develop	Small multiple yellow-white lesions that are gray when active; occur in posterior pole; may develop choroidal neo or subretinal fibrosis	Several small white dots in posterior pole with a granular macula. With resolution, granularity and dots fade	Hyperpigmented clusters with a white halo (1/4 DD) in macular area. With resolution, defects in RPE remain	Multiple creamy spots midperiphery; chronic vitritis, optic disc edema, vasculitis cystoid macular edema	Symmetrical circumpapillary RPE atrophy. Corridors of RPE atrophy along veins; bone-spicule cuffing of veins
Recurrence	Rare	Common	Common	No	Rare	Chronic	Chronic
Laterality	Bilateral	Bilateral	Unilateral or bilateral	Unilateral	Unilateral or bilateral	Bilateral	Bilateral
Management	No intervention except in anterior uveitis	Corticosteroids of questionable value; laser neovascular nets	Corticosteroids of value in active lesions	No intervention	No intervention	Possible corticosteroids Autoimmune?	No intervention

Pearls

Ocular Manifestations of Lyme Disease

Characteristics

Δ Peak occurrence in the summer months

Δ Spirochete transmitted by a tick bite. Tick most commonly associated with white-tailed deer

Δ Progresses through stages

   Stage 1—dermatological stage with flat erythematous bull's-eye lesion that spreads and flu-like symptoms; may have associated conjunctivitis and interstitial keratopathy

   Stage 2—neurologic stage with meningitis, cranial neuritis, encephalitis, peripheral radiculoneuropathy, and cardiac involvement; may have cranial palsies, optic disc edema, macular edema, vitritis, salt-and-pepper choroiditis, exudative retinal detachment, headaches, pain on eye movement, and photophobia

   Stage 3—rheumatological stage with rheumatoid arthritis and all associated eye signs

Management

Δ Proper differential diagnosis

   Order Lyme IFA, Lyme ELISA, FTA-ABS, MHA-TP, and RPR, but remember the cross-reactivity of the Lyme tests and the FTA-ABS. The Western blot test appears to be the most effective method of diagnosis

Δ Systemic antibiotic therapy is the cornerstone of management, with tetracycline the treatment of choice

Δ Ocular therapy may include topical antibiotics, topical steroids, therapy for exposure keratopathy, and punctal plugs

Δ Follow patient carefully, as many manifestations are delayed long after initial infestation

the initial infestation. Vitritis, choroiditis (salt-and-pepper or pigmented bone spicules very similar to syphilitic choroiditis), and exudative retinal detachment have also been reported. Likewise, a variable visual field presentation may occur.

Management. If there is the suspicion of Lyme disease, serologic tests should be ordered. The Lyme immunofluoroescent antibody test and FTA-ABS show cross-reactivity, as does the Lyme ELISA and the FTA-ABS, necessitating a negative MHA-TP and a RPR to confirm the diagnosis. A high positive FTA-ABS titer may produce a low false-positive antibody titer against the Lyme spirochete. The Western blot test appears to be the most sensitive test available for differential diagnosis. Antibiotic therapy is effective in the treatment of Lyme disease. The treatment of choice is tetracycline 250 mg po qid or doxycycline 100 mg po

bid for 10 to 20 days. Penicillin VK at 500 mg po qid for 10 to 20 days, or erythromycin at 250 mg po qid for 10 to 20 days, are alternatives in the initial stages of the disease. Very close follow-up is necessary to assure efficacy. The earlier the treatment, the more effective the control of potential complications.

The ocular manifestations must also be treated accordingly. The conjuntivitis may be responsive to the oral antibiotics but may require concomitant topicals. The interstitial keratopathy may require topical steroid management. Seventh-nerve palsies will create exposure keratopathy, which must be managed. The potential of keratoconjunctivitis sicca with stage 3 must be managed aggressively with tear substitutes and punctal implants.

The patient with confirmed Lyme disease must also be followed at routine intervals because of the delayed onset potential for a number of the ocular manifestations.

REFERENCES

Biochemical/Vitamin/Light Damage and Macular Degeneration

Alexander LJ. Ocular vitamin therapy. A review and assessment. *Optom Clin.* 1992;2:1–34.

Beutler E. Glutathione reductase: Stimulation in normal subjects by riboflavin supplementation. *Science.* 1969;165:613–615.

Bressler NM, et al. The grading and prevalence of macular degeneration in Chesapeake Bay watermen. *Arch Ophthalmol.* 1989;107:847–852.

Jury still out on nutritional supplementation. *Ophthalmol Times.* Dec. 1991:10.

Katz ML, Eldred GE. Failure of vitamin E to protect the retina against damage resulting from bright cyclic light exposure. *Invest Ophthalmol Vis Sci.* 1989;30:29–36.

Katz ML, Eldred GE, Robison WG. Lipofuscin autofluorescence: Evidence for vitamin A involvement in the retina. *Mech Ageing Dev.* 1987;39:81–90.

Katz ML, Robison WG. Light and aging effects on vitamin E in the retina and retinal pigment epithelium. *Vision Res.* 1987;27:1875–1879.

Liles MR, et al. Antioxidant enzymes in the aging human retinal pigment epithelium. *Arch Ophthalmol.* 1991;109:1285–1288.

Newsome DA, et al. Detection of specific extracellular matrix molecules in drusen, Bruch's membrane, and ciliary body. *Am J Ophthalmol.* 1987;104:373–381.

Newsome DA, et al. Oral zinc in macular degeneration. Arch Ophthalmol. 1988;106:192–198.

Prasad AS, et al. Hypocapremia induced by zinc therapy in adults. *JAMA.* 1978;240:2166–2168.

Sanders DR, moderator. Nutritional compliance and macular degeneration. *Ocular Surg News.* 1991(suppl):1–15.

Stephens RJ, et al. Vitamin E distribution in ocular tissues following long-term dietary depletion and supplementation as determined by microdissection and gas chromatography–mass spectrometry. *Exp Eye Res.* 1988;47:237–245.

Taylor HR. Ultraviolet radiation and the eye: An epidemiologic study. *Trans Am Ophthalmol Soc.* 1990;87:802–853.

Taylor HR, et al. Visible light and risk of age-related macular degeneration. *Trans Am Ophthalmol Soc.* 1990;88:163–173.

Tso MOM. Pathogenetic factors of aging macular degeneration. *Ophthalmology.* 1985;92:628–635.

Weiter JJ, et al. Relationship of senile macular degeneration to ocular pigmentation. *Am J Ophthalmol.* 1985;99:185–187.

West SK, et al. Exposure to sunlight and other risk factors for age-related macular degeneration. *Arch Ophthalmol.* 1989;107:875–879.

Young RW. Solar radiation and age-related macular degeneration. *Surv Ophthalmol.* 1988;32:252–269.

Macular Degeneration, Exudative and Nonexudative

Alexander LJ. The prevalence of macular drusen in a population of patients with known insulin-dependent diabetes mellitus. *J Am Optom Assoc.* 1985;56:806–809.

Anderson CJ, et al. Bilateral juxtapapillary subretinal neovascularization and pseudopapilledema in a three-year-old child. *J Pediatr Ophthalmol Strabismus.* 1978;15:296–299.

Aubsburger JJ, Benson WE. Subretinal neovascularization in chronic uveitis. *Albrecht von Graefes Arch Klin Ophthalmol.* 1980;215:32–51.

Blumenkranz MS, et al. Risk factors in age-related maculopathy complicated by choroidal neovascularization. *Ophthalmology.* 1986;93:552–558.

Bressler NM, et al. Age-related macular degeneration. *Surv Ophthalmol.* 1988;32:374–413.

Bressler NM, et al. Drusen characteristics in patients with exudative versus non-exudative age-related macular degeneration. *Retina.* 1988;8:109–114.

Bressler NM, et al. Natural course of poorly defined choroidal neovascularization associated with macular degeneration. *Arch Ophthalmol.* 1988;106:1537–1542.

Bressler NM, et al. Subfoveal neovascular membranes in senile macular degeneration: Relationship between membrane size and visual prognosis. *Retina.* 1983;3:7–11.

Chamberlin JA, et al. The use of fundus photographs and fluorescein angiograms in the identification and treatment of choroidal neovascularization in the macular photocoagulation study. *Ophthalmology.* 1989;96:1526–1534.

Ebert EM, et al. Functional vision in patients with neovascular maculopathy and poor visual acuity. *Arch Ophthalmol.* 1986;104:1009–1012.

Elman MJ, et al. The natural history of serous retinal pigment epithelium detachment in patients with age-related macular degeneration. *Ophthalmology.* 1986;93:224–230.

Ferris FL, Fine SL, Hyman L. Age-related macular degeneration and blindness due to neovascular maculopathy. *Arch Ophthalmol.* 1984;102:1640–1642.

Fine SL. Early detection of extrafoveal neovascular membranes by daily central field evaluation. *Ophthalmology.* 1985;92:603–609.

Folk JC. Aging macular degeneration clinical features of treatable disease. *Ophthalmology.* 1985;92:594–602.

Gass JDM. *Stereoscopic Atlas of Macular Diseases—Diagnosis and Treatment.* 3rd ed. St. Louis: Mosby; 1987.

Gass JDM. Retinal pigment epithelial rip during krypton red laser photocoagulation. *Am J Ophthalmol.* 1984;98:700–706.

Gass JDM. Pathogenesis of disciform detachment of the neuroepithelium, I–IV. *Am J Ophthalmol.* 1967;63:573–711.

Green SN, Yarian D. Acute tear of the pigment epithelium. *Retina.* 1983;3:16–20.

Green WR, et al. Pathologic features of senile macular degeneration. *Ophthalmology.* 1985;92:615–627.

Green WR, Wilson DJ. Choroidal neovascularization. *Ophthalmology.* 1986;93:1169–1176.

Guyer DR, et al. Subfoveal choroidal neovascular membranes in age-related macular degeneration. Visual prognosis in eyes with relatively good initial visual acuity. *Arch Ophthalmol.* 1986;104:702–705.

Haller J, et al. Retinal pigment epithelial tears: patterns and prognosis. *Ophthalmology.* 1988;95:8–13.

Kanski JJ, Morse PH. *Disorders of the Vitreous, Retina and Choroid.* Boston: Butterworths; 1983.

Lewis H, et al. Chorioretinal juncture. Multiple extramacular drusen. *Ophthalmology.* 1986;93:1098–1112.

Macular Photocoagulation Study Group. Krypton laser photocoagulation for idiopathic neovascular lesions: Results of a randomized clinical trial. *Arch Ophthalmol.* 1990;108:832–837.

Macular Photocoagulation Study Group. Krypton laser photocoagulation for neovascular lesions of age-related macular degeneration: Results of a randomized clinical trial. *Arch Ophthalmol.* 1990;108:816–824.

Macular Photocoagulation Study Group. Argon laser photocoagulation for neovascular maculopathy. Three year results from randomized clinical trials. *Arch Ophthalmol.* 1986;104:694–701.

Macular Photocoagulation Study Group. Recurrent choroidal neovascularization after argon laser photocoagulation for neovascular maculopathy. *Arch Ophthalmol.* 1986;104:503–512.

Macular Photocoagulation Study Group. Argon laser photocoagulation for idiopathic neovascularization: Results of a randomized clinical trial. *Arch Ophthalmol.* 1983;101:1358–1361.

Macular Photocoagulation Study Group. Argon laser photocoagulation for ocular histoplasmosis. *Arch Ophthalmol.* 1983;101:1347–1357.

Macular Photocoagulation Study Group. Argon laser photocoagulation for senile macular degeneration. Results of randomized clinical trial. *Arch Ophthalmol.* 1982;100:912–918.

Maguire P, Vine AK. Geographic atrophy of the retinal pigment eptihelium. *Am J Ophthalmol.* 1986;102:621–625.

Melrose MA, et al. Vision parameters in krypton laser photocoagulation of subfoveal neovascular membranes. *Ophthalmic Surg.* 1985;16:495–502.

Michelson JB, et al. Subretinal neovascular membrane and disciform scar in Behçet's disease. *Am J Ophthalmol.* 1980;90:182–185.

Miller H, et al. The role of pigment epithelium in the involution of subretinal neovascularization. *Invest Ophthalmol Vis Sci.* 1986;27:1644–1652.

Murphy RP. Age-related macular degeneration. *Ophthalmology.* 1986;93:969–971.

Olk RJ, Burgess DB. Treatment of recurrent juxtafoveal subretinal neovascular membranes with red laser photocoagulation. *Ophthalmology.* 1985;92:1035–1046.

Poliner LS, et al. Natural history of retinal pigment epithelial detachments in age-related macular degeneration. *Ophthalmology.* 1986;93:543–551.

Ryan SJ, et al. *Retinal Diseases.* Orlando: Grune & Stratton, 1985.

Schatz H, McDonald R. Atrophic macular degeneration: Rate of spread of geographic atrophy and visual loss. *Ophthalmology.* 1989;96:1541–1551.

Singerman LJ. Laser photocoagulation for choroidal new vessel membrane complicating age-related macular degeneration associated with pigment epithelial detachment. *Retina.* 1988;8:115–121.

Singerman LJ, et al. Spontaneous visual improvement in the first affected eye of patients with bilateral disciform scars. *Retina.* 1985;5:135–143.

Singerman LJ, Hionis R. Growth rate of subretinal neovascularization in age-related macular degeneration (discussion). *Ophthalmology.* 1989;96:1422–1429.

Singerman LJ, Kalski RS. Tunable dye laser photocoagulation for choroidal neovascularization complicating age-related macular degeneration. *Retina.* 1989;9:246–257.

Smiddy WE, Fine SL. Prognosis of patients with bilateral macular drusen. *Ophthalmology.* 1984;91:271–277.

Spencer WH. *Ophthalmic Pathology. An Atlas and Textbook.* Philadelphia: Saunders; 1985.

Strahlman ER, et al. The second eye of patients with senile macular degeneration. *Arch Ophthalmol.* 1983;101: 1191–1193.

Swanson DE, et al. Tears of the retinal pigment epithelium: Occurrence in retinal detachment and a chorioretinal scar. *Retina.* 1984;4:115–118.

Talbot JF. Age-related macular degeneration. *Semin Ophthalmol.* 1986;1:179–188.

Tso MO. Pathogenetic factors of aging macular degeneration. *Ophthalmology.* 1985;92:628–635.

Weiter JJ, et al. Relationship of senile macular degeneration to ocular pigmentation. *Am J Ophthalmol.* 1985;15:185–187.

Yanuzzi LA, et al. *The Macula. A Comprehensive Text and Atlas.* Baltimore: Williams & Wilkins; 1979.

Young NJA, et al. Pigment epithelial disease with abnormal choroidal perfusion. *Am J Ophthalmol.* 1980;90:607–608.

Young RW. Review: Pathophysiology of age-related macular degeneration. *Surv Ophthalmol.* 1987;31:291–306.

Choroidal Rupture

Alexander LJ. Choroidal rupture. *Rev Optom.* 1978;115: 33–34.

Gass JDM. *Stereoscopic Atlas of Macular Disease.* 3rd ed. St. Louis: Mosby; 1987.

Hart JCD, et al. Indirect choroidal tears at the posterior pole: A fluorescein angiographic and perimetric study. *Br J Ophthalmol.* 1980;64:59–67.

Pearlstone AD. Delayed loss of central vision following multiple posterior segment trauma. *Ann Ophthalmol.* 1980;12: 409–411.

Pruett RC, et al. Myopic cracks, angioid streaks, and traumatic tears in Bruch's membrane. *Am J Ophthalmol.* 1987; 103:537–543.

Spencer WH. *Ophthalmic Pathology. An Atlas and Textbook.* Philadelphia: Saunders; 1985.

Wyszynski RE, et al. Indirect choroidal rupture secondary to blunt ocular trauma: A review of eight cases. *Retina.* 1988;8:237–243.

Postsurgical and Trauma-induced Neovascular Development

Augsburger JJ, et al. Scatter photocoagulation for choriovitreal neovascularization. *Retina.* 1984;4:171–176.

Augsburger JJ, et al. Circumscribed choroidal hemangiomas: Long-term prognosis. *Retina.* 1981;1:56–61.

Berger AR, Boniuk I. Bilateral subretinal neovascularization after focal argon laser photocoagulation for diabetic macular edema. *Am J Ophthalmol.* 1989;108:88–90.

Carney MD, et al. Iatrogenic choroidal neovascularization in sickle cell retinopathy. *Ophthalmology.* 1986;93: 1163–1168.

Chandra SR, et al. Choroidal neovascular ingrowth after photocoagulation for proliferative diabetic retinopathy. *Arch Ophthalmol.* 1980;98:1593–1600.

Cialdini AP, et al. Photocoagulation of chorioretinal anastomoses in far-advanced age-related macular degeneration. *Ophthalmic Surg.* 1989;20:316–320.

Condon PI, et al. Choroidal neovascularization induced by photocoagulation in sickle cell disease. *Br J Ophthalmol.* 1981;65:192–197.

Dizon-Moore RV, et al. Chorioretinal and choriovitreal neovascularization: Their presence after photocoagulation of proliferative sickle cell retinopathy. *Arch Ophthalmol.* 1981;99:842–849.

Escoffery RD. Subretinal neovascularization following endophotocoagulation. *Retina.* 1981;1:211–215.

Gottlieb F, et al. Retinal angiomatous mass: A complication of retinal detachment surgery. *Retina.* 1984;4:152–157.

Holland PM. Postoperative subretinal neovascular membrane at the drain site of a scleral buckle. *Ophthalmic Surg.* 1985;16:174–177.

Lewen RM. Subretinal neovascularization complicating laser photocoagulation of diabetic maculopathy. *Ophthalmic Surg.* 1988;19:734–737.

Theodossiadis GP. Choroidal neovascularization after cryoapplication. *Albrecht von Graefes Arch Klin Ophthalmol.* 1981;215:203–208.

Trimble SN, Schatz H. Subretinal neovascularization following metallic intraocular foreign-body trauma. *Arch Ophthalmol.* 1986;104:515–519.

Varley MP, et al. Subretinal neovascularization after focal argon laser for diabetic macular edema. *Ophthalmology.* 1988;95:567–573.

Degenerative or Pathologic Myopia

Avila MP, et al. Natural history of choroidal neovascularization in degenerative myopia. *Ophthalmology.* 1984;91: 1573–1581.

Curtain BJ, Karlin DB. Axial length measurements and fundus changes of the myopic eye. *Am J Ophthalmol.* 1971;71: 42–53.

Gass JDM. *Stereoscopic Atlas of Macular Disease.* 3rd ed. St. Louis: Mosby; 1987.

Hotchkiss ML, Fine SL. Pathologic myopia and choroidal neovascularization. *Am J Ophthalmol.* 1981;91:177–183.

Jalkh AE, et al. Choroidal neovascularization in degenerative myopia: Role of laser photocoagulation. *Ophthalmic Surg.* 1987;18:721–725.

Klein RM, Curtain GJ. Lacquer crack lesions in pathologic myopia. *Am J Ophthalmol.* 1975;79:386–392.

Klein RM, Green S. The development of lacquer cracks in pathologic myopia. *Am J Ophthalmol.* 1988;106:282–285.

Levy JH, et al. The Fuch's spot: An ophthalmoscopic and fluorescein angiographic study. *Ann Ophthalmol.* 1977; 1433–1443.

Pruett RC, et al. Myopic cracks, angioid streaks, and traumatic tears in Bruch's membrane. *Am J Ophthalmol.* 1987; 103:537–543.

Angioid Streaks

Brancato R, et al. Laser treatment of macular subretinal neovascularization in angioid streaks. *Ophthalmologica.* 1987;195:84–87.

Cavallerano AA. Angioid streaks. *Clin Eye Vision Care.* 1991;3:34–38.

Cockburn DM. Angioid streaks: An illustrated medical and optometric review. *Clin Exp Optom.* 1991;74:120–124.

Coleman K, et al. Disk drusen and angioid streaks in pseudoxanthoma elasticum. *Am J Ophthalmol.* 1991;112: 166–170.

Federman JL, et al. Angioid streaks. *Arch Ophthalmol.* 1975;93:951.

Gass JDM, Clarkson JG. Angioid streaks and disciform macular detachment in Paget's disease. *Am J Ophthalmol.* 1973;75:576–586.

Geeraets WJ, Guerry D. Angioid streaks and sickle cell disease. *Am J Ophthalmol.* 1960;49:450.

Gelisken O, et al. A long-term follow-up study of laser coagulation of neovascular membranes in angioid streaks. *Am J Ophthalmol.* 1988;105:299–303.

Kayazawa F. A successful argon laser treatment in macular complications of angioid streaks. *Ann Ophthalmol.* 1981; 13:581–583.

Kothe AC, Bolduc M. Pseudoxanthoma elasticum: A clinical review and case study. *Clin Eye Vision Care.* 1991; 3:110–113.

Kreiser FE. Treatment of angioid streaks with neovascularization: Case report and clinical review. *S J Optom.* 1990;4:8–12.

Pruett RC, et al. Myopic cracks, angioid streaks, and traumatic tears in Bruch's membrane. *Am J Ophthalmol.* 1987;103:537–543.

Sigelman J. *Retinal Diseases. Pathogenesis, Laser Therapy, and Surgery.* Boston: Little, Brown; 1984.

Singerman LJ, Hatem G. Laser treatment of choroidal neovascular membranes in angioid streaks. *Retina.* 1981;1: 75–83.

Spencer WH. *Ophthalmic Pathology. An Atlas and Textbook.* Philadelphia: Saunders; 1985.

Idiopathic Central Serous Chorioretinopathy

Alexander LJ. Diseases of the retina. In: Bartlett JD, Jaanus SD, eds. *Clinical Ocular Pharmacology.* Boston: Butterworths; 1984.

Gass JDM. *Stereoscopic Atlas of Macular Diseases—Diagnosis and Treatment.* 3rd ed. St. Louis: Mosby; 1987.

Gomolin JES. Choroidal neovascularization and central serous chorioretinopathy. *Can J Ophthalmol.* 1989;24: 20–23.

Jalkh AE, et al. Retinal pigment epithelium decompensation, I. Clinical features and natural course. *Ophthalmology.* 1984;91:1544–1548.

Jalkh AE, et al. Retinal pigment epithelium decompensation, II. Laser treatment. *Ophthalmology.* 1984;91:1549–1553.

Levine R, et al. Long-term follow-up of idiopathic central serous chorioretinopathy by fluorescein angiography. *Ophthalmology.* 1989;96:854–859.

Mazzuca DE, Benson WE. Central serous retinopathy. *Surv Ophthalmol.* 1986;31:170–174.

Novak MA, et al. Krypton and argon laser photocoagulation for central serous choroidopathy. *Retina.* 1987;7:162–169.

Robertson DM. Argon laser photocoagulation treatment in central serous chorioretinopathy. *Ophthalmology.* 1986;93: 972–974.

Robertson DM, Ilstrup D. Direct, indirect, and sham laser photocoagulation in the management of central serous chorioretinopathy. *Am J Ophthalmol.* 1983;95:457–466.

Ryan SJ, et al. *Retinal Diseases.* Orlando: Grune & Stratton; 1985.

Slusher MM. Krypton red laser photocoagulation in selected cases of central serous chorioretinopathy. *Retina.* 1986;6: 81–84.

Spencer WH. *Ophthalmic Pathology. An Atlas and Textbook.* Philadelphia: Saunders; 1985.

Watzke RC, et al. Direct and indirect laser photocoagulation of central serous choroidopathy. *Am J Ophthalmol.* 1979; 88:914–918.

Yannuzzi IA. Type-A behavior and central serous chorioretinopathy. *Retina.* 1987;7:111–130.

Cystoid Macular Edema

Coscas G, Guadric A. Natural course of nonaphakic cystoid macular edema. *Surv Ophthalmol.* 1984;28(suppl):471–484.

Dugel PU, et al. Pars plana vitrectomy for intraocular inflammation-related cystoid macular edema unresponsive to corticosteroids. *Ophthalmology.* 1992;99:1535–1541.

Fisher DH, Schmidt EE. A variance of the vitreous wick syndrome and its relationship to cystoid macular edema. *S J Optom.* 1992;10:11–15.

Flach AJ, et al. Effectiveness of ketorolac tromethamine 0.5% ophthalmic solution for chronic aphakic and pseudophakic cystoid macular edema. *Am J Ophthalmol.* 1987;103: 479–486.

Jampol LM. Pharmacologic therapy of aphakic and pseudophakic cystoid macular edema. 1985 update. *Ophthalmology.* 1985;92:807–810.

Jampol LM, et al. Prophylaxis and therapy of aphakic cystoid macular edema. *Surv Ophthalmol.* 1984;28(suppl): 535–539.

Kanski JJ, Morse PH. *Disorders of the Vitreous, Retina and Choroid.* Boston: Butterworths; 1983.

Kraff MC, et al. Prophylaxis of pseudophakic cystoid macular edema with indomethacin. *Ophthalmology.* 1982;89: 886–889.

Loeffler KU, et al. Dominantly inherited cystoid macular edema. *Ophthalmology.* 1992;99:1385–1392.

Sigelman J. *Retinal Diseases. Pathogenesis, Laser Therapy, and Surgery.* Boston: Little, Brown; 1984.

Yanuzzi LA. A perspective on the treatment of aphakic cystoid macular edema. *Surv Ophthalmol.* 1984;28(suppl): 540–553.

Yanuzzi LA, et al. *The Macula. A Comprehensive Text and Atlas.* Baltimore: Williams & Wilkins, 1979.

Macular Holes

Aaberg TM. Macular holes: A review. *Surv Ophthalmol.* 1970;15:139–162.

Akiba J, et al. Risk of developing a macular hole. *Arch Ophthalmol.* 1990;108:1088–1090.

Bronstein MA, et al. Fellow eyes of eyes with macular holes. *Am J Ophthalmol.* 1981;92:757–761.

Buckner J. Solar retinopathy: A case report. *S J Optom.* 1989;7:23–25.

Chambers RB, et al. Modified vitrectomy for impending macular holes. *Ophthal Surg.* 1991;22:730–734.

Fish RH, et al. Macular pseudoholes: Clinical features and accuracy of diagnosis. *Ophthalmology.* 1992;99:1665–1670.

Gass JDM. Idiopathic senile macular hole: Its early stages and pathogenesis. *Arch Ophthalmol.* 1988;106:629–639.

Gass JDM, Joondeph BC. Observations concerning patients with suspected impending macular holes. *Am J Ophthalmol.* 1990;109:638–646.

Glaser BM, et al. Transforming growth factor-B2 for the treatment of full-thickness macular holes: A prospective randomized study. *Ophthalmology.* 1992;99:1162–1173.

Guyer DR, et al. Observations on patients with idiopathic macular holes and cysts. *Arch Ophthalmol.* 1992;110:1264–1268.

Jost BF, et al. Vitrectomy in eyes at risk for macular hole formation. *Ophthalmology.* 1990;97:843–847.

Kelly NE, Wendel RT. Vitreous surgery for idiopathic macular holes. *Arch Ophthalmol.* 1991;109:654–659.

Kothe AC, et al. Visual function in partial and full thickness macular holes. *Clin Eye Vision Care.* 1992;4:55–60.

Labelle P. Photocoagulation as the sole treatment for early posterior retinal detachment. *Retina.* 1981;184:26–29.

Morita H, et al. Causative factors of retinal detachment in macular holes. *Retina.* 1991;11:281–284.

Ogura Y, et al. Improved visualization of macular hole lesions with laser biomicroscopy. *Arch Ophthalmol.* 1991;109:957–961.

Poliner LS, Tornambe PE. Retinal pigment epitheliopathy after macular hole surgery. *Ophthalmology.* 1992;99:1671–1677.

Schocket SS, et al. Laser treatment of macular holes. *Ophthalmology.* 1988;95:574–582.

Sheta SM, et al. Cyanoacrylate tissue adhesive in the management of recurrent retinal detachment caused by macular hole. *Am J Ophthalmol.* 1990;109:28–32.

Presumed Ocular Histoplasmosis Syndrome

Aubsburger JJ, Benson WE. Subretinal neovascularization in chronic uveitis. *Albrecht von Graefes Arch Klin Ophthalmol.* 1980;215:32–51.

Beck RW, et al. Optic disc edema in presumed ocular histoplasmosis syndrome. *Ophthalmology.* 1984;91:183–185.

Burgess DB. Ocular histoplasmosis syndrome. *Ophthalmology.* 1986;93:967–968.

Dreyer RF, Gass DJ. Multifocal choroiditis and panuveitis. A syndrome that mimics ocular histoplasmosis. *Arch Ophthalmol.* 1984;102:1776–1784.

Fine SL, et al. Subretinal neovascularization developing after prophylactic argon laser photocoagulation of atrophic macular scars. *Am J Ophthalmol.* 1976;82:352–357.

Gass JDM. Follow-up study of presumed ocular histoplasmosis. *Trans Am Acad Ophthalmol Otolaryngol.* 1972;76:672–694.

Kanski JJ, Morse PH. *Disorders of the Vitreous, Retina and Choroid.* Boston: Butterworths; 1983.

Kleiner RC, et al. Subfoveal neovascularization in the ocular histoplasmosis syndrome: A natural history study. *Retina.* 1988;8:225–229.

Macular Photocoagulation Study Group. Persistent and recurrent neovascularization after krypton laser photocoagulation for neovascular lesions of ocular histoplasmosis. *Arch Ophthalmol.* 1989;107:344–352.

Macular Photocoagulation Study Group. Krypton laser photocoagulation for neovascular lesions of ocular histoplasmosis: Results of a randomized clinical trial. *Arch Ophthalmol.* 1987;105:1499–1507.

Macular Photocoagulation Study Group. Argon laser photocoagulation for neovascular maculopathy: Three-year results from randomized clinical trials. *Arch Ophthalmol.* 1986;104:694–701.

Macular Photocoagulation Study Group. Recurrent choroidal neovascularization after argon laser photocoagulation for neovascular maculopathy. *Arch Ophthalmol.* 1986;104:503–512.

Macular Photocoagulation Study Group. Argon laser photocoagulation for ocular histoplasmosis: Results of a randomized clinical trial. *Arch Ophthalmol.* 1983;101:1347–1357.

Olk RJ, et al. Subfoveal and juxtafoveal subretinal neovascularization in the presumed ocular histoplasmosis syndrome. *Ophthalmology.* 1984;91:1592–1602.

Ryan SJ, et al. *Retinal Diseases.* Orlando: Grune & Stratton; 1985.

Schlaegel TF. *Ocular Histoplasmosis.* New York: Grune & Stratton; 1977.

Schlaegel TF. Perspectives in uveitis. *Ann Ophthalmol.* 1981;13:799–806.

Schlaegel TF, Kenny D. Changes around the optic nerve head in presumed ocular histoplasmosis. *Am J Ophthalmol.* 1966;62:454.

Sigelman J. *Retinal Diseases. Pathogenesis, Laser Therapy, and Surgery.* Boston: Little, Brown; 1984.

Smith RE, et al. Ocular histoplasmosis: Significance of asymptomatic macular scars. *Arch Ophthalmol.* 1973;89:296–300.

Yanuzzi LA, et al. *The Macula. A Comprehensive Text and Atlas.* Baltimore: Williams & Wilkins; 1979.

Ocular Toxoplasmosis

Dobbie JG. Cryotherapy in the management of toxoplasmosis retinochoroiditis. *Trans Am Acad Ophthalmol Otolaryngol.* 1968;72:364–373.

Fitzgerald CR. Pars plana vitrectomy for vitreous opacity secondary to presumed toxoplasmosis. *Arch Ophthalmol.* 1980;98:321–323.

Gaynon MW, et al. Retinal neovascularization and ocular toxoplasmosis. *Am J Ophthalmol.* 1984;98:585–589.

Guldsten H. Clindamycin and sulphonamides in the treatment of ocular toxoplasmosis. *Acta Ophthalmol (Copenh).* 1983;61:51–57.

Holliman RE, et al. Serological investigation of ocular toxoplasmosis. *Br J Ophthalmol.* 1991;75:353–355.

Kanski JJ, Morse PH. *Disorders of the Vitreous, Retina and Choroid.* Boston: Butterworths; 1983.

Lakhanapal V, et al. Clindamycin in the treatment of toxoplasmic retinochoroiditis. *Am J Ophthalmol.* 1983;95:605–613.

Meredith JT. Toxoplasmosis of the central nervous system. *Am Fam Physician.* 1987;35:113–116.

Nobel KG, Carr RE. Toxoplasmic retinochoroiditis. *Ophthalmology.* 1982;89:1289–1290.

O'Connor GR. Protozoan diseases of the uvea. *Int Ophthalmol Clin.* 1977;17:163–176.

Perkins ES. Ocular toxoplasmosis. *Br J Ophthalmol.* 1973;57:1–17.

Rossini M. Acquired versus congenital ocular toxoplasmosis: A case report. *S J Optom.* 1992;10:28–33.

Ryan SJ, et al. *Retinal Diseases.* Orlando: Grune & Stratton; 1985.

Schlaegel TF. Perspectives in uveitis. *Ann Ophthalmol.* 1981;13:799–806.

Sigelman J. *Retinal Diseases. Pathogenesis, Laser Therapy, and Surgery.* Boston: Little, Brown; 1984.

Spencer WH. *Ophthalmic Pathology. An Atlas and Textbook.* Philadelphia: Saunders; 1985.

Steahy LP. Endolaser photocoagulation of toxoplasmosis. *Ann Ophthalmol.* 1988;20:463–465.

Tabbara KF, O'Connor GR. Treatment of ocular toxoplasmosis with clindamycin and sulfadiazine. *Ophthalmology.* 1980;87:129–134.

Ocular Parasititis

Brown DH. Ocular toxocara canis. *J Pediatr Ophthalmol.* 1970;7:182–191.

Cunha de Souza E, et al. Diffuse unilateral subacute neuroretinitis in South America. *Arch Ophthalmol.* 1992;110:1261–1263.

Forman AR, et al. Ophthalmomyiasis treated by argon laser photocoagulation. *Retina.* 1984;4:163–165.

Gass JDM, Braunstein RA. Further observations concerning the diffuse unilateral subacute neuroretinitis syndrome. *Arch Ophthalmol.* 1983;107:33–37.

Morris PD, Katerndahl DA. Human toxocariasis. Review with report of a probable cause. *Postgrad Med.* 1987;81:263–267.

O'Connor GR. Protozoan diseases of the uvea. *Int Ophthalmol Clin.* 1977;17:163–176.

Raymond LA, et al. Living retinal nematode (filarial-like) destroyed with photocoagulation. *Ophthalmology.* 1978;85:944–949.

Santos R, et al. Management of subretinal and vitreous cysticercosis: Role of photocoagulation and surgery. *Ophthalmology.* 1979;86:1501–1504.

Schlaegel TF. Perspectives in uveitis. *Ann Ophthalmol.* 1981;13:799–806.

Siam AL. Toxocaral chorioretinitis: Treatment of early cases with photocoagulation. *Br J Ophthalmol.* 1973;57:700–703.

Ocular Manifestations of Sarcoidosis

Doxanas MT, et al. Sarcoidosis with neovascularization of the optic nerve head. *Am J Ophthalmol.* 1980;99:842–849.

Duker JS, et al. Proliferative sarcoid retinopathy. *Ophthalmology.* 1988;95:1680–1686.

Galinos SD, et al. Choroido-vitreal neovascularization after argon laser photocoagulation. *Arch Ophthalmol.* 1975;93:524–530.

Gass JDM. *Stereoscopic Atlas of Macular Diseases—Diagnosis and Treatment.* 3rd ed. St. Louis: Mosby; 1987.

Graham EM, et al. Neovascularization associated with posterior uveitis. *Br J Ophthalmol.* 1987;71:826–833.

Jabs DA, Johns CJ. Ocular involvement in chronic sarcoidosis. *Am J Ophthalmol.* 1986;102:297–301.

Mizuno K, Takahashi J. Sarcoid cyclitis. *Ophthalmology.* 1986;93:511–517.

Obenauf CD, et al. Sarcoidosis and its ophthalmic manifestations. *Am J Ophthalmol.* 1978;86:648–655.

Schlaegel TF. Perspectives in uveitis. *Ann Ophthalmol.* 1981;13:799–806.

Spalton DJ, Sanders MD. Fundus changes in histologically confirmed sarcoidosis. *Br J Ophthalmol.* 1981;65:348–358.

Tingey DP, Gonder JR. Ocular sarcoidosis presenting as a solitary choroidal mass. *Can J Ophthalmol.* 1992;27:25–29.

Human Immunovirus and the Eye

AIDS Monthly Surveillance Report. Atlanta: Centers for Disease Control; June 1990:5.

Berger JR, et al. Neurologic disease as the presenting manifestation of acquired immunodeficiency syndrome. *South Med J.* 1987;80:683–686.

Bloom SM, et al. Posterior segment manifestations of human immunodeficiency virus (HIV) infection. *S J Optom.* 1992;10:13–22.

Bowen DL, et al. Immunopathogenesis of the acquired immunodeficiency syndrome. *Ann Int Med.* 1985;103:704–709.

Centers for Disease Control. Recommendations for prevention of HIV transmission in health care settings. *MMWR.* 1987;36(suppl 25):3–18.

Dalakas M, et al. AIDS and the nervous system. *JAMA.* 1989;261:2396–2399.

Den Beste BP, Hummer J. AIDS: A review and guide for infection control. *J Am Optom Assoc.* 1986;57:675–682.

Engstrom RE, et al. Hemorrheologic abnormalities in patients with immunodeficiency virus infection and ophthalmic microvasculopathy. *Am J Ophthalmol.* 1990;109:153–161.

Freeman WR, et al. Surgical repair of rhegmatogenous retinal detachments in immunosuppressed patients with cytomegalovirus retinitis. *Ophthalmology.* 1992;99:466–474.

Gallo RC, et al. Frequent detection and isolation of cytopathic retrovirus (HTLV-III) from patients with AIDS and at risk for AIDS. *Science.* 1984;224:500–503.

Gass JDM, et al. Acute syphilitic posterior placoid chorioretinitis. *Ophthalmology.* 1990;97:1288–1297.

Gottlieb MS, et al. Pneumocystis carinii pneumonia and mucosal candidiasis in previously healthy homosexual men: Evidence of a new acquired cellular immunodeficiency. *N Engl J Med.* 1981;305:1425–1431.

Harkins T, Maino JH. Cytomegalovirus retinitis complicated by optic neuropathy: A longitudinal study. *J Am Optom Assoc.* 1992;63:21–27.

Henderly DE, et al. Cytomegalovirus retinitis as the initial manifestation of the acquired immunodeficiency syndrome. *Ann Ophthalmol.* 1987;103:316–320.

Hennis HL, et al. Cytomegalovirus retinitis. *Surv Ophthalmol.* 1989;34:193–203.

Holland GN, et al. Acquired immune deficiency syndrome: Ocular manifestations. *Ophthalmology.* 1983;90:859–873.

Inslor MS. *AIDS and Other Sexually Transmitted Diseases and the Eye.* Orlando: Grune & Stratton; 1987.

Jabs DA, et al. Retinal detachments in patients with cytomegalovirus retinitis. *Arch Ophthalmol.* 1991;19: 794–799.

Jabs DA, et al. Treatment of cytomegalovirus retinitis—1992. *Arch Ophthalmol.* 1992;110:185–187.

Jaffe HW, et al. National case control study of Kaposi's sarcoma and pneumocystis carinii pneumonia in homosexual men, 1. Epidemiologic results. *Ann Int Med.* 1983;99: 145–151.

Lemp GF, et al. Projections of AIDS morbidity and mortality in San Francisco. *JAMA.* 1990;263:1497–1501.

Levy JA. Human immunodeficiency viruses and the pathogenesis of AIDS. *JAMA.* 1989;261:2997–3006.

Levy RM, et al. Neuroradiologic findings in AIDS: A review of 200 cases. *AJR.* 1986;147:977–983.

Macher A, et al. Disseminated bilateral chorioretinitis due to histoplasma capsulatum in a patient with acquired immunodeficiency syndrome. *Ophthalmology.* 1985;92: 1159–1164.

McLeish WM, et al. The ocular manifestations of syphilis in the human immunodeficiency virus type 1-infected host. *Ophthalmology.* 1990;97:196–203.

Miller AB, et al. Treatment of cytomegalovirus retinitis with zidovudine and ganciclovir in patients with AIDS: Outcome and toxicity. *Genitourin Med.* 1990;66:156–158.

Mills J. Pneumocystis carinii and toxoplasma gondii infections in patients with AIDS. *Rev Infect Dis.* 1986;8: 1001–1011.

Morbidity and Mortality Weekly Report. Update: Acquired immunodeficiency syndrome—United States, 1989. *MMWR.* 1990;39:81.

Price RW, et al. The brain in AIDS: Central nervous system HIV-1 infection and AIDS dementia complex. *Science.* 1988;239:586–591.

Redmond R, Wilson R. Neurological manifestations of AIDS. *J Am Optom Assoc.* 1990;61:760–767.

Roberts SP, Petrou Haefs TM. Central retinal vein occlusion in a middle-aged adult with HIV infection. *Optom Vis Sci.* 1992;69:567–569.

Sanborn GE, et al. Sustained-release ganciclovir therapy for treatment of cytomegalovirus retinitis. *Arch Ophthalmol.* 1992;110:188–198.

Schanzer MC, et al. Primary ocular malignant lymphoma associated with the acquired immune deficiency syndrome. *Ophthalmology.* 1991;98:88–91.

Sison RF, et al. Cytomegalovirus retinopathy as the initial manifestation of the acquired immunodeficiency syndrome. *Am J Ophthalmol.* 1991;112:243–249.

Smith TJ. Intravitreal sustained-release ganciclovir. *Arch Ophthalmol.* 1992;110:255–258.

Spaide RF, et al. Frosted branch angiitis associated with cytomegalovirus retinitis. *Am J Ophthalmol.* 1992;113: 522–528.

Specht CS, et al. Ocular histoplasmosis with retinitis in a patient with acquired immune deficiency syndrome. *Ophthalmology.* 1991;98:1356–1359.

Studies of Ocular Complications of AIDS Research Group. Mortality in patients with the acquired immunodeficiency syndrome treated with either foscarnet or ganciclovir for cytomegalovirus retinitis. *N Engl J Med.* 1992;326:213–220.

Tramont EC. Syphilis in the AIDS era. *N Engl J Med.* 1987; 316:1600–1601.

Acute Posterior Multifocal Placoid Pigment Epitheliopathy (APMPPE)

Ajamian PC, Coughran J. Acute posterior multifocal placoid pigment epitheliopathy. *S J Optom.* 1983;9:28–30.

Bauer JM, et al. Acute posterior multifocal placoid pigment epitheliopathy. *J Am Optom Assoc.* 1990;61:304–312.

Dreyer RF, Gass DJ. Multifocal choroiditis and panuveitis. A syndrome that mimics ocular histoplasmosis. *Arch Ophthalmol.* 1984;102:1776–1784.

Gass JDM. Acute posterior multifocal placoid pigment epitheliopathy. *Arch Ophthalmol.* 1968;80:177–185.

Goen TM, Terry JE. Acute posterior multifocal placoid pigment epitheliopathy. *J Am Optom Assoc.* 1987;58:112–117.

Hammer ME, et al. Death associated with acute multifocal placoid pigment epitheliopathy. *Arch Ophthalmol.* 1989; 107:170–171.

Isashiki M, et al. Acute posterior multifocal placoid pigment epitheliopathy associated with diffuse retinal vasculitis and late haemorrhagic macular detachment. *Br J Ophthalmol.* 1986;70:255–259.

Laatikan LT, Immonen IJR. Acute posterior multifocal placoid pigment epitheliopathy in connection with acute nephritis. *Retina.* 1988;8:122–124.

Sigelman J, et al. Acute posterior multifocal placoid pigment epitheliopathy associated with cerebral vasculitis and homonymous hemianopia. *Am J Ophthalmol.* 1979;88: 919–924.

Spaide RF, et al. Choroidal vasculitis in acute posterior multifocal placoid pigment epitheliopathy. *Br J Ophthalmol.* 1991;75:685–687.

Wilson CA, et al. Acute posterior multifocal placoid pigment epitheliopathy and cerebral vasculitis. *Arch Ophthalmol.* 1988;106:796–800.

Wolf MD, et al. HLA-B7 and HLA-DR2 antigens and acute posterior multifocal placoid pigment epitheliopathy. *Arch Ophthalmol.* 1990;108:698–700.

Wright BE, et al. Placoid pigment epitheliopathy and Harada's disease. *Br J Ophthalmol.* 1978;62:609–621.

Geographic Helicoid Peripapillary Choroidopathy

Annesley WH, et al. The clinical course of serpiginous choroidopathy. *Am J Ophthalmol.* 1979;87:133–142.

Blumenkranz MS, et al. Atypical serpiginous choroiditis. *Arch Ophthalmol.* 1982;100:1773–1775.

Brazitikos PD, Safran AB. Helicoid peripapillary chorioretinal degeneration. *Am J Ophthalmol.* 1990;109:290–294.

Chisholm IH, et al. The late stage of serpiginous (geographic) choroiditis. *Am J Ophthalmol.* 1976;82:343–351.

Hardy RA, Schatz H. Macular geographic helicoid choroidopathy. *Arch Ophthalmol.* 1987;105:1237–1242.

Jampol LM, et al. Subretinal neovascularization with geographic (serpiginous) choroiditis. *Am J Ophthalmol.* 1979; 88:683–689.

Laatikainen L, Erkkila H. A follow-up study of serpiginous choroiditis. *Acta Ophthalmol.* 1981;59:707–718.

Laatikainen L, Erkkila H. Serpiginous choroiditis. *Br J Ophthalmol.* 1974;58:777–783.

Lampariello DA. Geographic (serpiginous) choroiditis. *J Am Optom Assoc.* 1992;63:112–116.

Wajno T, Meredith TA. Unusual findings in serpiginous choroiditis. *Am J Ophthalmol.* 1982;94:650–655.

Weiss H, et al. The clinical course of serpiginous choroidopathy. *Am J Ophthalmol.* 1979;87:133–142.

Recurrent Multifocal Choroiditis

Callahan D, Gass JDM. Multifocal choroiditis and choroidal neovascularization associated with the multiple evanescent white dot and idiopathic blind spot enlargement syndrome. *Ophthalmology.* 1992;99:1678–1685.

Cantrill HL, Folk JC. Multifocal choroiditis associated with progressive subretinal fibrosis. *Am J Ophthalmol.* 1986;101: 170–180.

Cavallerano A. Punctate inner choroidopathy. *Clin Eye Vision Care.* 1989;1:75–79.

Dreyer RF, Gass DJ. Multifocal choroiditis and panuveitis. A syndrome that mimics ocular histoplasmosis. *Arch Ophthalmol.* 1984;102:1776–1784.

Frederick AR. Multifocal and recurrent (serous) choroidopathy (MARC) syndrome: A new variety of idiopathic central serous choroidopathy. *Doc Ophthalmol.* 1984;56: 203–235.

Joondeph BC, Tessler HH. Clinical course of multifocal choroiditis: Photographic and angiographic evidence of disease recurrence. *Ann Ophthalmol.* 1991;23:424–429.

Morgan CM, Schatz H. Recurrent multifocal choroiditis. *Ophthalmology.* 1986;93:1138–1147.

Palestine AG, et al. Progressive subretinal fibrosis and uveitis. *Br J Ophthalmol.* 1984;68:667–673.

Schlaegel TF. Perspectives in uveitis. *Ann Ophthalmol.* 1981;13:799–806.

Singerman LJ. Recurrent multifocal choroiditis. *Ophthalmology.* 1986;93:1143–1147.

Spaide RF, et al. Linear streaks in multifocal choroiditis and panuveitis. *Retina.* 1991;11:229–231.

Tiedeman JS. Epstein–Barr viral antibodies in multifocal choroiditis and panuveitis. *Am J Ophthalmol.* 1987;103: 659–663.

Watzke RC, et al. Punctate inner choroidopathy. *Am J Ophthalmol.* 1984;98:572–584.

Multiple Evanescent White Dot Syndrome

Aaberg TM, et al. Recurrences and bilaterality in the multiple evanescent white-dot syndrome. *Am J Ophthalmol.* 1985;100:29–37.

Callahan D, Gass JDM. Multifocal choroiditis and choroidal neovascularization associated with the multiple evanescent white dot and acute idiopathic blind spot enlargement syndrome. *Ophthalmology.* 1992;99:1678–1685.

Dodwell DG, et al. Optic nerve involvement associated with the multiple evanescent white-dot syndrome. *Ophthalmology.* 1990;97:862–868.

Gass JDM, Hamed LM. Acute macular neuroretinopathy and multiple evanescent white dot syndrome occurring in the same patients. *Arch Ophthalmol.* 1989;107:189–193.

Hamed LM, et al. Protracted enlargement of the blind spot in multiple evanescent white dot syndrome. *Arch Ophthalmol.* 1989;107:194–198.

Jampol LM, et al. Multiple evanescent white dot syndrome, I. Clinical findings. *Arch Ophthalmol.* 1984;102:671–674.

Khorram KD, et al. Blind spot enlargement as a manifestation of multifocal choroiditis. *Arch Ophthalmol.* 1991;109: 1403–1407.

Sieving PA, et al. Multiple evanescent white dot syndrome, II. Electrophysiology of the photoreceptors during retinal pigment epithelial disease. *Arch Ophthalmol.* 1984;102: 675–679.

Singh K, et al. Acute idiopathic blind spot enlargement. A spectrum of disease. *Ophthalmology.* 1991;98:497–502.

Wyhinny GJ, et al. Subretinal neovascularization following multiple evanescent white dot syndrome. *Arch Ophthalmol.* 1990;108:1384–1385.

Birdshot Retinochoroidopathy

Barondes MJ, et al. Peripheral retinal neovascularization in birdshot retinochoroidopathy. *Ann Ophthalmol.* 1989;21: 306–308.

Bloch-Michel E, Frau E. Birdshot retinochoroidopathy and HLA-A29$^+$ and HLA-A29$^-$ idiopathic retinal vasculitis: Comparative study of 56 cases. *Can J Ophthalmol.* 1991;26: 361–366.

Brucker AJ, et al. Subretinal choroidal neovascularization in birdshot retinochoroidopathy. *Am J Ophthalmol.* 1985;99: 40–44.

Fuerst DJ, et al. Birdshot retinochoroidopathy. *Arch Ophthalmol.* 1984;102:214–219.

Gass JDM. Vitiliginous chorioretinitis. *Arch Ophthalmol.* 1981;99:1778–1787.

Kaplan HJ, Aaberg TM. Birdshot retinochoroidopathy. *Am J Ophthalmol.* 1980;90:773–782.

Nussenblatt RB, et al. Birdshot retinochoroidopathy associated with HLA-A29 antigen and immune responsiveness to retinal S-antigen. *Am J Ophthalmol.* 1982;94:147–158.

Priem HA, Oosterhuis JA. Birdshot chorioretinopathy: Clinical characteristics and evolution. *Br J Ophthalmol.* 1988;72:646–659.

Rosenberg PR, et al. Birdshot retinochoroidopathy. *Ophthalmology.* 1984;91:304–306.

Ryan SJ, Maumenee AE. Birdshot retinochoroidopathy. *Am J Ophthalmol.* 1980;89:31–45.

Soubrane G, et al. Birdshot retinochoroidopathy and subretinal new vessels. *Br J Ophthalmol.* 1983;67:461–467.

Ocular Manifestations of Lyme Disease

Baum J, et al. Bilateral keratitis as a manifestation of Lyme disease. *Am J Ophthalmol.* 1988;105:75–77.

Bertuch AW, et al. Lyme disease: Ocular manifestations. *Ann Ophthalmol.* 1988;20:376–382.

Ferrari ND. Lyme disease: A review. *W Va Med J.* 1987;83: 16–20.

Ferris BK, Webb RM. Lyme disease and optic neuritis. *J Clin Neuro-ophthalmol.* 1988;8:73–78.

Finkel MF. Lyme disease and its neurological complications. *Arch Neurol.* 1988;45:99–102.

MacDonald AB. Lyme disease. *J Clin Neuro-ophthalmol.* 1987;17:1850–1854.

Pachener AR, Steere AC. The triad of neurological manifestations of Lyme disease: Meningitis, cranial neuritis, and radiculoneuritis. *Neurology.* 1985;35:47–53.

Park M. Ocular manifestations of Lyme disease. *J Am Optom Assoc.* 1989;60:284–289.

Sclecter SL. Lyme disease associated with optic neuropathy. *Am J Med.* 1986;81:143–145.

Steere AC, et al. Unilateral blindness caused by infection with the Lyme disease spirochete, *Borrelia burgdorferi. Ann Int Med.* 1985;103:382–384.

Steere AC. The early clinical manifestations of Lyme disease. *Ann Int Med.* 1983;99:76–82.

Wu G, et al. Optic disc edema and Lyme disease. *Ann Ophthalmol.* 1986;18:252–255.

Chapter Six ■ ■ ■ ■ ■ ■

Anomalies of the Vitreous and Peripheral Retina

THE HUMAN VITREOUS

The adult human vitreous is often overlooked in the analysis of diseases of the retina. It is, however, very important to understand the vitreous, diseases of the vitreous, and the vitreous connection to the retina. Vitreous–retina connections are extremely important in the genesis of the various diseases of the peripheral retina. It would be accurate to state that without the changes within the vitreous body over a lifetime and the potential vitreoretinal traction forces, very few rhegmatogenous retinal detachments would evolve. The combination of the actions of the vitreous and its connections to the retina make rhegmatogenous retinal detachments possible.

Anatomy and Attachments

The vitreous occupies about 67 to 75 percent of the ocular volume. The vitreous is a type of connective tissue that is semisolid to liquid in consistency and is composed of approximately 99 percent water. The vitreous is attached in a few places within the eye (Fig. 6–1). Among these attachments is the anterior vitreous attachment at the posterior lens surface. This anterior vitreous attachment is called Weiger's adhesion (the hyaloidocapsular ligament). Weiger's adhesion is very strong in a young person, creating potential complications should intracapsular extraction be performed for

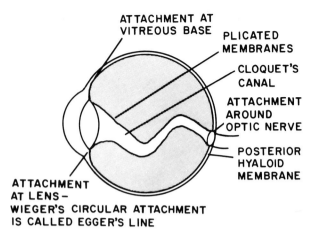

Figure 6–1. A schematic demonstrating the anatomy of the "normal" vitreous.

a congenital cataract. Weiger's adhesion weakens with age, enabling safe intracapsular cataract extraction. The line demarcated on the posterior lens capsule representing Weiger's adhesion is called Egger's line. The space immediately behind the crystalline lens but in front of the vitreous body is referred to as Berger's space. The anterior vitreous (anterior hyaloid membrane) also attaches at the vitreous base (vitreoretinal symphesis), which is a very strong connection, 2 to 3 mm wide, straddling the ora serrata. It holds the vitreous cortex, sensory retina, and pars plana together. This adhesion can be disturbed, usually by significant trauma, resulting in a giant retinal tear or perhaps a retinal dialysis. The posterior portion of the vitreous is attached at the optic disc margin in the form of a ring (the posterior base of Gartner in the area of Martegiani). This is most evident subsequent to a posterior vitreous detachment, because the attachment then becomes an annular opacity floating in front of the optic nerve head (Fig. 6–2).

Sometimes the force of the posterior vitreous detachment at the optic nerve head can result in preretinal hemorrhages occurring near the disc as well as in other areas of the retina where there may be attachments of the posterior hyaloid membrane near superficial retinal vessels. The posterior vitreous is also attached in the macular area in an oval form. This is usually a weak attachment that weakens even more with age. Detachment at the macula can create transient macular edema with metamorphopsia. This can be recurrent in a case of incomplete posterior vitreous detachment with repeated traction at the macular area. The posterior vitreous also may have weak connections at retinal vessels. This vascular connection is most evident in the case of posterior vitreous detachment with a subsequent preretinal bleed and retrovitreous hemorrhages as well as isolated superficial retinal hemorrhages (Fig. 6–3).

Pearls

Anatomy and Attachments of the Vitreous

Characteristics

Δ Attachments of the vitreous body to the retina include:

Weiger's adhesion at the anterior lens surface

2- to 3-mm zone at the vitreous base (vitreoretinal symphesis), which is very strong

Optic disc margins in the form of a ring (posterior, base of Gartner), which is very strong

Macular area that is loose, but detachment may precipitate tears and cystoid macular edema

Superficial retinal vessels that are usually loose, but detachment may precipitate rips in the vessels with superficial retinal hemorrhages and/or bleeding into the vitreous body

Δ 99 percent water occupying 67 to 75 percent of ocular volume

Δ Cloquet's canal bounded by plicated membranes runs from the crystalline lens to the optic disc and becomes more serpentine and mobile with age and in high myopia

Δ Anterior and posterior hyaloid membrane surrounds the vitreous cortex

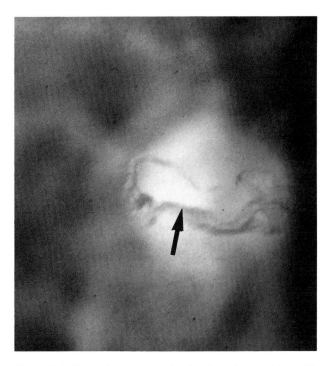

Figure 6–2. Example of an annular ring (*arrow*) associated with PVD.

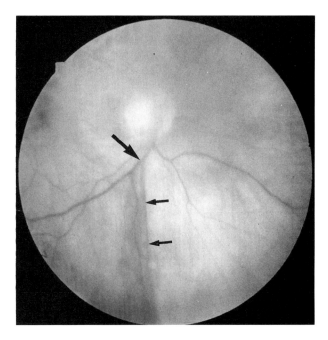

Figure 6–3. A preretinal and vitreous hemorrhage associated with the development of PVD. The large arrow points to the vessel tear and the small arrows point to the bleed into the inferior retino/vitreous space. Red blood cells create the haze over the optic nerve head.

One other aspect of the vitreous that must be considered is Cloquet's canal. Cloquet's canal (containing the primary vitreous) is a tubular structure running from the crystalline lens to the optic nerve head. Cloquet's canal is bounded by condensations of the vitreous, referred to as plicated membranes. At birth, Cloquet's canal runs straight from the lens to the optic disc, but with age the canal becomes more serpentine in appearance. With liquefaction of the vitreous, the canal then becomes mobile. Mittendorf's dot represents the primitive lenticular attachment of Cloquet's canal. A hyaloid membrane is a thin, glasslike structure that surrounds the cortex of the vitreous like a crust on bread. This hyaloid membrane is thought to be a modified collagen fiber structure from the outer layer of the cortex of the vitreous.

Vitreous Consistency and Transparency

The vitreous remains clear throughout most of the patient's life because the retinal vasculature is prevented from leaking into the vitreous cavity by the internal limiting membrane of the sensory retina and the hyaloid membrane of the vitreous cortex. Both of these structures act as selective barriers to prevent passage of blood components into the vitreous. Because the vitreous gel is approximately 99 percent water, it allows for maximum light transmission. The majority of the material within the vitreous that is considered to be solid is smaller than the wavelengths of visible light. As such, light scatter is minimized. Membrane sheets of vitreous material are scattered throughout the body of the vitreous and serve to reflect light contrasting with optically empty spaces. The play of these two components is sometimes referred to as luminous and dark substances.

Pearls

Vitreous Consistency

Characteristics

Δ Transparency is maintained by internal limiting membrane and hyaloid membrane

Δ Consistency is determined by vitrosin (V) concentration

Δ Viscosity is determined by hyaluronic acid (HA) macromolecule concentration: V + HA = elasticity

Δ Liquefaction occurs when HA macromolecules depolymerize
  Increases significantly with age
  Allows for rapid volume shifts
  Allows for movement of vitreous through breaks in the hyaloid membrane
  Allows for movement of vitreous through breaks in retina, which can break the bonds of the RPE

Δ Accumulation of fibril bodies also occurs in the aging vitreous, creating more visibility of the luminous and dark substances

The consistency of the vitreous is determined by the concentration of collagen-like material called vitrosin. The viscosity of the vitreous is about four times that of water because of the concentration of hyaluronic acid macromolecules. The combination of hyaluronic acid and vitrosin forms the elasticity of the vitreous. Liquefaction (synchysis senilis) or increased viscosity occurs when the hyaluronic acid macromolecules depolymerize. Before age 50 years, the liquid content of the vitreous is less than 25 percent, while after age 80 years the liquid content is over 62 percent. This liquefaction increases the chances of rapid volume shifts, movement of the vitreous through breaks in the hyaloid membrane, and movement of the vitreous through retinal tears and holes. The liquefied vitreous does create a change in the retinal pigment epithelium (RPE) once penetration of the retinal tissue occurs. The liquefied vitreous acts to break the mucopolysaccharide bonds of the RPE, allowing for escape of the pigment granules into the vitreous. This escape of the pigment granules into the vitreous is characteristically a sign of impending or active retinal detachment and is known as the tobacco dust (Shafer's) sign.

Degenerative changes of the vitreous also increase with age. Development of fibril patterns occurs in the adult eye related to a shift in the aggregation of collagen fibrils into formed bodies with settling of the hyaluronic acid into the intervening spaces.

Examination of the Vitreous

Clinical examination of the vitreous is difficult because it is a clear substance and as such makes standard examination techniques very difficult. The vitreous can, however, be examined under magnification with the use of a fundus contact lens or some other device coupled with the variable power of the slit lamp. The slit-lamp examination technique allows for microscopic examination of the vitreous. However, this is often an inadequate examination technique because the clinician must rely on subtle shadows and movement to properly diagnose vitreous alterations. Examination of the vitreous, and in fact the underlying peripheral retina, is often enhanced by dynamic rather than static examination techniques. It sometimes becomes necessary to incorporate the direct and binocular indirect ophthalmoscopy into the examination technique. The binocular indirect will often be unsuitable for examination of the vitreous contents. However, binocular indirect ophthalmoscopy can be used to pick up shadows of shifting vitreous that may be cast on the retina. The most effective examination technique of the vitreous, at least from a screening standpoint, is use of the direct ophthalmoscope. The direct ophthalmoscope held a few inches from the eye with proper magnification can be a very effective tool in *screening* for disorders of the vitreous. The clinician is using the backlit pupil while observing for breaks and shadows in the normal red reflex. Any examination technique of the vitreous is, however, enhanced by maximal dilation of the pupil in addition to proper dark adaptation of both the clinician and the patient.

■ ■ ■ ■ ■ ■

Clinical Note: Complete Examination of the Vitreous

Complete examination of the vitreous is both time consuming and requires a tremendous amount of skill. It uses all of the aspects available to the practitioner by way of the Goldmann three-mirror contact lens.

• The posterior portion of the Goldmann three-mirror contact lens can be used to scan the vitreous from immediately behind a crystalline lens to the retina interface. A wide beam in the slit lamp should be used, coupled with the lowest magnification possible. The beam should be variable, from vertical to oblique to a horizontal beam, to enhance total examination of the vitreous content. The slit is then narrowed, and the posterior portion of the Goldmann lens is used to examine the anterior vitreous more critically.

• While maintaining a narrow slit and low magnification, the central portion of the vitreous may now be examined. The slit should be focused very slowly and carefully as it is moved through the vitreous, which at this point includes Cloquet's canal. Again, for complete examination, vertical, oblique, and horizontal beams should be used to examine the entire vitreous.

• Still using the narrow slit beam, the posterior vitreous may now be evaluated. To properly examine the posterior vitreous, maintain a narrow slit beam and relatively low magnification. The red-free filter may also be used to attempt to enhance the view. It is important to remember that vitreous examination is a dynamic examination procedure. As such it is necessary to move the slit beam, practitioner's view, patient's fixation, and Goldmann three-mirror lens. Movement enhances a situation known as the ascension phenomenon. The ascension phenomenon refers to the movement of the plicated Cloquet's canal. It is important to remember that anything viewed within the vitreous is going to be seen because of reflection of light from the beam. In theory the vitreous is optically empty, and as such one must remember that all things seen are obstructions to this free passage of light.

• To examine the vitreous using the mirrors, the practitioner must remember that the widest mirror is the equatorial mirror and should be used first. To come forward into the retina (the anterior retina), the clinician must use the more squared mirror. The U-shaped gonioscopy mirror may be tilted to examine pars plana and the vitreous base. It is extremely important to remember when using the mirrors that minimal magnification is necessary to enhance the view. In addition to that, it is necessary to manipulate the beam and mirror considerably to get to the area of interest. An indenter is available on some three-mirror lenses to enhance the view.

THE AGING VITREOUS

Introduction and Description. The aging vitreous becomes more easily viewed because of an increased density of fibers usually occurring after the age of 40 years. There is also an increase in the mobility of Cloquet's canal (the structure surrounding the primary vitreous). As mentioned before, this is known as the ascension phenomenon. The mobility of the structure within the vitreous becomes much more apparent with age because of liquefaction of the vitreous. This increased liquefaction with age manifests as the development of lacunae, or optically empty spaces. These lacunae are usually in the midvitreous area and begin to coalesce with time, developing into larger cavities. It is important to remember that liquefaction of the vitreous does occur at a slightly earlier age in myopic patients than in other patients, increasing the potential for development of retinal tears and subsequent detachment. It is also very important to remember that extensive liquefaction at a young age is usually an indication of a pathologic condition. In addition to an increase in liquefaction, there is also a condition known as syneresis, or shrinkage (inward collapse) of the vitreous, caused by separation of the liquids and solids. Age-related vitreous liquefaction and syneresis together are known as fibrillary degeneration. It is important to recognize the fact that fibrillary degeneration is a crucial prerequisite to the genesis of posterior vitreous detachment. The retinal manifestations of aging vitreous—liquefaction and syneresis—are many. They include white without pressure, retinal edema, and retinal tears. Figure 6–4 shows an illustration of the aging vitreous.

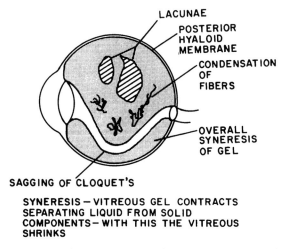

Figure 6–4. A schematic demonstrating vitreous changes typical of the aging vitreous.

POSTERIOR VITREOUS DETACHMENT (PVD)

Introduction and Description. Posterior vitreous detachment (PVD) is undoubtedly one of the more common occurrences that a clinician will experience in practice. It is, however, an extremely difficult process to view clinically. From an epidemiologic standpoint, PVD rarely occurs until the age of 45 years but after that age occurs more frequently in women than in men. It does occur very commonly in up to 90 percent of aphakic eyes. PVD definitely increases in frequency with age, with a prevalence approximately equal to the person's age over 50 years. PVD can occur in younger patients and is usually related to trauma or an inflammatory process that causes a localized alteration in the vitreous structure. PVD occurs as a result of several factors associated with aging. Figure 6–5 illustrates a flow pattern for the genesis of posterior vitreous detachment.

PVD implies that the vitreous behind the vitreous base and hyaloid membrane is separated from the sensory retina. There can be several different categories of PVD. Under most circumstances, vitreous detachment is classified as complete or incomplete PVD. This can be further broken down into subcategories with collapse or without collapse of the vitreous gel. Figures 6–6 to 6–10 illustrate various types of PVD.

Clinically, the most frequently occurring PVD is a PVD with collapse of the vitreous gel. In this variety of PVD the vitreous is completely separated from the sensory retina up to the vitreous base. The vitreous base collapses on itself but remains attached at the very strong anterior oral attachment. Clinically this creates the appearance of the posterior hyaloid membrane and vitreous cortex hanging down from the vitreous base. This also creates the common annular opacity (separation of the ring of Gartner) floating in

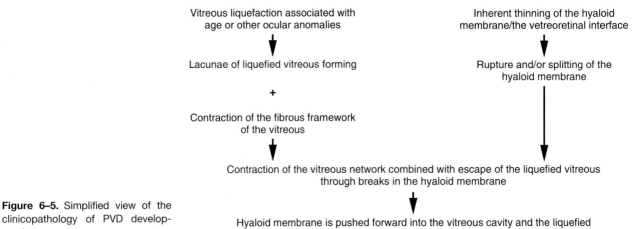

Figure 6–5. Simplified view of the clinicopathology of PVD development.

front of the optic nerve head. The incomplete posterior vitreous detachment does not represent a complete separation of the vitreous cortex from the sensory retina. This variation may occur with or without collapse of the vitreous gel, and may result in continued tugging in the macular area, resulting in macular edema.

Symptoms of PVD are fairly classical but do vary from patient to patient. Floaters are common, especially those of sudden onset with well-outlined shadows cast on the retina from debris. If insect-shaped and multiple, these floaters may indicate an operculated retinal tear. If they are cobweb or hazy in appearance, they may indicate an associated vitreous

hemorrhage. Multiplicity of floaters and a haze over the vision are both strongly suggestive of an associated retinal break or a hemorrhage associated with either the tear or the PVD. Photopsia is reported to occur in 25 to 50 percent of cases but is also a symptom associated with retinal breaks. Photopsia usually occurs as lightning streaks in the far periphery of the field of vision and represents the separation of the hyaloid membrane from the oral zone of the retina. These lightning streaks are due to vitreoretinal traction that causes physical stimulation of the photoreceptors. Photopsia may continue for weeks to years. The cessation of photopsia usually indicates that there is no longer traction and tugging on that vitreoretinal adhesion. Metamorphopsia, or distorted vision, may also result from macular edema secondary to the tugging of the vitreoretinal adherence at the macula. In addition, the practitioner must remember that the vitreoretinal adherence in oval form at the macula may tug with enough strength to precipitate transient macular edema and may help to create a macular hole. The classical shower of floaters that may occur is either a

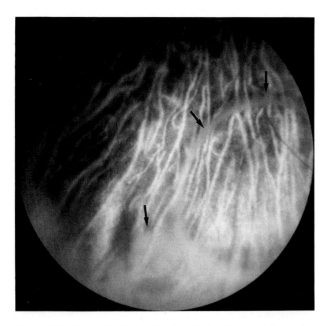

Figure 6–6. Example of a localized posterior vitreous detachment associated with trauma. This is known as vitreous veils (*arrows*).

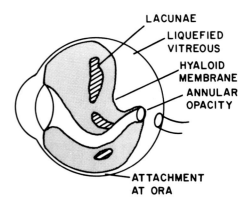

Figure 6–7. A schematic demonstrating vitreous changes typical of complete PVD with collapse.

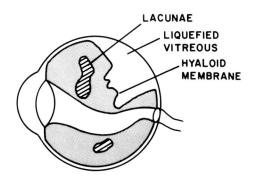

Figure 6–8. A schematic demonstrating vitreous changes typical of incomplete PVD with collapse.

vitreous hemorrhage or possibly a retinal tear associated with the vitreous detachment.

The signs of PVD include vitreous opacities, the most common and classical being the annular ring in front of the optic nerve head. This annular ring represents the previous adherence of the vitreous face around the optic nerve. It must be remembered, however, that vitreous opacities may occur in any shape. Hemorrhages may occur around the disc associated with mild tears of the loosely adherent vitreous face to retinal vessels. These hemorrhages are transient. These hemorrhages may also occur elsewhere in the retina where a strong vitreoretinal connection may have been. Vitreous hemorrhages may also occur associated with PVD and classically occur in the retrovitreous space. As mentioned previously, PVD may cause transient retinal edema (especially in the macula area), white without pressure, retinal tears, macular holes, and the long-term effects of traction (folds of the retina). The actual detection of the corrugated hyaloid membrane collapsed forward into the cortex is also a reasonably good sign of a posterior vitreous detachment. The corrugated hyaloid membrane is often more visible when using the red-free illumination feature of the binocular indirect ophthalmoscope or slit lamp.

Acute symptomatic PVD is associated with the

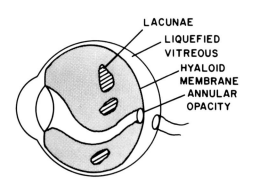

Figure 6–9. A schematic demonstrating vitreous changes typical of complete PVD without collapse.

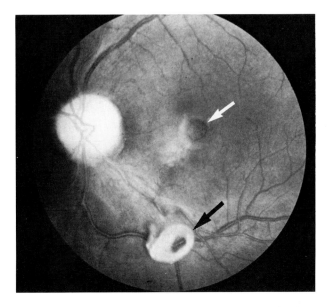

Figure 6–10. PVD as evidenced by the annular opacity (*dark arrow*) associated with a through-and-through macular hole (*white arrow*).

onset of retinal breaks in anywhere from 8 to 46 percent of cases. More conservative estimates put the association of retinal breaks with posterior vitreous detachment at 15 to 30 percent of cases. Although the percentage association of retinal breaks with symptomatic PVD is arguable, the lesson to learn is that there is an association and this association must be carefully investigated. It is also important to note that a high percentage of patients with retinal detachments do not have any history of flashes or floaters. About one third to one half of symptomatic retinal breaks progress on to retinal detachments. The more recent the break, the more likely that the break will progress toward retinal detachment. Fresh breaks are characterized by pigment granules in the anterior vitreous, vitreous hemorrhage, and the absence of RPE hyperplasia around the tear. Hemorrhage into the vitreous occurring with a PVD is associated with a retinal break in 75 percent of cases. About 2.5 percent of symptomatic PVDs have traction at the posterior pole and may result in transient macular edema. It is also important to note that retinal detachment is highly unlikely 6 months after a PVD has occurred, as the traction has usually been relieved and any breaks that have occurred have developed RPE hyperplasia to seal the wound.

Cataract extraction often will precipitate vitreous detachment because of the shift of ocular contents. Extracapsular cataract extraction with maintenance of the posterior capsule has the potential to minimize the shift forward of the vitreous, but this effect is somewhat negated by the use of YAG capsulotomy to clear an opaque posterior capsule. A

Posterior Vitreous Detachment

Characteristics

△ Increases in frequency with age—90 percent of aphakic patients

△ When occurring in younger patients, may be associated with inflammatory processes or trauma

△ Presents with sudden-onset floaters—not a shower of small floaters, which is more characteristic of a retinal break

△ Often associated with photopsia in the form of peripherally appearing lightning streaks that may continue for years

△ May have metamorphopsia due to macular edema that presents as the result of the detachment of the loose adherence in the macular area

△ Appearance of annular ring floating over optic nerve is the classic sign

△ May have short-lived preretinal hemorrhages around the optic nerve or in the retinal periphery

△ May have retrovitreous hemorrhages associated with a PVD, but 75 percent of these have an associated retinal break

△ With time may see corrugated hyaloid membrane in the cortex that is enhanced with the use of red-free light

△ May be retinal signs such as retinal breaks that occur in 15 to 30 percent of symptomatic PVDs. Fresh breaks are characterized by pigment granules, hemorrhage, and absence of RPE hyperplasia around wound

△ More common in postsurgical cataract patients

Management

△ Maximal dilation investigating peripheral retina with scleral indentation for tears—patients with acute retinal tears usually detach within 6 weeks after the onset of symptoms

△ Advise of signs/symptoms of retinal detachment which is unlikely 6 months after onset of PVD

△ Follow up in 1 to 4 weeks depending on signs and symptoms, then 1 month later as PVD is a dynamically evolving process

△ With all fresh retinal breaks, ask for a consultation with a retinal specialist

and flare in the anterior chamber are important as well as tonometry (at times decreased intraocular pressure with retinal detachment). Screening full-field age-related perimetry prior to dilation may also give some information regarding the status of the retina early in the process. Central visual field testing would, however, be of limited value. The patient should then be maximally dilated. As discussed before, the practitioner must use a combination of the direct ophthalmoscope, binocular indirect ophthalmoscope, and Goldmann-type fundus lens. In addition, it is obligatory to investigate the peripheral retina carefully for tears using scleral indentation. It is important to realize that patients with acute retinal tears usually will present a retinal detachment within 6 weeks after the onset of symptomatology. Should the media be cloudy, it may be necessary to incorporate B-scan ultrasonography into the diagnostic protocol to eliminate the possibility of a retinal detachment as a cause of the onset of photopsia.

Assuming that there are no retinal tears, the practitioner must educate the patient about the signs and symptoms of retinal detachment. Because the posterior vitreous detachment is a dynamic, evolving process, it is important to realize that after the initial examination, the possibility of further detachment and development of a retinal tear exists (Fig. 6–11). As such, it is important to schedule a follow-up examination depending on the patient's signs and symptoms. Subsequent evaluations should be scheduled at between 1 to 4 weeks, and then 1 month later to assure that a retinal tear does not develop. **See color plates 87 and 88.**

break secondary to a PVD in a postsurgical cataract patient usually occurs within 6 to 8 weeks after the vitreous detachment.

Management. Management of the posterior vitreous detachment is somewhat complex and must be tailored to match the patient's situation. Develop a case history and perform a visual acuity test. Important points to consider in the history include the presence and duration of symptoms, associated trauma, and the use of miotic therapy for the treatment of glaucoma. Pupillary evaluation and evaluation for cells

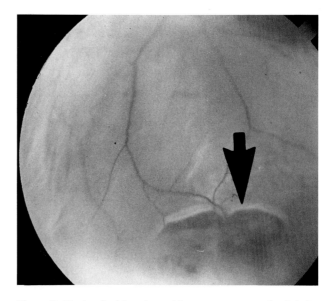

Figure 6–11. A retinal tear (*arrow*) in an area surrounding inferior lattice degeneration associated with an evolving PVD.

SYSTEMIC CONDITIONS ASSOCIATED WITH VITREOUS AND RETINAL DEGENERATION

Introduction

There are several systemic conditions that have been associated with vitreous degeneration, including diabetes mellitus, sickle-cell hemoglobinopathy, Wagner–Jensen–Stickler vitreoretinal dystrophy, Marfan syndrome, homocystinuria, Ehlers–Danlos syndrome, pseudoxanthoma elasticum, and retinitis pigmentosa. The pseudoxanthoma elasticum complex presents with vitreous liquefaction, PVD, and brown cells liberated into the vitreous. Retinitis pigmentosa presents with vitreous liquefaction, PVD, and brown cells in the vitreous. All retinal vascular diseases with proliferative potential can compromise the overlying vitreous, creating liquefaction; and can likewise grow forward into the vitreous, creating bands that can then precipitate traction retinal detachment. All of the associate conditions carry potentially severe systemic disease implications and as such must be carefully diagnosed and managed.

Marfan Syndrome

Marfan syndrome is created by an unknown genetic defect that is autosomal dominant and is characterized by the ocular manifestation of superior temporal lens luxation in 50 to 80 percent of cases, axial myopia greater than 7D in about 20 percent of cases, vitreous degeneration, decreased corneal diameter, iris transillumination defects, retinal detachment, and a high incidence of vitreous loss during cataract surgery. Skeletal abnormalities and cardiac abnormalities characterize the systemic features, creating a risk in general anesthesia and a 50 percent mortality rate by age 50.

Ehlers–Danlos Syndrome

Ehlers–Danlos syndrome is characterized by high myopia, microcornea, glaucoma, angioid streaks, vitreous and retinal degeneration (prevalence of lattice degeneration) and detachment, ptosis, and strabismus. Tissue fragility, elasticity of the skin, and hemorrhagic diathesis are the most prevalent systemic abnormalities, and increase risk under general anesthesia.

Homocystinuria

Homocystinuria is a genetic defect transmitted in an autosomal recessive fashion. Homocystinuria is characterized by inferior lens luxation and possible dislocation into the anterior chamber (high percentage), and vitreous and retinal degeneration and detachment. Systemic manifestations include skeletal abnormalities similar to Marfan syndrome, cardiovascular abnormalities, and thrombotic vascular occlusions

TABLE 6–1. THE DIFFERENTIAL DIAGNOSTIC FEATURES OF HOMOCYSTINURIA AND MARFAN SYNDROME

Feature	Homocystinuria	Marfan Syndrome
Inheritance	Autosomal recessive	Autosomal dominant
Skeletal abnormalities	Osteoporosis, fractures, rarely arachnodactyly	Arachnodactyly and loose joints
Vascular disease	Dilatation with thrombosis in intermediate-sized arteries and veins	Dilatation or dissection of aorta
Ectopia lentis	Often observed in children; lens displaced inferiorly and often dislocated into anterior chamber or vitreous cavity	Often detected in children; lens displaced superiorly and seldom dislocated into anterior chamber or vitreous cavity

that increase risk of death under general anesthesia. Table 6–1 illustrates some of the differentiating features of Marfan syndrome and homocystinuria.

ANTERIOR VITREOUS DETACHMENT

Introduction and Description. Anterior vitreous detachment is a relatively rare condition. Spontaneous anterior vitreous detachment is rare because of the very strong attachment of the vitreous to the oral area of the retina. As such, most anterior vitreous detachments are typically associated with trauma or lens dislocation secondary to conditions such as Marfan

---

Pearls

Anterior Vitreous Detachment

Characteristics

△ Usually associated with trauma and/or lens dislocation

△ Symptoms include floaters and veils of sudden onset

△ Signs include an increase in visibility of vitreous fibers and the appearance of cells

Management

△ Rule out retinal tears and/or retinal dialysis, especially near ora

△ If signs/symptoms of continued retinal traction present, follow up in 3 months and advise of signs/symptoms of retinal detachment

△ If asymptomatic and no signs of traction, follow up yearly and advise of signs/symptoms of retinal detachment

△ Differentiate from avulsion of the vitreous base

△ Ask for a retinal consultation if retinal breaks or retinal dialysis is present

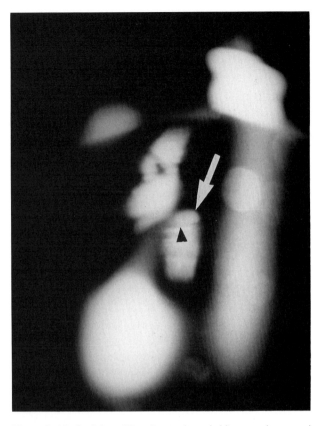

Figure 6–12. Avulsion of the vitreous base (*white arrow* is ora and *black dart* is edge of avulsed base) associated with trauma but without the development of a retinal dialysis.

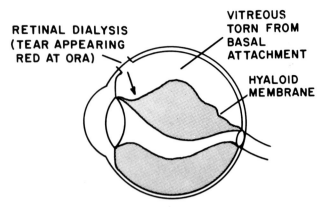

Figure 6–13. A schematic demonstrating vitreous changes typical of a basal vitreous detachment.

ated from retinal dialysis by the observation that the area under the cleft is not the typical red coloration characteristic of retinal tears and dialysis. This observation is enhanced with a three-mirror fundus lens evaluation and scleral indentation. When the differentiation is difficult, a retinal consultation is in order.

■ ■ ■ ■ ■ ■

Clinical Note: Basal Vitreous Detachment

Basal vitreal detachment (Fig. 6–13) is extremely rare, but again is associated with trauma and retinal dialysis occurring at the ora serrata. It is important to manage the retinal dialysis by a retinal consultation for the consideration of surgical intervention. Again the practitioner must differentiate basal vitreous detachment from the more benign avulsion of the vitreous base.

syndrome and homocystinuria. The symptoms of anterior vitreous detachment include sudden appearance of floaters appearing as veils coming in front of the line of sight. The signs that the practitioner may observe are cells out into the vitreous cortex and an increase in the visibility of fibers.

Management. Management of anterior vitreous detachment would include assuring that there are no retinal tears or retinal dialysis at the oral boundary. Retinal tears are highly likely because trauma that would cause an anterior vitreous detachment would more than likely also cause a retinal tear. If there are signs and symptoms of retinal traction, recheck the patient in 3 months and have the patient report at the onset of any new or changing symptoms. If a patient is asymptomatic and there are no retinal tears, the patient may be rechecked in 1 year. It is of course necessary in all of these cases to make the patient aware of the signs and symptoms of retinal detachment. Any indication of a retinal break or retinal dialysis requires a retinal consult for the consideration of surgical intervention.

Avulsion of the vitreous base may also occur associated with trauma (Fig. 6–12). This is differenti-

ASTEROID BODIES

Introduction and Description. Asteroid bodies are a relatively common finding in the vitreous. Asteroid bodies are classically described as Benson's bodies. They usually occur in patients over the age of 60 years, with approximately 90 percent unilaterality. Although arguable, most studies point to the fact that there is no particular association with systemic-based diseases other than diabetes mellitus. There certainly have been frequent reports relating asteroid bodies to diabetes, citing that about 30 to 33 percent of patients with asteroid bodies have diabetes. There is also a relationship to systemic hypertension in 60 percent of individuals with asteroid bodies, and a 30 percent occurrence of atherosclerotic vascular disease. From a

Asteroid Bodies

Characteristics

△ Usually present over the age of 60 years and most often unilateral

△ Composed of calcium soaps

△ The patient may complain of floaters

△ Small yellow-white spheres adherent to vitreous framework; return to original position when the eyes are moved from one position to another

△ Increased vitreous density in the eye with asteroid bodies

△ Several reports relate asteroid bodies to diabetes (30 to 33 percent)

△ Also a relationship to systemic hypertension (60 percent) and atherosclerotic vascular disease (30 percent)

Management

△ Although clinically remarkable, asteroid bodies are self-limiting and benign

△ The patient should be cautioned that an increase in the appearance of floaters necessitates a dilated fundus evaluation

△ Routine eye examinations are in order

△ If there are associated signs and symptoms of diabetes, order a fasting blood sugar level test

△ Perform brachial blood pressure assessment and consider the relationship to atherosclerotic disease

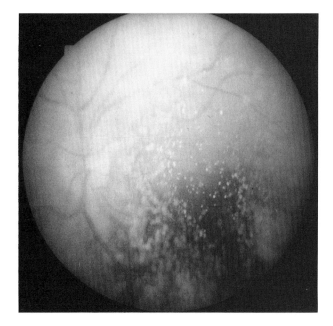

Figure 6–14. Asteroid hyalosis filling the vitreous cavity while only slightly reducing visual acuity.

Because there is a relationship to diabetes, atherosclerotic vascular disease, and hypertension, consider questioning the patient regarding signs and symptoms of diabetes; if the answers are equivocal or if there are other eye signs, order a fasting blood sugar test. Certainly brachial blood pressure assessment should be performed.

histopathologic standpoint, it is known that asteroid bodies are composed of calcium soaps that are 0.01 to 0.1 mm in diameter. The patients are often symptomless; however, the author has personally observed patients who complain of floaters in some of the more dramatic cases. From a clinical standpoint, the practitioner can observe small yellow-white spheres within the vitreous body. These spheres are adherent to the vitreous framework and always return to their original position after asking the patient to look up and then to return to a straight-ahead gaze (Fig. 6–14). When comparing the affected eye to the other, there is an increase in the vitreous density in the eye with the asteroid bodies.

Management. From a management standpoint, it is only important that the patient be aware of the fact that he or she has asteroid bodies and realize that asteroid bodies are a benign self-limited condition that will not lead to blindness. Patients must also be told to be aware of the floaters common in this condition but that any increase in floaters warrants a dilated fundus evaluation. Routine eye examinations are in order.

■ ■ ■ ■ ■ ■
Clinical Note: Synchisis Scintillans

Synchisis scintillans is classically described as a bilateral vitreous disorder in the young. Synchisis scintillans is thought to be an accumulation of flat crystals of cholesterol (cholesterolosis bulbi). It is thought that these flat crystals sink to the bottom of the vitreous. Synchisis scintillans probably only occurs in blind, severely damaged eyes. The condition is probably very rare.

PARAVASCULAR VITREOUS ATTACHMENTS

Introduction and Description. Paravascular vitreous attachments may be acquired or congenital. They are also known as retinal tufts and will be discussed in more detail under the heading of vitreoretinal traction tufts. It is important to recognize, however, that they represent a strong adhesion of the posterior vit-

Paravascular Vitreous Attachments

Characteristics

△ Strong adhesion of vitreous cortex (hyaloid membrane) to equatorial zone of retina

△ Presents as white granular tissue that may demonstrate vitreous strands with potential for retinal tear

△ Often symptomless unless there is a vitreous detachment or an impending retinal break

△ A phosphene noted by a patient may be a sign of an impending tear associated with a paravascular vitreous attachment

Management

△ Advise on signs/symptoms of retinal detachment

△ Advise on the signs and implications of phosphenes

△ Document and follow up in 6 to 12 months with routine eye examinations

Amyloid Degeneration of the Vitreous

Characteristics

△ Primary form is not inherited and does not have systemic manifestations

△ Secondary form is a rare systemic disease with dominant inheritance pattern

△ Usually presents after second decade and runs 20 years

△ Ocular involvement in 8 percent of both primary and secondary types resulting from amyloid deposition in ocular tissues
  Diplopia
  Photophobia and blepharospasm
  Progressive loss of vision
  Ophthalmoplegia
  Vitreous opacities, retinal hemorrhages, and perivascular exudates

Management

△ Supportive management, as there is no cure

△ Genetic counseling is indicated in the secondary type

△ Consultation with a vitreoretinal specialist may be necessary at times but vitrectomy results in rapid reformation of the amyloid deposits in the vitreous

△ Routine eye examinations are necessary

△ Evaluation of the systemic manifestations are necessary on a routine basis

reous cortex (the hyaloid membrane) to the equatorial zone of the retina in the form of granular tissue. These adhesions are considered to be proliferated glial cells. They are typically asymptomatic; however, they may have an associated phosphene, indicating a localized or generalized vitreous detachment with the possibility of an impending retinal break.

Management. Management protocol for vitreoretinal tufts should be followed. Examinations every 6 to 12 months are indicated, with advice to the patient regarding the appearance of phosphenes as being a herald of vitreous detachment and/or retinal breaks. Signs and symptoms of retinal detachment should be given.

HEREDITARY VITREORETINAL DYSTROPHIES AND DEGENERATIONS

Although the hereditary vitreoretinal dystrophies and degenerations are relatively rare, the ocular and systemic implications can be devastating. From the view of a primary eye care practitioner, it is important to recognize these anomalies to provide proper intervention at an opportune time.

Amyloid Degeneration of the Vitreous— Primary Heredofamilial Amyloidosis

Introduction and Description. Amyloidosis is a very rare systemic disease with multiple manifesta-

tions. The disease can mimic several other conditions. Often amyloidosis is classified into the primary and secondary type. In the primary type, there is no particular hereditary pattern and no systemic disease debilitation. In the secondary type the amyloid substance is deposited in the liver, spleen, kidneys, and adrenal glands, and is associated with chronic debilitating diseases. Primary heredofamilial amyloidosis associated with the eye is the type more often seen clinically. The secondary type of amyloidosis is transmitted as a dominant trait involving an extra chromosome. The condition typically presents after the second decade of life and runs a course of approximately 20 years. From the ocular standpoint, it must be realized that ocular involvement is present in 8 to 10 percent of primary and secondary cases including diplopia, progressive loss of vision, photophobia, blepharospasm, ophthalmoplegia, exophthalmos, vitreous opacities, retinal hemorrhages, and exudates. The vitreous may be the first area of involvement within the eye and may be a predecessor to organ involvement of the remainder of the body.

The amyloid is typically deposited in the vessels of the choroid, optic nerve, and retina. The amyloid in the vitreous results from a break through the internal limiting membrane from retinal vessel foci. This presence in the vitreous results in fibrillar deposits within the vitreous content. The ocular signs are then vitreous opacities, typically being bilateral and slowly progressive, accompanied by retinal hemorrhages and perivascular exudates. Along with the ocular symptoms and signs, there may be the systemic manifestations of fatigue, loss of weight, progressive peripheral neuropathy, gastrointestinal disorders, and endocrine and cardiovascular compromise. Serum protein electrophoresis and vitreous biopsy may confirm the diagnosis.

Management. As there is no cure for primary heredofamilial amyloidosis, management consists of supportive treatment for the systemic manifestations of the disease. Should severe vision loss occur, vitrectomy may be necessary to clean the debris from the vitreous. Unfortunately, the amyloid deposits recur rapidly after vitrectomy. It is important to realize, however, that vitrectomy may cause retinal and vitreous bleeds because of the adhesion and close association of the vitreous to the foci of amyloid involvement of the retinal vessels. Certainly, vision-threatening changes within the vitreous deserve a consultation with a vitreoretinal specialist.

Provision of the best possible prescription, routine eye examinations, and a systemic evaluation are all necessary.

Congenital Hereditary Retinoschisis (CHRS)

Introduction and Description. Congenital hereditary retinoschisis (CHRS) is sometimes known as juvenile retinoschisis. The disease is transmitted as a recessive X–linked Mendelian trait affecting male offspring. In rare cases, however, females may contract the disease as an autosomal recessive disease. CHRS may present between the ages of 7 months to 28 years. The condition is more often than not bilateral and may be either progressive or stationary.

Congenital hereditary retinoschisis occurs as a result of the splitting of the retina at the nerve fiber layer. Associated with this splitting of the retina is vitreous liquefaction. The patient complains of poor vision, strabismus, nystagmus (if the condition occurs at a young enough age), and floaters. The condition is often stationary, with periods of slow progression that alternate with periods of spontaneous remission. Signs of progression are an increase in the extent or volume of the retinoschisis, an increase in the size or number of inner layer or outer layer breaks, decreased visual acuity, and vitreous hemorrhage. Progression of the disease is fairly rapid in the initial stages, slowing at later stages. There is a deep scotoma in the area of the retinoschisis.

Congenital Hereditary Retinoschisis

Characteristics

△ Bilateral with slow progression and periods of remission

△ X-linked recessive transmission but some sporadic cases reported involving females

△ May present between 7 months and 28 years of age

△ Schisis of retina at nerve fiber layer with early-onset vitreous liquefaction

△ In 50 percent of the cases there is the presentation of the retinoschisis in the inferotemporal quadrant with a veil membrane that does not run to ora

△ Macular cystic changes may present as depigmented star on mottled background that is also identified as striate

△ Macular involvement in 98 to 100 percent of cases

△ Deep scotoma in area of retinoschisis

△ Color and night vision are typically unaffected

△ Development of retinal breaks is common

△ Vitreous liquefaction, vitreous detachment, and vitreous traction membranes are common

△ Retinal detachment in about 25 percent of cases and vitreous hemorrhage in about 40 percent of patients

Management

△ Advise of signs/symptoms of retinal detachment

△ Provision of the best refractive correction, documentation of the vitreoretinal status, and yearly follow-up

△ Consultation with retinal specialist for retinal breaks, the presentation of vitreoretinal traction bands and rhegmatogenous retinal detachment

△ Consultation with a retinal specialist for progression of the retinoschisis toward the macular zone

△ Genetic counseling is in order

△ Low-vision rehabilitation when necessary

Usually congenital hereditary retinoschisis occurs in the inferotemporal quadrant but generally not all the way out to the ora. The schisis is often accompanied by a veil membrane coursing out into the vitreous carrying retinal vasculature in the elevation. To differentiate congenital from acquired retinoschisis, the practitioner must remember that acquired retinoschisis usually runs all the way to the ora serrata and usually occurs in older patients. There are inner layer and outer layer breaks, or holes, that can develop within the schisis and are often multiple. The clinician may also notice pigmented demarcation lines along the posterior border of the retinoschisis, indicating progression and remission. There may be associated optic nerve changes in the form of pseudopapilledema, dragging of the disc vasculature, and in some instances, descending optic atrophy. Neovascular glaucoma and hemorrhagic retinal cysts may also occur in CHRS.

Macular changes usually involve a cystic kind of alteration, giving a depigmented star on the background of mottled pigment. This has been described as stellate or striate and becomes more atrophic and pigmented with age. Macular retinoschisis is present in almost all affected patients and is the only sign in 50 percent of the patients. The retinoschisis in the periphery is only present in about 50 percent of the patients with CHRS.

Liquefaction of the vitreous is also a characteristic that may allow for vitreous cortex bands to be attached to the retinoschisis. Other vitreous changes include free-floating strands, vitreous detachment, and the above-cited vitreoretinal traction bands. Retinal detachment occurs in about 25 percent of affected eyes while vitreous hemorrhage presents in about 40 percent of individuals with the vitreoretinal traction associated with CHRS.

Other characteristics include possible alteration of the ERG, subnormal EOG, and delayed filling or hypoperfusion of the retinal vasculature in the affected areas.

Management. There is no especially good treatment for congenital hereditary retinoschisis. Treatment of the breaks in the retinoschisis and/or the associated retinal detachment are indicated once those lesions appear. Suggestions have been offered indicating that the retinoschisis approaching the macula may be treated by photocoagulation or cryopexy along the margin to prevent progression. Both positive and negative results have been reported in the literature. Surgical intervention with vitrectomy and/or scleral buckling have been successful in the repair of retinal detachments. Vitrectomy has also been suggested as a prophylactic measure when vitreoretinal traction bands threaten the retina.

It is absolutely necessary that a patient with congenital hereditary retinoschisis have yearly examinations to ascertain times of progression. Should the condition progress, it is necessary to recognize complications as early as possible. Genetic counseling is indicated. The patient often becomes a candidate for low-vision rehabilitation. **See color plate 89.**

Wagner's Hereditary Vitreoretinal Degeneration

Introduction and Description. Wagner's hereditary vitreoretinal degeneration is autosomal dominant with 100 percent penetrance but variable expressivity. This assures that 50 percent of the offspring of an affected parent will have the disease. Wagner's degeneration is bilateral and progressive and may present with either prominent vitreous or chorioretinal changes. At birth the infant may have an entirely normal fundus. The children with Wagner's typically develop some degree of myopia of moderate or high amounts. As the child ages, the tessellation of the central and peripheral fundus becomes more prominent. Along with tessellation, the choroidal vessels along the distribution pattern of

---

Pearls

Wagner's Hereditary Vitreoretinal Degeneration

Characteristics

Δ Bilateral progressive autosomal dominant condition with 100 percent penetrance but variable phenotypic presentation

Δ Often normal-appearing fundus at birth

Δ Tessellation of central and peripheral fundus along with atrophy of the choroidal vessels associated with myopia in the child

Δ With progression there is fibrillary degeneration of the vitreous with development of a preretinal membrane and vitreous strands

Δ The large lacunae in the vitreous cavity create a situation of an optically empty vitreous cavity

Δ Contraction of membrane and strands creates retinal changes, including RPE clumping around vessels and paravascular sheathing

Δ With further vitreous shrinkage retinal breaks (75 percent) and retinal detachment (50 percent) occur

Δ 60 percent incidence of early-onset cataract and most patients have lenticular opacities by age 10 years

Δ Primary open angle glaucoma in over 33 percent of patients over the age of 30 years

Δ Possible altered ERG, EOG, visual field defects, and fluorescein angiography anomalies

Δ Color vision and dark adaptation are typically normal

Management

Δ Advise of signs/symptoms of retinal detachment

Δ Follow up every 6 months with a dilated fundus evaluation

Δ Consultation with a retinal specialist for development of retinal breaks and retinal detachment

Δ Management of retinal detachment is difficult because of the combination of vitreoretinal conditions

Δ Cataract surgery is often a procedure needed in early life

Δ Genetic counseling is indicated

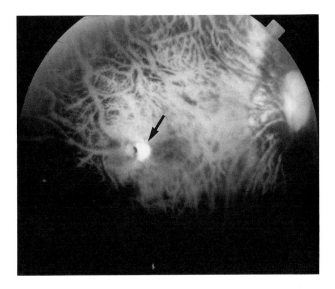

Figure 6–15. Retinal view of a patient with Wagner's vitreoretinal degeneration (*arrow* points to a fibrotic scar).

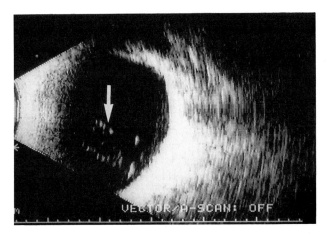

Figure 6–16. B-scan of the patient with Wagner's degeneration (Figure 6–15), demonstrating vitreous strands and debris.

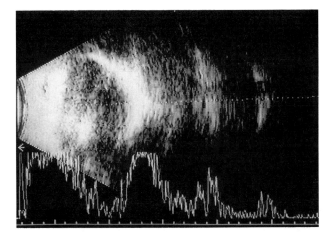

Figure 6–17. B-scan of the fellow eye of the patient in Figures 6–15 and 6–16, demonstrating the pthisical reaction to a long-standing retinal detachment.

the retinal vessels become atrophic (Figs. 6–15 to 6–17). **See color plate 90.**

Progressive vitreous changes are observed in most patients and typically occur earlier in life. Initially there is liquefaction and fibrous condensation of the vitreous. This will eventually create a large lacuna in the posterior vitreous that appears optically empty. Vitreous detachment is common in this condition. Preretinal avascular gray-white membranes from the equator to the retinal periphery (reported to join the anterior hyaloid membrane) form to then develop on the surface of the retina. Contracture of these preretinal membranes causes kinking of the vessels and edema of the retina. Associated with this there are often peripheral clumps of RPE, peripheral paravascular sheathing, pigment accumulation, and choroidal atrophy. During adolescence and early adulthood there is shrinkage of the vitreous body resulting in the development of retinal tears with or without posterior vitreous detachment. Seventy-five to 85 percent of these patients do develop retinal tears, and 50 percent develop retinal detachment. Along with the retinal changes there is an increased incidence of cataract to more than 60 percent as the patient matures, and lenticular opacities occur in most patients prior to the age of 10 years. After the age of 40 years almost all patients have cataracts. Primary open-angle glaucoma is a finding in over one-third of patients over age 30 years.

There are no particular symptoms until the retinal or lenticular complications ensue. There may be an altered electroretinogram and EOG associated with Wagner's. There may be associated visual field constrictions and ring scotomas. The fluorescein angiogram will show areas of hyperfluorescence associated with the RPE abnormalities, and may demonstrate areas of choriocapillaris and retinal nonperfusion.

Color vision and dark adaptation are usually normal while visual acuity may be reduced associated with retinal detachment.

Management. Management of this condition, once identified, consists of dilated fundus examinations every 6 months and routine provision of the best possible correction. Advice regarding signs and symptoms of retinal detachment are also in order. As retinal breaks or detachments develop, it is important to intervene with photocoagulation, cryopexy, vitrectomy, or scleral buckling. Unfortunately, prognosis for reattachment of the retina in Wagner's is relatively poor because of the combination of vitreous degeneration, vitreoretinal traction, and multiple retinal breaks. Cataract surgery is often indicated at an early age. Genetic counseling is also an important consideration.

Goldmann–Favre's Vitreoretinal Degeneration

Introduction and Description. Goldmann–Favre's vitreoretinal degeneration is a rare autosomal recessive condition that seems to be a combination of the signs and symptoms of Wagner's vitreoretinal degeneration and congenital hereditary retinoschisis. Goldmann–Favre's degeneration should always be a consideration with the complaint of night blindness. The condition affects almost all retinal layers and structures within the eye. In Goldmann–Favre's degeneration there is a progressive loss of vision associated with retinoschisis and pigmented (often bone spicule in nature) chorioretinal degeneration. The condition is more often than not bilateral, with no particular predilection for sex.

Associated with a progressive loss of vision are areas of scotomas. The central and peripheral retinoschisis look entirely different. The central retinoschisis appears as it does in congenital hereditary retinoschisis as a beaten metallic stellate alteration. The peripheral schisis will be elevated, and there can be inner layer and outer layer breaks. There may also be RPE clumping—bone-corpuscular-like—along the vessels. There is a subnormal to extinguished electroretinogram and a subnormal EOG as well as night blindness. Variable visual field defects may be present with capillary leakage and areas of capillary nonperfusion on fluorescein angiography. Color vision may be abnormal. An early-onset cataract may be present associated with considerable liquefaction of the vitreous that may be accompanied by traction and vitreous detachment. The patient also often complains of poor day vision (hemeralopia).

Management. There is no known effective management for Goldmann–Favre's vitreotapetoretinal degeneration. The best the clinician can hope to do is perform routine eye examinations at least every 6 months on this patient, advise on the hereditary aspect of the disease, and ask for a retinal consultation to treat complications as they occur. Advice regarding signs and symptoms of retinal detachment are also in order. Retinal breaks may be treated prophylactically and vitrectomy, photocoagulation, cryopexy, and buckling may be beneficial in cases of retinal detachment.

Familial Exudative Vitreoretinopathy (FEVR)

Introduction and Description. Familial exudative vitreoretinopathy (FEVR) is inherited in an autosomal dominant pattern with approximately 100 percent penetrance but variable phenotypic presentation. FEVR occurs bilaterally in relatively young patients presenting primarily in the temporal retina and simulating retinopathy of prematurity. There is, however, no history of prematurity or oxygen supplementation at birth. There are no associated systemic manifestations, and the disease process involves primarily the vitreous and the retina. Visual loss is slow and progressive. There is no particular association reported with refractive errors and night blindness is not a typical symptom.

Patients with exudative vitreoretinopathy may run the full gamut of fundus signs. In *stage 1*, the patients are usually asymptomatic with good visual acuity. There can be excessive white without pressure or white with pressure, unusual peripheral vessels, and vitreous shrinkage with band formation. In addition, this stage may be characterized by an abrupt termination of peripheral vessels at a scalloped border (a peripheral avascular zone greater than 2 DD) with associated fine pigmentation and, at times, intraretinal yellowish deposits. The avascular zone is enhanced on fluorescein angiography and may even have leakage between the vascular and avascular zone. *Stage 2* resembles the cicatricial stage of ROP with severe, dilated tortuous peripheral vessels present with neovascularization. Traction may occur, creating an ectopic macula. Associated with the neovasculariza-

---

Pearls

Goldmann–Favre's Vitreoretinal Degeneration

Characteristics

△ Bilateral progressive loss of vision with the characteristic of complaints of night blindness
△ Autosomal recessive inheritance
△ Central and peripheral retinoschisis with RPE clumping along vessels in the form of bone spicules
△ Vitreous liquefaction accompanied by traction and vitreous detachment
△ Abnormal to extinguished ERG and subnormal EOG
△ Variable visual field defects and areas of capillary leakage and nonperfusion on fluorescein angiography
△ Possible early-onset cataract

Management

△ Advise of signs/symptoms of retinal detachment
△ Documentation of the condition and follow up every 6 months or sooner depending on signs/symptoms
△ Consultation with a retinal specialist for complications such as retinal breaks and retinal detachment
△ Vitrectomy may be necessary for traction bands
△ Genetic counseling is indicated
△ Low-vision rehabilitation when necessary

Familial Exudative Vitreoretinopathy

Characteristics

Δ Bilateral presentation in young patients with slowly progressive loss of vision

Δ Autosomal dominant inheritance with 100 percent penetrance and variable phenotypic presentation

Δ No particular association with refractive error and no night blindness

Δ Stages of development:

Stage 1

Usually asymptomatic with good acuity

Excessive white without pressure (WWOP)

Vitreous shrinkage and band formation

Peripheral avascular zone larger than 2 DD

Possible peripheral avascular zone fine pigmentation and intraretinal yellow deposits

Stage 2

Dilated tortuous peripheral vessels

Peripheral neovascularization

Possible hemorrhages

Ectopic macula from temporal dragging

Stage 3

Fibrotic scaffolding with traction

Subretinal exudates

Cataracts

Rubeosis iridis

Vitreous detachment and vitreous hemorrhage

Traction (most common under age 10 years) and rhegmatogenous retinal detachment (most common in the 20s)

Δ Often stability after age 30 years

Δ Fluorescein angiographic findings include leakage of capillaries in the disc and macular area, in the fibrovascular tuft area and at the vascular/avascular border in the periphery

Δ Possible defective platelet anomaly

Management

Δ Treatment of retinal breaks

Δ Treatment of neovascularization

Δ Vitrectomy, photocoagulation, cryopexy, and buckling procedures for the retinal reattachment

Δ Genetic counseling is necessary

Δ Routine reexaminations based on the stage of the disease

Δ Provision of the best possible prescription

---

tion may be recurrent hemorrhages. *Stage 3* is characterized by the fibrotic scaffolding with the formation of traction retinal detachments and/or retinal breaks. In this stage there may be the accumulation of subretinal exudates, cataracts, rubeosis, and anterior chamber anomalies. There is a minimal liquefaction of the vitreous, and vitreous haze occurs as the result of

cells that may have been liberated. Vitreous detachment and vitreous hemorrhage are also possible.

In the end stages the patient can develop both traction and rhegmatogenous retinal detachments and optic atrophy. The incidence of traction retinal detachment is most common under age 10 years whereas rhegmatogenous retinal detachment is more common over age 20 years. It is believed that after age 30 years, FEVR stabilizes with minimal reduction in vision function.

Fluorescein angiographic findings may include leakage from capillaries near the disc and fovea secondary to the physical dragging toward the temporal periphery. The fibrovascular masses may also demonstrate leakage. Electrodiagnostic testing is of no particular benefit.

The development of the temporal proliferation may be associated with defective platelet aggregation precipitating hypoxia in the temporal zone similar to sickle cell disease and retinopathy of prematurity.

Management. Familial exudative vitreoretinopathy demonstrates relatively poor results with attempts at prophylactic treatment. The accepted mode of management at this time is treatment of the retinal detachment and/or breaks when they do occur and treatment of the vitreous hemorrhage when it occurs. Prophylactic therapy for the associated neovascularization may be of benefit. Vitrectomy and retinal reattachment surgery are indicated at the appropriate time.

It is, of course, necessary to provide genetic counseling to these patients as well as routine ocular examinations that are based on the stage of the disease. Provision of the best possible correction is always indicated.

Snowflake Vitreoretinal Degeneration

Introduction and Description. Snowflake vitreoretinal degeneration is considered to be a genetically inherited anomaly that may have a relationship to retinitis pigmentosa. Some consider that snowflake vitreoretinal degeneration is inherited as an autosomal dominant disease with variable expressivity. Snowflake vitreoretinal degeneration seems to progress through four stages of development. In *stage 1*, occurring under the age of 15 years, there seems to be white without pressure throughout the peripheral retina in which small yellow dot opacities are observed. At *stage 2*, ages 15 to 25 years, yellow-white crystalline dots occur in the inner retinal layers in the area of white without pressure. This combination gives focally elevated appearance to the affected retina. These yellow-white dots occur most frequently in the superior temporal quadrant. These dots may appear par-

Snowflake Vitreoretinal Degeneration

Characteristics

Δ Considered to be autosomal dominant with variable expressivity

Δ Occurs in the inner retinal layers, ora to equator

Δ Stage 1 (under 15 years)—white without pressure throughout periphery with the occasional appearance of yellow dots in the WWOP

Δ Stage 2 (15 to 25 years)—crystalline yellow dots in oval patches within the white without pressure and fibrillary vitreous degeneration

Δ Stage 3 (25 to 50 years)—vessel sheathing and RPE changes with condensed vitreous strands; possible early cataract and retinal break

Δ Stage 4 (over 50 years)—increased fundus pigmentation and chorioretinal atrophy with cataract and retinal breaks. In addition, there may be obliteration of the peripheral vasculature and the development of retinal neovascularization

Δ Electrodiagnosis is normal to abnormal and visual fields show variable constriction

Δ Fluorescein angiography demonstrates both capillary leakage and nonperfusion

Management

Δ Advise of signs/symptoms of retinal detachment

Δ Arrange a retinal consultation for retinal breaks, retinal detachment or retinal neovascularization

Δ Watch for the development of associated cataracts

Δ Autosomal-dominant inheritance, therefore genetic counseling

Δ Follow up according to signs and symptoms but at least every 6 months

allel to the equator in oval patches similar to the appearance of lattice degeneration. Additionally, there is fibrillary degeneration of the vitreous.

At *stage 3*, ages 25 to 50 years, sheathing of the vessels appears in the affected area and RPE clumping in the area of the snowflakes. Condensed vitreous strands also appear at this particular stage, indicating concomitant vitreal changes. Often at this stage there is development of an early-onset cataract. During *stage 4* there appears to be increased fundus pigmentation and chorioretinal atrophy as well as obliteration of the peripheral vasculature. There have been reports of peripheral retinal neovascularization associated with the vascular obliteration during this stage. At this point cataracts progress to the point where visualization of the posterior pole becomes difficult. Visual field changes occur at this stage as well as low-amplitude scotopic b-wave electroretinogram changes and altered dark adaptation without the

complaint of night vision problems. Fluorescein angiography will demonstrate both leaking capillaries and areas of capillary nonperfusion.

The layers involved in snowflake vitreoretinal degeneration include primarily the inner retinal layers. This presents from the ora to anterior to the equator. The condition progresses through stages and may develop retinal breaks.

Management. It is important that you educate patients as to the genetics of the situation and make them aware of signs and symptoms of changes that occur as they progress through the stages. A referral for a retinal consultation is indicated at approximately stage 2 to stage 3 if and when retinal breaks, retinal detachment, or peripheral retinal neovascularization occur. Cataract surgery is often necessary in these patients.

With the progressive nature of the disease, it is important to provide the best possible correction and examine the patient at least every 6 months.

Stickler Syndrome (Wagner–Jensen–Stickler Vitreoretinal Dystrophy)

Introduction and Description. Stickler syndrome (Wagner–Jensen–Stickler vitreoretinal dystrophy) is a hereditary condition characterized by vitreous membranes, vitreous degeneration, vitreous detachment, a lightly pigmented fundus, RPE abnormalities, myopia, lattice retinal degeneration with a 60 to 70 percent incidence of retinal breaks, retinal detachment, and cataracts. There is also a relationship to primary open-angle glaucoma. Stickler syndrome is the most common autosomal-dominant connective tissue disorder in North America with incomplete penetrance and variable expressivity. Systemic features include dwarfism in some cases; skeletal abnormalities, especially irregularity of many joints; and arthropathy, prominent epicanthal folds, palate anomalies, and hearing deficit. There is considerable confusion regarding Stickler syndrome, as there are many reports in the literature attributing its characteristics to other syndromes.

Management. Early recognition of patients with Stickler syndrome is important because of the relationship of the disease to retinal breaks, vitreous degeneration, and retinal detachment. The associated poor prognosis for retinal reattachment with late discovery makes early diagnosis critical to at least attempt prophylaxis and to provide early surgical intervention. Relatives of patients with Stickler syndrome should also be examined to provide early interventive care. Because of the progressive nature of the disease, signs and symptoms of retinal detachment should be provided, and routine examinations at least every 6 months are in order. At the first sign

Stickler Syndrome (Wagner–Jensen–Stickler Vitreoretinal Dystrophy)

Characteristics

△ Most common autosomal dominant connective tissue disorder in North America with incomplete penetrance and variable expressivity

△ Ocular characteristics include:

Vitreous membranes, vitreous degeneration, and vitreous detachment

Lightly pigmented fundus and RPE anomalies

Myopia

Lattice degeneration

60 to 70 percent chance of retinal breaks

Retinal detachment

Cataracts and primary open-angle glaucoma

△ Systemic manifestations include:

Irregularity of the joints and arthropathy

Orofacial disorders

Dwarfism in some cases

Hearing deficit in some cases

Management

△ Signs and symptoms of retinal detachment

△ Routine examinations at least every 6 months with provision of best possible correction

△ Examine relatives of the patients for early detection of ocular anomalies

△ Ask for a retinal consultation at the first sign of retinal breaks, retinal detachment, or vitreous traction

△ Request a consultation with a rheumatologist if the patient is not under care

HEMORRHAGE INTO THE VITREOUS

Retrovitreous Hemorrhage

Introduction and Description. Vitreous hemorrhages occur in two categories, retrovitreous and intravitreous hemorrhages. Retrovitreous hemorrhages may occur in eyes with PVD. Retrovitreous hemorrhages are also associated with trauma, retinal vein occlusion, age-related macular degeneration, sickle-cell disease, intraocular tumors, subarachnoid or subdural hematoma, diabetic retinopathy, retinal breaks without a detachment, and rhegmatogenous retinal detachment. Retrovitreous hemorrhages can occur in any retinal vascular disease that creates neovascularization of the retina, optic nerve head, or choroid. The patient who presents with a retrovitreous hemorrhage will typically complain of floaters and/or loss of vision, depending on the particular location of the hemorrhage.

Retrovitreous hemorrhages present as bright red, unclotted blood that shifts readily with eye movements. They are often keel shaped or boat shaped when they settle. It is always possible to view the vitreous base when a retrovitreous hemorrhage occurs. The clinician may also notice red blood cells perfused into the vitreous gel. Retrovitreous hemorrhages occur as a result of vitreous strands that pull on retinal vessels when a posterior vitreous detachment occurs. It is believed that there is a normal, loose adherence of the vitreous base to retinal blood vessels in addition

of vitreous traction or the development of retinal breaks a retinal consultation should be ordered. A consultation with a rheumatologist is also a consideration if the patient is not already under care.

■ ■ ■ ■ ■ ■

Clinical Note: Autosomal Dominant Vitreochoroidopathy (ADVIRC)

Autosomal dominant vitreochoroidopathy is a rare progressive dystrophy with a variable expressivity. There is an area of abnormal pigment clumping between the equatorial zone of the retina and the ora. Early-onset cataracts and yellowish dots in the retina may also occur. Retinal neovascularization may occur as well as other alterations of the blood retinal barrier. Vitreous opacities, cells, and fibrillary changes may also be present. Vision may be lost by either vitreous hemorrhage or cystoid macular edema. There is no complaint of night vision problems. Treatment is photocoagulation of the vascularly compromised areas and vitrectomy when necessary.

Retrovitreous Hemorrhage

Characteristics

△ May occur in eyes associated with PVD

△ Associated with trauma, diabetic retinopathy, retinal breaks without retinal detachment, rhegmatogenous retinal detachment, retinal vein occlusion, and any other retinal vascular disease that may create retinal, disc, or choroidal neovascularization

△ Presents as bright red blood that is keel shaped with settling and shifts readily with eye movements

△ It is almost always possible to view the vitreous base

Management

△ Ascertain the underlying cause. B-scan and ultrasonography are necessary at times

△ In some instances hospitalization is necessary to facilitate settling of the blood

△ Discontinue antiplatelet drugs if possible

△ A retinal consultation should be strongly considered

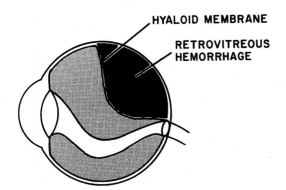

Figure 6–18. A schematic illustrating a retrovitreous hemorrhage.

to the standard zones of attachment at the ora, optic nerve head, and macula (Figs. 6–18 and 6–19).

It is imperative that the cause of the hemorrhage be determined. If the hemorrhage obstructs the underlying retina it is important to perform B-scan ultrasonography. If possible, a fluorescein angiography may assist in the differential diagnosis of the cause.

Management. Retrovitreous hemorrhages eventually disappear with hemolysis and phagocytosis. It is important, however, to ascertain the cause of a retrovitreous hemorrhage should there be a threat of repeat hemorrhage. The patient must be hospitalized in some instances with the consideration of the possibility of vitrectomy. The patient should discontinue all antiplatelet drugs such as aspirin if at all possible. A con-

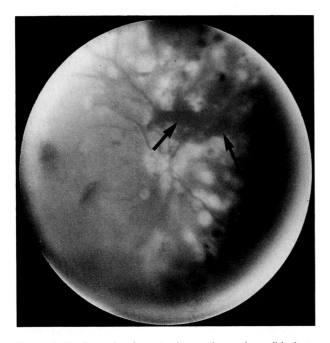

Figure 6–19. Example of a retrovitreous hemorrhage (*black arrows*) in a patient with long-standing diabetic retinopathy. Note the photocoagulative scars.

sultation with a qualified retinal specialist in cases of retrovitreous hemorrhage is usually a judicious approach, especially with the evidence that early vitrectomy with repair of the causative factor has proven to be of distinct benefit in some cases such as those associated with diabetic retinopathy.

Intravitreous Hemorrhage

Introduction and Description. Intravitreous hemorrhage (Figs. 6–20 and 6–21) may or may not have a posterior vitreous detachment associated with it. Intravitreous hemorrhage is secondary to trauma and proliferative diabetic retinopathy (34.1 percent), retinal breaks without detachment (22.4 percent), rhegmatogenous retinal detachments (14.9 percent), and retinal vein occlusion (13.0 percent). Again, any condition predisposing to the development of retinal, disc, and choroidal neovascularization may set the stage for intravitreal hemorrhage. Intravitreous hemorrhage usually occurs secondary to a ruptured blood vessel (neovascularization) that may have associated vitreous traction. The blood within the vitreous gel clots very quickly, forming fixed projections. Blood may collect within lacunae, which are more liquefied than the cortex and as a result of that appear as a denser red. The blood in the lacunae changes to a grey coloration more rapidly than the clotted blood within the cortex. The patient with an intravitreous hemor-

Pearls

Intravitreous Hemorrhage

Characteristics

△ Associated with proliferative diabetic retinopathy (34 percent), retinal break without retinal detachment (22 percent), rhegmatogenous retinal detachment (15 percent), and retinal vein occlusion (13 percent)

△ Any retinal vascular condition lending to the development of retinal, disc, or choroidal neovascularization may precipitate the development of a vitreous hemorrhage

△ Blood clots quickly forming fixed projections within cortex but stays very red within the liquefied lacunae

△ There is slow resorption of the hemorrhage from superior to inferior with formation of dense membranes inferiorly

Management

△ Ascertain cause and assess the underlying retina with B-scan ultrasonography

△ Consultation with a retinal specialist should be strongly considered as some cases may benefit from early vitrectomy and endophotocoagulation

△ Hospitalization is necessary at times to assist in the settling of the blood

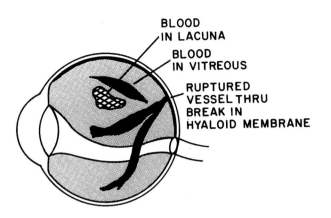

Figure 6–20. A schematic illustrating the possibilities associated with an intravitreous hemorrhage.

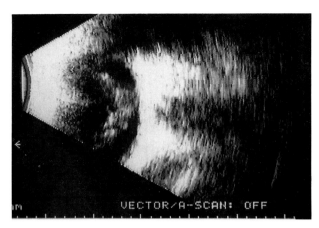

Figure 6–21. B-scan of an eye with an intravitreous hemorrhage.

rhage may complain of floaters or sudden loss of vision of variable degree.

Signs of intravitreous hemorrhage vary considerably according to the extent of the hemorrhage. A long-standing intravitreous hemorrhage will present with intravitreal membranes projecting out into the vitreous cortex. These intravitreal grey membranes occur in the inferior portion of the vitreous body. Intravitreous hemorrhages take a long time to resorb and with resorption change color from the top to the bottom of the vitreous cavity. Gravity will pull most of the coagulated blood down into the inferior vitreous, creating a longer resorption time in that particular area.

Management. It is important to attempt to ascertain the cause for an intravitreal hemorrhage. This is often difficult because the extent of the blood within the cavity will prevent effective evaluation of the retina. B-scan ultrasonography is often necessary to assess the underlying retina in cases of intravitreal hemorrhage. Patients with intravitreal hemorrhages often need hospitalization, with the consideration of vitrectomy once enough blood has cleared from the cavity to evaluate the retina. Certain patients with diabetic vitreous hemorrhage benefit from early vitrectomy intervention with consideration of endophotocoagulation. It is important to consult a qualified retinal specialist concerning patients with intravitreal hemorrhages. It is also important to note that it is possible to have a combination of retrovitreous and intravitreous hemorrhages and that the combinations are often associated with trauma.

PERSISTENT HYPERPLASTIC PRIMARY VITREOUS (PHPV)

Introduction and Description. Persistent hyperplastic primary vitreous (PHPV), shown in Figures 6–22 and 6–23, occurs in full–term infants that have had no exposure to oxygen therapy. Histopathologically, PHPV represents a failure of regression of the

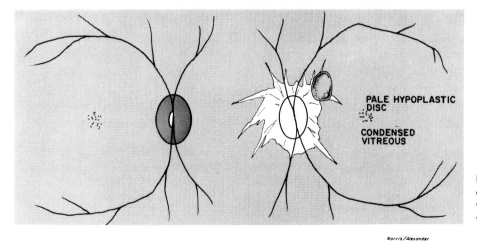

Figure 6–22. A schematic illustrating optic-nerve head changes associated with persistent hyperplastic primary vitreous.

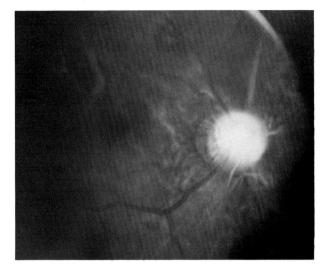

The posterior form presents with unilateral microcornea, often a pale hypoplastic disc, a normal crystalline lens, vitreous membranes containing hyaloid artery remnants, vitreoretinal adhesions, and peripapillary RPE changes. The most prominent abnormality is the presence of a dense vitreous condensation coursing from the disc, forming a retinal fold and then extending to the nasal periphery. In the posterior form it is important to remember that the vitreous membranes that remain have the potential to cause retinal folds and subsequent decrease in visual acuity.

Management. Management of the anterior form is early surgical intervention when the visual axis is occluded, the anterior chamber is shallow, or if there is

OD

A. PIGMENT DYSTROPHY
B. VITREAL CONDENSATION
C. VITREO-RETINAL MEMBRANE
D. TORTUOUS VESSELS
E. HYPOPLASTIC DISC
F. MACULA DRAGGED TOWARD
   DISC

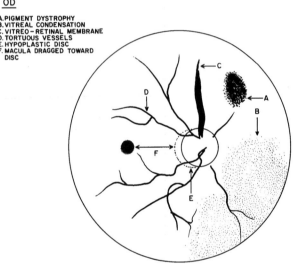

Figure 6–23. A black-and-white photograph of PHPV with the schematic illustrating the changes. (*Photo and figure from T. Madgar.*)

structures of the primary vitreous. There are two basic forms of PHPV, anterior and posterior. Within the framework of these two forms several variations may occur. The anterior form of PHPV presents with leukocoria, unilateral affliction, microcornea, occasionally strabismus, a retrolental membrane that may progress to a cataract, congenital glaucoma, microophthalmia, and a normal retina. The ciliary processes may be drawn to the periphery of the crystalline lens and are easily seen with dilation. The traction on the ciliary body by the retrolental mass may eventually compromise aqueous formation and create hypotony leading to the development of a phthisical globe. Additionally, rubeosis may present with subsequent neovascular glaucoma and possibly bleeding into the anterior chamber.

Pearls

Persistent Hyperplastic Primary Vitreous

Characteristics

△ Failure in the regression of the structures of the primary vitreous

△ Full-term gestation with no oxygen supplementation in the neonatal history

△ Anterior form—leukocoria, unilateral, strabismus, retrolental membrane, cataract, microcornea, shallow anterior chamber, congenital glaucoma, normal retina, alterer ciliary body that may create hypotony and a pthisical globe, and iris neovascularization

△ Posterior form—microcornea, unilateral, vitreous membranes and vitreoretinal adhesions usually in the nasal retina, nasal retinal folds, peripapillary RPE changes, and pale hypoplastic disc

Management

△ Anterior—early surgical intervention when the visual axis is occluded, when there is a shallow angle, or if there is documented progression of traction

△ Anterior—lensectomy after determining retinal status with ultrasonography

△ Anterior—patient education

△ Posterior—monitor yearly for the development of retinal breaks, traction retinal detachment, or glaucoma

△ Posterior—patient education

△ Differentiate from other causes of leukocoria that may be both vision and life threatening; computed tomography may be of value in the differentiation

△ Differentiate from Norrie's disease because of the hereditary implications

△ Retinal consultation is indicated when vitrectomy or retinal repair is necessary

indication of progressive traction that may precipitate retinal breaks or retinal detachment. There is the possibility of blindness and possible loss of the eye. Surgical intervention in the anterior form actually may result in improvement of vision, but vision improvement in the posterior variation is highly unlikely. In the posterior form it is important to watch the patient yearly for the development of glaucoma and/or retinal breaks. Lensectomy may also be necessary after B-scan ultrasonography determines the retinal status. Vitrectomy and retinal procedures may be necessary to attempt to correct retinal damage. Prognosis for vision is typically poor with surgery, but success is maintenance of the structure of the globe.

Perhaps the most important feature of PHPV is the differentiation of this condition from other ocular disease anomalies. Computed tomography (CT) may be of use to differentiate PHPV from other more vision and life-threatening causes of leukocoria. The CT findings include increased density of the retrolental soft tissue, absence of calcification, microphthalmia, and indications of detached retina. It is important to differentiate PHPV in the anterior form from retinoblastoma. In the posterior form, PHPV may simulate retinopathy of prematurity. The primary differentiating feature from retinopathy of prematurity is the fact that PHPV occurs in full-term infants who have had no oxygen therapy. The leukocoria of the anterior form becomes a bit more of a diagnostic dilemma, perhaps necessitating the implementation of higher-level diagnostic procedures. When in doubt, consult a retinal specialist concerning the differential diagnosis of PHPV, retinoblastoma, and retinopathy of prematurity.

Clinical Note: Norrie's Disease

Norrie's disease is a condition that may be confused with PHPV. Norrie's disease is an X-linked disorder associated with a hearing impairment, ocular appearance similar to PHPV, and cerebral dysplasia (retardation). The ocular disorder is characterized by leukocoria, retinal folds, shallow anterior chambers, synechiae, retinal detachment, micro-ophthalmos, corneal degeneration, cataract, and pthisis bulbi. Differentiation of Norrie's disease from PHPV is important because of the genetic implications.

ANATOMIC CHARACTERISTICS OF THE PERIPHERAL RETINA

Figure 6–24 is a schematic representation of retinal layers in the posterior pole. Variations in these layers occur in the peripheral retina. The retinal periphery is defined as the zone from the equator to the ora serrata and is approximately 3 disc diameters (DD) or 1 condensing lens (20 D) in width. This retinal periphery has several anatomic landmarks that can guide the practitioner in the examination and location of various lesions.

Vortex Vein Ampullae. The vortex vein ampullae mark the equator of the eye (Fig. 6–25). There is usually one vortex vein per quadrant, but there may be up to ten in each eye. These vortex vein ampullae vary in appearance from reddish to orange, take on the shape of an octopus, and often have a significant

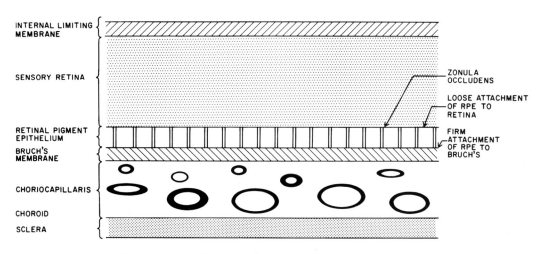

Figure 6–24. A schematic retinal cross section of a normal retina.

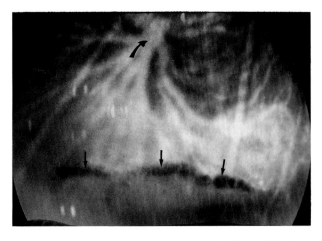

Figure 6–25. Example of a vortex vein ampulla (*curved black arrow*) that serves as an anatomic marker for the retinal equator. The small black arrows point to RPE hyperplasia associated with lattice degeneration.

amount of pigment surrounding them. There may be several tributaries emptying into a single ampulla. The ampullae may dilate with pressure created in changing direction of gaze or by making a postural change. When they dilate they assume a darker color and become elevated. These variations are known as vortex vein varices.

Posterior Ciliary Nerves. The long posterior ciliary nerves and arteries often serve as a good anatomic landmark in the peripheral retina. The long posterior ciliary nerves and arteries run at the 3-o'clock and 9-o'clock positions from the ora to the equator of the posterior pole. The long posterior ciliary nerves are typically yellowish to white in color, often with pigmented borders. The artery usually runs above the ciliary nerve in the nasal retina and below the ciliary nerve in the temporal retina.

The short posterior ciliary nerves may number 10 to 20 in the peripheral retina and have a tendency to congregate near the vertical meridians. As with the long posterior ciliary nerves and arteries, the short posterior ciliary nerves are yellowish to white, again often with pigmented borders. The short posterior ciliary arteries may be scattered anywhere on the horizontal meridian and may have associated pigment margins. **See color plate 95.**

Peripheral Retinal Vessels. Peripheral retinal vessels typically run a much different course than those in the posterior pole. Peripheral retinal vessels often run parallel to the ora serrata. The area close to the ora serrata, however, is usually devoid of any apparent retinal vasculature. This avascular zone is enlarged in familial exudative vitreoretinopathy.

Ora Serrata. The ora serrata is the anterior limit of the neural retina. The ora serrata is scalloped more nasally than temporally. The practitioner can distinguish the temporal from the nasal ora serrata because the temporal ora serrata is usually narrower. The rounded areas extending from the pars plana, which is brown in color, are called oral bays. The whitish retinal extensions into these bays are called oral teeth. The oral bays and oral teeth together are called dentate processes, of which there are 20 to 30 per eye. Dentate processes are usually absent in the temporal aspect of the peripheral retina. Deep or large oral bays may occur as anatomical variants in the ora serrata region. Bridging oral teeth with no particular contact with the pars plana can also occur as an anatomic variance.

Pars Plana. The pars plana is an anatomic landmark that is chocolate in color, running from the ora serrata to the ciliary processes. The ciliary processes number 60 to 70 and are cream colored in indirect view but pigmented with the slit-lamp view. As in the sensory retina, one can have separation of layers of the epithelium of the pars plana, which are pars plana cysts.

Vitreous Base. The vitreous base is also considered an anatomic landmark of the peripheral retina. The vitreous base is a strong connection of the vitreous to the retinal tissue, running in a 2- to 4-mm band that straddles the ora serrata. The vitreous base band is typically wider nasally than it is temporally. The posterior limit of the vitreous base is usually invisible but is the anatomic limit of a posterior vitreous detachment. The anterior limit of the vitreous base may be seen as a whitish haze on the pars plana. The entire vitreous base band may be marked by an increase in pigmentation beneath the base itself, especially if there is excessive vitreoretinal traction. This increased pigmentation is nothing more than an RPE hyperplasia that is a reaction to insult to the retina. It is interesting to note that about 15 percent of retinal breaks can be seen along the posterior extensions of the vitreous base.

SCLERAL INDENTATION

Mastering scleral indentation elevates the clinician to the highest level of diagnostic skill in peripheral retinal evaluation. In reality, it is close to impossible to discern subtleties of the retina near the ora without the benefit of scleral indentation. Not only does scleral indentation push retinal structural alterations into view, but it also increases the contrast between intact retina and retinal breaks and places elevations in profile (Fig. 6–26). The indented retinal/choroidal structure is darker than the surrounding retina, which increases

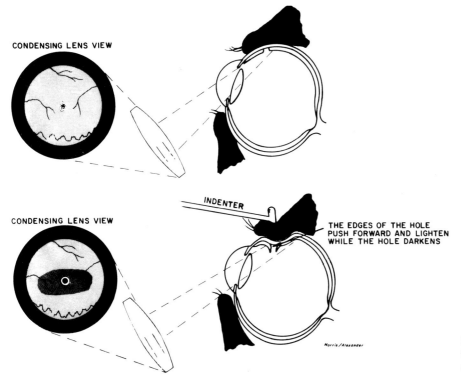

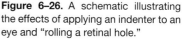

Figure 6–26. A schematic illustrating the effects of applying an indenter to an eye and "rolling a retinal hole."

the contrast. It is also important to realize that there is decreased retinal translucency with indentation because the examiner is viewing the retina at a more oblique angle. Scleral indentation is a kinetic procedure as well, which enhances the discovery of subtle changes. It is far easier to see changes when the retinal structures are moving. The discovery of retinal breaks (tears and holes) is facilitated with indentation as the edges roll upward and lighten while the hole darkens. The rolling of holes is illustrated in Figure 6–26.

Scleral indentation is indicated with patient complaints of flashes, floaters, and decreased vision when the cause is elusive. A history of any trauma, even remote by a few months, is also an indication for scleral indentation. Previous retinal detachment in the fellow eye, high myopia, vitreous hemorrhage, and pigment cells in the vitreous are also indications to consider scleral indentation.

It is important to orient oneself to retinal structure prior to the performance of scleral indentation. Figure 6–27 gives the basic ocular dimensions from the corneal limbus to facilitate orientation with common retinal landmarks. It is also important to realize that to indent the equator it is only necessary to place the indenter 13 mm or about ½ inch posterior to the limbus. The distance back from the limbus to most structures that need to be viewed is almost always less than 13 mm.

Scleral indentation can be performed safely in most patients. Patients with active glaucoma or in-

traocular lenses should be indented with great care. Patients with recent intraocular surgery or those suspected of having penetrating trauma should not be indented. Choice of the type of indenter is at the discretion of the practitioner.

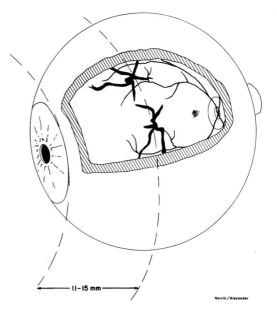

Figure 6–27. A schematic illustrating the relatively short distance from the limbus to the equator.

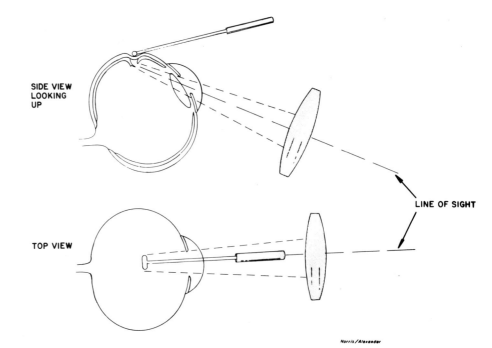

SIDE VIEW
LOOKING
UP

TOP VIEW

LINE OF SIGHT

Norris/Alexander

Figure 6–28. A schematic illustrating the proper alignment of the scleral indenter, condensing lens, and line of sight.

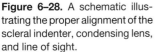

Clinical Note: Technique for Scleral Indentation

1. Topical anesthesia may be applied to the eye prior to indentation, but remember that this may cause mild corneal edema and sloughing. This will obviously compromise the view. Most of the time indentation is performed through the lids, which eliminates the need for anesthesia.

2. Maximal dilation is an absolute necessity. This is usually best achieved by a combination of 1 percent tropicamide and 2.5 percent phenylephrine given twice.

3. Educate the patient as to the mild discomfort (pressure) experienced during the procedure.

4. Recline the patient and tilt the head forward, backward, and side to side to maximize the view. An example of this would be tilting the head back (chin up) to facilitate the view of the superior retina.

5. To view the 12-o'clock position (the easiest zone to view), ask the patient to gently close his or her eyes and to look down. Place the tip of the indenter on the upper lid at the upper margin of the tarsal plate (do not attempt to indent through the tarsal plate).

6. While maintaining the position of the indenter, have the patient slowly look up—the practitioner must move the indenter tip back as the eye rolls upward.

7. Remember that the indenter tip should always be tangential to the globe—not perpendicular, as this would be painful. Also remember to keep line of sight, condensing lens, and shaft of the indenter aligned. Figure 6–28 illustrates proper alignment. If any component is out of alignment the retinal orientation is quickly lost.

8. When all components are aligned, exert gentle pressure and view the mound created by the indentation.

The necessary pressure can only be attained through practice.

9. Remember that indentation is intended to be a kinetic procedure. Move the indenter gently, remembering to keep the entire observation system aligned. Also recall that the indenter must be moved opposite to what appears to be necessary when viewing through the condensing lens. Said another way, move the indenter toward the cornea to view the retina inferior in the condensing lens. Once the accessible area has been examined, move to the next quadrant.

10. To depress the 3-o'clock and 9-o'clock quadrants, it may be necessary to drag the lids up or down into position. If there is not enough laxity of the lids, it may be necessary to anesthetize and depress directly on the bulbar conjunctiva. Application of a viscous nonpreserved artificial tear may facilitate the procedure.

PERIPHERAL RETINAL CHANGES THAT USUALLY POSE NO IMMEDIATE THREAT TO VISION

Peripheral Senile Pigmentary Degeneration

Introduction and Description.   Peripheral senile pigmentary degeneration (Figs. 6–29 and 6–30), also known as peripheral tapetochoroidal degeneration, appears as granular pigment between the ora serrata and the equator in approximately 20 percent of the population over the age of 40 years and has a tendency to progressively increase in prominence with age. The condition is usually bilateral but often is more apparent in the nasal quadrant. The pigment often cuffs or

Peripheral Senile Pigmentary Degeneration

Characteristics

△ Granular pigment between equator and ora in 20 percent of patients over 40 years of age
△ Usually bilateral
△ Often accompanied by peripheral degenerative drusen
△ The pigment may cuff venules or may be bone spicule-like
△ The cause is degenerating RPE scattered in sensory retina with loss of photoreceptors and sclerosis of the choriocapillaris
△ No night blindness, electrodiagnostic alterations, or vascular attenuations

Management

△ Self-limiting and benign
△ Routine eye examinations with the provision of the best possible prescription

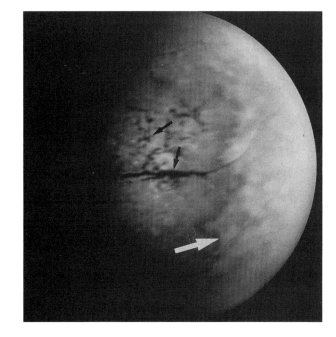

Figure 6–30. Example of peripheral senile pigmentary degeneration (*black arrows*), which can simulate retinal changes associated with retinitis pigmentosa. The white arrow points to a zone of scalloped retinal white without pressure.

surrounds the venules as macrophages carry the pigment toward the retinal vessels. This pigment may take on a reticular or bone spicule appearance, simulating the appearance of retinitis pigmentosa. This degeneration is often accompanied by benign peripheral retinal

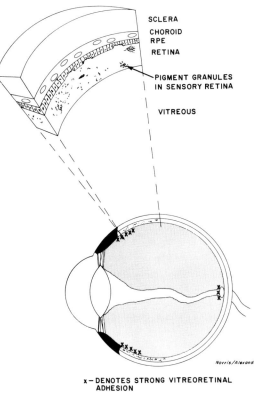

SCLERA
CHOROID
RPE
RETINA

— PIGMENT GRANULES IN SENSORY RETINA

VITREOUS

x – DENOTES STRONG VITREORETINAL ADHESION

Norris/Alexander

Figure 6–29. A schematic illustrating the clinicopathologic changes associated with peripheral senile pigmentary degeneration.

drusen. The pigmentary degeneration has also been likened to a honeycomb appearance. **See color plate 91.**

The differential diagnosis between this and retinitis pigmentosa is made by considering patient characteristics such as night vision problems and vascular attenuation as well as performing routine visual field analysis. The layers involved in peripheral senile pigmentary degeneration are degenerating RPE scattering pigment throughout the sensory retina. There is ultimately loss of photoreceptors and sclerosis of the choriocapillaris, implicating the possibility of vascular compromise associated with aging. The prognosis of this condition is usually benign. There is typically no compromise of visual fields or dark adaptation, and the electroretinogram (ERG) and electro-oculogram (EOG) are normal. Electrodiagnostic characteristics do help to differentiate this condition from retinitis pigmentosa or pigmented paravenous retinochoroidal atrophy.

Management. Peripheral senile pigmentary degeneration is an age-related change that requires no particular treatment except for routine visual examinations every 2 years. Figure 6–29 illustrates the specific histopathologic changes associated with peripheral senile pigmentary degeneration. The practitioner can see that there is a breakdown in the RPE with deposition of the pigment granules in the sensory retina. Loss of the RPE does imply that there will eventually be loss or compromise of overlying photoreceptors.

Primary Chorioretinal Atrophy (Pavingstone or Cobblestone)

Introduction and Description. Primary chorioretinal atrophy (Figs. 6–31 and 6–32) is also known as cobblestone degeneration or pavingstone degeneration. Primary chorioretinal atrophy occurs in over 27 percent of patients above 20 years of age. It is bilateral in 30 to 70 percent of patients. Primary chorioretinal atrophy usually appears as small (0.5 to 1.5 mm) pale yellow or depigmented nonelevated areas in the peripheral retina that are often surrounded by RPE hyperplasia. Nearly 80 percent of the lesions are in the inferotemporal quadrant. These changes are typically separated from the ora serrata. The lesions may be larger when they coalesce, and they will certainly have associated pigmentary changes. The choroidal vessels may be seen within the lesion because of loss of overlying RPE. This is a fairly common age-related change with prevalence increasing with age. **See color plate 92.**

The layers involved are the loss or attenuation of the choriocapillaris, with subsequent atrophy of the

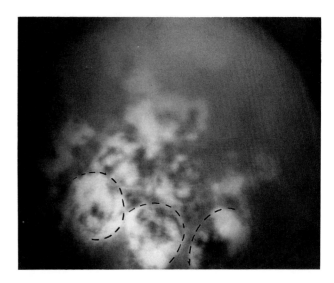

Figure 6–32. Areas of primary chorioretinal atrophy outlined by the dotted lines.

overlying RPE and outer retina within the area of the lesion. This process is thought to occur as a result of occlusion of compartments of the choriocapillaris. There is a resultant depression in the area because of retinal tissue loss. This depression may be enhanced by scleral indentation. As far as prognosis is concerned, the involvement may increase with age, but it is of no long-term significance, as the inner retinal layers stay intact. There is no particular potential toward the development of retinal holes in primary chorioretinal atrophy. Should a retinal detachment occur elsewhere, the detachment would proceed more rapidly in the area of primary chorioretinal atrophy

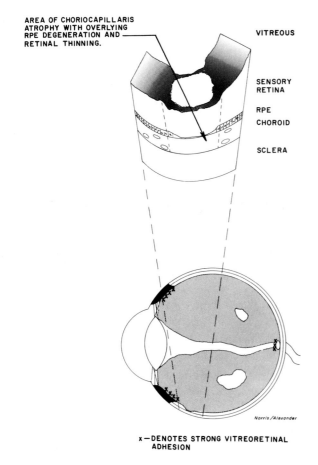

AREA OF CHORIOCAPILLARIS ATROPHY WITH OVERLYING RPE DEGENERATION AND RETINAL THINNING.

VITREOUS

SENSORY RETINA

RPE
CHOROID

SCLERA

Norris / Alexander

x — DENOTES STRONG VITREORETINAL ADHESION

Figure 6–31. A schematic illustrating the clinicopathologic changes associated with primary chorioretinal atrophy.

Pearls

Primary Chorioretinal Atrophy

Characteristics

△ 0.5- to 1.5-mm nonpigmented areas between the equator and ora that usually are inferior favoring the 5- to 7-o'clock areas

△ Often the lesions will have an RPE hyperplasia surrounding

△ As the lesions coalesce one may see underlying choroidal vessels

△ Aging change with 30 to 70 percent bilaterality

△ Thought to be an occlusion of the choriocapillaris with subsequent RPE and retinal tissue loss

Management

△ Self-limiting and benign

△ Routine eye examinations are in order, with provision of the best possible spectacle prescription because of the inherent thinning of the retina in the affected zones.

Management. From a management standpoint, the primary concern is differential diagnosis including postinflammatory scars, retinal holes, and lattice degeneration. It is only necessary to examine the patient with primary chorioretinal atrophy every 2 years unless there are other extenuating circumstances. Figure 6–31 demonstrates primary chorioretinal atrophy. The clinician can see that there is a basic underlying infarct in the choriocapillaris. This infarct compromises blood flow to the RPE and thus the sensory retina. This action causes degeneration and atrophy of those structures, allowing for depigmentation and the genesis of the whitish circular-to-oval lesion.

Postinflammatory Chorioretinal Scar

Introduction and Description. Postinflammatory chorioretinal scars (Figs. 6–33 and 6–34) can present in many different ways. The scar is usually a white to yel-

low area of fibrosis within the retina, with reactive RPE proliferation. This proliferation scatters dark pigmentation throughout the lesion and is nothing more than a reaction of the RPE to insult. In the majority of chorioretinal scars there is overlying vitreous condensation with some strand-like attachments to the scar. **See color plate 88.**

The layers involved in chorioretinal scars can vary as well. Depending on the severity of the lesion, one may have involvement of the choriocapillaris, RPE, and the sensory retina.

The prognosis is fairly good for a chorioretinal scar. The chorioretinal scar usually is a benign finding, but there may be a retinal break associated with a posterior vitreous detachment because of the vitreoretinal condensation at the scar. One must also note that in certain chorioretinal or retinal scars there can be a reactivation of the lesion. The best example of reactivation is ocular toxoplasmosis.

Management. In the management of chorioretinal scars, it is important that the practitioner watch for possible retinal breaks in the area of the scar, especially at the edge of the lesion. This is especially a concern when a PVD occurs. In the case of toxoplasmosis, the patient must be notified about the possibility of reactivation and the signs and symptoms of reactivation because of the importance of early incorporation of treatment in this condition. Patients with chorioretinal scars should be rechecked at yearly intervals. A schematic of a chorioretinal scar demonstrates fibrosis of the scar tissue deep into the retina and actually often penetrating out into the vitreous. There is also the presence of an overlying vitreous condesate and

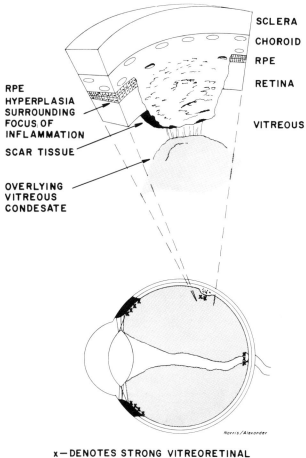

Figure 6–33. A schematic illustrating the clinicopathologic changes associated with a chorioretinal scar.

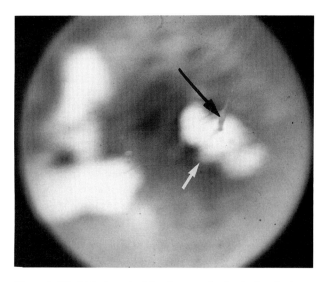

Figure 6–34. A black-and-white photograph of a chorioretinal scar (*white arrow*) with an overlying vitreous condensation (*black arrow*).

Postinflammatory Chorioretinal Scar

Characteristics

Δ Usually white to yellow intraretinal fibrosis with accompanying RPE hyperplasia

Δ There may be overlying vitreous condensation strands

Δ The scar may involve choroid through the retina to the vitreous

Δ Possible traction-induced tears. If they occur, tears are usually secondary to a PVD and occur at the edge of the lesion

Δ Scars may reactivate if they are secondary to ocular toxoplasmosis

Management

Δ Monitor yearly and provide best possible prescription

Δ If a toxoplasmosis scar is suspected, employ home monitoring

Δ Carefully investigate for retinal tears, especially in cases of PVD

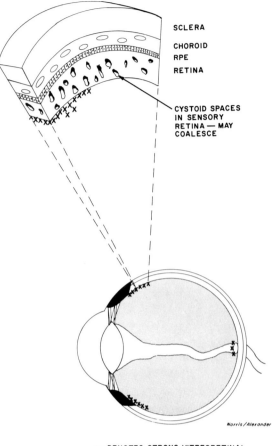

x—DENOTES STRONG VITREORETINAL ADHESION

Figure 6–35. A schematic illustrating the clinicopathologic changes associated with peripheral cystoid degeneration.

the vitreoretinal adhesions that are present in many of these inflammatory conditions. The vitreous condesate occurs because of an overlying inflammatory condition of the vitreous called vitritis.

Peripheral Cystoid Degeneration—Typical

Introduction and Description. Microcystoid peripheral retinal degeneration is the most prevalent of the benign peripheral retinal conditions. Typical peripheral cystoid degeneration (Fig. 6–35) appears as an area of thickened retina extending about ½ disc diameter from the ora serrata. Peripheral cystoid can, however, extend all the way to the equator. The cystoid area appears hazy gray with enclosed hazy red dots. Vitreous strands and dots may be present above the affected area. Peripheral cystoid degeneration appears more dramatically temporally and inferiorly within the retina. The extent of peripheral cystoid, at least the appearance of the changes, appears to increase with age.

Peripheral cystoid degeneration involves cystoid-like changes in the outer plexiform layer of the retina that can eventually extend to involve the entire sensory retina. These cysts may coalesce and are thought by some to be precursors to retinoschisis. **See color plate 93.**

Typical peripheral cystoid degeneration occurs bilaterally in virtually all patients over 8 years of age. There may be the associated finding of formation of inner-layer retinal holes. The presence of typical peripheral cystoid degeneration appears to increase

Typical Peripheral Cystoid Degeneration

Characteristics

Δ Usually a hazy gray area near the ora but may extend to equator

Δ Most evident temporally and inferiorly, and is bilateral in virtually everyone over 8 years of age—it is just easier to see in some patients than others

Δ May have small red dots within the cystoid area and strands in vitreous over the cystoid

Δ Intraretinal cysts may form that may coalesce to form retinoschisis—no substantial proof as to this evolution

Management

Δ Self-limiting and benign, with occasional inner-layer holes

Δ Routine eye examinations are indicated with provision of the best possible prescription

with age. It is important to remember, however, that this is a very common condition and is usually of no threat to the patient whatsoever.

The holes that potentially develop within typical peripheral cystoid degeneration are usually limited to inner-layer atrophic holes. As such, the holes are of no threat to the development of retinal detachment. In the evaluation of the patient with peripheral cystoid degeneration, remember that cystoid degeneration is considered by some to be a precursor to the development of retinoschisis. The accompanying schematic will demonstrate the changes at a histopathologic level associated with peripheral cystoid degeneration. It is to be noted that the cystoid spaces that develop within the sensory retina may coalesce and form larger cystic spaces, causing a true splitting or schisis of the sensory retina, although there is no substantial proof as to this occurrence.

Management. Management of peripheral cystoid degeneration is nothing more than routine eye examinations, as there is no immediate or long-term threat to retinal or visual status.

Peripheral Cystoid Degeneration—Reticular

Introduction and Description. Reticular peripheral cystoid degeneration presents as an area posterior to but continuous with typical cystoid degeneration. Reticular cystoid degeneration is far less common than typical peripheral cystoid degeneration, occurring most commonly in the inferotemporal portion of the retina. The retinal changes present closer to the equatorial region of the retina than typical cystoid degeneration. These areas are hazy and may be irregular, with a reticular pattern that appears like sclerotic retinal vessels. This appearance can simulate the development of the fishbone or sclerotic retinal vessel appearance of lattice degeneration. There is also an accompanying stippled appearance to the inner surface of the retina. These posterior margin changes are often angulated and well demarcated to give the practitioner some means of differential diagnosis from typical cystoid degeneration.

The layers involved are slightly different than those of typical cystoid degeneration. The cystoid spaces in reticular peripheral cystoid degeneration occur in the nerve fiber layer, and this may eventually extend into the inner plexiform layer.

Usually reticular peripheral cystoid degeneration is of no threat to vision, occurring commonly in 13 to 18 percent of adults with bilateral presentation in 41 percent of affected adults. Again, the only association with a vision-threatening problem is the possibility that reticular cystoid is a precursor to degenerative retinoschisis.

Pearls

Reticular Peripheral Cystoid Degeneration

Characteristics

△ Hazy irregular areas continuous with but posterior to typical peripheral cystoid degeneration

△ Areas are reticular, appearing as fishbone sclerotic vessels, and the inner retinal layer has a stippled appearance

△ The posterior border is angulated and well demarcated

△ Occurs as cystoid spaces in the nerve fiber layer that may extend into the inner plexiform layer

△ Occurs in 13 to 18 percent of adults with 41 percent bilaterality

△ Possible association to the development of degenerative retinoschisis

Management

△ Usually benign and self-limiting, but must watch for hole development and the development of degenerative retinoschisis

△ Routine eye examinations with the provision of the best possible correction are indicated

---

Management. Reticular peripheral cystoid degeneration can be managed by routine eye examinations, again looking for the potential development of breaks in the retina, which may be the precursor to the development of retinal detachment. The practitioner must also be alert to the potential development of degenerative retinoschisis in the area of reticular degeneration that may progress toward loss of vision function.

Retinal Pigment Epithelial Window Defect

Introduction and Description. The RPE window defect (Figs. 6–36 and 6–37) is a relatively common occurrence in the normal population. RPE window

---

Pearls

RPE Window Defect

Characteristics

△ White to yellow, round, well-circumscribed areas in the retina with no surrounding of reactive RPE hyperplasia

△ The lesion is the result of absence of melanin in the RPE

△ Benign but may appear to increase in size over the years

△ To be differentiated from reddish to reddish brown retinal holes

Management

△ Routine eye examinations with provision of the best possible prescription

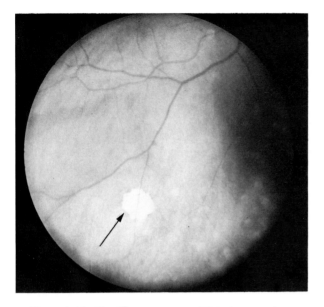

Figure 6–36. The arrow points to an RPE window defect.

defects appear as white to yellow, round, well-circumscribed areas often occurring in the equatorial region. The window defects may, however, occur at any point within the retina. There is usually no associated reactive RPE hyperplasia surrounding the area as there would be with a chorioretinal scar. It is important to note that the RPE is not absent in this particular defect; however, there is an absence of melanin within the RPE cell. The RPE window defect is in and of itself no concern. Clinically they may enlarge over the years. This enlargement is of no direct threat to vision.

Management. The management of RPE defects includes differential diagnosis and patient education. The primary concern is the differential diagnosis from a retinal hole. This differential is very straight forward when considering that an RPE window defect is yellowish to white in color and is well circumscribed, whereas a retinal hole is always reddish or reddish brown in color and often has a surrounding cuff of white retinal edema and may have a cuff of reactive RPE hyperplasia.

Routine eye examinations should be conducted on patients with RPE window defects.

Congenital Hypertrophy of the RPE (CHRPE)

Introduction and Description. Congenital hypertrophy of the RPE (CHRPE) is also known as a halo nevus (Figs. 6–38 and 6–39). Also one other variant of this is the presentation of multiple isolated areas of CHRPE, called "bear tracks" (Fig. 6–40). CHRPE often

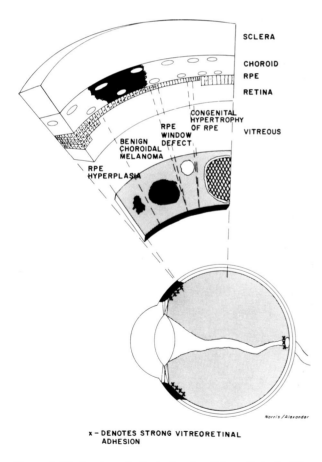

x – DENOTES STRONG VITREORETINAL ADHESION

Figure 6–37. A schematic illustrating the clinicopathologic differences between RPE hyperplasia, benign choroidal melanoma, RPE window defect, and congenital hypertrophy of the RPE.

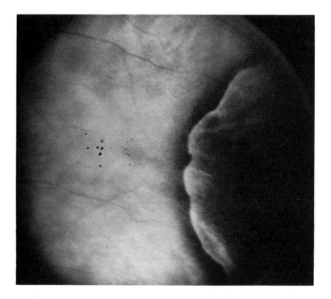

Figure 6–38. Congenital hypertrophy of the RPE, also known as the "halo" nevas. Note the scalloped edges.

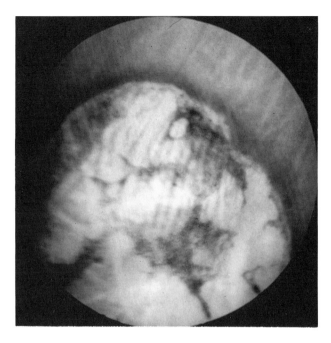

Figure 6–39. Congenital hypertrophy of the RPE. Note the significant chorioretinal atrophy within the confines of the lesion.

presents as a dark gray to black area of variable size, and can occur anywhere in the retina. The lesions typically are flat, with an area of depigmentation or the variant of pigmentation surrounding the lesion. This area of depigmentation, sometimes actually clinically appearing as hyperpigmentation, is known as the

halo. Often there are associated areas of chorioretinal atrophy within the lesion, known as lacunae. This chorioretinal atrophy becomes more apparent as the patient ages and can actually simulate chorioretinal scarification.

The layers involved in CHRPE are primarily the RPE cells and the choriocapillaris (Fig. 6–37). In this condition the RPE cells are enlarged with essentially the same amount of melanin pigment. There is an associated choriocapillaris atrophy in this condition that creates the clinical picture of the lacunae.

CHRPE is a benign condition. There is, however, a scotoma corresponding to the area of hypertrophy, especially when tested at threshold. As this lesion ages, the scotoma becomes more absolute because of the associated underlying chorioretinal atrophy and overlying sensory retinal degenerative changes.

Pearls

Congenital Hypertrophy of the RPE

Characteristics

△ Also known as halo nevus and bear tracks
△ Flat gray to black area with a surround of depigmentation (often a contrast of hyperpigmentation) and internal areas of chorioretinal atrophy known as lacunae that become more evident with age
△ The histopathology is enlarged RPE cells and choriocapillaris atrophy and ultimate retinal degeneration
△ Scotomas occur in the affected areas that become more dense with age
△ Association with familial adenomatous polyposis (FAP), a hereditary colerectal disease with a strong tendency for malignant conversion
    FAP has an autosomal dominant inheritance
    This association is arguable, but it is recognized that 4 or more lesions in both eyes in a person with a family history of FAP is strongly suggestive of the disorder

Management

△ Self-limiting and benign unless there are multiple lesions in both eyes in a person with a family history of FAP
△ All family members of persons with the hereditary history of FAP should receive annual dilated fundus evaluations, and if 4 or more lesions of CHRPE appear, the patient should have annual sigmoidoscopy
△ If there is a family history of FAP, the patient and family should receive genetic counseling
△ Routine yearly eye examinations with the provision of the best possible prescription is indicated

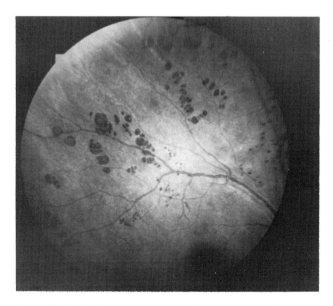

Figure 6–40. A clinicopathologic variation of congenital hypertrophy of the RPE, often referred to as "bear tracks."

Although controversial, there is the reported association of CHRPE with familial adenomatous polyposis (FAP), a hereditary bowel disorder with a propensity for malignancy. FAP is inherited as an autosomal dominant trait with the causative gene on the long arm of chromosome 5. FAP presents as the development of numerous adenomatous polyps in the large intestine around puberty. The majority of the patients will progress to colon cancer before the 50s if untreated. Recent reports have varied considerably as to the association of FAP to CHRPE. One study suggests that 4 or more CHRPE lesions distributed in both eyes seems to be a congenital marker for FAP, and when present in a family it is found in all diagnosed patients in that family. Another study recommends that all patients at risk of inheriting FAP should undergo dilated fundus examinations as early as possible and that all patients with 4 or more CHRPE lesions should undergo annual sigmoidoscopic examinations beginning before age 10 years. Other studies support the fact that if there is a family history of FAP, ophthalmoscopic evaluation for CHRPE is of value as an additional screening test for colerectal cancer. There is the suggestion that a difference exists between CHRPE associated with FAP (these are hamartomas of the RPE) and the CHRPE not associated with FAP. Latest works confirm this suggestion by denying the existence of a relationship between multiple presentations of CHRPE and FAP. Certainly isolated lesions and minimal group pigmentations are not suggestive of FAP when there is no reportable family history of FAP. Nevertheless, the practitioner must be aware of the relationship.

Management. The clinician should observe, record, and differentiate this condition from a malignant melanoma. The practitioner must also be aware of the association of 4 or more lesions of CHRPE to familial adenomatous polyposis in patients with a family history of this autosomal dominant inherited condition. When a patient has a family history of FAP, dilated fundus evaluation is crucial, with the recommendation that all family members have a dilated fundus evaluation at as young an age as possible, with special attention placed on the dilated fundus evaluation at puberty. Should 4 or more lesions be found in each eye with a positive family history of FAP, annual sigmoidoscopy is recommended. Routine visual examinations about every year with a positive family history are in order. The patient and family members with a hereditary history of FAP should receive genetic counseling. The CHRPE lesion that is isolated, or grouped pigmentation that is not suggestive of FAP, need only be examined at a routine interval. **See color plates 95 to 97.**

RPE Hyperplasia

Introduction and Description. RPE hyperplasia occurs most often as a result of insult to the retina or the components of the supportive system of the retina. The clinician will see RPE hyperplasia in many different conditions, including chorioretinal scars, circumpapillary choroiditis, choroidal neovascularization, vitreoretinal traction, traumatic contrecoup injuries, and isolated areas of RPE hyperplasia (Fig. 6–41). RPE hyperplasia appears jet black with irregularly shaped areas that are variable in size. The appearance is the result of invasion of the sensory retina by replicating RPE cells (Fig. 6–37). The RPE hyperplasia is actually an attempt at repair in many conditions such as the development of choroidal neovascular nets, atrophic retinal holes, and the retinal pigmentary demarcation lines of retinal detachment. The pigment is an indication of a process that has been developing over 60 to 90 days. The RPE hyperplasia often indicates relative stability, but likewise may indicate a very ominous condition such as the melanoma bodies that may present on the dome of a malignant choroidal melanoma. RPE hyperplasia may cause an area of an isolated scotoma but is usually nonprogressive.

Management. It is important for the clinician to ascertain the cause for the RPE hyperplasia. If the cause is not currently active, the clinician may just follow the patient on a routine basis. If there is an active inflammatory lesion causing the RPE hyperplasia, it is important to provide the proper therapeutic interven-

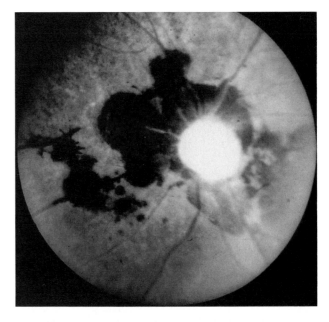

Figure 6–41. Non-descript RPE hyperplasia surrounding the optic nerve head associated with trauma to the eye.

RPE Hyperplasia

Characteristics

△ Very dense black area that does not disappear with red-free illumination

△ Usually a reaction of the retinal tissue and retinal supportive tissue to insult with the RPE cells subsequently invading the sensory retina

△ Results in a scotoma at threshold

△ Multiple causative factors that may indicate both stability (the pigment around a retinal break) or activity (the pigment on the dome of a malignant choroidal melanoma)

Management

△ Self-limiting, but must ascertain the cause of the retinal insult

△ Routine eye examinations are indicated if the cause of the RPE hyperplasia is determined to be benign and stable

△ A retinal consultation is indicated for conditions demonstrating activity

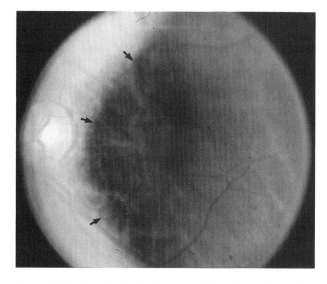

Figure 6–43. Example of a benign choroidal melanoma (nevus) totally occupying the posterior pole. The small arrows delineate the proximity to the optic nerve head.

tion. The list of causative factors for RPE hyperplasia is exhaustive. The practitioner must consider each presentation of RPE hyperplasia in an isolated manner when determining differential diagnosis.

Benign Choroidal Melanoma (Choroidal Nevus)

Introduction and Description. Benign choroidal melanoma (Figs. 6–42 and 6–43) is also known as a choroidal nevus and occurs in up to 30 percent of patients. The choroidal nevus or benign choroidal melanoma usually is a flat slate-gray lesion with indistinct margins usually 1 to 5 mm in size. These lesions may have overlying drusen (up to 80 percent) as well as other alterations in the RPE that are a result of poor vascular supply from the choriocapillaris. The overlying alterations of the RPE increase in prevalence and intensity with age. The reduced blood supply occurs as the result of the physical barrier created by the lesion. There also may be an associated serous sensory retinal detachment overlying the drusen. The benign choroidal melanoma is the result of accumulation of melanocytes within the choroid (Fig. 6–37). Some believe that this nevus may convert to malignancy, but the growth occurring in 5 to 10 percent of lesions over a 5-year period should not be considered an absolute sign of conversion to malignancy. Assuming that it is a relatively small lesion, under 5 DD, one can be relatively well assured that it is benign and nonprogressive. Ninety-five percent of benign choroidal melanomas are under 2 DD in size. **See color plate 98.**

Table 6–2 will help make the differential diagnosis and suggest a decision as to the proper management of this condition. It is, however, prudent to at least document the size of the lesion, preferably with photography, and to follow the patient on a routine basis to assure that there is no progression toward malignancy. It has been documented that a choroidal nevus not only changes at the onset of pregnancy, but may progress to malignancy. If there is any indication of the possibility of malignancy, a consultation with a retinal specialist

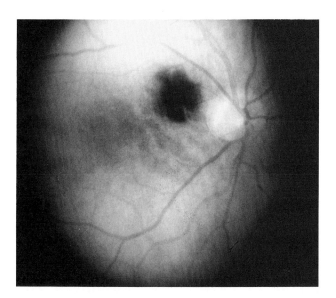

Figure 6–42. Example of a one-disc diameter benign choroidal melanoma (nevus) near the optic nerve head.

**TABLE 6–2. DIFFERENTIAL DIAGNOSIS OF
MALIGNANT CHOROIDAL MELANOMA**

Size (DD)	Associated Findings	Classification
0.5–2	None	Benign
2–5	Elevated lesion, overlying drusen, subretinal fluid	Suspicious—consider ultrasound, fluorescein angiography; photodocument, recall 6 months
5 or larger	Elevated lesion, overlying drusen, overlying orange pigmentation, photopsia, large feeder vessels	Malignant until proven otherwise

trained in ocular oncology is indicated. Should a serous elevation be associated with the benign choroidal melanoma and be threatening to vision, a retinal consultation for possible photocoagulative intervention is indicated. Choroidal neovascular membranes may also occur in the area of the nevus, necessitating the consideration for photocoagulative intervention. Photocoagulative intervention in cases of neovascular membranes associated with nevi follows the same guidelines as for any other neovascular situation.

Figure 6–37 gives a schematic representation of retinal epithelial hyperplasia, benign choroidal melanoma, RPE defects, and congenital hypertrophy of the RPE. The practitioner can see that an RPE hyperplasia presents because there is true proliferation of the RPE, which appears as a blackish lesion within the retina. The benign choroidal melanoma presents because of the melanocytes within the choroid and appears grayish because it is filtered by the RPE and sensory retina. The RPE window defect appears white because of the absence of melanin within the RPE. The congenital hypertrophy of the RPE presents as a grayish lesion because of swelling of the RPE cells.

Management. Management of benign choroidal melanomas varies considerably with the clinical presentation. All benign choroidal melanomas should be recorded in the chart with either a drawing of the size and location or a photodocumentation of the lesion. Photocoagulation by a qualified retinal specialist may be of value in the management of associated serous retinal elevations and in situations where neovascular membranes develop in zones of benign choroidal melanomas.

Malignant Choroidal Melanoma

Introduction and Description. Malignant choroidal melanoma is the most common primary ocular malignancy with peak incidence in the 60s. There are approximately 1500 new cases reported each year in the

Benign Choroidal Melanoma (Choroidal Nevus)

Characteristics

△ Flat, slate-gray lesions of variable size (usually 1 to 5 mm) with indistinct margins

△ May have overlying drusen as well as other RPE changes that have a tendency to increase in prevalence and intensity with age

△ Isolated sensory retinal detachment may occur near the lesion associated with leakage through the altered RPE–Bruch's membrane network

△ Neovascular membranes may occur near or within the nevus associated with the altered RPE–Bruch's membrane network

△ The lesion represents an accumulation of melanocytes in choroid

△ 5 to 10 percent of the lesions grow without conversion to malignancy

△ Both growth and conversion to malignancy may occur with the onset of pregnancy

Management

△ Up to 2 DD—document and follow

△ 2 DD to 5 DD—suspicious. Consider special tests and careful follow-up

△ Over 5 DD—assume malignancy until proven otherwise

△ Always document with either a drawing or a photograph

△ If serous elevations or choroidal neovascular membranes develop in the area of the lesion, ask for a retinal consultation for the possibility of photocoagulative intervention

△ Routine eye examinations with provision of the best prescription are indicated with patient education

United States. Unfortunately, the presentation of the lesion can occur at any point in time, even during pregnancy. The primary lesion is most prevalent in lightly pigmented individuals with only a rare occurrence in blacks. Often the patient is asymptomatic but blurred vision, visual field defects, floaters, or pain may be the presenting symptoms. Not only can the condition create loss of vision, but choroidal melanoma is known to metastasize with high mortality.

Malignant choroidal melanoma can assume many different clinical appearances (Figs. 6–44 and 6–45). More often the lesion appears as a pigmented mottled elevated lesion varying from whitish to a grayish-green color. The melanoma is usually confined to the choroidal or subretinal space. The lesion is usually over 10 DD when it is discovered. The Collaborative Ocular Melanoma Study classifies choroidal melanomas according to the size of the lesion (Table 6–3).

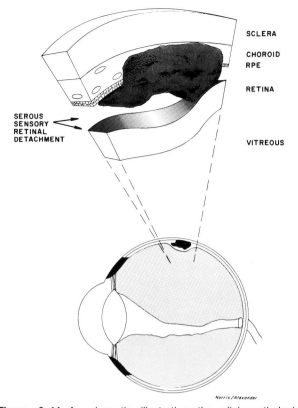

Figure 6–44. A schematic illustrating the clinicopathologic changes associated with the development of a malignant choroidal melanoma.

TABLE 6–3. COLLABORATIVE OCULAR MELANOMA STUDY CLASSIFICATION SYSTEM

Tumor Type	Largest Basal Diameter (mm)	Height (mm)
Small	5 or less	1–3
Medium	5–16	4–8
Large	Over 16	Over 8

The mottling associated with the lesion may be orange due to lipofuscin deposition on the surface of the lesion or may be drusen. There may be an accompanying RPE hyperplasia on the surface of the tumor. This RPE hyperplasia is known as melanoma bodies, and is pathognomonic of a malignancy. After the lesion breaks through Bruch's membrane, it may be lobular in nature, taking on the formation of a collar button. There is often an associated serous retinal elevation over the top of the malignancy. This is due to the leaking of fluid through the compromised RPE–Bruch's membrane barrier. Other variations include fibrous metaplasia, cystoid degeneration, retinoschisis, exudative retinal detachment, vitreous hemorrhage, extrascleral tumor presentation, and vitreous seeding of the tumor.

The malignant choroidal melanoma originates in the choroid as malignant melanocytes but may extend well into the vitreous. The extent of involvement is totally dependent upon the elapsed time of the development of the lesion. The histologic classification is spindle-cell nevus, spindle-cell melanoma, mixed-cell melanoma, and necrotic melanoma. The histologic classification is important to the survival prognosis but is, unfortunately, only attainable through surgical removal.

The prognosis is relatively poor in malignant choroidal melanomas. The prognosis is closely related to the type of tumor cell, the size of the tumor at presentation, and is somewhat dependent on the type of intervention chosen. Five-year survival for a spindle-cell nevus is 100 percent, for a spindle-cell melanoma 97 percent, and for a mixed-cell melanoma 87 percent. Survival percentages decrease with advancing years and drop to 45 percent for mixed-cell over a 15-year period. The five-year survival rate for pregnant women with posterior uveal melanomas is 71 percent. Tumors under 10 mm have a 19 percent 10-year death rate, tumors 11 to 15 mm a 40 percent 10-year death rate, and tumors over 15 mm a 65 percent death rate. There is a potential spread to the liver, lungs, bone, lymph nodes, gastrointestinal tract, subcutaneous tissues, and brain. With documented metastasis, the 10-year death rate is 100 percent. Metastases usually occur within 4 years of enucleation. A diffuse growth pattern and extrascleral extension are also poor prognostic signs. There appears

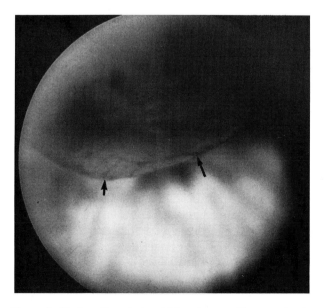

Figure 6–45. A malignant choroidal melanoma. The grossly elevated edge is demarcated by the black arrows.

Malignant Choroidal Melanoma

Characteristics

△ Most common primary ocular malignancy with peak incidence in the 60s

△ Approximately 1500 new cases per year in the United States

△ Must watch for conversion of benign melanomas during pregnancy

△ Patient is usually asymptomatic but may experience visual symptoms

△ Usually over 10 DD when discovered; the larger the tumor the poorer the local and systemic metastatic prognosis

△ Mottled, elevated lesion varying from whitish to gray-green color

△ Lobullar or collar-button appearance after breaking through Bruch's membrane

△ Overlying orange lipofuscin, melanoma bodies, and serous sensory retinal detachment may occur as well as other isolated signs

△ Accumulation of malignant melanocytes in the choroid

△ B-scan ultrasonography, fluorescein angiography, and radioactive uptake studies may assist in the diagnosis

Management

△ Rule out metastases, especially to the liver (95 percent of cases of metastases)

    0.5 to 3.5 percent have metastases at presentation

△ Arrange consultation with a retinal specialist trained and skilled in the management of ocular malignancies

    Possible observation without intervention in small tumors

    Possible intervention with:

        Photocoagulation

        Localized radiotherapy

        External beam irradiation

        Local surgical excision

        Enucleation

△ Metastases carry a very poor prognosis, with average survival times of 2 months untreated and 5 months treated

△ Continue to provide the best possible prescription and follow for the development of other ocular conditions that may develop secondary to management techniques

to be the possibility of determining tendencies for uveal melanomas by assessment of chromosomal abnormalities but the clinical development is in its infancy.

Diagnostic techniques that are of value in the determination of the differential diagnosis include fluorescein angiography, ultrasonography, and ra-

dioactive phosphorus uptake. The internal tumor vascularity is very apparent on fluorescein angiography. On B-scan ultrasonography there is a solid mass with a smooth anterior surface, an acoustic hollowing (echo free), and an associated orbital shadowing from the tumor mass. Fine-needle aspiration biopsy may be effective in diagnosing some cases.

Management. Proper management of a malignant choroidal melanoma would include differential diagnosis of the lesion and the performance of laboratory studies to determine whether or not there have been metastases of the lesion. These studies include carcinoembryonic antigen (CEA), liver studies, brain scans, and chest radiographs.

Localized management of the malignant melanoma is attempted to retain vision, preserve the globe, and attempt to minimize metastases. Currently there are several methods of ocular management of malignant choroidal melanomas. The size of the tumor again becomes an important factor. Small or medium-sized tumors exhibiting signs of slow growth in the elderly, ill, or one-eyed patients are often followed closely without intervention. Medium-sized tumors are often subjected to radioactive plaque radiotherapy, whereas larger tumors are treated by external beam radiation. Small posterior pole tumors less than 10 mm in diameter and less than 3 mm high may be destroyed by photocoagulation applied over several visits. A tumor that has been treated adequately with photocoagulation will appear as a depressed scar with fibrotic scarification overlying the bare sclera and a flat pigmented area within. Unfortunately, even the "ideal" clinical picture does not ensure a cure of the tumor. Cryotherapy may also be used for small peripheral melanomas. Local resection of the tumor, exenteration, and enucleation are also options available for management of the tumor. There is the belief, however, that surgical removal of the globe may enhance metastasis, and this technique is usually reserved for tumors that are not treatable with other forms of therapy. Localized sclerouvectomy for ciliary body and choroidal tumors may preserve the globe but significant ocular complications may result.

Results of iodine 125 localized plaque radiation indicate a retention of acuity at 20/100 or better in 45 percent of patients, with a 4 to 18 percent localized recurrence and a mortality rate of 17 percent related to metastases. The localized effects of radiation include radiation retinopathy, cataract, and neovascular glaucoma.

Proton beam irradiation is reported to result in 20/200 vision or better in 60 percent of patients with death from metastasis at 14 to 20 percent. The 5-year probability of localized control of the tumor with proton beam is 97 percent. Regrowth of the tumor is strongly related to the development of metastases. Helium ion irradiation creates similar mortality rates of 13 to 16 percent from metastases.

In spite of the presence of metastases with all forms of radiation therapy, it still appears that 5-year survival time is better with radiotherapy than enucleation (this is arguable according to some studies). Within 2 to 5 years after enucleation, 40 to 70 percent of patients develop clinically detectable metastases. Once the tumor has metastasized, regardless of the treatment modality, the survival is 2 to 11 months after diagnosis of hepatic involvement (up to 95 percent of cases of metastasis). Treatment for the metastases improves the survival time from 2 to 5 months. Between 0.5 and 3.5 percent of patients with uveal melanoma have metastatic involvement at presentation.

Regardless of outcome, all suspect uveal melanomas deserve a consultation with a retinal oncology specialist with experience in the management of patients with this vision- and life-threatening condition.

Figure 6–44 shows that the lesion is space occupying and can cause an overlying serous sensory retinal detachment. It is important that any lesion that is large, elevated, and dark in the peripheral retina have specialized studies applied to it such as ultrasound, fluorescein angiography, and photography to ascertain whether or not the lesion is malignant. **See color plates 99 and 100.**

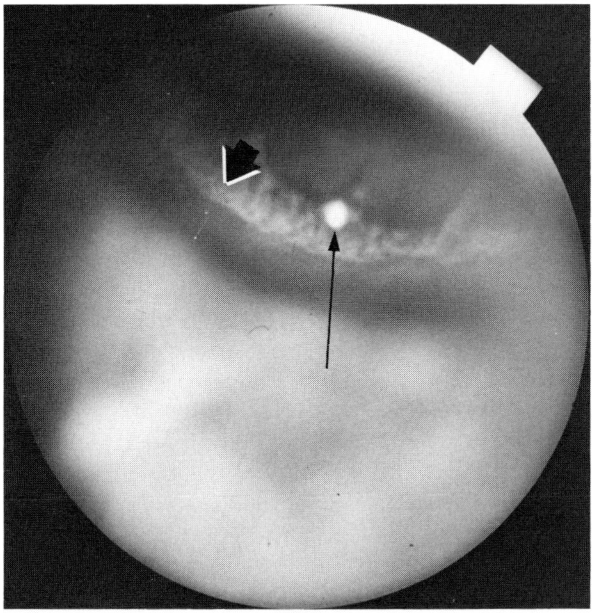

Figure 6–46. An oral pearl (*long arrow*) on an indenter in an area of cystoid degeneration (*short wide arrow*). (*Photo courtesy of W. Townsend.*)

Pearls

Oral Pearls

Characteristics

△ White spheres between base and tip of the dentate processes

△ Occur between RPE and Bruch's membrane, and are the histopathologic equivalent of retinal drusen

Management

△ Self-limiting and benign

△ Routine eye examinations

Oral Pearls

Introduction and Description. Oral pearls (Fig. 6–46) are also known as pearls of the ora serrata. These usually appear as single white spheres between the base and tip of the dentate processes. They occur between the RPE and Bruch's membrane, thus making them the histopathologic correlates to drusen in the retina of the posterior pole. Oral pearls occur in approximately 20 percent of the population. These are benign and typically show no progression whatsoever. In fact, these would be close to impossible to find in a routine eye examination unless scleral indentation were applied. **See color plate 93.**

Management. Management consists of routine eye examinations with no particular indication of predilection toward progression or development of retinal breaks or localized detachments.

Enclosed Oral Bays

Introduction and Description. The enclosed oral bay is a brownish depression surrounded by sensory

---

Pearls

Enclosed Oral Bays

Characteristics

△ Brown depression surrounded by sensory retina near ora—a discontinuity in the normal outline of the ora serrata

△ Perform scleral indentation to assess for breaks

△ Examine yearly if there is a retinal break at posterior edge of oral bay

Management

△ Educate patient regarding signs and symptoms of retinal detachment

△ If no retinal break, routine eye examinations are indicated with the provision of the best possible prescription

△ If associated retinal break or detachment, a consultation with a retinal specialist is indicated

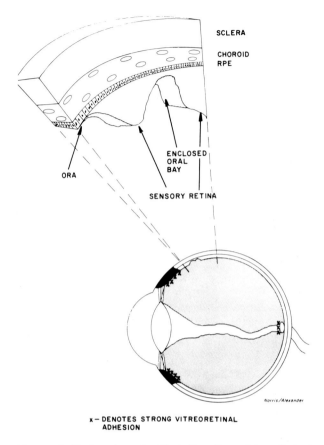

Figure 6–47. A schematic illustrating the clinicopathologic changes associated with an enclosed oral bay.

retina near the ora serrata. The enclosed oral bay is found in approximately 6 percent of the population. Enclosed oral bays are areas of nonpigmented ciliary epithelium of the pars plana surrounded by sensory retina. The schematic in Figure 6–47 demonstrates an enclosed oral bay with the surrounding of sensory retinal tissue. There is a 15 to 20 percent chance of associated retinal breaks at the posterior edge of the enclosed oral bay. These breaks rarely progress to retinal detachment and are best found with indentation.

Management. Yearly examinations, or a consultation with a retinal specialist (if a very conservative approach is desired), are indicated for the patient with an enclosed oral bay if there is an associated break. In addition, educate the patient regarding signs and symptoms of retinal detachment. Otherwise, routine eye examinations are the rule for patients with uncomplicated enclosed oral bays.

Retinal White Without Pressure (WWOP)

Introduction and Description. Retinal white without pressure (WWOP; Figs. 6–48 and 6–49) is a fairly common occurrence, having been found in 2.5 per-

cent of white and 23 percent of black individuals (it has been reported in up to 30 percent of the general population). WWOP has been estimated to occur in approximately 5 percent of eyes under the age of 20 years and in 66 percent of eyes over the age of 70 years. Retinal WWOP appears as an area of the retina that is translucent white to gray, often bounded posteriorly by a reddish-brown line. WWOP can be very dramatic in blacks, actually appearing thickened, and often convoluted or elevated. This elevation is actually an optical illusion, as the retina is flat when viewed with three-mirror lenses or scleral indentation. The translucent gray area often just fades toward the ora serrata and rarely extends posteriorly to the equator in whites but may extend posteriorly in blacks. WWOP may have scalloped borders (suggested to be a sign of possible progression), and has been noted to be migratory in nature. There may also be WWOP that surrounds an area of normal-appearing retina, and there does appear to be a direct association of increases in appearance with aging. WWOP occurs at a higher incidence in myopic pa-

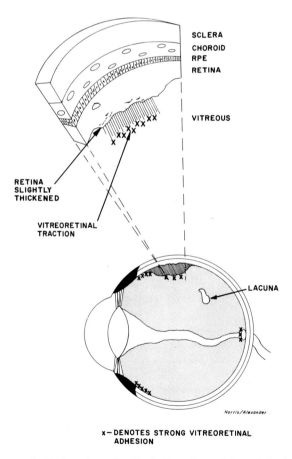

Figure 6–48. A schematic illustrating the clinicopathologic changes associated with WWOP.

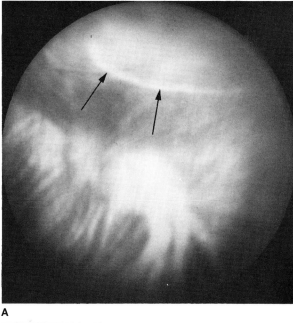

A

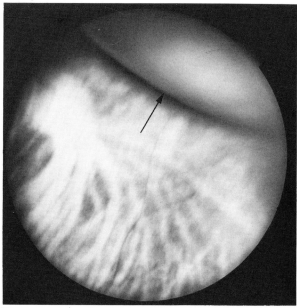

B

Figure 6–49. A. WWOP near a vortex vein without indentation. **B.** Same area under indentation. (*Photos courtesy of W. Townsend.*)

Retinal White Without Pressure

Characteristics

△ Area of translucent white to gray retina usually between the ora and equator bounded posteriorly by a reddish line

△ Variable reported incidence, but minimally 2.5 percent in whites and 23 percent in blacks; also more easily seen in blacks

△ May appear thickened but is not and may extend posteriorly to the equator in blacks

△ May be migratory

△ Higher incidence in black patients and myopic patients, with overall incidence increasing with age

△ Vitreoretinal traction causing disorganization of sensory retina

△ Often found at the borders of lattice degeneration and posterior staphylomas; associated with localized retinal detachments and PVD

△ May have associated traction retinal tears, which are most frequent at ages 40 to 50 years

△ Retinal dark without pressure is more common in the posterior pole and may be associated with sickle-cell disease

Management

△ Indent to rule out breaks

△ 6-month follow-up if any of the following associated factors leading to retinal tear development
  WWOP near lattice degeneration
  WWOP with scalloped borders
  WWOP with elevated traction membrane
  WWOP with progressive vitreous degeneration

△ If no associated risk factors, 12 to 24 month follow-up

△ Watch carefully for tears when there is an associated posterior vitreous detachment

△ Inform of the signs/symptoms of retinal detachment

△ Consultation with retinal specialist if there are signs or symptoms threatening retinal tears

△ Manage retinal white with pressure in the same manner

△ Consider the possibility of sickle-cell disease in retinal dark without pressure
  Ask about family history and consider ordering screening blood test (Sickledex)

tients and is reported as 10 times as high in black patients. There may be areas of WWOP seen surrounding lattice degeneration, at the borders of posterior staphylomas, associated with local retinal detachments, and in focal areas of the retina in posterior vitreous detachment. In these instances the argument for the vitreoretinal traction theory of the genesis of WWOP gains credence. WWOP may be circumferential and usually occurs bilaterally.

WWOP appears to represent an unusual vitreo-

retinal relationship that causes disorganization of the nerve fiber layer of the sensory retina even down to the RPE. Some clinicians think there may even be an associated development of retinal edema. The actual cause–effect relationship in WWOP is controversial.

Usually WWOP is associated with vitreous degeneration and PVD. There is, however, a relatively low incidence of retinal tears, considering this particular relationship. Horseshoe or linear retinal tears can develop along the posterior border of white with pressure or white without pressure, and these tears are associated with the traction of PVD. If retinal tears occur at the posterior border of retinal WWOP in patients in their 40s or 50s, there is a slight risk of the associated development of retinal detachment because of the coincident increase in the likelihood of vitreous liquefaction and detachment with an increase in age. **See color plate 101.**

Management. In the management of the patient with WWOP, it is important to consider factors that are contributory to the development of retinal breaks. These factors are listed in Table 6–4.

Patients with WWOP should be followed at 1- to 2-year intervals depending on the presence of associated risk factors. In general, WWOP is not a very ominous sign for the development of serious retinal problems. The patients should be reexamined every 6 months if the posterior borders of the WWOP are scalloped and there is extensive vitreous degeneration. As patients get into their 40s and 50s, there is also the increased risk of associated retinal breaks and detachment because of the increased incidence of vitreous liquefaction and detachment. The clinician must also take more precautions in patients with high myopia. It is necessary to make the patients aware of signs and symptoms of retinal detachment as well as to watch for breaks that may develop at the posterior border of the lesion. Scleral indentation should be used in patients at risk to rule out retinal breaks.

It should be noted in the patient exhibiting WWOP that the retina is thickened and that there is some associated cystic development. The most important aspect of this is the vitreoretinal traction that occurs with WWOP. This vitreoretinal traction is strongly implicated in the genesis of retinal tears and subsequent retinal detachments.

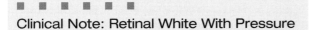

■ ■ ■ ■ ■ ■
Clinical Note: Retinal White With Pressure

White *with* pressure is an optical phenomenon of the retina similar to white without pressure. The retina appears translucent white to gray on scleral indentation, and is thought to be histologically similar to white without pressure. White with pressure has the same prognosis and management as white without pressure, yet white without pressure is considered by some to be the more severe form.

TABLE 6–4. FACTORS ASSOCIATED WITH RETINAL TEARS IN CASES OF WHITE WITHOUT PRESSURE

White without pressure along posterior margins of lattice degeneration

White without pressure with scalloped borders

Presence of an elevated tractional membrane adherent to the posterior margin of white without pressure

Progressive pathologic shrinkage of vitreous

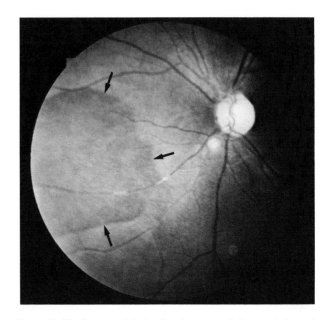

Figure 6–50. An area of dark without pressure in the posterior pole (*outlined by arrows*).

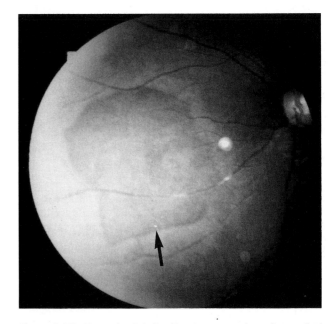

Figure 6–51. Example of dark without pressure (*arrow*), or retinal toast in the posterior pole.

Clinical Note: Retinal Dark Without Pressure

Dark without pressure (Figs. 6–50 and 6–51) appears as islands of homogeneous, flat, brown areas in the fundus of black patients. These areas may be migratory in nature, and typically occur near the posterior pole of the eye. The retinal change often looks like a piece of bread or toast. This is the opposite of what one would expect with WWOP, which has more of a tendency to occur between the equator and the ora. There appears to be no particular vitreous connection in dark without pressure, but there does appear to be a relationship to sickle-cell disease. Patients with dark without pressure should be considered as potential sickle-cell patients, and this diagnosis should be ruled out.

Pars Plana Cysts

Introduction and Description. Pars plana cysts (Fig. 6–52) are the histopathologic equivalent of a retinal detachment within the sensory retina. Pars plana cysts appear as ¼- to 3-DD cysts that are oval to oblong. Pars plana cysts usually have a smooth, rigid, semitransparent surface, and may have a small amount of pigment on the inner surface. The cavities are thought to contain hyaluronic acid similar to that contained in a retinoschisis. Pars plana cysts may extend from the

SCLERA
CHOROID
PIGMENTED EPITHELIUM
SENSORY RETINA
ORA
VITREOUS
NON-PIGMENTED EPITHELIUM
FILLED WITH HYALURONIC ACID

Norris/Alexander

x – DENOTES STRONG VITREORETINAL ADHESIONS

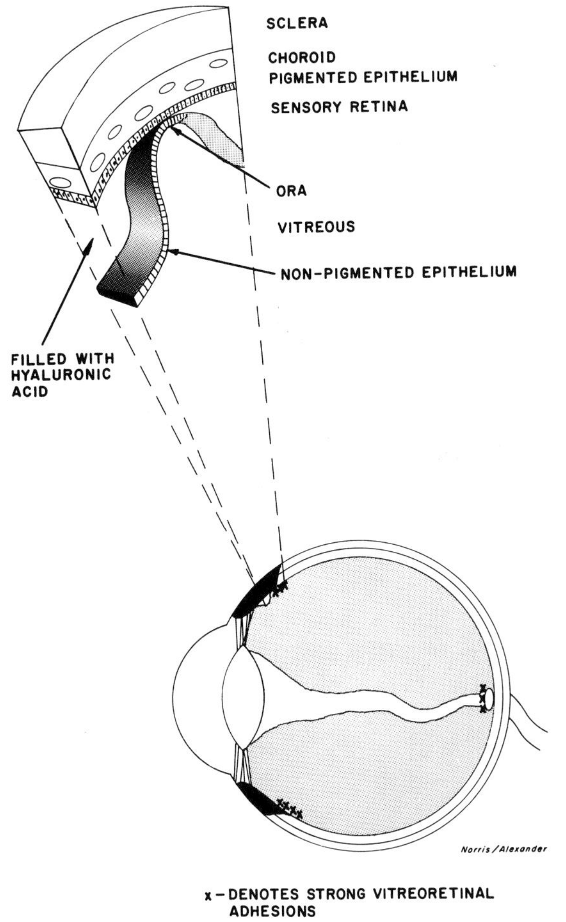

Figure 6–52. A schematic illustrating the clinicopathology of a pars plana cyst.

Pearls

Pars Plana Cysts

Characteristics

△ One-fourth to 3-DD cysts that are oval, occurring from the ora to the ciliary processes

△ Transparent, taut, smooth surfaces

△ Thought to be filled with hyaluronic acid similar to retinoschisis

△ Separation of nonpigmented and pigmented epithelium of the pars plana—histopathologic equivalent of retinal detachment

△ Often associated with a traumatic retinal detachment and posterior uveitis, and reported to be associated with multiple myeloma

△ Important to differentiate from macrocystic development associated with retinal (oral) dialysis

Management

△ Pars plana cysts are self-limiting and benign, assuming no other complications that may lend to retinal detachment such as basal vitreous detachment

△ Routine eye examinations and patient education are indicated

△ If there is the possibility of macrocysts, a dialysis is likely, necessitating a retinal consultation

ora serrata to the ciliary processes. According to various studies, these cysts are present in 3 to 18 percent of all patients. Because of the location, it is obvious that pars plana cysts are seen best with scleral indentation.

Pars plana cysts are an acquired separation of the nonpigmented epithelium from the pigmented epithelium of the pars plana. It is important to remember that the sensory retina becomes nonpigmented epithelium at the pars plana, so that this condition is the histopathologic equivalent of a retinal detachment.

Pars plana cysts are often associated with traumatic retinal detachment and posterior uveitis, and have been reported with multiple myeloma. In and of themselves, pars plana cysts are relatively benign.

It is important to distinguish pars plana cysts from the macrocysts that often present up to 8 DD in size associated with oral dialysis. The macrocysts become an important diagnostic tool in the detection of the elusive retinal dialysis.

Management. No treatment is indicated in isolated pars plana cysts, assuming that all other retinal problems such as tears have been ruled out. Routine eye examinations are indicated.

Macrocysts associated with retinal dialysis, on the other hand, are important because dialysis inevitably results in an insidious development of retinal detachment.

Figure 6–52 demonstrates the actual splitting of the nonpigmented epithelium from the pigmented epithelium. This simulates a retinal detachment but has none of its implications.

PERIPHERAL RETINAL CHANGES THAT MAY POSE A THREAT TO VISION

Vitreoretinal Traction Tufts

Introduction and Description. Vitreoretinal traction tufts (Figs. 6–53 to 6–55) are also known as retinal tufts or granular tissue. Vitreoretinal tufts appear as grayish-white pieces of tissue at the vitreoretinal interface usually located between the equator and the ora serrata. Tufts occur more often nasally and have the tendency to accumulate within the vitreous base.

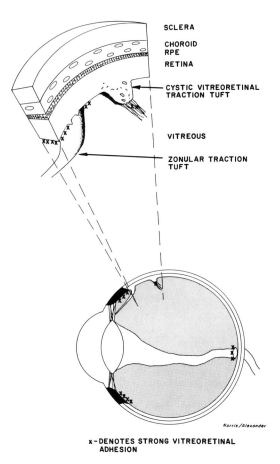

Figure 6–53. A schematic illustrating the clinicopathology of vitreoretinal traction tufts.

Pearls

Vitreoretinal Traction Tufts

Characteristics

△ Grayish white tufts of tissue at the vitreoretinal interface between the equator and ora

△ Often have RPE hyperplasia near or within the traction tuft

△ Often nasal within the vitreous base

△ Noncystic tufts occur in 72 percent of population, while cystic tufts occur in 5 percent and zonular traction tufts in 15 percent of population

△ Scleral indentation may be needed to assess for retinal breaks

△ Retinal breaks may occur associated with vitreous liquefaction, syneresis, or vitreous detachment

Management

△ Advise on signs/symptoms of retinal detachment

△ Arrange a consultation with a retinal specialist when retinal breaks occur

△ Monitor according to presence of other potentiators of retinal detachment

△ Advise on importance of the appearance of phosphenes

△ Routine examinations with the provision of the best possible correction are indicated

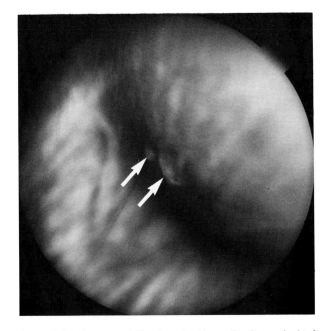

Figure 6–54. Arrows pointing to a double cystic vitreoretinal tuft on indentation. (*Photo courtesy of W. Townsend.*)

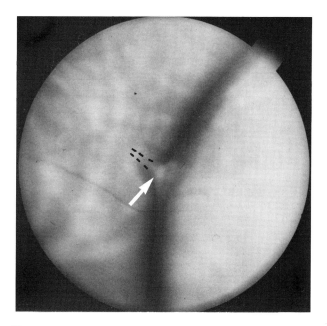

Figure 6–55. A zonular traction tuft on indentation. The dotted lines follow the traction. (*Photo courtesy of W. Townsend.*)

There is by definition a connection to the vitreous body, and as such tufts have tendencies toward changes as the vitreous body liquefies and shrinks. The tufts are often identifiable by the associated occurrence of RPE hyperplasia at or near the traction point. Noncystic vitreoretinal tufts occur in about 72 percent of the population, with about a 50 percent chance of bilaterality. In spite of the high incidence, the noncystic tufts are often not seen in the clinical setting. Cystic tufts, on the other hand, are larger and only occur in about 5 to 7 percent of the population, with a rare incidence of bilaterality. Zonular traction tufts run anterior into the vitreous with a triangular base and occur in about 15 percent of the population, with a low incidence of bilaterality. **See color plate 102.** Again, RPE hyperplasia is a common occurrence in these variations of vitreoretinal adhesions.

Vitreoretinal tufts are considered to be accumulations of proliferated glial cells on the surface of the retina, causing retinal degeneration. The tufts are often benign but may be associated with retinal tears when vitreous liquefaction and detachment do occur. Approximately 7 percent of retinal detachments in one report were associated with cystic retinal traction tufts. Cystic retinal traction tufts represent a 1 percent chance of association with a retinal detachment.

Management. The management of vitreoretinal tufts consists of monitoring tufts when they are associated with other potentiators of retinal detachment. Indentation may be needed to assess for retinal breaks. The clinician must realize the importance of the vitreoretinal adhesion in the genesis of a retinal de-

tachment, as a tug on a vitreoretinal tuft during a PVD may precipitate a retinal break. The clinician must make the patient aware of signs and symptoms of retinal detachment and also that a localized phosphene associated with a stressed vitreoretinal tuft may be a sign of an impending retinal tear. Special observation must be made during an evolving PVD. Retinal breaks may need photocoagulation or cryotherapy. A retinal consultation is advised at the first sign of a retinal break associated with cystic retinal traction tufts. Prophylaxis is not indicated in virtually all cases of vitreoretinal traction tufts. The only exception may be the consideration of the fellow eye to a retinal detachment.

Figure 6–53 illustrates that the zonular traction tufts actually run forward toward the ciliary body process and are often attached to the zonules of the crystalline lens. There is also a cystic vitreoretinal traction tuft present in this figure. It can be seen from the figure that should a PVD occur with the strong vitreoretinal traction tuft connections, there is a potential for a tear at the site of the tuft.

Meridional Fold or Complex

Introduction and Description. Meridional folds (Figs. 6–56 and 6–57) are elevated retinal tissue redundancies that develop in the area of the ora serrata. **See color plate 94.** The folds may extend up to 4 DD posteriorly toward the equator and are perpendicular

---

Pearls

Meridional Folds

Characteristics

△ 0.5- to 4-DD grayish elevated tissue perpendicular to the ora (run radial to the ora serrata)
△ Occur in about 25 percent of the population
△ Occur most frequently in the superior nasal quadrant
△ Associated vitreoretinal traction may produce posterior border tears
△ Meridional complexes in about 15 percent of population, often associated with peripheral retinal excavations posterior to the complex
△ Peripheral retinal excavations are reddish brown and may have an associated RPE hyperplasia surrounding them

Management

△ Routine 12- to 24-month follow-up examinations assessing carefully for the development of retinal breaks
△ Patient education as to signs and symptoms of retinal detachment is in order as necessary
△ Arrange consultation with a retinal specialist for retinal breaks that are found

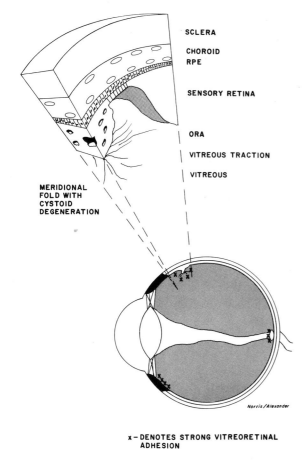

x – DENOTES STRONG VITREORETINAL ADHESION

Figure 6–56. A schematic illustrating the clinicopathology of a meridional fold.

(run radial) to the ora serrata. They appear grayish white and are best seen with scleral indentation. Meridional folds occur in about 25 percent of the population, with a 50 percent incidence of bilaterality. Meridional folds occur in males more frequently than in females. Multiple folds may present. Folds occur most often in the superior nasal quadrant, originating most frequently at dentate processes. Vitreoretinal traction may be present, running both anteriorly and posteriorly. Meridional folds are often associated with enclosed oral bays.

Meridional folds are altered retinal tissue composed of a proliferation of glial cells. The inner layer of the retina in these cases is degenerated and may have cystic-like changes. Retinal breaks may occur at the posterior edge of the fold secondary to traction, but there is only a rare retinal detachment secondary to these folds.

Figure 6–56 demonstrates the genesis of a meridional fold with associated cystoid degeneration. It can be seen that meridional folds do occur at the ora serrata and set up potential for a retinal tear because of compromised retina as well as vitreous traction occurring in this area.

Management. Management of patients with meridional folds consists of routine 12- to 24-month follow-up examinations with assessment for retinal breaks. It is also important to make the patient aware of signs and symptoms of retinal detachment. Meridional folds only rarely predispose to retinal breaks and/or detachment. As a result, prophylactic treatment is not indicated. A retinal consultation is indicated for a retinal break or an associated retinal detachment.

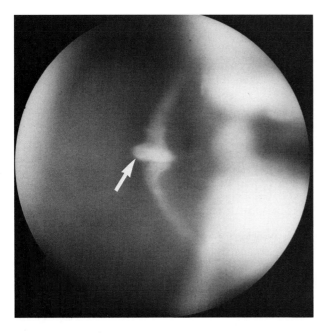

Figure 6–57. A meridional fold (*arrow*). (*Photo courtesy of W. Townsend.*)

■ ■ ■ ■ ■ ■

Clinical Note: Meridional Complex

A meridional complex is an enlarged dentate and ciliary process aligned in the same meridian with a meridional fold extending from the dentate to the ciliary process. A peripheral retinal excavation may be located posterior to the complex. A peripheral retinal excavation is an area of thinned retina that is perpendicular to the ora and can occur as an isolated incident in 10 percent of the population. An excavation can mimic a retinal hole and must be indented to properly differentiate. A peripheral retinal excavation may assume a reddish-brown coloration and may be surrounded by RPE hyperplasia. Meridional complexes occur most commonly in the superior nasal quadrant in approximately 15 percent of the population. Because of the compromise of the retina—that is, the retinal excavation—it is important to realize that there is potential for the development of a retinal tear in these particular conditions.

Degenerative Retinoschisis (RS)

Introduction and Description. Degenerative retinoschisis (RS) is usually a bilateral (38 to 82 percent of cases) condition with no particular predilection for sex. The condition is relatively rare, occurring in 1.5 to 7 percent of persons over the age of 40 years. The degeneration occurs most frequently in the inferior temporal quadrant, with a high percentage (over 70 percent) of the lesions attaining postequatorial borders. Retinoschisis is most often asymptomatic, but will show as an absolute scotoma on field testing. It appears that a very low percentage (under 10 percent) of RS lesions demonstrate progression, expansion, development of retinal breaks outside of the schisis, or progression toward retinal detachment. RS may develop in previously uninvolved areas of retina in an eye with retinoschisis.

See color plates 103 and 104. Two forms of degenerative RS have been described, flat (typical) and bullous (reticular). Typical, or flat, RS is believed to represent an advanced form of cystoid degeneration. Flat RS is usually confined to an area anterior to the equator and only rarely has associated retinal holes. The inner layer of a flat RS is typically smooth, thin, and has a beaten metallic appearance. The pathologic correlate of the typical retinoschisis is a splitting of the retina at the outer plexiform layer. The outer retinal layers are usually well preserved (Fig. 6–58).

Reticular or bullous RS appears as a thin, transparent, ballooning forward of retinal tissue most often in the inferior temporal quadrant. The surface is very taut and typically does not move with eye movements. This is a direct contrast with rhegmatogenous retinal detachment that undulates freely with eye movements. There is about a 70 percent incidence of "snowflakes" or whitish bodies deposited on the surface of the reticular RS. There is also an association with sclerotic or white-appearing vessels on the surface of the schisis, which gives the appearance of the

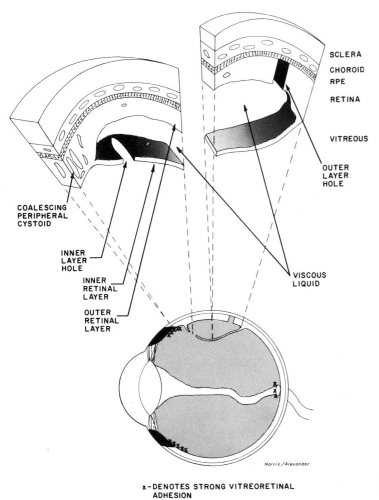

x–DENOTES STRONG VITREORETINAL
ADHESION

Figure 6–58. A schematic illustrating the clinicopathology of acquired RS.

Pearls

Degenerative Retinoschisis

Characteristics

△ Usually bilateral (38 to 82 percent) with increased incidence with aging

△ Appears most often in inferior temporal quadrant, with over 70 percent attaining postequatorial borders

△ Usually asymptomatic but shows as a scotoma on threshold visual field testing

△ Under 10 percent of degenerative retinoschisis demonstrates progression, expansion, development of retinal breaks outside of the schisis, or development of associated retinal detachment

△ Flat RS or typical RS is usually confined to area anterior to equator and is nonthreatening to vision
   Pathologic correlate is splitting of the retina at the outer plexiform layer

△ Bullous or reticular RS
   Taut ballooning of tissue
   70 percent incidence of "snowflake" bodies on surface
   Reticular (honeycomb) surface and dimmed choroidal detail
   May have clear inner-layer breaks; small, pink, outer-layer breaks (23 percent of cases)
   Sclerotic vessels on the surface give the reticular appearance
   May have associated hemorrhage at the edge of the cavity, hemorrhage into the cavity, vitreous hemorrhage, and peripheral neovascularization
   Pathologic correlate is splitting of the nerve fiber layer
   Cavity thought to be filled with hyaluronic acid
   33 percent have associated retinal detachments usually limited to the area of the schisis

△ Pigmented demarcation line strongly suggestive of schisis detachment

△ 60 percent have associated vitreous liquefaction

△ 25 percent of patients have breaks in at least one layer, with breaks in both layers in 40 percent of those patients

△ Incidence of asymptomatic localized retinal detachment is 6 percent, while the incidence of symptomatic detachment is 0.5 percent

△ 13.5 percent of patients show progression

Management

△ Keep in mind that a retinal detachment can develop

△ If RS without breaks, observe every 12 months for progression and educate patient as to signs/symptoms of retinal detachment
   A 60-degree visual field test should be part of the follow-up management of the patient with reticular retinoschisis

△ If RS with progression that is threatening vision, consult with a retinal specialist—possibility of photocoagulative intervention

△ If RS with inner-layer break anterior to the equator, observe every 6 months, and educate patient as to signs/symptoms of retinal detachment

△ If RS with demonstrable outer layer breaks, ask for a retinal consultation

△ If RS with inner and outer layer breaks, ask for a retinal consultation

△ If RS with an associated progressive retinal detachment, ask for a retinal consultation

△ If RS scheduled for intraocular operative procedure such as lensectomy or YAG capsulotomy, ask for a retinal consultation prior to the procedure

△ Provision of the best correction and patient education is critical in the care of the patient

reticular pattern. With indirect types of illumination, the inner and outer layers of the RS may take on a honeycomb appearance, which helps significantly in the differential diagnosis from retinal detachment. The posterior leading edge of an RS may appear serrated but usually does not have a pigmented line of demarcation. The presence of a pigmented demarcation line is suggestive of the presence of a secondary detachment of the outer schisis layer, which has been stationary long enough to produce the change (typically considered at 3 months). There is always an area of cystoid degeneration between RS and the ora serrata. This zone of cystoid may not present in cases of retinal detachment, which helps in the differentiation of the two situations. With reticular RS there are visible choroidal features, yet they are dim. This is an important differential diagnosis from retinal detachment, in

which choroidal features are significantly compromised.

RS may develop breaks in the inner layer of the schisis, which are oval and clear. Retinal breaks in the outer layers of a reticular RS are present in about 23 percent of cases, and are small and pink with rolled edges. Some clinicians refer to a group of small outer-layer breaks as frog's eggs, because of the appearance and color. These breaks usually occur from the center to the posterior portion of the RS. A hemorrhage may occur at the edge of an RS or actually may bleed into the schisis cavity with a layered appearance. Vitreous hemorrhage and peripheral neovascularization have also been reported associated with degenerative retinoschisis. Both the outer and inner layers of a reticular retinoschisis have a propensity to form holes, which may lead to the development of rhegmatoge-

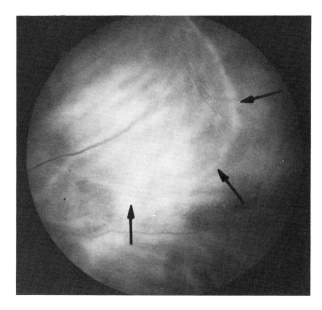

Figure 6–59. The arrows outline a zone of acquired RS.

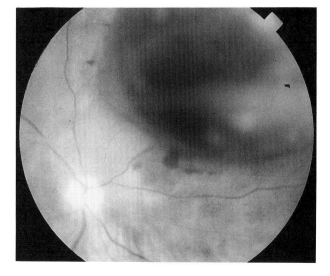

Figure 6–60. A retinal detachment with an overlying retinoschisis. The vessel tear associated with the retinal detachment bled into the schisis cavity.

nous retinal detachment (Figs. 6–59 to 6–61). The pathologic correlate of a reticular schisis is a splitting of the retina in the nerve fiber layer, resulting in a very thin inner retinal layer. The thin layer may make the reticular schisis more difficult to identify in the clinical setting.

The cavity of the retinoschisis is thought to be filled with hyaluronic acid, which is typically very viscous. This viscous fluid is responsible for making the RS so taut. The viscous fluid is also the reason that the RS does not undulate as does a typical retinal detachment. The cavity of a retinal detachment is filled with liquefied vitreous, which is not nearly as viscous as hyaluronic acid.

Sixty percent of patients with RS have vitreous liquefaction. Over 25 percent of patients with RS have a break in at least one layer of the schisis and 40 percent of those patients have breaks in both layers. Approximately 33 percent of patients with bullous retinoschisis have associated retinal detachments usually limited to the area of the schisis. This detachment is often identifiable by the associated presence of RPE hyperplasia. The incidence of a localized asymptomatic RS retinal detachment is 6 percent, whereas the expected incidence of a symptomatic RS retinal detachment is 0.5 percent. Visual field defects are present secondary to the RS, but typically do not become evident until the RS progresses toward the posterior pole. Progression of an RS is very rare, with only about 13.5 percent of patients showing progression. If progression does occur, it is both circular in nature and moves toward the posterior pole. If a vitreous detachment occurs, progress usually stops because the traction on the schisis is actually relieved. Flashes and

floaters can occur associated with the vitreous traction of an RS. As the schisis progresses toward the posterior pole there may be an associated cystoid maculopathy.

Management. In the management of RS it is important to note that approximately 6 percent of patients with RS develop asymptomatic retinal detachment. It should also be noted that some cases of retinoschisis may actually regress. In spite of the overwhelming support of the minimal risk of detachment and progression in the literature, the author has seen a number of retinal detachments secondary to retinoschisis as well as progression of the schisis toward the poste-

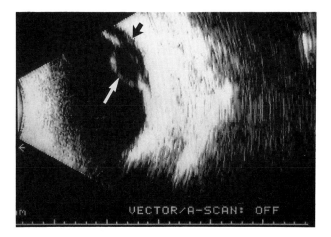

Figure 6–61. B-scan of the retinal detachment (*black arrow*) with the overlying blister of the retinoschisis (*white arrow*) shown in Figure 6–60.

rior pole in a number of patients. This author is not particularly comfortable with retinoschisis and takes a very conservative management approach with these patients. A false sense of security associated with schises can result in devastating visual results. The importance of following specific guidelines in the management of patients with RS cannot be overemphasized. The following guidelines represent a very conservative approach; as the clinician becomes more comfortable with managing retinoschisis, the patient with some of the following changes may be followed within the primary care setting.

1. A patient with an RS without breaks should be observed annually for progression. He or she also should be made aware of the signs and symptoms of progression of RS as well as the signs and symptoms of retinal detachment. A 60-degree visual field should be part of the routine management of the patient with a reticular retinoschisis.
2. A patient with RS that is progressing and that is threatening vision deserves a retinal consultation in spite of reports suggesting a very low incidence of vision loss even with progression. In these instances, photocoagulation of the progressing border or of the entire schisis may result in flattening of the RS in about 50 percent of these cases. This type of management is, however, very controversial.
3. A patient with RS with an inner-layer break anterior to the equator should be observed semiannually, as there is no particular potential to allow liquefied vitreous under the retina. Again, this patient should be made aware of the signs and symptoms of progression of retinoschisis as well as the signs and symptoms of retinal detachment.
4. A patient with retinoschisis with outer-layer breaks should be referred to a retinal specialist. Although the prevalence of retinal detachment in these cases is variable, there is some controversy as to whether or not these patients should be treated. It is well known that the viscous RS fluid usually does not leak in underneath the retina, but it must be remembered that it may and there may be liquefied vitreous lurking around. Where there is a controversy it is best to take the conservative approach to the management of these patients and to ask for a consultation with a retinal specialist.
5. If there is a patient with RS with outer- and inner-layer breaks, this is an indication for immediate consultation with a retinal specialist even though progression to a detachment is not inevitable.
6. A patient with RS with an associated progressive retinal detachment (schisis detachment) deserves a retinal consultation for treatment with photocoagulation, cryotherapy, and/or possible scleral buck-

ling. This is the only absolute indication for intervention.
7. A patient with a traction RS deserves a retinal consultation for proper management.
8. Any patient with RS scheduled for an intraocular procedure such as cataract extraction or YAG capsulotomy deserves a retinal consultation prior to the surgical procedure.

Figure 6–58, degenerative bullous RS, demonstrates the actual splitting of the retinal tissue with viscous fluid in the resultant cavity. The schematic also demonstrates the presence of an inner-layer and outer-layer retinal hole.

Lattice Degeneration

Introduction and Description. Lattice degeneration (Figs. 6–62 to 6–64) is also known as equatorial or circumferential retinal degeneration or perivascular lattice degeneration (radial lattice). Lattice degeneration affects the inner retinal layers appearing as a demarcated area of retinal atrophy with a reported tendency toward retinal breaks. Lattice degeneration often appears in young patients, usually reaching maximum incidence by the 20s, after which new lesions occur in less than 1 percent of affected patients. Lattice degeneration is typically found in 6 to 10 percent of the general population and occurs bilaterally in approximately 50 percent of eyes. There is the suggestion that there is an hereditary aspect to some cases of lattice degeneration, but the precise nature of inheritance is very difficult to interpret. **See color plate 105.**

Lattice degeneration occurs most frequently in

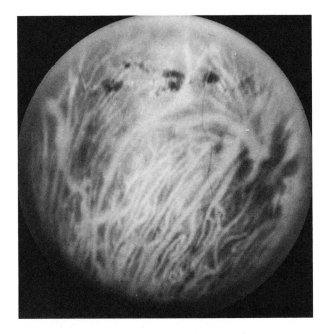

Figure 6–62. A typical presentation of lattice degeneration.

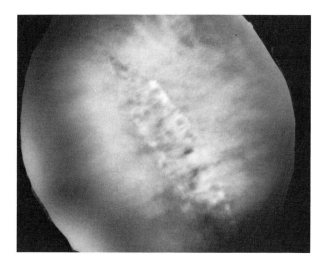

Figure 6–63. A variation of lattice degeneration known as snail-track degeneration.

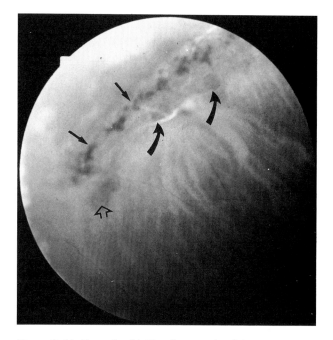

Figure 6–64. Example of lattice degeneration (*black arrows*) in a circumferential pattern. The curved black arrows point to a tear at the posterior border of the lattice and the open arrow points to an associated retinal bleed.

the superior and inferior retina (usually 11 to 1 o'clock and 5 to 7 o'clock positions), is usually 1 to 4 DD in length, and ½ to 2 DD in width. The presentation is usually discontinuous but some more advanced cases show a continuous single or multiple row of lesions throughout the retinal periphery. About 7 percent of lattice lesions are radial and are usually associated with larger retinal vessels (perivascular lattice; Fig. 6–65). The more posterior the lesion occurs, the wider the lesion. There is associated RPE hyperplasia in about 80 percent of the lesions, and tiny glistening yellowish flecks occur in about 80 percent of these lesions as well. The sclerosis of the white vessels, or fishboning, often attributed to these lesions increases in frequency with age, but is thought to occur in only about 10 to 12 percent of lesions. If new fishboning occurs, it is typically in patients over age 35 years and occurs in the superior quadrant lesions. White without pressure may also occur along the borders of the lesions, with a lacunae of liquefied vitreous overlying the lesion. Chorioretinal atrophy occurs quite frequently inside the borders of the lesions. Atrophic holes occur in the base of about 18 percent (14 to 32 percent) of lattice lesions and are usually not associated with the development of retinal detachment.

The various stages that are often associated with the development of lattice degeneration follow. It is important to remember that lattice degeneration usually does not increase in prevalence with age but does increase in severity of clinical presentation.

Stage 1: The lattice degeneration presents as a grayish, granular-appearing retinal thinning usually along a vessel. This can occur at a relatively young age in the equatorial region.

Stage 2: At this stage the vessels become sheathed but are still patent. The vessels take on the fishbone appearance or sclerotic branching appearance often attributed to lattice degeneration. Also in this stage is the presentation of reactive RPE hyperplasia.

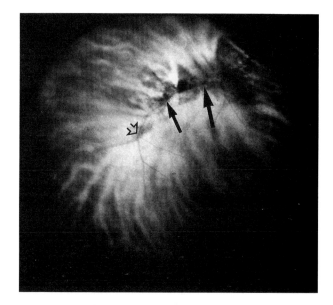

Figure 6–65. Example of the radial alignment characteristic of paravascular lattice degeneration (*dark arrows*) with the open arrow pointing at the blood vessel.

Stage 3: At this stage there is an affectation of the larger vessels in the lattice degeneration. There is also an increase in pigment at this stage and an enlargement of the lesion. During this stage there may be the development of holes and tears. It is important to note that these holes are nothing more than the result of extreme thinning of the retinal tissue that occurs associated with lattice degeneration. The tears occur as a result of the vitreoretinal adhesions to these particularly thinned areas of the retina. The tears occur when there is a change in this vitreoretinal interface, such as that occurring with a posterior vitreous detachment. At this stage there is continual retinal thinning. Breaks inside of lattice degeneration are relatively common and present as round holes. These holes are reddish in color in contrast to the surrounding translucency of the lattice degeneration. If breaks occur outside the lesion, they are usually flat linear breaks or horseshoe tears at the posterior border of the lattice degeneration. **See color plates 105 and 109.**

Lattice degeneration occurs as the result of loss of inner retinal layers down to the outer nuclear layer. The precise pathogenesis is controversial but is attributed to various conditions including vitreous traction, retinal ischemia, and an inherent internal limiting membrane anomaly. There is overlying vitreal liquefaction plus vitreoretinal adhesions and often white without pressure at the borders of the lesion. The holes that occur within the lattice are a result of either continual degeneration of the retinal layers or the particular vitreoretinal adhesions that occur associated with these lesions.

Pearls

Lattice Degeneration

Characteristics

Δ Usually occurs from the ora to equator in young patients, reaching maximum incidence by age 20 years
  Increases in severity with age but not in incidence
Δ Suggestion that some lattice degeneration is hereditary
Δ Occurs in 6 to 10 percent of general population
Δ Usually 1 to 4 DD long and 1/2 to 2 DD wide in a discontinuous fashion circumferentially—most often just a single row
Δ About 7 percent are radial in presentation with an affinity for the larger vessels
Δ Bilateral in about 50 percent of patients and presenting most often in vertical meridians
Δ The more posterior the lesion in the fundus, the wider the lesion
Δ The lesion is an area of retinal thinning with an overlying lacunae of liquefied vitreous—etiology is questionable
Δ Characteristics include:
  RPE hyperplasia (80 percent)
  Yellow glistening flecks (80 percent)
  Fishbone (sclerosed) vessel formation (10 percent) that increases with age
  Chorioretinal atrophy within the lesion is possible
  Surround of white without pressure commonly occurs in lattice
  Atrophic holes within the base of the lesion (14 to 32 percent)
  Flap tears at the border in 1.5 to 2.5 percent
    10 percent of asymptomatic tears lead to retinal detachment
    33 percent of symptomatic tears lead to retinal detachment
Δ Overall risk of retinal detachment associated with lattice degeneration is 0.05 to 0.1 percent, and risk decreases with age

Management

Δ Always consider other risk factors for the development of retinal breaks and retinal detachments
Δ Risk for retinal detachment is greater in youth, in cases with vitreoretinal traction, and in higher degrees of myopia
Δ Lattice degeneration only—document lesion, indent when indicated, advise of signs/symptoms of retinal detachment, and examine in 1 year
Δ Lattice degeneration with symptoms—document lesion, indent for holes, advise of signs/symptoms of retinal detachment, and re-examine in 6 months
Δ Lattice degeneration with asymptomatic atrophic holes but no associated risk factors—document lesion, advise of signs/symptoms of retinal detachment, and re-examine in 6 months
Δ Lattice degeneration with significant risk factors for retinal detachment such as symptomatic lattice with atrophic holes or signs of progression—a retinal consultation is indicated
Δ Lattice degeneration with retinal breaks at the margin of the lesion—a retinal consultation is indicated
Δ Retinopathy of prematurity with lattice degeneration should have the consideration of prophylactic treatment
Δ Fellow eyes of retinal detachment with lattice degeneration should have the consideration of prophylactic treatment
Δ Special consideration should be made for patients with lattice degeneration who are to undergo intraocular procedures and YAG capsulotomy
Δ Special considerations should be made for patients with lattice degeneration who are being considered for long-term miotic therapy
Δ Protection in eye hazard situations

Lattice degeneration is complex as far as prognosis is concerned. The more posterior the lattice, the more of a tendency to develop breaks. Breaks rarely develop in older, more heavily pigmented lesions. Twenty to 45 percent of eyes operated on for retinal detachment have lattice degeneration. If an eye has lattice degeneration, the chances of a retinal detachment are only about 0.05 to 0.1 percent. If an eye has lattice degeneration, the chance of atrophic retinal holes within that lesion is 18 to 32 percent. If an eye has lattice degeneration, the overall chance of retinal breaks in or around this lesion is approximately 25 percent. Flap tears occur along the lateral or posterior border of the lesion in 1.5 to 2.5 percent of the eyes. Ten percent of asymptomatic tears associated with lattice lead to retinal detachment, whereas 33 percent of symptomatic tears associated with lattice lead to retinal detachment. The frequency of retinal detachment associated with atrophic holes in lattice degeneration is 3 to 14 percent. These figures vary considerably in the literature but are usually accepted more toward the lower percentage of incidence. The risk of retinal detachment associated with lattice degeneration decreases with increasing age. It is estimated that approximately 0.05 to 0.1 percent of persons with lattice degeneration will develop a retinal detachment. Table 6–5 lists the signs of progression of lattice degeneration.

Management. Management of lattice degeneration can be complex. It is very important to understand that all patients with lattice degeneration should be educated to the signs and symptoms of retinal-detachment just because the area of lattice represents an area of retinal thinning with the potential for the development of retinal detachment. The other considerations in the management of the patient with lattice degeneration are the risk factors for retinal detachment. Table 6–6 lists specific risk factors in all peripheral retinal diseases that may contribute to the development of retinal detachment. Table 6–7 lists photopsia presenting as a clinical sign associated with retinal lesions.

With the risk factors for retinal detachment in mind, the practitioner can properly manage the patient with lattice degeneration. Lattice degeneration can be broken down into the following categories in regard to

TABLE 6–6. RISK FACTORS ASSOCIATED WITH THE DEVELOPMENT OF RETINAL DETACHMENT

Vitreous degeneration in the form of vitreous liquefaction or shrinkage

Younger patients have more of a tendency toward retinal detachments than older patients

Patients with myopia over 3 D have more of a tendency toward retinal detachment

Patients with a fellow eye with retinal detachment have a significantly higher rate of associated retinal detachment

Patients with a strong family history of retinal detachment have more of a tendency toward detachment

Patients with symptomatic breaks of the retina have a much higher frequency of associated retinal detachment

Patients with aphakia have a significantly higher rate of retinal detachments than phakic patients

Progression of retinal thinning or other signs in young patients has more of a tendency toward retinal detachments

The presence of significant vitreoretinal traction in elderly patients has more of a tendency toward retinal detachment

management. In spite of the fact that lattice degeneration is present in 20 to 45 percent of cases of retinal detachment, the risk of retinal detachment with lattice degeneration is estimated at 0.05 to 0.1 percent.

1. *Lattice degeneration as the only sign or symptom.* Examine this patient on a yearly basis and try to draw the size and location of the lesion. Also educate the patient as to signs and symptoms of retinal detachment. Scleral indentation is indicated when tears are suspected.
2. *Lattice degeneration with symptoms of flashes and floaters.* Examine this patient every 6 months, drawing the location and size of the lesion. Also educate the patient as to the signs and symptoms of retinal detachment. Scleral indentation is indicated.
3. *Lattice degeneration with associated asymptomatic atrophic holes but no associated risk factors.* Examine this patient at 6-month intervals, drawing the size and location of the lattice lesion. Young myopic patients, inferior holes, and vitreoretinal adhesions also contribute to increased risk. Myopia over 5.00 D significantly increases the risk in these

TABLE 6–5. SIGNS OF PROGRESSION OF LATTICE DEGENERATION

1. Enlargement of the lattice lesion
2. Appearance of holes or further thinning within the lattice lesion
3. Prominence of vitreous traction presenting at the border of the lesion, especially conducive to the development of linear tears at the posterior border
4. Alteration of the vitreous body in the form of liquefaction, shrinkage, and PVD

TABLE 6–7. PHOTOPSIA PRESENTING AS A CLINICAL SIGN ASSOCIATED WITH RETINAL LESIONS

Lattice alone	41%
Lattice with holes	31%
Snail track	10%
White with and without pressure	14%
Round holes	14%
Horseshoe tear	10%
Acute posterior vitreous detachment	14%

patients. Also educate the patient as to the signs and symptoms of retinal detachment.

4. *Lattice degeneration with any of the other risk factors* (*such as symptomatic lattice with atrophic holes*) *for retinal detachment.* Request a consultation with a retinal specialist.

5. *Lattice with observed breaks at the margin of the lesion.* Request a consultation with a retinal specialist.

In addition to the commonly outlined features in the management of patients with lattice degeneration, the clinician must also consider environmental factors. An example of this would be a 15-year-old myopic football player with lattice degeneration and isolated asymptomatic atrophic holes. In this particular case a retinal consultation may be indicated for the possibility of intervention with cryopexy as a prophylactic measure in spite of the fact that lattice degeneration does not seem to have a negative effect in traumatized eyes. Certainly protective eyewear is indicated. Clinical judgment will dictate the best line of attack in these particular conditions. It is generally considered that lattice degeneration with or without holes is a condition that should not be treated prophylactically unless the fellow eye has a retinal detachment. The prophylactic treatment of these lesions may actually increase the risk of retinal detachment. Observation is the overwhelming consensus by the majority of retinal practitioners.

Retinopathy of prematurity with lattice degeneration poses an increased risk for retinal breaks and detachment and as such the lattice is often prophylactically treated. Two other conditions that must be carefully considered in patients with lattice degeneration are the use of strong topical miotics, which inherently increase the risk of retinal detachment, and the possibility of intraocular surgery. Prior to intraocular surgery, a patient with lattice degeneration, especially with holes or no history of posterior vitreous detachment, should have a retinal consultation. In addition, it is important to recognize the fact that YAG posterior capsulotomy increases the risk of retinal detachment in all cases, especially in those patients with inherently compromised retinas.

Snail-Track Degeneration

Introduction and Description. Snail-track degeneration (Fig. 6–63) is also known as Scheckenspuren. Snail-track degeneration is in reality nothing more than lattice degeneration without the fishbone appearance. The lesion appears slick or slimy, like the trail left by a snail or slug. The layers involved are the same as lattice degeneration, with the exception that microglial cells containing lipoprotein material appear to be present.

Management. The prognosis and management of snail-track degeneration is essentially the same as lattice degeneration. Because of the retinal thinning and the overlying vitreous liquefaction, there is certainly the concern for the development of retinal holes and tears. **See color plate 106.**

Atrophic Retinal Holes (Retinal Breaks)

Introduction and Description. Any break in the continuity of the retinal structure represents an opportunity for liquefied vitreous to percolate underneath the retina, alter the bonds of the RPE, and create the potential for a rhegmatogenous retinal detachment. For any retinal break to become a potential problem, however, there must be associated vitreous liquefaction and traction. The vitreous base classification of retinal breaks will be used throughout the discussion and is described in Table 6–8.

It is important to recognize the fact that the majority of retinal detachment occurs associated with retinal tears rather than retinal holes. A retinal hole is considered to be a round retinal break without accompanying vitreoretinal traction. Atrophic retinal holes (Figs. 6–66 to 6–69) appear as pinpoint to 2-DD round, red lesions. These holes occur in about 2 to 3 percent of the general population. The redness of the lesion is nothing more than the RPE–choroidal structure showing through an area that used to be occupied by retinal tissue. These atrophic retinal holes are often surrounded by a cuff of whitish edema or pigment. The whitish edema is nothing more than intraretinal edema or a subclinical sensory retinal detachment surrounding the lesion. The pigment associated with the lesion usually indicates that the lesion has been present for approximately 3 months and is a sign for most clinicians of relative stability. The pigment is reactive RPE hyperplasia. The whitish cuff indicates vitreoretinal traction. When an atrophic hole is viewed with scleral indentation, the hole becomes volcano-like or fishmouth—that is, when the indenter is applied, the surrounding of the hole actually puckers. Atropic holes are seen in a variety of conditions, including peripheral cystoid degeneration, lattice degeneration, snail-track degeneration, and pars planitis, and isolated within the

TABLE 6–8. THE VITREOUS BASE CLASSIFICATION OF RETINAL BREAKS

Classification	Description
Oral	Retinal break (dialysis) at the ora serrata
Intrabasal	Retinal break within the vitreous base
Juxtabasal	Retinal break along the posterior border of the vitreous base
Extrabasal	Retinal break posterior to the vitreous base

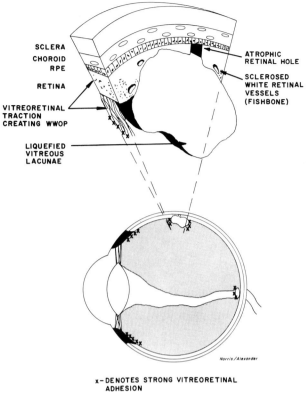

SCLERA
CHOROID
RPE

RETINA

VITREORETINAL
TRACTION
CREATING WWOP

LIQUEFIED
VITREOUS
LACUNAE

ATROPHIC
RETINAL HOLE

SCLEROSED
WHITE RETINAL
VESSELS
(FISHBONE)

Norris/Alexander

x-DENOTES STRONG VITREORETINAL
ADHESION

Figure 6–66. A schematic of the clinicopathology of lattice degeneration with an enclosed atrophic hole.

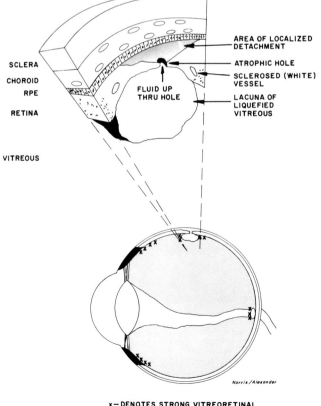

SCLERA

CHOROID
RPE

RETINA

VITREOUS

FLUID UP
THRU HOLE

AREA OF LOCALIZED
DETACHMENT

ATROPHIC HOLE

SCLEROSED (WHITE)
VESSEL

LACUNA OF
LIQUEFIED
VITREOUS

Norris/Alexander

x-DENOTES STRONG VITREORETINAL
ADHESION

Figure 6–67. A schematic of the clinicopathology of a localized retinal detachment at an atrophic hole within an area of lattice degeneration.

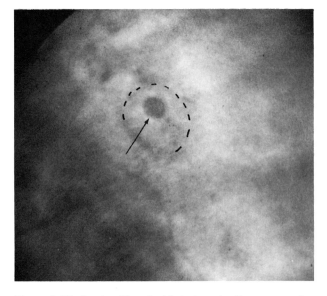

Figure 6–68. An atrophic retinal hole (*arrow*) with a surrounding subclinical detachment (*dotted line*).

retina. Atrophic holes are the most common of the retinal breaks (over 70 percent). If atrophic holes are present in one eye there is about a 20 percent chance that holes will be present in the fellow eye.

Atrophic retinal holes are round, full-thickness breaks in the retina due to progressive retinal thinning rather than true vitreoretinal traction. The atrophy is thought to be secondary to underlying vascular insufficiency that compromises the retina to the point where a break actually develops. Figures 6–66 and 6–67 demonstrate the clinicopathology of atrophic

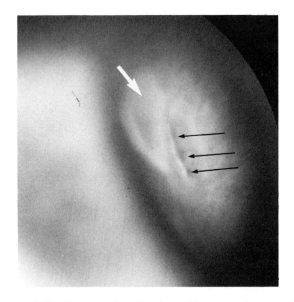

Figure 6–69. Three atrophic retinal holes (*black arrows*) near a retinal cyst (*white arrow*). The area is indented. (*Photo courtesy of W. Townsend.*)

retinal holes associated with lattice degeneration. Overlying the thinning of the retina manifest as lattice degeneration is a lacunae of liquefied vitreous. In this area of retinal thinning, there is a punched-out or atrophic retinal hole down to the RPE. It should be noted that in this particular example there is no associated retinal detachment, but there is vitreoretinal traction creating white without pressure at the edge of the lesion. In Figure 6–66 there are sclerosed white retinal vessels giving the fishbone appearance to lattice degeneration. In Figure 6–67 there is a localized retinal detachment at an atrophic hole within the lattice. The only difference between this and the previous lesion is that the liquefied vitreous has gained access through the atrophic hole into the area between the RPE and the sensory retina. This intrusion of fluid creates a localized retinal detachment that may progress to become a full rhegmatogenous retinal detachment. **See color plate 107.**

Management. The atrophic retinal hole represents an access line for liquefied vitreous to seep underneath the sensory retina. When fluid accumulates between sensory retina and the RPE, it is known as a sensory retinal detachment. However, it is known that fewer than 7 percent of atrophic holes develop progressive retinal detachment. Atrophic holes in the superior retina and those holes exposed to large volumes of liquefied vitreous are more prone to the development of rhegmatogenous retinal detachment. Also the association of strong vitreoretinal traction increases the propensity toward retinal detachment. The greater the number of holes in an eye, the greater the risk of retinal detachment. Location of the hole within the vitreous base (intrabasal) carries a minimum risk for detachment, whereas a hole along the border of the vitreous base (juxtabasal) carries an increased risk of detachment.

Management of patients with atrophic holes is as multifaceted as is lattice degeneration. Certainly all patients with atrophic holes should be educated as to the signs and symptoms of retinal detachment. Remember the risk factors relative to the development of retinal detachment when deciding on management strategies in patients with atrophic retinal holes. Management of atrophic holes can be broken into the following categories.

1. *Patients with isolated asymptomatic atrophic holes.* Monitor these patients on a yearly basis, and educate them as to the signs and symptoms of retinal detachment.
2. *Patients with isolated asymptomatic atrophic holes with a cuff of edema or focal detachment less than 1 DD and no indication of RPE hyperplasia.* Monitor these patients every 6 months, drawing the location and

Atrophic Retinal Holes

Characteristics

Δ A retinal break without vitreoretinal traction

Δ Pinpoint to 2-DD round, red lesion, often with a surrounding whitish cuff of retinal edema (subclinical detachment) and/or RPE hyperplasia

Δ Occur in about 2 to 3 percent of the population

Δ Usually ora to equator in a number of conditions associated with retinal thinning

Δ May be of choroidal vascular insufficiency origin creating retinal thinning

Δ Represent full-thickness retinal breaks—an access line for liquefied vitreous under the sensory retina which by definition typically have no associated vitreoretinal traction

Δ RPE hyperplasia surrounding the lesion indicates presence for 60 to 90 days

Δ Atrophic holes fishmouth on scleral indentation

Δ Risk factors which increase the likelihood of detachment

    Superior location

    Proximity to liquefied vitreous

    Multiple numbers

    Juxtabasal location

Δ Fewer than 7 percent of atrophic holes develop retinal detachment

Management

Δ Isolated asymptomatic atrophic holes—document, advise of signs/symptoms of retinal detachment, and examine in 1 year

Δ Isolated asymptomatic atrophic holes with cuff of edema or focal detachment less than 1 DD and no RPE hyperplasia—document, advise of signs/symptoms of retinal detachment, and examine in 1 to 3 months

Δ Isolated asymptomatic atrophic holes with a cuff of edema or focal detachment less than 1 DD and RPE hyperplasia—document, advise of signs/symptoms of retinal detachment, and examine in 3 to 6 months

Δ Isolated asymptomatic atrophic holes with cuff of edema larger than 1 DD—consultation with a retinal specialist is indicated

Δ Isolated symptomatic atrophic holes—consultation with a retinal specialist is indicated

Δ Isolated atrophic holes with flap tear or demonstrable vitreoretinal adhesions—consultation with a retinal specialist is indicated

Δ Modify above strategies based on risk factors for retinal detachment

size of the lesion. Also educate these patients as to the signs and symptoms of the development of retinal detachment.

3. *Patients with isolated asymptomatic atrophic holes with a cuff edema larger than 1 DD.* These patients deserve a retinal consultation, as 30 percent of patients with atrophic holes with cuffs of edema over 2 DD progress to retinal detachment.

4. *Patients with symptomatic atrophic retinal holes.* These patients should have a retinal consultation in spite of the fact that the retinal specialist may not opt to treat at that particular point in time.

5. *Patients with strong vitreoretinal adhesions associated with atrophic holes.* An atrophic hole with a flap tear indicates a strong vitreoretinal adhesion. Such patients should be considered at risk to develop a significant retinal tear with ensuing retinal detachment. These patients deserve a retinal consultation.

All of these modes of management should be tempered with clinical judgment regarding associated risk factors for retinal detachment. For example, juxtabasal holes deserve a more judicious follow-up than intrabasal holes, and multiple holes, especially if superior, are more prone to the development of detachment. In general, however, atrophic retinal holes do not represent the threat to detachment that retinal tears carry.

Operculated Retinal Holes (Retinal Breaks)

Introduction and Description. Operculated retinal holes (Figs. 6–70 to 6–72) typically occur from the equator to the ora serrata. These appear as round red holes with an overlying free-floating plug of retinal tissue attached to the vitreous. This free-floating plug is called the operculum and represents the vitreoretinal adhesion that has freed itself. The plug often appears smaller than the hole it came from because of atrophy of this retinal tissue secondary to removal from the nutritional supply of the retina. A fresh plug is larger than a plug that has aged and atrophied. When an operculated retinal hole occurs, there may be an associated hemorrhage. This hemorrhage occurs when a retinal vessel is torn near the site of the break. Inside of the retinal holes may be yellowish bodies called pathologic drusen. Operculated holes may be surrounded by white with pressure or white without pressure as well as a localized subclinical retinal detachment (the cuff of edema). As with an atrophic retinal hole, an operculated hole may develop a pigmented demarcation line. The operculated hole is similar in nature to the atrophic hole. The primary difference between an atrophic and an operculated hole is the associated plug of retinal tissue. In both conditions there is thinned atrophic retina that breaks down to the point where a hole occurs. The opercu-

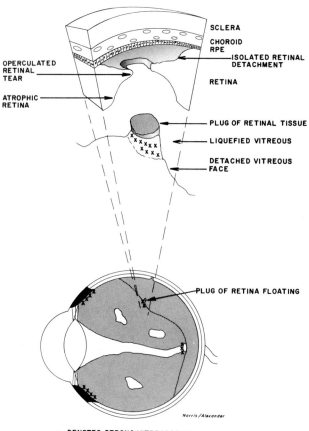

Figure 6–70. A schematic of the clinicopathology of an operculated retinal tear.

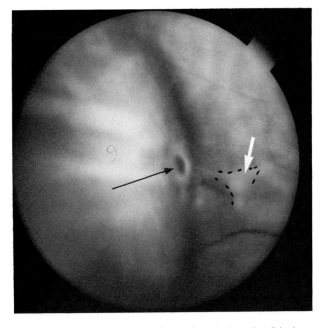

Figure 6–71. An operculated retinal hole on indentation (*black arrow*). Note the surrounding edema. The blurred plug is indicated by the white arrow. (*Photo courtesy of W. Townsend.*)

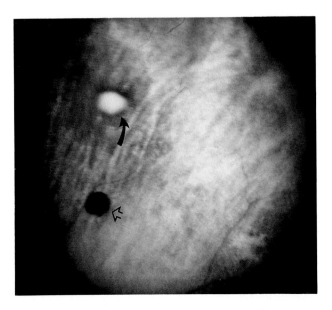

Figure 6–72. Example of an operculated retinal tear. The open arrow points to the hole while the curved arrow points to the plug.

lated hole just has the association of vitreoretinal traction forcing the development of the hole. **See color plate 108.**

Management. The operculated hole occurs as a result of an abnormal vitreoretinal adhesion that is tugged away by a change in the vitreous, often a vitreous detachment, creating a hole in the atrophic retinal tissue. The operculated hole may be the result of a freed vitreoretinal traction tuft. The prognosis is usually good with an operculated hole, as the abnormal vitreoretinal traction has been relieved. The positive prognosis would have to be modified if there is nearby liquefied vitreous and if there is nearby vitreoretinal traction. The fresh break is more likely to cause a retinal detachment than a long-standing break.

As with the operculated hole and lattice degeneration, the management of a patient with an operculated retinal hole can be somewhat complex. At all points in the management the primary care practitioner must consider extenuating risk factors. It is important to educate the patient as to the signs and symptoms of retinal detachment. The variations in operculated retinal holes may be managed according to the following guidelines.

1. *If a patient has a fresh single operculated hole,* the patient should be educated as to the signs and symptoms of retinal detachment and examined again within 6 weeks. The patient may then be followed in 6 to 12 months. Scleral indentation is indicated.
2. *If a patient has an asymptomatic single operculated retinal hole and you are seeing the patient for the first time,* monitor the patient at 6- to 12-month intervals, educating as to the signs and symptoms of retinal detachment. Scleral indentation may be indicated.
3. *If a patient has asymptomatic multiple operculated retinal holes,* monitor this patient every 6 months, educating the patient as to the signs and symptoms of retinal detachment. Indentation may be indicated.
4. *If the patient has an asymptomatic single operculated break with a cuff of surrounding edema and no RPE hyperplasia,* monitor the patient in 3 months; if there is pigment, in 6 months; and educate the patient as to the signs and symptoms of retinal detachment.
5. *If the patient is symptomatic, aphakic, or there is a retinal detachment in the fellow eye or continued traction surrounding the operculated retinal tear,* a consultation with a retinal specialist is indicated.
6. Again, remember other risk factors regarding retinal detachment.
7. *If surrounding cuff of edema exceeds 2 DD,* a consultation with a retinal specialist is indicated.

Pearls

Operculated Retinal Holes

Characteristics

△ Result of an abnormal vitreoretinal adhesion being tugged forward
△ Round, red holes with an overlying floating plug of tissue that is usually smaller in appearance than the hole because of tissue atrophy
△ Possibility of an associated vitreous hemorrhage resulting from a tear in a retinal vessel that may be bridging the retinal break
△ Occur between ora and equator
△ Possible pathologic drusen inside of holes
△ May have associated white without pressure surrounding the lesion
△ May have associated localized retinal detachment (cuff of edema)
△ The fresher the break, the more likely the development of an associated retinal detachment

Management

△ If fresh single operculated hole—document, advise of signs and symptoms of retinal detachment, and examine again in 6 weeks
△ If asymptomatic single operculated hole seen for the first time—document, advise of signs/symptoms of retinal detachment, and re-examine in 6 to 12 months
△ If asymptomatic multiple operculated holes—document, advise of signs/symptoms of retinal detachment, and re-examine every 6 months
△ If asymptomatic single operculated break with a cuff of surrounding edema less than 1 DD and no RPE hyperplasia—document and re-examine in 3 months while educating on signs and symptoms of retinal detachment
△ If symptomatic operculated hole, if in an aphakic eye, if there is a retinal detachment in the fellow eye, or if there is continued traction around the hole—a retinal consultation is indicated
△ If surrounding of edema exceeds 2 DD—a retinal consultation is indicated

Figure 6–70 demonstrates the histopathology of operculated retinal tears. It can be seen that there is a plug of retinal tissue that is attached to the vitreous face. This vitreous face has fallen forward and has pulled the plug out of the retina. With this hole in the sensory retina there is potential for the liquefied vitreous to have access between the RPE and the sensory retina, allowing for sensory retinal detachment.

The operculated tear is considered to be a retinal break that is not an indication for interventive treatment without the occurrence of associated findings such as a retinal tear or threatening vitreoretinal traction.

PERIPHERAL RETINAL CHANGES THAT POSE A DIRECT THREAT TO VISION

Linear Retinal Tear (Retinal Break With Vitreoretinal Traction)

Introduction and Description. A linear retinal tear is a retinal break associated with vitreoretinal traction and often appears as a horseshoe tear (Figs. 6–73 to 6–75). Up to 10 to 15 percent of posterior vitreous detachments will have at least one retinal tear. A linear retinal tear appears red (more red in older lesions), surrounded by atrophic gray retinal tissue (increases in density with age of the lesion). If the torn retina remains attached to the detached vitreous, the break is usually referred to as a flap tear. A fresh retinal break is often difficult to identify as the tissue changes have yet to occur to enhance the contrast between the atrophic surrounding tissue and the "red" tear. This retinal tissue may also be edematous in the early phases of the tear. The flap of retinal tissue that has detached typically shrinks over time because of lack

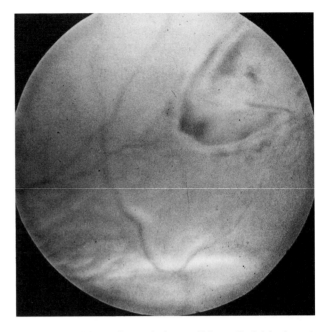

Figure 6–74. A horseshoe retinal tear within a retinal detachment.

of nutritional blood supply. This shrinkage or atrophy is similar to that occurring in the retinal plug of an operculated retinal tear.

A linear tear may be in the shape of a horseshoe with the apex or rounded end usually but not always pointing toward the posterior pole. These tears often occur near the posterior border of the vitreous base, around lattice, around retinal tufts, around snowflake degeneration, and around white without pressure.

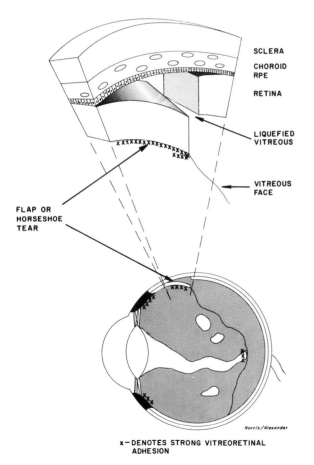

Figure 6–73. A schematic of the clinicopathology of a linear or horseshoe retinal tear.

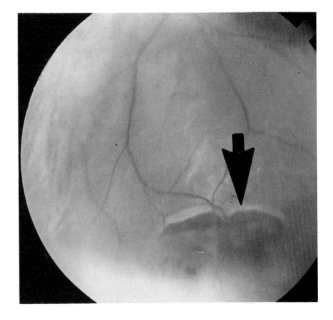

Figure 6–75. A retinal tear (*arrow*) associated with a PVD. The area previously surrounded lattice degeneration.

Linear Retinal Tear

Characteristics

△ A retinal break associated with vitreoretinal traction

△ 10 to 15 percent of vitreous detachments have an associated retinal break

△ A tear in the retina is red, with a surrounding of gray retinal tissue—if the adhesion remains it is called a flap tear

△ The detached flap shrinks over time

△ If in the shape of a horseshoe, the apex (rounded point) usually points toward posterior pole because of the downward pull of the associated vitreous detachment

△ Result of strong vitreoretinal adhesion in an area of thin retina

△ The retinal break plus the associated liquefied vitreous increase the likelihood of a rhegmatogenous retinal detachment

△ The retinal break may have a bleed into the vitreous because of an associated break in a bridged vessel

△ The blood or liberated pigment may produce floaters while the physical rip will produce photopsia

△ Fresh breaks are more prone to detachment than older breaks

△ Other risk factors should be considered when assessing the management of the retinal tear

Management

△ Thirty percent chance of retinal detachment—a retinal consultation is indicated

△ Treatment of:
   Symptomatic retinal tears
   Asymptomatic retinal tears in fellow eyes with a retinal detachment
   Juxtabasal and oral tears
   Retinal detachments greater than 1 DD surrounding a break
   Remaining flap attachments

△ Consider treatment if a cataract is to be removed or if a YAG capsulotomy is being considered

△ Re-examine the treated patient within 1 week assuring that fluid is not extending and that no new tears have developed

△ Re-examine every few weeks until scarification has occurred

Horseshoe tears are the direct result of an abnormally strong vitreoretinal adhesion. This vitreoretinal adhesion typically occurs in an area of atrophic retina often in the form of a vitreoretinal traction tuft. When vitreous collapse occurs, the strong vitreoretinal adhesion pulls on the already compromised atrophic retina, creating a tear. This break coupled with the liquefied vitreous significantly increases the risk for rhegmatogenous retinal detachment. Should a retinal vessel be involved in the tear, there may be an associated hemorrhage into the vitreous. Also, there may be retinal tissue bridging the gap of the tear as well as vitreoretinal traction bands. As with many other tears, holes, and other alterations in retinal tissue, RPE hyperplasia may occur over a period of time. The genesis of the horseshoe or flat retinal tear is demonstrated in Figure 6–73. **See color plate 109.**

It should be noted that traction remains after the tear, allowing for further development of retinal detachment. Linear retinal tears usually occur superiorly, creating even more difficulty because of gravity pulling on the retinal tissue. Linear retinal tears occur most commonly in situations where the retina is thin, there is trauma, or there is a condition associated with vitreous degeneration. The tears occur most commonly in patients over 40 years of age, in those with myopia, in patients with lattice degeneration, in patients with aphakia, and often secondary to trauma.

The patient will often experience a flash of light or multiple bouts of photopsia at the time of the break, with the possible subsequent appearance of floaters from liberated blood cells or pigment cells. Fresh retinal breaks are more prone to develop associated detachment than older breaks.

Management. Linear retinal tears are the leading cause of rhegmatogenous retinal detachment. There is approximately a 30 percent chance of retinal detachment associated with a horseshoe or flap retinal tear. Management of patients with retinal tears of any kind in any location calls for consultation with a retinal specialist. Judgment regarding therapeutic intervention is at the discretion of the retinal surgeon. Risk factors for the development of retinal detachment (Table 6–9) weigh into the decision to intervene with prophylactic treatment. Indications for treatment with laser photocoagulation include symptomatic flap tears, asymptomatic tears in eyes opposite a retinal detachment, juxtabasal and oral tears, prevention of the spread of small retinal detachments surrounding a retinal break (greater than 1 DD), and YAG severing of vitreoretinal flaps associated with a break. Consideration for treatment should be extended to all patients contemplating cataract surgery or YAG capsulotomy. Typically a photocoagulated break is treated with two to three confluent rows of burns up to the margin of the break extending to the ora. Cryotherapy is the treatment of choice in these situations when breaks occur anterior to the equator or the media is too opaque to carefully visualize the retina.

After prophylactic intervention, the patient should be examined within 1 week to assure no extension of subretinal fluid and to assure that no additional breaks occurred associated with the treatment.

TABLE 6–9. RISK FACTORS FOR THE DEVELOPMENT OF RETINAL DETACHMENT ASSOCIATED WITH RETINAL BREAKS

Fellow phakic eyes to a retinal detachment have a 10% risk of developing a detachment

Fellow aphakic eyes to a retinal detachment have a 21 to 36% risk of developing a retinal detachment

Intrabasal tears rarely progress; juxtabasal tears are at greatest risk

Symptomatic flap tears result in a high incidence (25 to 90%) of retinal detachment

Symptomatic operculated tears result in retinal detachment in 15% of eyes

YAG capsulotomy in an eye with pseudophakia increases the risk of retinal detachment (see patients day after surgery and then in 6 months)

Aphakia (2 to 3%) increases the risk of retinal detachment versus phakic eyes (0.01%)

Use of strong miotics increases the risk of retinal detachment

Axial myopia greater than 25 mm increases the risk of retinal detachment

Liquefied, syneretic vitreous increases the risk of retinal detachment

Family history of retinal detachment increases the risk

Blunt and penetrating trauma increases the risk of retinal detachment

Males have an increased incidence of retinal detachment, especially at a younger age

Other predisposing lesions such as lattice degeneration and vitreoretinal traction tufts

Complete dilated fundus examinations should then be repeated every few weeks until there is total assurance of effective scarification.

Retinal Dialysis (Retinal Breaks)

Introduction and Description. Retinal dialysis (Fig. 6–76) is a retinal break (tear) occurring near the ora serrata less than 90 degrees in size. The dialysis typically occurs in males under the age of 40 years with no particular tendencies in myopia. The incidence of dialysis in the general population is less than 0.01 percent whereas it accounts for 8 to 17 percent of detachments for all age groups and 19 to 51 percent of detachments in young patients. The patients are asymptomatic in about 60 percent of cases, symptoms developing when the fovea is ultimately detached. The evolution of the detachment is slow, taking 125 to 140 days for evolution from the time of the initial tear. The inferior temporal quadrant is involved in 50 percent of the cases. Retinal dialysis appears as any other tear or hole in the retina. The hole or tear in a dialysis is red with grayish retina surrounding it, but differs from a giant retinal tear in that there are typically no radial tears in the dialysis. This grayish retina is either atrophic or edematous, depending upon elapsed time. The dialysis is often only observable in early stages with scleral indentation. It is therefore important to carefully investigate the oral area in patients who have suffered recent trauma, keeping in mind that at times scleral indentation is contraindicated in trauma.

A three-mirror examination is often of benefit when scleral indentation is contraindicated. There is no particular vitreous connection in the genesis of retinal dialysis except an occasional concurrent vitreous hemorrhage. Intraocular pressure is increased in about 20 percent of eyes with dialysis and decreased in about 25 percent of eyes with retinal dialysis. The transient increase in IOP associated with dialysis and detachment is referred to as Schwartz syndrome and is thought to be due to accumulation of released rod outer segments in the trabecular meshwork. Retinal macrocysts (4 to 8 DD) are also a characteristic feature of retinal dialyses.

It is important to recognize the fact that there is controversy regarding the etiology of retinal dialysis. One report states that 87 percent of unilateral nasal

Pearls

Retinal Dialysis

Characteristics

△ Red retinal tear at the ora less than 90 degrees

△ Usually occurs in males under age 40 and is asymptomatic in approximately 60 percent of patients

△ Inevitable evolution of retinal detachment in 125 to 140 days

△ IOP increases in 20 percent (Schwartz syndrome) and decreases in 25 percent of cases of dialysis-related detachment

△ Pigmented demarcation lines and retinal macrocysts are more prevalent in the nontraumatic variety

△ Associated signs of trauma such as hyphema, angle recession, vitreous hemorrhage, and others are more common in the traumatic variety

△ Need to indent cases of trauma unless contraindicated by the type of trauma to pick up early retinal dialysis

△ If spontaneous in the young, they are bilateral in some cases, and there is the suggestion that there may be a hereditary tendency

Management

△ Slow progression toward retinal detachment—a retinal consultation is indicated

△ Surgical repair is usually successful if intervention occurs prior to macular involvement

△ All cases of ocular trauma should be followed in 60 to 90 days to assure that there is not a previously undetected retinal dialysis evolving toward detachment

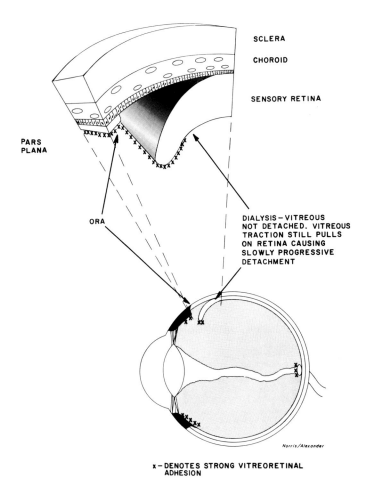

SCLERA

CHOROID

SENSORY RETINA

PARS PLANA

ORA

DIALYSIS – VITREOUS NOT DETACHED. VITREOUS TRACTION STILL PULLS ON RETINA CAUSING SLOWLY PROGRESSIVE DETACHMENT

Norris/Alexander

x – DENOTES STRONG VITREORETINAL ADHESION

Figure 6–76. A schematic of the clinicopathology of a retinal dialysis.

and superior dialyses were attributable to trauma. Other reports state that trauma plays an insignificant role in the genesis of any inferior temporal dialysis, whereas another study concludes that all dialyses result from trauma. If the classification of the dialysis is broken down to traumatic and nontraumatic, the characteristics of the patients are different. The characteristics are outlined in Table 6–10.

Management. In either the spontaneous or the traumatic retinal dialysis there can be the slow progression toward retinal detachment because of the fact that strong vitreoretinal adhesions remain attached to the sensory retina. The typical delay from the onset of the tear in a traumatic dialysis is 125 days, and in a nontraumatic dialysis is 140 days. The strong vitreoretinal adhesions are subject to continued pull and stress by the vitreous. Because there is a relatively slow progression toward retinal detachment, retinal dialysis may have multiple demarcation lines. It is safe to say that with retinal dialysis one may assume eventual

retinal detachment. Management for retinal dialysis is a request for a retinal consultation. The urgency of the consult depends on the proximity of the retinal detachment to the posterior pole. Some dialyses may be treated with cryopexy and photocoagulation; some of them may necessitate the employment of a scleral buckle.

Figure 6–76 demonstrates a retinal dialysis, which is nothing more than a retinal tear or detachment at the ora serrata. It is important to note that the vitreous is not detached in these instances and that the strong vitreoretinal traction at the base of the vitreous still remains. This can cause a continual pull on the retina with the genesis of a slowly progressive retinal detachment (Figures 6–77 and 6–78).

Long term follow-up of the postsurgical detachment patient is outlined in the section on retinal detachment later in the chapter.

All cases of ocular trauma should be followed in 60 to 90 days to assure that a previously undetected dialysis is not evolving into a retinal detachment.

TABLE 6–10. CHARACTERISTICS OF PATIENTS WITH TRAUMATIC VERSUS NONTRAUMATIC RETINAL DIALYSIS

	Traumatic	Nontraumatic
Sex/average age	Males 84%/28 years	Males 60%/26 years
Location	Superior nasal 46%, inferior temporal 30%, anterior to ora in 74%	Inferior temporal 66%, superior nasal 14%, posterior to ora in 91%
Presence of pigmented demarcation lines	25–50%	45–80%
Presence of retinal macro-cysts	13–14%	25–30%
Presence of primary open-angle glaucoma	12–16%	Under 5%
Other character-istics	Other signs of trauma such as hemorrhage, cataracts, avulsed vitreous base, angle recession, hypema, lens subluxation, iridodialysis	More of a tendency to-ward bilaterality, possible suggestion of hereditary pattern (AR)

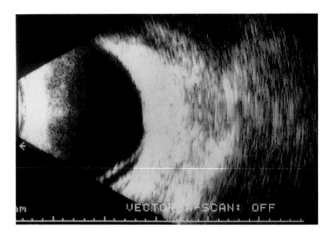

Figure 6–78. B-scan of the retinal detachment shown in Figure 6–77.

Giant Retinal Tear (Retinal Breaks)

Introduction and Description. A giant retinal tear (Figs. 6–79 and 6–80) is a form of a retinal break that by definition involves over 90 degrees of the oral zone of the retina. The tear usually starts at the posterior edge of the vitreous base and is often 360 degrees. The giant retinal tear typically occurs four times as frequently in males as females and is associated with myopia over 8 D. Giant retinal tears are also very symp-

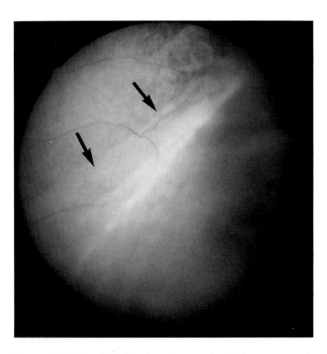

Figure 6–77. A retinal detachment secondary to trauma associated with a retinal dialysis. The arrows point to the advancing edge of the detachment, which is characterized by folds.

Pearls

Giant Retinal Tear

Characteristics

△ Retinal tear at ora greater than 90 degrees with retina folding over onto itself like a taco shell
△ Four times more frequent in males
△ Usually associated with myopia over 8 D
△ 70 percent are idiopathic, 20 percent associated with trauma, 10 percent associated with chorioretinal degeneration, some association with intraocular surgery, may occur in Stickler syndrome
△ Considerable vitreoretinal traction at edge of tear leading to the inevitable retinal detachment and producing significant symptomatology in the form of photopsia and floaters

Management

△ Fellow eyes have:
   12.8 percent giant tears
   11.9 percent retinal tears
   10.2 percent retinal holes
   15.9 percent retinal detachment
△ Consultation with a very good retinal specialist is indicated
△ In comanaging the patient watch for development in the fellow eye and the development of proliferative vitreoretinopathy postsurgically

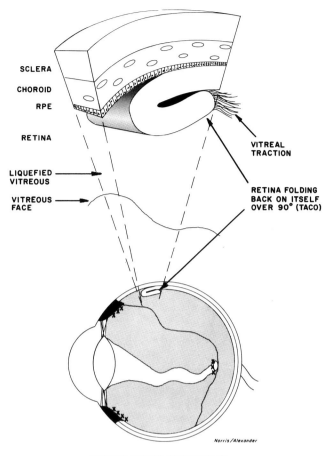

SCLERA
CHOROID
RPE
RETINA
LIQUEFIED VITREOUS
VITREOUS FACE

VITREAL TRACTION

RETINA FOLDING BACK ON ITSELF OVER 90° (TACO)

Norris/Alexander

x—DENOTES STRONG VITREORETINAL ADHESION

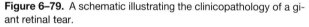

Figure 6–79. A schematic illustrating the clinicopathology of a giant retinal tear.

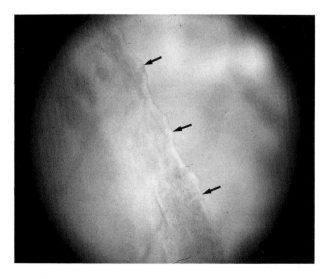

Figure 6–80. The edge of a giant retinal tear (*arrows*).

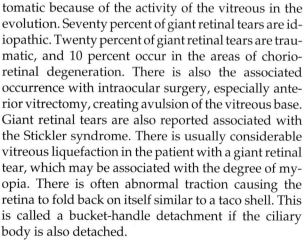

tomatic because of the activity of the vitreous in the evolution. Seventy percent of giant retinal tears are idiopathic. Twenty percent of giant retinal tears are traumatic, and 10 percent occur in the areas of chorioretinal degeneration. There is also the associated occurrence with intraocular surgery, especially anterior vitrectomy, creating avulsion of the vitreous base. Giant retinal tears are also reported associated with the Stickler syndrome. There is usually considerable vitreous liquefaction in the patient with a giant retinal tear, which may be associated with the degree of myopia. There is often abnormal traction causing the retina to fold back on itself similar to a taco shell. This is called a bucket-handle detachment if the ciliary body is also detached.

A giant retinal tear may occur along the posterior margin of white without pressure (Stickler syndrome), in extensive areas of lattice degeneration, and in areas of previous cryopexy therapy or photocoagulated retina. Giant retinal tears often occur at the ora serrata involving the ciliary body epithelium. A giant retinal tear is a sensory retinal detachment with vitreoretinal traction at the rolled edge of the tear.

Management. The prognosis for a giant retinal tear is very poor. There is invariable progression toward retinal detachment. Of more importance is the fellow eye. Over 12 percent of fellow eyes to giant retinal tears have giant breaks as well. Nearly 12 percent of fellow eyes have retinal tears, about 10 percent of fellow eyes have retinal holes, 0.4 percent have retinal dialysis, and nearly 16 percent of fellow eyes to giant retinal tears have retinal detachment.

Giant retinal tears have a variable surgical prognosis. However, the sooner the tear is discovered the better the prognosis. An immediate retinal consultation is indicated. A number of surgical techniques have been employed to correct giant tears including scleral buckling, photocoagulation, cryopexy, vitrectomy, gas tamponade, and injection of healon and heavy oils. It is also important to be aware of the associated complications in the fellow eye. The overall prognosis is worsened postsurgically by the high incidence of proliferative vitreoretinopathy. The giant retinal tear is shown in schematic cross section (Fig. 6–79) demonstrating persistence of vitreal traction and progression of the retinal detachment.

In postsurgical comanagement watch for the development of problems in the fellow eye and take care to watch for the development of proliferative vitreoretinopathy in the operated eye.

Commotio Retinae

Introduction and Description. Commotio retinae is the result of blunt trauma to the eye or surrounding area, creating contrecoup shock waves that disturb the retina (Fig. 6–81). Commotio retinae may occur any-

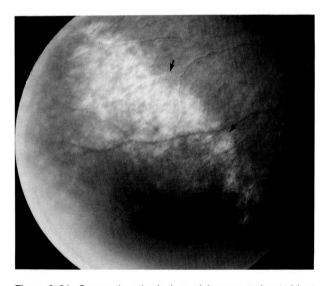

Figure 6–81. Commotio retina in the periphery secondary to blunt trauma to the eye. The area of retinal swelling appears white and is demarcated by the arrows.

Commotio Retinae

Characteristics

△ Secondary to blunt trauma—may be called Berlin's edema in posterior pole

△ Opaque whitish retina due to disorganization of the outer retinal layers

△ May result in reactive RPE hyperplasia, RPE atrophy, macular breaks, choroidal neovascular development

△ May have reduced acuity or field defects depending on the area affected

△ Trauma is the cause of unilateral rhegmatogenous retinal detachment in 12 to 20 percent of younger patients

Management

△ Educate the patient on signs/symptoms of retinal detachment

△ Carefully examine the retina with scleral indentation especially investigating for retinal dialysis

△ Monitor for the development of vision-threatening retinal changes associated with trauma

△ Follow up dilated fundus examination within 2 weeks

where in the retina. When it occurs in the posterior pole, it is often referred to as Berlin's edema. Blunt ocular trauma is reported to be the cause of unilateral rhegmatogenous retinal detachment in 12 to 20 percent of patients, especially younger patients, and as such must always be a concern. Retinal dialysis is the most common precipitating factor in detachment in younger patients.

Immediately after the trauma, the retina maintains its transparency. Within a few hours the traumatized area becomes opaque—retinal whitening. The swelling and disorganization that creates this opaque appearance is believed to be confined to the outer retinal layers. The opaque retina blocks background choroidal fluorescence on fluorescien angiography. If the trauma is severe enough, choroidal rupture as well as retinal dialysis may occur.

The long-term appearance may vary from no observable changes, to reactive hyperplasia mixed with RPE atrophy, to traumatic macular breaks (holes), and to the remote possibility of choroidal neovascular development.

Symptoms depend on the section of the retina that is involved. If the posterior pole is involved, visual acuity is reduced to variable levels. If the peripheral retina is affected, visual field defects will occur when tested with perimetry.

Management. Little can be done to facilitate the course of the natural healing process of commotio retinae. The best that can be done is to carefully investigate with scleral indentation for other vision-threatening signs associated with trauma that might be amendable to intervention. A follow-up dilated fundus examination should be performed within 2 weeks and the patient should be made aware of the signs and symptoms of retinal detachment.

Choroidal Detachment

Introduction and Description. Choroidal detachment is commonly associated with penetrating ocular trauma but may be associated with inflammatory conditions (such as Vogt–Koyanagi–Harada syndrome), tumor, postsurgical complications, retinal detachment, scleral buckling after retinal detachment, spontaneous secondary to rapid ocular decompression, and rupture of a choroidal neovascular membrane. The detachment may be serous or hemorrhagic, each having very distinct clinical signs and symptoms. The association with trauma is the result of hypotony causing an alteration of the sclera and a transudation of serous fluid. There is a smooth bullous elevation of the retina and choroid which is orange brown and extends around the periphery up to 360 degrees. The elevation is lobular, simulating a nonrhegmatogenous detachment secondary to a melanoma.

With a serous choroidal detachment, the patient has decreased vision or may be asymptomatic. The intraocular pressure is lower in the affected eye (as low as 4 to 6 mm Hg) with a shallow anterior chamber and cells and flare.

With a hemorrhagic choroidal detachment, the patient complains of severe pain, a red eye, and decreased vision. There is high intraocular pressure with a shallow anterior chamber and cells and flare.

Management. The choroidal detachment is a situation managed best by the retinal specialist. The differential diagnosis is difficult at best, often necessitating the use of B-scan and CTs. The anterior chamber reaction can be controlled by cycloplegics and topical prednisone forte 1% four to six times a day. Surgical drainage of the fluid may be necessary in addition to repair of the causative factor.

Pars Planitis

Introduction and Description. Pars planitis is a chronic inflammatory disease of the peripheral retina that is characterized by remissions and exacerbations over 20 to 30 years. It has been reported to be the primary disease in between 7 to 8 percent of patients with uveitis. It is bilateral in 60 to 80 percent of patients and has no sexual predilection. The etiology of pars planitis is uncertain, although an autoimmune origin and a relationship to demyelinizing disease have been suggested.

The age of onset is thought to be in the childhood years, but this is obscure, as most patients are asymptomatic at this stage. The disease usually becomes apparent in young adulthood.

Initially, dirty, yellowish exudates aggregate near small-sheathed vessels in the extreme periphery. These early "snowbanks" lie on the retina and move easily into the vitreous as cells and flare in the retrolental space. In the early phases of the disease, the snowbanks can only be seen with scleral indentation. This process occurs most frequently in the inferior retina. Should the process continue, the globular exudates coalesce and may form a large plaque (snowbank) covering the ora serrata. This plaque has fuzzy, raised edges when active, and appears to be membranous with a hard covering when inactive. The fibrovascular membrane may eventually develop neovascularization in the anterior chamber; yellowish gelatinous exudates may also deposit over the trabecular meshwork and iris surface.

The patient with pars planitis may enter with complaints of hazy vision or floaters from the cells and flare in the retrolental space. The patient may also complain of reduced visual acuity secondary to the cystoid macular edema. Remissions and exacerbations are characteristic. There is the remote relationship of pars planitis to demyelinizing disease.

Other complications of pars planitis include secondary glaucoma, posterior subcapsular cataract, posterior vitreous detachment, vitreous hemorrhage, retinal breaks, retinal detachment, optic disc edema,

Pars Planitis

Characteristics

△ Chronic inflammatory process, bilateral in 60 to 80 percent, characterized by remissions and exacerbations

△ Early age of onset but may be asymptomatic at presentation

△ Thought to be a retinal vasculitis rather than a posterior uveitis

△ Symptoms are hazy vision, with possible vision reduction secondary to cystoid macular edema

△ Dirty yellow exudates appear in periphery near sheathed vessels often only visible with scleral indentation

△ Exudates may coalesce to form snowbanks that may break off into vitreous—may also form a large plaque

△ Complications include posterior subcapsular cataracts, glaucoma, retinal breaks, retinal detachment, optic disc edema, vitreous detachment, vitreous hemorrhage, choroidal neovascularization, and peripheral retinal neovascularization

Management

△ Control vision-threatening inflammatory process with steroids
  Methylprednisolone acetate 40 mg subconjunctivally every 2 to 6 weeks, then tapered
  Oral prednisone at 50 to 100 mg every other day over 4 to 6 weeks, then tapered
  Topical prednisone forte q 1 to 2 hours, then tapered, for the anterior chamber reaction

△ Provide routine follow-up care every 1 to 4 weeks during the active phase, and patient education—watch for steroid responders

△ Retinal consultation for the possible application of cryotherapy, as this is known to minimize the inflammatory process and maximize visual results

△ Retinal consultation for the possible need for photocoagulation for peripheral retinal neovascularization and choroidal neovascularization and for possible vitrectomy

velopment of the snowbanks and to minimize the cystoid macular edema. Methylprednisolone acetate 40 mg injected subconjunctivally every 2 to 6 weeks may be used with compromised vision then tapered. Oral steroids at 50 to 100 mg by mouth may be given every other day over a 4- to 6-week period, and then tapered to help in suppression of the inflammation. Topical prednisone forte every 1 to 2 hours is used to quiet the anterior chamber reaction. Patients should be reevaluated every 1 to 4 weeks during the active treated phase of the disease with special emphasis on detecting "steroid responders." Improvement is slow, and often the best that can be expected is to hold the process down while it runs the course.

Cryotherapy applied to active snowbank lesions is a successful treatment in a number of patients and appears to minimize recurrence while improving vision. If the condition is unresponsive to steroids or cryotherapy, immunosuppressive agents may be attempted.

Photocoagulation for the accompanying development of peripheral retinal neovascularization and choroidal neovascularization is also of benefit. Elimination of the neovascularization will minimize the risk of the development of vitreous hemorrhage. Vitrectomy may be necessary in cases of vitreous hemorrhages, retinal traction, and the development of preretinal macular fibrosis.

Because of the prolonged use of corticosteroids, posterior subcapsular cataracts develop in many patients. The associated cystoid macular edema is the cause of reduced acuity in many patients. Other complications include band keratopathy and vitreoretinal changes that can precipitate RS, retinal detachment, peripheral neovascularization, and hemorrhage.

The patient should be on routine follow-up care and should be educated as to the signs of exacerbation. Careful investigation should be performed for associated retinal breaks. Up to 80 percent of patients with pars planitis have very good visual prognosis with no intervention whatsoever. There is, however, the occasional need for surgical intervention to clear vitreous hemorrhage and to repair retinal detachment.

and choroidal neovascularization. Peripheral retinal neovascularization is thought to result from the intraocular inflammation rather than retinal hypoxia. Because of the patchy staining of the major retinal veins, the macular edema and the optic disc edema on fluorescein angiography, the disease process is believed to be the result of peripheral retinal vasculitis.

Management. Pars planitis is a chronic disease that runs a prolonged course. Because the condition is inflammatory, steroids in the form of sub-Tenon injections or oral forms are indicated to "control" the de-

Rhegmatogenous Retinal Detachment

Introduction and Description. Rhegmatogenous detachment is to be contrasted with tractional detachment secondary to other retinal diseases such as retinopathy of prematurity, proliferative diabetic retinopathy, and a number of other processes. The tractional detachment is usually in the posterior pole and the surface is often concave rather than the characteristic convexity of the rhegmatogenous detachment (Fig. 6–82). The exudative retinal detachment is solid and is the result of the accumulation of exudative ma-

uefied vitreous (which breaks the bonds of the RPE) into the wound. There is a strong bond between RPE and Bruch's membrane. As such, most retinal detachments occur between the RPE and the sensory retina. It is also very important to realize that the immediate cause of rhegmatogenous retinal detachment is vitreoretinal traction in areas of atrophic or thinned retina or in an area of strong vitreoretinal adhesion such as the juxtabasal zone. In the area of thinned retina, a hole or a tear is created for the ingress of liquefied vitreous between the sensory retina and RPE. This ingress of liquefied vitreous in addition to the continued vitreoretinal traction is the beginning of the retinal detachment. Symptoms of a retinal detachment are presented in Table 6–11.

One of the symptomatic consequences of the retinal detachment is the presence of floaters and flashes of light indicating the initial tear as well as the evolution of the ripping away of the retina. The majority of retinal detachments are asymptomatic. Often the patient will have floaters in the anterior vitreous (retrolental space) resulting from liberated red blood cells and pigment granules when the break occurs. This is known as tobacco dust or Shaffer's sign. Any sign of floaters or flashes should be considered indicative of a retinal detachment until proven otherwise. Peripheral field loss occurs with retinal detachment and is a very important sign.

A rhegmatogenous retinal detachment is the result of a retinal break. Retinal detachment occurs in 0.005 to 0.01 percent of the general population. Retinal detachment occurrence peaks between ages 50 and 60 years. Only 1 to 3 percent of patients with high myopia develop retinal detachment. Between 1.7 and 3 percent of aphakic patients develop retinal detachment, 50 percent of those occurring 1 year postsurgically. Up to 23 to 40 percent of retinal detachments occur in patients with aphakia and pseudophakia. Most retinal detachments result from retinal tears rather than retinal holes, and most retinal breaks occur associated with posterior vitreous detachment. The fresh break is also more likely to cause a rhegmatogenous detachment than an older break. The lack of RPE hyperplasia, presence of vitreous hemorrhage secondary to a ripping of a bridging vessel, and presence of pig-

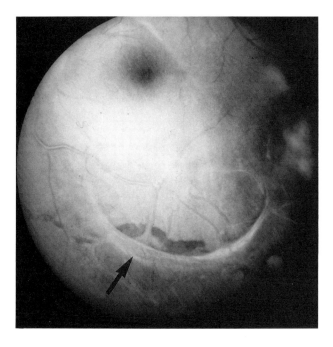

Figure 6–82. Example of a traction retinal detachment (*arrow*) without the occurrence of a retinal tear and infusion of subretinal liquefied vitreous. Blood lies under the detached area.

terial, serous fluid, hemorrhage, or a neoplasm underneath the sensory retina (Fig. 6–83). The clinician must realize that there is a very weak bond between the sensory retina and the RPE.

A rhegmatogenous retinal detachment is the result of breaks in the peripheral retina often secondary to a collapsing vitreous with the percolation of the liq-

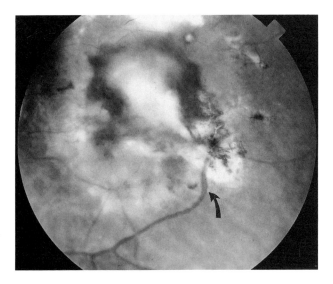

Figure 6–83. Example of a solid exudative retinal detachment without the occurrence of a retinal tear and infusion of subretinal liquefied vitreous. This is secondary to angiomatosis retinae with the feeder vessel identified with the curved arrow.

TABLE 6–11. RETINAL DETACHMENT: SYMPTOMS

Any sudden onset of or increase in the number of floaters

Any sudden shower of small floaters like gnats

Any dramatic onset of flashes of light or a change in the pattern of flashes normally seen or flashes of light that do not go away

Any sudden change in vision

Any loss of peripheral or side vision when one eye is covered

The appearance of a curtain, cloud, or discoloration over your vision

Rhegmatogenous Retinal Detachment

Characteristics

Δ Contrast with tractional detachments and exudative detachments

Δ Occurrence in 0.005 to 0.01 percent of the population with peak occurrence near 60 years of age but occurrence in aphakic patients approaches 3 percent

Δ 23 to 40 percent of retinal detachments in aphakic patients

Δ Fellow eyes to a retinal detachment in phakic eyes have an 11 to 31 percent chance of detachment

Δ Fresh breaks are most likely to cause a detachment and are characterized by:
  Vitreous hemorrhage
  Symptoms
  Absence of surrounding RPE hyperplasia
  Pigment granules in the anterior vitreous

Δ Strong vitreoretinal adhesion in area of thin or weak retina allowing for a tear or hole, creating a tunnel for intrusion of liquefied vitreous under the sensory retina

Δ Vitreous breaks mucopolysaccharide bonds liberating RPE and allowing for sensory retinal separation

Δ If a bridging retinal vessel is torn during the process there is a resultant vitreous hemorrhage

Δ The majority of retinal detachments are asymptomatic

Δ SYMPTOMS OF A RETINAL DETACHMENT
  Any sudden onset of or increase in the number of floaters
  Any sudden shower of small floaters like gnats
  Any dramatic onset of flashes of light or a change in the pattern of flashes normally seen or flashes of light that do not go away
  Any sudden change in vision
  Any loss of peripheral or side vision when one eye is covered
  The appearance of a curtain, cloud, or discoloration over your vision

Δ Key diagnostic sign is obscuration of underlying choroidal detail

Δ Must use scleral indentation to discover shallow retinal detachment—a 60-degree visual field will also assist in the diagnosis of hard-to-see detachments

Δ Always consider associated risk factors when following for the development of detachment and for assessing for the possibility of detachment

Δ Appears as semitransparent undulating elevation when fresh that becomes more opaque with age—examine the patient while seated to assure that the detachment falls forward

Δ May use B-scan to assist in diagnosis, especially using the kinetics of eye movement to enhance the view

Δ Billowing folds of retina indicate a lot of subretinal fluid

Δ A pigmented demarcation line, retinal macrocysts, folded whitish lines, and proliferation of glial cells on the surface and accumulation of intraretinal exudates indicate aging of the detachment

Δ Intraocular pressure may be both elevated (Schwartz syndrome) or decreased

Management

Δ A fresh retinal detachment is a medical emergency calling for an immediate retinal consultation

Δ Long-standing detachments can wait for a 1- to 2-day retinal consultation

Δ Surgical success:
  90 percent anatomical success rate for reattachment
  55 percent vision to 20/50 success rate
  10 to 20 percent require multiple surgical procedures

Δ In comanagement of the postsurgical patient, watch for the early and late complications

Δ COMPLICATIONS FOLLOWING RHEGMATOGENOUS RETINAL DETACHMENT REPAIR

Up to 6 Months Postop	After 6 Months Postop
• Cystoid macular edema in 30 to 40 percent of eyes	• Cystoid macular edema
• Endophthalmitis	• Endophthalmitis
• Preretinal macular fibrosis (proliferative vitreoretinopathy) in up to 25 percent of patients having scleral buckles	• Preretinal macular fibrosis (proliferative vitreoretinopathy) in up to 25 percent of patients having scleral buckles
• Redetachment of the retina	• Cataract
• Glaucoma	• Subretinal fluid
• Conjunctival adhesions causing symblepharon	• Strabismus
• Strabismus in up to 55 percent of patients having scleral buckles	• Severe anisometropia and aniseikonia
• Severe anisometropia and aniseikonia	• Cataract formation secondary to intraocular manipulation
• Severe vitreous floaters	• Pthisis bulbi
• Anterior segment ischemia and necrosis	• Buckle movement, exposure and intrusion
• Choroidal detachment	• Keratoconjunctivitis sicca
• Movement and exposure of the buckle	• Ptosis
• Keratoconjunctivitis sicca	

Δ Comanagement of the refractive error requires careful consideration for the aniseikonia and anisometropia

Δ Prior to initiation of miotic therapy on any glaucoma patient, carefully evaluate the peripheral retina and examine the retina under dilation on a yearly basis in all patients on miotic therapy

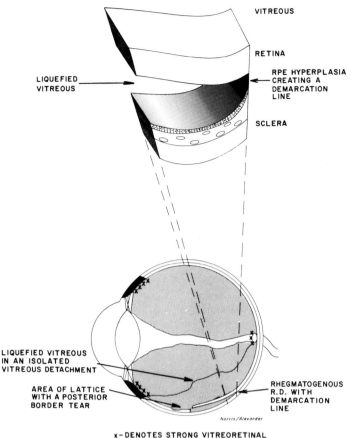

VITREOUS

RETINA

RPE HYPERPLASIA
CREATING A
DEMARCATION
LINE

SCLERA

LIQUEFIED
VITREOUS

LIQUEFIED VITREOUS
IN AN ISOLATED
VITREOUS DETACHMENT

AREA OF LATTICE
WITH A POSTERIOR
BORDER TEAR

RHEGMATOGENOUS
R.D. WITH
DEMARCATION
LINE

Norris/Alexander

x — DENOTES STRONG VITREORETINAL
ADHESION

Figure 6–84. A schematic illustrating the clinicopathology of a rhegmatogenous retinal detachment with a pigmented demarcation line.

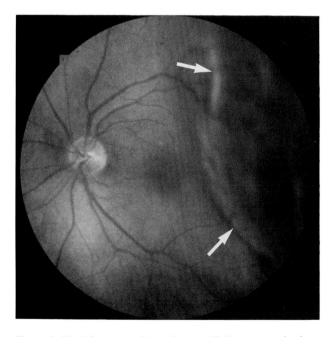

Figure 6–85. A fresh retinal detachment with the progressing border approaching the macula.

ment granules in the vitreous, are signs of recent occurrence of the break. The presence of pigment hyperplasia around a break is a good prognostic sign. The occurrence of the vitreous shift in cataract surgery is thought to be partially responsible for the increased incidence of rhegmatogenous retinal detachment. In phakic eyes the incidence of detachment in the fellow eye is between 11 and 31 percent. Bilaterality is a very important consideration in the diagnosis and management of retinal detachment. Risk factors associated with retinal detachment are given in Table 6–9. **See color plates 110 and 111.**

A retinal detachment (Figs. 6–84 to 6–88) appears as an undulating elevation that is transparent in the early stage evolving to semitransparency with time. The older the detachment, the more opaque the detached area. The undulation is enhanced by having the patient move the eye around. This facilitates viewing the detachment both with the binocular indirect ophthalmoscope and with B-scan ultrasonography when viewing through an opaque media. Examination of the patient in the seated position often enhances the billowing and undulation effect, as the

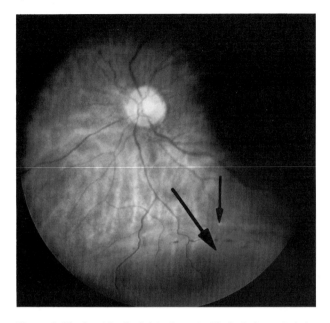

Figure 6–86. An old retinal detachment with dual pigmented demarcation lines (*arrows*).

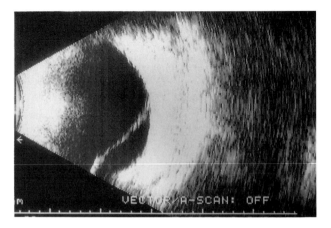

Figure 6–88. B-scan of the retinal detachment shown in Figure 6–87.

retina has a tendency to settle back when the patient is in a supine position. This elevation contains retinal vessels and is known to obscure underlying choroidal detail. A shallow retinal detachment is more difficult to see, and often the clinician must use the scleral in-

denter to discover this subtlety. When symptoms indicate a possible detachment but the view is not confirmatory, visual fields and B-scan ultrasonography (Fig. 6–88) can be of assistance. When performing the visual field test, take care to perform 60-degree fields to encompass the peripheral retina. Billowing folds of retina indicate a significant accumulation of subretinal fluid.

Progression of a retinal detachment is determined by location, size, and number of breaks in the retina, and the strength of the remaining vitreoretinal adhesions (Table 6–12). If a retinal detachment remains stationary for about 3 months, a pigment hyperplasia line develops at its posterior border. This is known as a demarcation line or a high-water line. Demarcation lines occur more frequently in inferior retinal detachments because of the slower progression. **See color plate 111.** Superior retinal detachments will evolve at a faster rate because of the involvement of gravity. Demarcation lines may be multiple in appearance and indicate chronicity. A long-standing retinal detachment is taut and often folded with irregular white lines because of hydration and proliferation of glial and connective tissues on its surface.

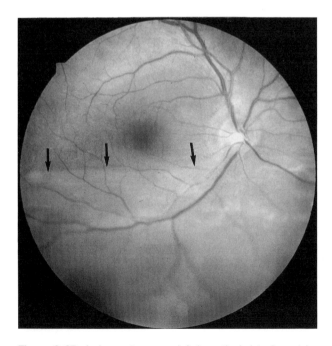

Figure 6–87. A rhegmatogenous inferior retinal detachment intruding just slightly inferior to the macula. The small arrows represent the advancing edge.

TABLE 6–12. INDICATORS OF DURATION OF RETINAL DETACHMENT

1. Pigmented demarcation line—3 months
2. Taut surface and connective tissue on surface—long-standing
3. Balloons of subretinal fluid inferior—4 weeks in superior retina
4. Thinned retina—long-standing
5. Intraretinal cysts and fixed retinal folds—long-standing
6. Shifting subretinal fluid—long-standing with breaks in detached retina
7. Intraretinal exudates—long-standing

Contraction of these tissues can produce folds, and undulation with movement is minimized. Pigment may accumulate, and eventually the retinal tissue becomes necrotic. Massive preretinal proliferation may occur with chronicity, but it is more commonly characteristic of postsurgical retinal detachment complications. In chronic retinal detachments the intraocular pressure may be elevated (Schwartz syndrome) or decreased, and there may be cells and flare in the anterior chamber. The retinal detachment is due to abnormal vitreoretinal traction, causing a break in compromised sensory retina. This break allows access of liquefied vitreous into the subretinal space. Continuing traction with increased liquefied vitreous in the space will allow for a progression in the development of the retinal detachment. Figure 6–84, a rhegmatogenous retinal detachment with the demarcation line, demonstrates the liquefied vitreous in the subsensory retinal space. This figure also demonstrates the reactive hyperplasia creating the demarcation line.

Management. Rhegmatogenous retinal detachment is caused by a retinal break with the ingress of liquefied vitreous and continued vitreoretinal traction. The detachment has the potential to progress to include the macula at a relatively rapid rate. It must be remembered that the longer the macula is detached, the poorer the prognosis.

There are indicators of the duration of a retinal detachment. These could be useful in determining the general prognosis of a patient as well as how soon the patient should be seen by a retinal specialist. It should be remembered that when a retinal detachment has been present in the upper quadrant for over 4 weeks, the subretinal fluid often sinks into the lower half of the fundus, where large balloons of detachment present. Another indicator of the duration is the pigmented demarcation line. A pigmented demarcation line usually takes approximately 3 months to form. Other pigmentary changes also occur over a longer period of time. Marked retinal atrophy or thinned retina results from a long-standing retinal detachment. The longer the retina is detached, the more prone this retina is toward the development of intraretinal cysts and fixed retinal folds. The intraretinal macrocysts are characteristic of retinal dialysis, which creates a slowly evolving rhegmatogenous retinal detachment. Also, it should be noted that shifting subretinal fluid indicates a retina that has been detached for a while with small breaks in that area of detached retina. Another sign of duration of the retinal detachment is the presence of intraretinal yellowish exudates. These exudates appear in an area of detached retina after a prolonged period. These yellowish intraretinal exudates disappear once the retina is reattached.

The management of all rhegmatogenous retinal detachments is a consultation with a fellowship-trained retinal specialist. A recent onset detachment deserves an immediate consultation whereas a consultation for a chronic detachment may be delayed by a couple of days. This author is adamant about same-day consultations, as a delay often will severely compromise outcome. The anatomic success rate of reattachment approaches 90 percent of surgical cases. Unfortunately, visual results of 20/50 or better are achieved in only 55 percent of eyes. Approximately 10 to 20 percent of eyes require multiple surgical procedures to achieve reattachment. Surgical procedures are numerous and the reader interested in the techniques can consult a number of texts concerning this issue.

The primary care practitioner is often concerned with the comanagement of the post surgical detachment patient and should be aware of complications following the procedures. Complications are listed in Table 6–13.

Of special interest is the refractive challenge following retinal detachment repair requiring a buckling procedure. The correction of the patient brings a new challenge, as there is usually a significant anisometropia and often an image size difference between the two eyes. This necessitates alterations in both the base curves and thickness of the spectacle

TABLE 6–13. COMPLICATIONS FOLLOWING RHEGMATOGENOUS RETINAL DETACHMENT REPAIR

Up to 6 Months Postop	After 6 Months Postop
Cystoid macular edema in 30 to 40% of eyes	Cystoid macular edema
Endophthalmitis	Endophthalmitis
Preretinal macular fibrosis (proliferative vitreoretinopathy) in up to 25% of patients having scleral buckles	Preretinal macular fibrosis (proliferative vitreoretinopathy) in up to 25% of patients having scleral buckles
Redetachment of the retina	Cataract
Glaucoma	Subretinal fluid
Conjunctival adhesions causing symblepharon	Strabismus
Strabismus in up to 55% of patients having scleral buckles	Severe anisometropia and aniseikonia
Severe anisometropia and aniseikonia	Cataract formation secondary to intraocular manipulation
Severe vitreous floaters	Pthisis bulbi
Anterior segment ischemia and necrosis	Buckle movement, exposure and intrusion
Choroidal detachment	Keratoconjunctivitis sicca
Movement and exposure of the buckle	Ptosis
Keratoconjunctivitis sicca	

lenses and manipulation of the refractive indices of the spectacle lenses. The use of a contact lens postoperatively is the ideal solution to the globe elongation problem; unfortunately, the patient often has keratoconjunctivitis sicca in the operated eye, complicating successful wear of the contact lens.

One other clinical note concerns the patient with glaucoma. It is incumbent on the primary care practitioner to always carefully evaluate the fundus for risk factors associated with retinal detachment prior to initiating miotic therapy. After initiation of miotic therapy, it is important to carefully evaluate the retina under dilation on a yearly basis.

REFERENCES

Human Vitreous and Posterior Vitreous Detachment

Avila MP, et al. Biomicroscopic study of the vitreous in macular breaks. *Ophthalmology.* 1983;90:1277–1283.

Balazs EA. Fine structure of the developing vitreous. *Int Ophthalmol Clin.* 1975;15:53–63.

Berman ER, Michelson IC. The chemical composition of the human vitreous body as related to age and myopia. *Exp Eye Res.* 1964;3:9–15.

Boldrey EE. Risk of retinal tears in patients with vitreous floaters. *Am J Ophthalmol.* 1983;96:783–787.

Cibis GW, et al. Retinal hemorrhages in posterior vitreous detachment. *Am J Ophthalmol.* 1975;80:1043–1046.

Davis MD. Natural history of retinal breaks without detachment. *Arch Ophthalmol.* 1974;92:183–194.

Fine B, Tousimis A. The structure of the vitreous body and the suspensory ligaments of the lens. *Arch Ophthalmol.* 1961;65:95–110.

Foos RY. Vitreoretinal juncture: Topographical variations. *Invest Ophthalmol.* 1972;11:801–808.

Forrester JV, Grierson I. The cellular response to blood in the vitreous: An ultrastructural study. *J Pathol.* 1979;129:43–52.

Foulds WS. The vitreous in retinal detachment. *Trans Ophthalmol Soc UK.* 1975;95:412–416.

Hagler WS. Pseudophakic retinal detachment. *Trans Am Acad Ophthalmol Soc.* 1982;80:45–63.

Hirokawa H, et al. Role of the vitreous in idiopathic preretinal macular fibrosis. *Am J Ophthalmol.* 1986;101:166–169.

Hogan MJ. The vitreous, its structure, and relation to the ciliary body and retina. *Invest Ophthalmol.* 1963;2:418–445.

Jack R. Regression of the hyaloid vascular system. *Am J Ophthalmol.* 1972;74:261–272.

Jaffe NS. Complications of acute posterior vitreous detachment. *Ophthalmology.* 1968;79:568–571.

Jaffe NS, et al. Retinal detachment in myopic eyes after intracapsular and extracapsular cataract extraction. *Am J Ophthalmol* 1984;97:48–52.

Jalkh A, et al. Prognostic value of vitreous findings in diabetic retinopathy. *Arch Ophthalmol.* 1982;100:432–434.

Kanski JJ. Complications of acute posterior vitreous detachment. *Br J Ophthalmol.* 1975;80:44–46.

Linder B. Acute posterior vitreous detachment and its retinal complications. A clinical biomicroscopic study. *Acta Ophthalmol.* 1966;87:1–108.

McDonnel PJ, et al. Comparison of intracapsular and extracapsular cataract surgery. Histopathologic study of eyes obtained postmortem. *Ophthalmology.* 1985;92:1208–1212.

Morse PH, et al. Light flashes as a clue to retinal disease. *Arch Ophthalmol.* 1974;91:179–185.

Murakami K, et al. Vitreous floaters. *Ophthalmology.* 1983;90:1271–1276.

Novak M, Welch RB. Complications of acute symptomatic posterior vitreous detachment. *Am J Ophthalmol.* 1984;97:308–314.

Schepens CL, Marden D. Data on the natural history of retinal detachment: Further characterization of certain unilateral nontraumatic cases. *Am J Ophthalmol.* 1966;61:213–226.

Schepens CL, et al. Role of the vitreous in cystoid macular edema. *Surg Ophthalmol.* 1984;28:499–504.

Sebag J. Aging of the vitreous. *Eye.* 1987;1:254–262.

Sebag J, et al. Fibrous structure of the human vitreous. *Ophthalmology.* 1981;88:62.

Tasman WS. Posterior vitreous detachment and peripheral retinal breaks. *Trans Am Acad Ophthalmol Otolaryngol.* 1968;72:217–224.

Asteroid Hyalosis

Bergren RL, et al. Prevalence and association of asteroid hyalosis with systemic diseases. *Am J Ophthalmol.* 1991;111:289–293.

Hampton GR, et al. Viewing through the asteroids. *Ophthalmology.* 1981;88:669–672.

Topilow HW, et al. Asteroid hyalosis: Biomicroscopy, ultrastructure, and composition. *Arch Ophthalmol.* 1982;100:964–968.

Amyloid Degeneration of the Vitreous

Cohen AS. Amyloidosis. *N Engl J Med.* 1967;277:522–530.

Hitchings RA, Tripathi RC. Vitreous opacities in primary amyloid disease: A clinical, histochemical, and ultrastructural report. *Br J Ophthalmol.* 1976;60:41–54.

Kaufman HE, Thomas LB. Vitreous opacities diagnostic of familial primary amyloidosis. *N Engl J Med.* 1959;261:1267–1271.

Paton D, Duke JR. Primary familial amyloidosis: Ocular manifestations with histopathologic observations. *Am J Ophthalmol.* 1966;61:736–747.

Savage DJ, et al. Amyloidosis of the vitreous: Fluorescein angiographic findings and association with neovascularization. *Arch Ophthalmol.* 1982;100:1776–1779.

Schwartz MF, et al. An unusual case of ocular involvement in primary systemic nonfamilial amyloidosis. *Ophthalmology.* 1982;89:394–401.

Wong VG, McFarlin DE. Primary familial amyloidosis. *Arch Ophthalmol.* 1967;78:208–213.

Congenital Hereditary Retinoschisis

Balian JV, Falls HF. Congenital vascular veils in the vitreous. *Arch Ophthalmol.* 1960;63:92–101.

Bengtsson B, Linder B. Sex-linked hereditary juvenile retinoschisis: Presentation of two affected families. *Acta Ophthalmol.* 1967;45:411–423.

Brockhurst RJ. Photocoagulation in congenital retinoschisis. *Arch Ophthalmol.* 1970;84:158–165.

Burns RP, et al. Juvenile sex-linked retinoschisis: Clinical and genetic studies. *Trans Am Acad Ophthalmol Otolaryngol.* 1971;75:1011–1021.

Conway BP, Welch RB. X-chromosome-linked juvenile retinoschisis with hemorrhagic retinal cyst. *Am J Ophthalmol.* 1977;83:853–855.

Forsius H, et al. Visual acuity in 183 cases of X-chromosomal retinoschisis. *Can J Ophthalmol.* 1973;8:385–393.

Harris GS. Retinoschisis: Pathogenesis and treatment. *Can J Ophthalmol.* 1968;3:312–317.

Harris GS, Yeung JW. Maculopathy of sex-linked juvenile retinoschisis. *Can J Ophthalmol.* 1976;11:1–10.

Hirose T, et al. Congenital retinoschisis with night blindness in two girls. *Ann Ophthalmol.* 1980;12:848–856.

Hung JY, Hilton GF. Neovascular glaucoma in a patient with X-linked juvenile retinoschisis. *Ann Ophthalmol.* 1980;12:1054–1055.

Lisch W. Hereditary vitreoretinal degenerations. *Dev Ophthalmol.* 1983;8:1–90.

Odland M. Congenital retinoschisis. *Acta Ophthalmol.* 1981; 59:649–658.

Sabates FN. Juvenile retinoschisis. *Am J Ophthalmol.* 1966;62: 683–688.

Schulman J, et al. Indication for vitrectomy in congenital retinoschisis. *Br J Ophthalmol.* 1987;69:482–486.

Yanoff M, et al. Histopathology of juvenile retinoschisis. *Arch Ophthalmol.* 1968;1:30–33.

Wagner's Hereditary Vitreoretinal Degeneration

Alexander RL, Shea M. Wagner's disease. *Arch Ophthalmol.* 1965;74:310–318

Brown GC, Tasman WS. Vitrectomy and Wagner's vitreoretinal degeneration. *Am J Ophthalmol.* 1978;86:485–488.

Hirose T, et al. Wagner's hereditary vitreoretinal degeneration and retinal detachment. *Arch Ophthalmol.* 1973;89: 176–185.

Manning LM. Wagner's hereditary vitreoretinal degeneration. *Aust J Ophthalmol.* 1980;8:29–33.

Manschot WA. Pathology of hereditary conditions related to retinal detachment. *Ophthalmologica.* 1971;162:223–224.

Takahashi M, et al. Biomicroscopic evaluation and photography of posterior vitreous detachment. *Arch Ophthalmol.* 1980;98:665–668.

Van Nouhuys CE. Chorioretinal dysplasia in young subjects with Wagner's hereditary vitreoretinal degeneration. *Int Ophthalmol.* 1981;3:67–77.

Goldmann–Favre Vitreoretinal Degeneration

Carr RE, Siegel JM. The vitreo-tapeto-retinal degenerations. *Arch Ophthalmol.* 1970;84:436–445.

Fishman GA, et al. Diagnostic features of the Favre–Goldmann syndrome. *Br J Ophthalmol.* 1976;60:345–353.

Green JL, Jampol LM. Vascular opacification and leakage in X-linked (juvenile) retinoschisis. *Br J Ophthalmol.* 1979;63: 368–373.

Peyman GA, et al. Histopathology of Goldmann–Favre syndrome obtained by full-thickness eye-wall biopsy. *Ann Ophthalmol.* 1977;9:479–484.

Familial Exudative Vitreoretinopathy

Boldrey EE, et al. The histopathology of familial vitreoretinopathy. A report of two cases. *Arch Ophthalmol.* 1985; 103:238–241.

Brockhurst RJ, et al. Pathological findings in familial exudative vitreoretinopathy. *Arch Ophthalmol.* 1981;99: 2143–2146.

Canny CLB, Oliver GL. Fluorescein angiographic findings in familial exudative vitreoretinopathy. *Arch Ophthalmol.* 1976;94:1114–1120.

Chaudhuri PR, et al. Familial exudative vitreoretinopathy associated with familial thrombocytopathy. *Br J Ophthalmol.* 1983;67:755–758.

Criswick VG, Schepens CL. Familial exudative vitreoretinopathy. *Am J Ophthalmol.* 1969;68:578–594.

Feldman EL, et al. Autosomal dominant exudative vitreoretinopathy. *Arch Ophthalmol.* 1983;101:1532–1535.

Gow J, Oliver GL. Familial exudative vitreoretinopathy. An expanded view. *Arch Ophthalmol.* 1971;86:150–155.

Jampol LM, Goldbaum MH. Peripheral proliferative retinopathies. *Surv Ophthalmol.* 1980;25:1–14.

Miyakubo H, et al. Retinal vascular pattern in familial exudative vitreoretinopathy. *Ophthalmology.* 1984;91: 1524–1530.

Miyakubo H, et al. Retinal involvement in familial exudative vitreoretinopathy. *Ophthalmologica.* 1982;185: 125–135.

Ober RR, et al. Autosomal dominant exudative vitreoretinopathy. *Br J Ophthalmol.* 1980;64:112–120.

Tasman W, et al. Familial exudative vitreoretinopathy. *Trans Am Ophthalmol Soc.* 1981;79:211–225.

Van Nouhuys CE. Dominant exudative vitreoretinopathy and other vascular developmental disorders of the peripheral retina. *Doc Ophthalmol.* 1982;54:1–14.

Snowflake Vitreoretinal Degeneration

Hirose T, et al. Snowflake degeneration in hereditary vitreoretinal degeneration. *Am J Ophthalmol.* 1974;77:143–153.

Pollack A, et al. Prophylactic laser photocoagulation in hereditary snowflake vitreoretinal degeneration. A family report. *Arch Ophthalmol.* 1983;101:1536–1539.

Robertson DM, et al. Snowflake degeneration of the retina. *Ophthalmology.* 1982;89:1513–1539.

Stickler Syndrome

Blair JV, et al. Hereditary progressive arthro-ophthalmopathy of Stickler. *Am J Ophthalmol.* 1979;88:876–888.

Hall JG, Herrod H. The Stickler syndrome presenting as dominantly inherited cleft palate and blindness. *J Med Genet.* 1975;12:397–400.

Herrmann J, et al. The Stickler syndrome (hereditary arthroophthalmopathy). *Birth Defects.* 1975;11:76–103.

Liberfarb RM, Hirose T. The Wagner–Stickler syndrome. *Birth Defects.* 1982;18:525–538.

Maumenee IH. Vitreoretinal degeneration as a sign of generalized connective tissue disease. *Am J Ophthalmol.* 1979; 88:432–449.

Nielsen CE. Stickler's syndrome. *Acta Ophthalmol.* 1981; 59:286–295.

Autosomal Dominant Vitreochoroidopathy

Blair NP, et al. Autosomal dominant vitreoretinochoroidopathy. *Br J Ophthalmol.* 1984;68:2–9.

Kaufman SJ, et al. Autosomal dominant vitreo-retinochoroidopathy. *Arch Ophthalmol.* 1982;100:272–278.

Persistent Hyperplastic Primary Vitreous

Federman JL, et al. The surgical and nonsurgical management of persistent hyperplastic primary vitreous. *Ophthalmology.* 1982;89:20–24.

Gass JDM. Surgical excision of persistent hyperplastic primary vitreous. *Arch Ophthalmol.* 1970;83:163–168.

Goldberg MF, Mafee M. Computed tomography for diagnosis of persistent hyperplastic primary vitreous (PHPV). *Ophthalmology.* 1983;90:442–451.

Mann I. Congenital retinal fold. *Br J Ophthalmol.* 1935;19: 641–658.

Moazed K, et al. Rubeosis iridis in "pseudogliomas." *Surv Ophthalmol.* 1980;25:85–90.

Nankin SJ, Scott WE. Persistent hyperplastic primary vitreous: Roto-extraction and other surgical experience. *Arch Ophthalmol.* 1977;95:240–243.

Pollard Z. Results of treatment of persistent hyperplastic primary vitreous. *Ophthalmic Surg.* 1991;22:48–52.

Pruett RC, Schepens CL. Posterior hyperplastic primary vitreous. *Am J Ophthalmol.* 1970;69:535–543.

Renz B, Vygantas C. Embryonic intraocular vasculature and associated developmental anomalies including persistent hyperplastic primary vitreous. *Perspect Ophthalmol.* 1979; 3:121–128.

Stark WJ, et al. Persistent hyperplastic primary vitreous: Surgical treatment. *Ophthalmology.* 1983;90:452–457.

Peripheral Senile Pigmentary Degeneration

Bastek JV, et al. Chorioretinal juncture. Pigmentary patterns of the peripheral fundus. *Ophthalmology.* 1982;89: 1455–1463.

Rutnin U, Schepens CL. Fundus appearance in normal eyes, III. Peripheral degenerations. *Am J Ophthalmol.* 1967;64: 1040–1062.

Primary Chorioretinal Atrophy

Jones WL, Reidy RW. *Atlas of the Peripheral Fundus.* Boston: Butterworths; 1985.

O'Malley PO, Allen RA, Strattsma BR, O'Malley CC. Pavingstone degeneration of the retina. *Arch Ophthalmol.* 1965;73:169–182.

Rutnin U, Schepens CL. Fundus appearance in normal eyes, III. Peripheral degenerations. *Am J Ophthalmol.* 1967;64: 1040–1062.

Typical and Reticular Peripheral Cystoid Degeneration

Bastek JV, et al. Chorioretinal juncture. Pigmentary patterns of the peripheral fundus. *Ophthalmology.* 1982;89: 1455–1463.

Hines JL, Jones WC. Peripheral microcystoid retinal degeneration and retinoschisis. *J Am Optom Assoc.* 1982;53: 541–545.

Rutnin U, Schepens CL. Fundus appearance in normal eyes, III. Peripheral degenerations. *Am J Ophthalmol.* 1967;64: 1040–1062.

Congenital Hypertrophy of the RPE

Heyen F, et al. Predictive value of congenital hypertrophy of the retinal pigment epithelium as a clinical marker for familial adenomatous polyposis. *Dis Col Rect.* 1990;33: 1003–1008.

Kasner L, et al. A histopathologic study of the pigmented fundus lesions in familial adenomatous polyposis. *Retina.* 1992;12:35–42.

Morton DG, et al. Role of congenital hypertrophy of the retinal pigment epithelium in the predictive diagnosis of familial adenomatous polyposis. *Br J Surg.* 1992;79:689–693.

Romania A, et al. Retinal pigment epithelium lesions as a biomarker of disease in patients with familial adenomatous polyposis. A follow-up report. *Ophthalmology.* 1992; 99:911–913.

Shields JA, et al. Lack of association among typical congenital hypertrophy of the retinal pigment epithelium, adenomatous polyposis, and Gardner syndrome. *Ophthalmology.* 1992;99:1709–1713.

Benign Choroidal Melanoma

Augsburger JJ, et al. Macular choroidal nevi. *Int Ophthalmol Clin.* 1981;21:99–106.

Folk JC, et al. The treatment of serous macular detachment secondary to choroidal melanomas and nevi. *Ophthalmology.* 1989;96:547–551.

Gass JDM. Problems in the differential diagnosis of choroidal nevi and malignant melanomas. The 33rd Edward Jackson memorial lecture. *Am J Ophthalmol.* 1977;87: 299–323.

Lim H. Choroidal melanocytic growth: A review of the common clinical procedures for diagnosis. *S J Optom.* 1992;10: 16–19.

Mims J, Shields JA. Follow-up studies of suspicious choroidal nevi. *Ophthalmology.* 1978;85:929–943.

Mines JA, et al. Choroidal (subretinal) neovascularization secondary to choroidal nevus and successful treatment with argon laser photocoagulation: Case reports and review of the literature. *Ophthalmologica.* 1985;190:210–218.

Pro M, et al. Serous detachment of the fovea associated with choroidal nevi. *Arch Ophthalmol.* 1978;96:1374–1377.

Shields CL, et al. Uveal melanoma and pregnancy. *Ophthalmology.* 1991;98:1667–1673.

Shields JA. *Diagnosis and Management of Intraocular Tumors.* St. Louis: Mosby; 1983.

Malignant Choroidal Melanoma

Albert DM, et al. Treatment of metastatic uveal melanoma: Review and recommendations. *Surv Ophthalmol.* 1992;36: 429–438.

Brancato R, et al. Enucleation after argon laser photocoagulation for choroidal melanoma. *Ann Ophthalmol.* 1988;20: 296–298.

Coleman DJ, et al. Ultrasonic tissue characterization of uveal melanoma and prediction of patient survival after enucleation and brachytherapy. *Am J Ophthalmol.* 1991;112: 682–688.

Davidorf FH, et al. Choroidal malignant melanoma. An 18-year experience with radon. *Arch Ophthalmol.* 1987; 105:352–355.

Earl J, et al. Selection of iodine 125 for the Collaborative Ocular Melanoma Study. *Arch Ophthalmol.* 1987;105:763–764.

Egan KM, et al. Epidemiologic aspects of uveal melanoma. *Surv Ophthalmol.* 1988; 32:239–251.

Favilla I, et al. Phototherapy of posterior uveal melanomas. *Br J Ophthalmol.* 1991;75:718–721.

Francois J. Treatment of malignant choroidal melanomas by photocoagulation. *Ophthalmologica.* 1982;184:121–130.

Gragoudas ES. Proton beam therapy of uveal melanomas. *Arch Ophthalmol.* 1986;104:349–351.

Gragoudas ES, et al. Survival of patients with metastases from uveal melanoma. *Ophthalmology.* 1991;98:383–390.

Gragoudas ES, et al. Intraocular recurrence of uveal melanoma after proton beam irradiation. *Ophthalmology.* 1992;99:760–766.

Haas BD, et al. Diffuse choroidal melanoma in a child. A lesion extending the spectrum of melanocytic hamartomas. *Ophthalmology.* 1986;93: 1632–1638.

Jalkh AE, et al. Treatment of small choroidal melanomas with photocoagulation. *Ophthalmic Surg.* 1988;19:738–742.

Lincoff H, et al. The cryosurgical treatment of intraocular tumors. *Am J Ophthalmol.* 1967;63:389–399.

Lommatzsch PK, Lommatzsch R. Treatment of juxtapapillary melanomas. *Br J Ophthalmol.* 1991;75:715–717.

McLean IW, et al. Reappraisal of Callender's spindle: A type of malignant melanoma of the choroid and ciliary body. *Am J Ophthalmol.* 1978;86:557–564.

Meyer-Schwickerath G. Photocoagulation of choroidal melanomas. *Doc Ophthalmol.* 1980;50:57–61.

Nowakowski VA, et al. Uveal melanoma: Development of metastases after helium ion irradiation. *Radiology.* 1991; 178:277–280.

Packer S, et al. Long-term results of iodine 125 irradiation of uveal melanoma. *Ophthalmology.* 1992;99:767–774.

Park WL. The collaborative ocular melanoma study. *J Am Optom Assoc.* 1992;63:609–610.

Prescher G, et al. Nonrandom chromosomal abnormalities in primary uveal melanoma. *J Nat Cancer Inst.* 1990; 82:1765–1769.

Seddon JM, et al. Relative survival rates after alternative therapies for uveal melanomas. *Ophthalmology.* 1990;97: 769–777.

Shields CL, et al. Uveal melanoma and pregnancy. *Ophthalmology.* 1991;98:1667–1673.

Shields JA. Counseling the patient with a posterior uveal melanoma. *Am J Ophthalmol.* 1988;106:88–91.

Shields JA. Current approaches to the diagnosis and management of choroidal melanomas. *Surv Ophthalmol.* 1977; 21:443–463.

Shields JA, et al. Partial lamellar sclerouvectomy for ciliary body and choroidal tumors. *Ophthalmology.* 1991;98: 971–983.

Straatsma BR, et al. Enucleation versus plaque irradiation for choroidal melanoma. *Ophthalmology.* 1988;95:1000–1004.

Oral Pearls and Enclosed Oral Bays

Jones WL, Reidy RW. *Atlas of the Peripheral Fundus.* Boston: Butterworths; 1985.

Rutnin U, Schepens CL. Fundus appearance in normal eyes. *Am J Ophthalmol.* 1967;64:840.

Sigelman J. Vitreous base classification of retinal tears: Clinical application. *Surv Ophthalmol.* 1980;25:59–74.

Tasman W, Shields JA. *Disorders of the Peripheral Fundus.* Hagerstown, MD: Harper & Row; 1980.

Retinal White With Pressure

Hunter JE. Retinal white without pressure: review and relative incidence. *Am J Optom Physiol Opt.* 1982;59:293–296.

Nagpal KC, et al. Dark without-pressure fundus lesions. *Br J Ophthalmol.* 1975;59:476–479.

Rutnin U, Schepens CL. Fundus appearance in normal eyes, III. Peripheral degenerations. *Am J Ophthalmol.* 1967;64: 1040–1062.

Tolentino FI, et al. *Vitreoretinal Disorders. Diagnosis and Management.* Philadelphia: Saunders; 1976:334–339.

Vitreoretinal Traction Tufts

Byer NE. Cystic retinal tufts and their relationship to retinal detachment. *Arch Ophthalmol.* 1981;99:1788–1790.

Meridional Folds

Tasman W, Shields JA. *Disorders of the Peripheral Fundus.* Hagerstown, MD: Harper & Row; 1980.

Degenerative Retinoschisis

Byer NE. Long-term natural history study of senile retinoschisis with implications for management. *Ophthalmology.* 1986;93:1127–1137.

Byer NE. The natural history of senile retinoschisis. *Trans Am Acad Ophthalmol Otolaryngol.* 1976;81:458–471.

Byer NE. Spontaneous regression of retinoschisis. *Arch Ophthalmol.* 1972;88:207–209.

Campo RV, et al. Vascular leakage, neovascularization, and vitreous hemorrhage in senile bullous retinoschisis. *Am J Ophthalmol.* 1983;95:826–832.

Foos RY. Senile retinoschisis: Relationship to cystoid degeneration. *Trans Am Acad Ophthalmol Otolaryngol.* 1970; 74:433–450.

Hauch TL, et al. Macular function in typical and reticular retinoschisis. *Retina.* 1981;1:293–295.

Landers MB, Robinson CH. Photocoagulation in the diagnosis of senile retinoschisis. *Am J Ophthalmol.* 1977;84: 18–23.

Straatsma BR. Clinical features of degenerative retinoschisis. *Aust J Ophthalmol.* 1980;8:201–206.

Yassur Y, et al. Argon laser treatment of senile retinoschisis. *Br J Ophthalmol.* 1983;67:381–384.

Lattice Degeneration

Bastek JV, et al. Chorioretinal juncture. Pigmentary patterns of the peripheral fundus. *Ophthalmology.* 1982;89: 1455–1463.

Burton TC. The influence of refractive error and lattice degeneration on the incidence of retinal detachment. *Trans Am Ophthalmol Soc.* 1989;87:143–157.

Byer NE. Long-term natural history of lattice degeneration of the retina. *Ophthalmology.* 1989;96:1396–1402.

Byer NE. Lattice degeneration of the retina. *Surv Ophthalmol.* 1978;23:213–248.

Byer NE. Changes in and prognosis of lattice degeneration of the retina. *Trans Am Acad Ophthalmol Otolaryngol.* 1974; 78:114–125.

Byer NE. Clinical study of lattice degeneration of the retina. *Trans Am Acad Ophthalmol Otolaryngol.* 1965;69:1064–1081.

Celorio JM, Pruett RC. Prevalence of lattice degeneration and its relation to axial length in severe myopia. *Am J Ophthalmol.* 1991;111:20–23.

Folk JC, et al. The fellow eye of patients with phakic lattice retinal detachment. *Ophthalmology.* 1989;96:72–79.

Foos RY, et al. Comparison of lesions predisposing to rhegmatogenous retinal detachment by race of subjects. *Am J Ophthalmol.* 1983;96:644–649.

Foos RY, Simons KB. Vitreous in lattice degeneration of the retina. *Ophthalmology.* 1984;91:452–457.

Halpern JI. Routine screening of the retinal periphery. *Am J Ophthalmol.* 1966;62:99–102.

Kraushar MF, Steinberg JA. Miotics and retinal detachment: Upgrading the community standard. *Surg Ophthalmol.* 1991;35:311–316.

Leff SR, et al. Rhegmatogenous retinal detachment after YAG capsulotomy. *Ophthalmology.* 1987;94:1222–1225.

Lewkonia I, et al. Lattice degeneration in a family with retinal detachment and cataract. *Br J Ophthalmol.* 1973;57: 566–577.

MacEwan CJ, Baines PS. Retinal detachment following YAG laser capsulotomy. *Eye.* 1989;3:759–763.

Michaelson IC, et al. A study in the prevention of retinal detachment. *Ann Ophthalmol.* 1969;1:49–55.

Murakami F, Ohba N. Genetics of lattice degeneration of the retina. *Ophthalmologica.* 1982;185:136–140.

Okinami S, et al. Juvenile retinal detachment. *Ophthalmologica.* 1987;194:95–102.

Parelhof ES, et al. Radial perivascular lattice degeneration of the retina. *Ann Ophthalmol.* 1980;12:25–32.

Robinson MR, Streeten BW. The surface morphology of retinal breaks and lattice degeneration. A scanning electron microscopic study. *Ophthalmology.* 1986;93:237–246.

Semes LP. Lattice degeneration of the retina and retinal detachment. *Optom Clin.* 1992;2:71–91.

Straatsma BR, et al. Lattice degeneration of the retina. *Trans Am Acad Ophthalmol Otolaryngol.* 1974;78:87–113.

Tasman WS. Pseudophakic retinal detachment after YAG laser capsulotomy. *Aust NZ J Ophthalmol.* 1989;17:277–279.

Tasman WS. Late complications of retrolental fibroplasia. *Ophthalmology.* 1979;86:1724–1740.

Snail-track Degeneration

Byer NE. Lattice degeneration of the retina. *Surv Ophthalmol.* 1978;23:213–248.

Shukla M, Ahuja OP. A possible relationship between lattice and snail track degenerations of the retina. *Am J Ophthalmol.* 1981;92:482–485.

Straatsma BR, et al. Lattice degeneration of the retina. *Trans Am Acad Ophthalmol Otolaryngol.* 1974;78:87–113.

Atrophic Retinal Holes

Foos RY. Retinal holes. *Am J Ophthalmol.* 1978;86:354–358.

Foos RY. Tears of the peripheral retina: Pathogenesis, incidence, and classification in autopsy eyes. *Mod Probl Ophthalmol.* 1975;15:68–81.

Jones WL, Reidy RW. *Atlas of the Peripheral Fundus.* Boston: Butterworths; 1985.

Kanski JJ. *Retinal Detachment. A Colour Manual of Diagnosis and Treatment.* Boston: Butterworths; 1986.

Rutnin U, Schepens CL. Fundus appearance in normal eyes. *Am J Ophthalmol.* 1967;64:840.

Schepens CL. *Retinal Detachment and Allied Diseases.* Philadelphia: Saunders; 1983.

Sigelman J. Vitreous base classification of retinal tears: Clinical application. *Surv Ophthalmol.* 1980;25:59–74.

Operculated Retinal Holes

Foos RY. Tears of the peripheral retina: Pathogenesis, incidence, and classification in autopsy eyes. *Mod Probl Ophthalmol.* 1975;15:68–81.

Jones WL, Reidy RW. *Atlas of the Peripheral Fundus.* Boston: Butterworths; 1985.

Kanski JJ. *Retinal Detachment. A Colour Manual of Diagnosis and Treatment.* Boston: Butterworths; 1986.

Rutnin U, Schepens CL. Fundus appearance in normal eyes. *Am J Ophthalmol.* 1967;64:840.

Schepens CL. *Retinal Detachment and Allied Diseases.* Philadelphia: Saunders; 1983.

Linear Retinal Tears

Benson WE. Prophylactic therapy of retinal breaks. *Surv Ophthalmol.* 1977;22:41–47.

Berglin I, et al. A new technique of treating rhegmatogenous retinal detachment using the Q-switched Nd:YAG laser. *Ophthalmic Surg.* 1987;18:890–892.

Byer NE. The natural history of asymptomatic retinal breaks. *Ophthalmology.* 1982;89:1033–1039.

Fleck BW, et al. Nd:YAG laser augmented pneumatic retinopexy. *Ophthalmic Surg.* 1988;19:855–858.

Folk JC, et al. The fellow eye of patients with phakic lattice retinal detachment. *Ophthalmology.* 1989;96:72–79.

Kain HL. Chorioretinal adhesions after argon laser photocoagulation. *Arch Ophthalmol.* 1984;102:612–615.

Machemer R. The importance of fluid absorption, traction, intraocular currents, and chorioretinal scars in the therapy of rhegmatogenous retinal detachments. XLI Edward Jackson memorial lecture. *Am J Ophthalmol.* 1984;98: 681–693.

Sigleman J. Laser therapy of peripheral retinal diseases, I. Breaks and detachments. *Ophthalmic Laser Ther.* 1985;1: 35–49.

Sigleman J. Vitreous base classification of retinal tears: Clinical applications. *Surv Ophthalmol.* 1980;25:59–74.

Smith PW, et al. Retinal detachments after extracapsular cataract extraction with posterior chamber intraocular lens. *Ophthalmology.* 1987;94:495–504.

Retinal Dialysis

Assaf AA. Traumatic retinal detachment. *J Trauma.* 1985;25: 1085–1089.

Chignell AH. Retinal dialysis. *Br J Ophthalmol.* 1973;57: 572–577.

Goffstein R, Burton TC. Differentiating traumatic from nontraumatic retinal detachment. *Ophthalmology.* 1982;89: 361–364.

Hagler WS. Retinal dialysis: A statistical and genetic study to determine pathogenic factors. *Trans Am Ophthalmol Soc.* 1980;78:687–733.

Hagler WS, North AW. Retinal dialyses and retinal detachment. *Arch Ophthalmol.* 1968;79:376–388.

Hamrick KE, Helgeson MK. Retinal dialysis. *Optom Clinics.* 1992;2:93–112.

Johnston PB. Traumatic retinal detachment. *Br J Ophthalmol.* 1991;75:18–21.

Kinyoun JL, Knobloch WH. Idiopathic retinal dialysis. *Retina.* 1984;4:9–14.

Matsuo N, et al. Photoreceptor outer segments in the aqueous humor in rhegmatogenous retinal detachment. *Am J Ophthalmol.* 1986;101:673–679.

Ross WH. Traumatic retinal dialyses. *Arch Ophthalmol.* 1981;99:1371–1374.

Schwartz A. Chronic open-angle glaucoma secondary to rhegmatogenous retinal detachment. *Am J Ophthalmol.* 1973;75:205–211.

Smiddy WE, Green WR. Retinal dialysis: Pathology and pathogenesis. *Retina.* 1982;2:94–116.

Verdaguer TJ, et al. Genetical studies in nontraumatic retinal dialysis. *Mod Probl Ophthalmol.* 1975;15:34–39.

Zion VM, Burton TC. Retinal dialysis. *Arch Ophthalmol.* 1980;98:1971–1974.

Giant Retinal Tears

Ando F, Kondo J. Surgical techniques for giant retinal tears with retinal tacks. *Ophthalmic Surg.* 1986;17:408–411.

Billington BM, et al. Management of retinal detachment in the Wagner–Stickler syndrome. *Trans Ophthalmol Soc UK.* 1985;104:875–879.

Chung H, et al. Use of high-density silicone oil for giant retinal tear. *Retina.* 1987;7:180–182.

Fitzgerald CR. The use of Healon in a case of rolled-over retina. *Retina.* 1981;1:227–231.

Freeman HM. Fellow eyes of giant retinal breaks. *Trans Am Ophthalmol Soc.* 1978;76:643–682.

Hoffman ME, Sorr ELM. Management of giant retinal tears without scleral buckling. *Retina.* 1986;6:197–204.

Kanski JJ. Giant retinal tears. *Am J Ophthalmol.* 1975;79: 846–852.

McLeod D. Giant retinal tears after central vitrectomy. *Br J Ophthalmol.* 1985;69:96–98.

Peyman GA, Schulman JA. *Intravitreal Surgery.* Norwalk, CT: Appleton-Century-Crofts; 1986:294–303.

Peyman GA, Smith RT. Use of fluorosilicone to unfold a giant retinal tear. *Int Ophthalmol.* 1987;10:149–150.

Commotio Retinae

Crouch ER, Apple DJ. Posttraumatic migration of retinal pigment epithelial melanin. *Am J Ophthalmol.* 1974;78: 251–254.

Goffstein R, Burton TC. Differentiating traumatic from nontraumatic retinal detachment. *Ophthalmology.* 1982;89: 361–368.

Goldberg MF. Choroidoretinal vascular anastomoses after blunt trauma to the eye. *Am J Ophthalmol.* 1976;82:892–895.

Ross WH. Traumatic retinal dialyses. *Arch Ophthalmol.* 1981;99:1371–1374.

Schepens CL, Marden D. Data on the natural history of retinal detachment: Further characterization of certain unilateral nontraumatic cases. *Am J Ophthalmol.* 1966;61: 213–226.

Smith RE, et al. Late macular complications of choroidal ruptures. *Am J Ophthalmol.* 1974;77:650–658.

Winslow RL, Tasman W. Juvenile rhegmatogenous retinal detachment. *Ophthalmology.* 1978;85:607–618.

Choroidal Detachment

McCulloch C. Pathological and surgical examination of the handling of the lacerated eyeball. *Can J Ophthalmol.* 1983; 18:178–184.

Peyman GA, et al. Computed tomography in choroidal detachment. *Ophthalmology.* 1984;91:156–159.

Zakov ZN, et al. Ultrasonographic mapping of vitreoretinal abnormalities. *Am J Ophthalmol.* 1983;96:622–631.

Pars Planitis

Aaberg TM. The enigma of pars planitis. *Am J Ophthalmol.* 1987;103:828–830.

Aaberg TM, et al. Treatment of pars planitis, I. Cryotherapy. *Surv Ophthalmol.* 1977;22:120–125.

Aaberg TM, et al. Treatment of peripheral uveoretinitis by cryotherapy. *Am J Ophthalmol.* 1973;75:685–688.

Akiyama K, et al. Retinal vascular loss in idiopathic central serous chorioretinopathy with bullous retinal detachment. *Ophthalmology.* 1987;94:1605–609.

Arkfeld DF, Brockhurst RJ. Peripapillary subretinal neovascularization in peripheral uveitis. *Retina.* 1985;5:157–160.

DeVenyi RG, et al. Cryopexy of the vitreous base in the management of peripheral uveitis. *Am J Ophthalmol.* 1988;106: 135–138.

Felder KS, Brockhurst RJ. Neovascular fundus abnormalities in peripheral uveitis. *Arch Ophthalmol.* 1982;100: 750–754.

Mieler WF, et al. Vitrectomy in the management of peripheral uveitis. *Ophthalmology.* 1988;95:859–864.

Nussenblatt RB, et al. Cyclosporin A therapy in the treatment of intraocular inflammatory disease resistant to systemic corticosteroids and cytotoxic agents. *Am J Ophthalmol.* 1983;96:275–282.

Pederson JE, et al. Pathology of pars planitis. *Am J Ophthalmol.* 1978;86:762–774.

Schlaegel TF, Weber JC. Treatment of pars planitis, II. Corticosteroids. *Surv Ophthalmol.* 1977;22:120–125.

Shorb SR, et al. Optic disc neovascularization associated with chronic uveitis. *Am J Ophthalmol.* 1976;82:175–178.

Towler HMA, et al. Low-dose cyclosporin A therapy in chronic posterior uveitis. *Eye.* 1989;3:282–287.

Retinal Detachment

Benson WE. *Retinal Detachment. Diagnosis and Management.* Hagerstown, Md: Harper & Row; 1980.

Benson WE. Prophylactic therapy of retinal breaks. *Surv Ophthalmol.* 1977;22:41–47.

Bradford JD, et al. Pseudophakic retinal detachments. The relationships between retinal tears and the time following cataract surgery at which they occur. *Retina.* 1989;9: 181–186.

Cavallerano AA. Retinal detachment. *Optom Clin.* 1992;2: 25–69.

Charteris DG, et al. Proliferative vitreoretinopathy. Lymphocytes in epiretinal membranes. *Ophthalmology.* 1992; 99:1364–1367.

Chignell AH, et al. Failure in retinal detachment surgery. *Br J Ophthalmol.* 1973;57:525–530.

Coonan P, et al. The incidence of retinal detachment following extracapsular cataract extraction. A ten-year study. *Ophthalmology.* 1985;92:1096–1101.

Cox MS, et al. Traumatic retinal detachment due to ocular contusion. *Arch Ophthalmol.* 1965;76:678–685.

DeJuan E, McCuen BW, Machemer R. The use of retinal tacks in the repair of complicated retinal detachments. *Am J Ophthalmol.* 1986;102:20–24.

Delaney WV, Oates RP. Retinal detachment in the second eye. *Arch Ophthalmol.* 1978;96:629–634.

Eagling EM, Roper-Hall MJ. *Eye Injuries. An Illustrated Guide.* Philadelphia: Lippincott; 1986.

Glaser BM. Treatment of giant retinal tears combined with proliferative vitreoretinopathy. *Ophthalmology.* 1986;93: 1193–1197.

Glaser BM, et al. Proliferative vitreoretinopathy. The mechanism of development of vitreoretinal traction. *Ophthalmology.* 1987;94:327–337.

Hagler WS. Pseudophakic retinal detachment. *Trans Am Acad Ophthalmol Soc.* 1982;80:45–63.

Haimann MH, et al. Epidemiology of retinal detachment. *Arch Ophthalmol.* 1982;100:289–292.

Hamilton AM, Taylor W. Significance of pigment granules in the vitreous. *Br J Ophthalmol.* 1972;56:700–702.

Jones WL, Reidy RW. *Atlas of the Peripheral Fundus.* Boston: Butterworths; 1985.

Kanski JJ. *Retinal Detachment. A Colour Manual of Diagnosis and Treatment.* Boston: Butterworths; 1986.

Kraushar MF. Miotics and retinal detachment. *Arch Ophthalmol.* 1991;109:1659.

Kraushar MF, Steinberg JA. Miotics and retinal detachment: Upgrading the community standard. *Surv Ophthalmol.* 1991;35:311–316.

Laatikainen L. The fellow eye in patients with unilateral retinal detachment: Findings and prophylactic treatment. *Acta Ophthalmologica.* 1985;63:546–551.

Laatikainen L, Harju H. Bilateral rhegmatogenous retinal detachment. *Acta Ophthalmol.* 1985;63:541–545.

Lobes LA, Grand MG. Incidence of cystoid macular edema following scleral buckling procedure. *Arch Ophthalmol.* 1980;98:1230–1232.

Lobes LA, Grand MG. Subretinal lesions following scleral buckling procedures. *Arch Ophthalmol.* 1980;98:680–683.

Machemer R. Pathogenesis and classification of massive preretinal proliferation. *Br J Ophthalmol.* 1978;62:737–747.

Machemer R, et al. An updated classification of retinal detachment with proliferative vitreoretinopathy. *Am J Ophthalmol.* 1991;112:159–165.

Marmor MR, et al. The effect of metabolic inhibitors on retinal adhesion and subretinal fluid resorption. *Invest Ophthalmol Vis Sci.* 1980;19:893–903.

McPherson A, et al. Retinal detachment following late posterior capsulotomy. *Am J Ophthalmol.* 1983;95:593–597.

Merin S, et al. The fate of the fellow eye in retinal detachment. *Am J Ophthalmol.* 1971;71:477–481.

Merin S, et al. The fate of the fellow eye in retinal detachment. *Am J Ophthalmol.* 1971;71:477–481.

Negi A, et al. Effects of intraocular pressure and other factors on subretinal fluid resorption. *Invest Ophthalmol Vis Sci.* 1987;28:2099–2102.

Novak M, Welch RB. Complications of acute symptomatic posterior vitreous detachment. *Am J Ophthalmol.* 1984;97: 308–314.

Ober RR, et al. Rhegmatogenous retinal detachment after neodymium–YAG capsulotomy in phakic and pseudophakic eyes. *Am J Ophthalmol.* 1986;101:81–89.

Peyman GA, Schulman JA. *Intravitreal Surgery.* Norwalk, CT: Appleton-Century-Crofts; 1986.

Phelps CD, Burton TC. Glaucoma and retinal detachment. *Arch Ophthalmol.* 1977;95:418–422.

Pierro L, et al. Peripheral retinal changes and axial myopia. *Retina.* 1992;12:12–17.

Rickman-Barger L, et al. Retinal detachment after neodymium: YAG laser posterior capsulotomy. *Am J Ophthalmol.* 1989;107:531–536.

Schepens CL. *Retinal Detachment and Allied Diseases.* Philadelphia: Saunders; 1983.

Shulka M, Ahuja OP. Photopsia—due to retinal disease. *Ind J Ophthalmol.* 1982;30:91–93.

Sigelman J. *Retinal Diseases. Pathogenesis, Laser Therapy and Surgery.* Boston: Little, Brown; 1984.

Spalton DJ, Hitchings RA, Hunter PA. *Atlas of Clinical Ophthalmology.* London: Gower; 1984.

Tani P, et al. Prognosis for central vision and anatomic reattachment in rhegmatogenous retinal detachment with macula detached. *Am J Ophthalmol.* 1981;92:611–620.

Tasman W, Shields JA. *Disorders of the Peripheral Fundus.* Hagerstown, MD: Harper & Row; 1980.

Transactions of the New Orleans Academy of Ophthalmology Symposium on Medical and Surgical Disease of the Retina and Vitreous. St. Louis: Mosby; 1985.

Wilke SR, et al. The incidence of retinal detachment in Rochester, Minnesota, 1979–1978. *Am J Ophthalmol.* 1982; 94:670–673.

Chapter Seven ■ ■ ■ ■ ■ ■

*H*ereditary Retinal–Choroidal Dystrophies

A CLINICAL GUIDE TO UNDERSTANDING VISUAL ELECTRODIAGNOSIS

In addition to standard differential diagnostic testing techniques such as visual acuities, visual fields, color vision testing, and objective observation technique, the clinician has visual electrodiagnosis to assist in differential diagnosis of hereditary retinal and choroidal diseases. Visual electrodiagnosis is a complex issue and is covered in great detail in several texts. This section is intended to briefly explain electrodiagnostic tests and to relate these tests to hereditary retinal and choroidal disease. The intent is to sensitize the clinician to the indications for electrodiagnostic testing procedures and to provide the clinician with an understanding of the results and how the results apply to the patient.

Electroretinogram (ERG)

The electroretinogram (ERG) is a measurement of the electrical response of the eye to a flash of light. The test is nonspecific, as the stimulus is presented throughout the retina by ganzfeld illumination. In spite of nonspecificity, the ERG is of value in diagnosing ocular disease in which rods or cones are altered in a generalized fashion. The rod–cone dystrophy, retinitis pigmentosa, is the best example of a generalized disease process that affects the ERG.

The Test. The ERG is performed on a patient whose eyes have been maximally dilated. The patient must be light adapted for the photopic ERG and dark adapted for a scotopic ERG. A ground electrode (earclip) is attached to the earlobe that has been appropriately cleaned to enhance contact. A skin electrode is then attached to either the mastoid process or the forehead, after the area has been appropriately cleaned. The skin electrode is the reference against the potential created when the retina is stimulated by light. A contact lens electrode is then placed on the patient's anesthetized cornea, and the fellow eye is occluded. All of the electrode leads are then attached to a preamplifier, and the impedance of the system is checked. The patient then places the chin on a chinrest in a ganzfeld (hemispherical) bowl that assures uniform distribution of the light flash so that the retina is uniformly stimulated. Flashes of light are presented at specified intervals, and the system averages the eye's response, creating a waveform on the oscilloscope. This waveform and its alterations offer a means of analyzing components of retinal function. The ERG is then repeated on the fellow eye. After dark adaptation, the process is repeated to generate a scotopic ERG.

Waveform. Figure 7–1 illustrates a typical waveform generated during an ERG, and describes the various components. Although variable and complex, the a-b amplitude is the most frequently measured component and is reduced in diseases such as rod–cone dystrophy.

One extremely useful variation of the ERG is the flicker ERG. The patient is set up in the same manner, and a flashing light of increasing frequency creates a measured response. The macular cones can respond to a flicker of around 30 Hz, whereas the peripheral rods and cones will cease to function at around 20 Hz. The

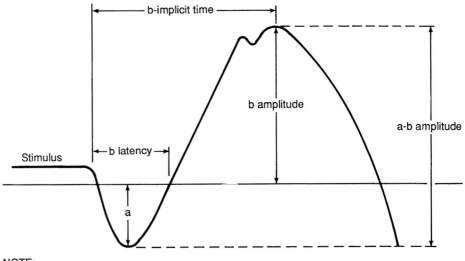

NOTE:
- a-b amplitude (major interest) is measured in uv.
- Average 80-150 uv photopic 300-500 uv scotopic with high intensity flash (photopic is usually 30% of scotopic).
- Average b implicit is 30 ms photopic and 50 ms scotopic.

WAVEFORM	RETINAL COMPONENT	ALTERED IN
Photopic A	Cones	Cone dystrophies
Scotopic A	Rods	Congenital stationary night blindness
Photopic B	Inner nuclear layer (cones)	
Scotopic B	Inner nuclear layer (rods)	
Flicker ERG	Macular cones	Cone dystrophies (macular degeneration)

Figure 7–1. Components of the photopic clinical ERG.

flicker ERG will therefore be especially useful in patients suspected of having macular cone dysfunction.

Electro-oculogram (EOG)

The electro-oculogram (EOG) is a measure of the electrical potential generated by the retinal pigment epithelium (RPE)/photoreceptor complex. The measure of this potential is achieved by setting up a system to measure the electrical potential difference between the "voltage-positive" cornea as it is related to the posterior pole. A comparison is then made between the potential difference in the dark and the potential difference in the light. If there is disease of the RPE, this light peak–dark trough ratio is reduced. The light rise in the potential is generated by light stimulation of the RPE/photoreceptor complex (electrical activity is created by light). It is important to note, however, that midretinal layers must also be functioning properly.

The Test. It is not necessary that the patient be maximally dilated for the performance of an EOG. Electrodes must be placed on the medial and lateral canthi of the patient's eyes after the areas have been appropriately cleaned. An earclip electrode is then placed to serve as a ground. A correction may be worn if necessary. The electrode leads are then attached to a preamplifier and the impedance is checked. The patient then places the chin in the chinrest of the ganzfeld and is instructed to look from right to left as the targets alternate flashes.

The test takes approximately 30 minutes, including a brief training period. Recordings are typically made for about 15 seconds of each minute. The test is started with the lights on and is run for about 10 minutes. The lights are then turned off, and the test is run for 10 minutes in the dark. The lights are then turned on again, and the test is run for the final 10 minutes. The test generates light and dark amplitudes.

Waveform. The ratio of the amplitudes is called the Arden ratio, which is around 2 to 1 in normal eyes and is less than 1.6 to 1 in abnormal conditions. Figure 7–2 illustrates a typical EOG waveform showing light and dark amplitudes. The EOG test will be altered in diseases such as vitelliform dystrophy and the later stages of retinitis pigmentosa. The EOG is most specific for vitelliform dystrophy.

Visually Evoked Cortical Potential (VECP)

The visually evoked cortical potential (VECP, or VEP), also known as visually evoked response (VER), is a measure of the very small electrical potential at the visual cortex when the eye is stimulated by either flashes of light or more defined, alternating, checkerboard patterns on a television monitor at a fixed distance. When using the checkerboard patterns, an indirect measure of foveal acuity is being determined. The patient should always wear the best possible refraction for performance of this test.

Because the waveform is dependent on an intact

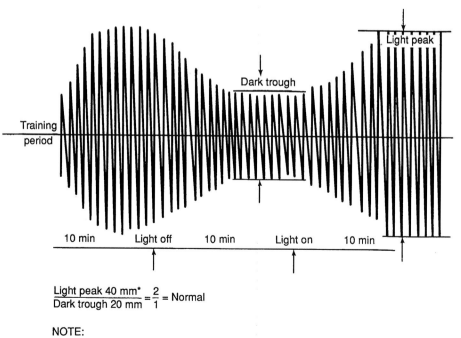

$$\frac{\text{Light peak 40 mm*}}{\text{Dark trough 20 mm}} = \frac{2}{1} = \text{Normal}$$

NOTE:
*Example only

Figure 7–2. Components of the clinical EOG.

visual pathway from the cornea to the cortex, it is possible that the waveform could be altered by disease anywhere in this pathway. The results are therefore nonspecific.

The Test. Initially a skin electrode (reference) is placed on the mastoid process or forehead, and a ground electrode is attached to the earlobe after the skin has been properly prepared. Another skin electrode is placed about 1.5 cm above the inion overlying the visual cortex. The electrode leads are then attached to the preamplifier, and the impedance of the system is checked. Most commercial systems are produced for neurology and will create an upside-down waveform unless the reference and active electrode leads are switched at the preamp. The patient then views a point on a television monitor from a fixed distance (1 m) with best corrected vision. The response to an alternating checkerboard pattern is then recorded according to the established protocol. It is often necessary to run through several alternative patterns to create a large enough summated waveform to be clinically useful. The amplitude of the waveform can be increased to a point by enlarging the size of the checkerboard squares.

The difficulty in measuring the VEP arises because the amplitude of the wave is so small, and it must be amplified by summation. The extraneous electrical noise from the brain and the environment must also be filtered to create a usable waveform. The only way to overcome the problems of recording usable waveforms is the use of a computer system to selectively filter the noise and to summate the multiple waveform. Fortunately technology has decreased the cost and size of the equipment necessary to accomplish the job.

Another stimulus may be used in pediatric patients and in nonattentive or noncommunicative patients. A flash stimulus or a light emitting diode (LED) flash in goggles will create a waveform. The LED goggles may even be used with the eyes closed.

Waveform. Figure 7–3 illustrates a typical VECP waveform. As with ERG and EOG, interpretation is subject to many factors. All of these tests are but a part of the diagnostic puzzle. It may be said that a reduction in amplitude indicates a reduction in acuity levels. This interpretation is not absolute, however, as there are reports of "normal" VECP patterns in patients who are legally blind. Interpretations and advice must be given with caution so as not to be misinterpreted. Interpretation of the implicit time is also of value, as delays indicate altered nerve fiber conductivity, as one would expect in cases of demyelinizing diseases. A change in target contrast, which decreases waveform amplitude, is also a sensitive test for eyes with nerve-fiber conduction defects.

A CLINICAL GUIDE TO UNDERSTANDING GENETICS

The purpose of this section is to familiarize the clinician with inheritance patterns and application of these patterns to patient management. The topic of genetics is far too complex to address in a text about posterior segment disease; but it is hoped that armed with the basics presented here, the clinician will at least be able

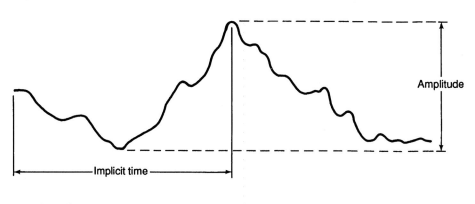

EXPECTEDS:

	TARGET/CHECK SIZE		
	7.5' arc	15' arc	30' arc
Implicit time	115 ms	100 ms	30 ms
Amplitude	5 uv	12 uv	10 uv

Figure 7–3. Components of the typical VECP waveform.

TABLE 7–1. DEFINITIONS OF BASIC GENETIC TERMINOLOGY

Alleles—Alternate forms of a gene located at corresponding points on homologous chromosomes

Autosome—Any chromosome other than the sex (X or Y) chromosome. Man has 22 pairs of autosomes and 1 pair of sex chromosomes, or a diploid total of 46

Carrier—A phenotypically normal person who is heterozygous for a normal gene and an abnormal gene

Chromosome—A structure composed of DNA and protein located in the nucleus of all cells and that functions as the genetic blueprint of the person

    Hemizygous—A term that applies to the genes on the X chromosome in a male. Males have only one X; therefore males are hemizygous with respect to X-linked genes

    Heterozygous—A term that applies to an individual with two different alleles on corresponding points on homologous chromosomes, that is, one allele is normal

    Homozygous—A term that refers to an individual with identical alleles at corresponding loci on homologous chromosomes

Congenital—Present at birth, may or may not be genetically determined

Consanguinity—Mates being genetically related, literally by blood lines

Dominant (gene)—A gene that may produce an expression of its phenotype in a single dose

Expressivity—The degree to which a trait is manifested; may vary from mild to severe

Familial—Refers to any trait that is more commonly expressed in relatives of an affected individual than in the general population

Gene—A segment of a DNA molecule that codes the synthesis of a polypeptide chain or RNA molecule

Genotype—The genetic constitution; more specifically, the alleles present at one locus

Homologous chromosomes—A pair of chromosomes, one from each parent, having the same gene loci in the same order

Multiplex—Refers to a pedigree in which there is more than one case of a particular disease

Pedigree—A variety of a family tree established to study genetic characteristics

Penetrance—The frequency of expression of a gene or pair of genes

Phenotype—The physical expression of genetic characteristics (genotype)

Proband (propositus)—The index case if they are affected; the case from which the pedigree is generated

Recessive (gene)—A gene that is only expressed phenotypically if homozygous. Identical alleles must be present at the same loci

Sibs (siblings)—Brothers or sisters

Simplex—Refers to no known family history

Trait—A transmitted genetic condition

X-linked—Genes on the X-chromosome or traits determined by such genes

---

to generate a pedigree and know when genetic counseling is necessary. Definition of basic terminology is necessary to the understanding of clinical genetics. Table 7–1 provides a brief definition of some of these terms.

Genetic disorders can be classified into three basic categories: single-gene disorders, chromosome disorders, and multifactorial disorders. Single-gene disorders are the result of mutations that may be on one or both pairs of chromosomes. The single-gene disorders occur at the frequency of 1 in 2000. Chromosome disorders are due to excesses or deficiencies of chromosomes or segments of chromosomes. Down syndrome is an example of a chromosome disorder. The frequency of chromosome disorders is 7 in 1000 live births, and accounts for about 50 percent of first-trimester abortions. Multifactorial disorders result from a combination of many small variations that together create a major defect. These disorders recur in families, but usually no specific pedigree pattern can be established.

Because of the complexity of hereditary retinal disease, the establishment of a good family history (pedigree) when considering specific conditions is crucial. The family history can assist in diagnosis. The pedigree can give some guidance as to whether the condition is genetic, and can assist the clinician in ed-

ucating the patient as to prognosis and the likelihood of passing the condition to future generations.

Generating a Pedigree

Generating a pedigree involves nothing more than establishing a very basic family tree to look for specific characteristics. A step-by-step procedure will be presented below to examine a hypothetical 38-year-old male complaining of night blindness of recent onset. Figure 7–4 defines the symbols that will be used in pedigree analysis.

Step 1. Ask your patient with night blindness to list his brothers and sisters in descending order of birth, and to state if any of them are affected with night blindness or if they are deceased. He has a sister, aged 57 years, who is night blind; a brother, aged 43 years, who is not night blind; and a sister who died at the age of 19 years in an automobile accident.

    Draw:

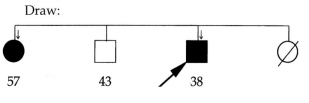

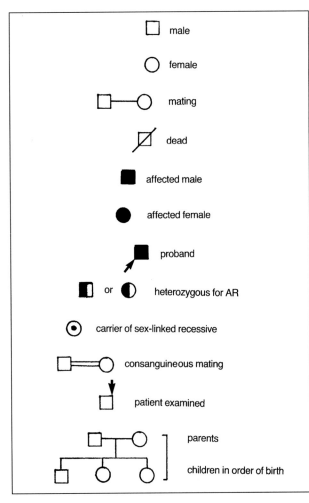

Figure 7–4. Standardized symbols used in the generation of a pedigree.

Step 2. Ask if parents or aunts or uncles were affected with night blindness, and draw them on the tree. The father is night blind, the mother is not. The paternal aunt is not affected, and the maternal aunt and uncle are not affected.
Draw:

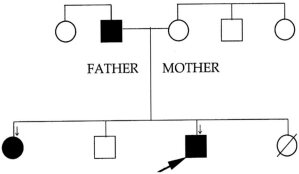

Step 3. Ask if grandparents were affected with night blindness, and add them to the tree. The maternal grandparents were not night blind, but are deceased. The paternal grandfather is not

night blind, but the grandmother was night blind and is now deceased.
Draw:

I. Grandparents
II. Parents
III. Siblings

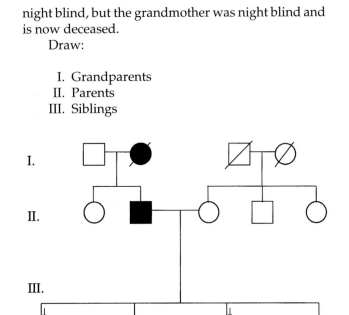

Although simplistic, this exercise covers the basics for generating a pedigree. There are many variations that occur in a pedigree because of variability in phenotypic expression of the gene. Table 7–2 and Figures 7–5 to 7–8 represent the classical pedigree presentations encountered in hereditary ocular disease. When referring to these, the clinician should remember that variability of expression and spontaneous mutation can "break all the rules" in effective pedigree analysis. In fact, the rules are usually broken.

TABLE 7–2. EXPECTED OUTCOMES OF X-LINKED RECESSIVE MATING

Mating Types	Phenotype Offspring
Normal male = Normal female	All normal
Normal male = Recessive heterozygous female	Daughters—50% normal 50% carriers
	Sons—50% normal 50% affected
Normal male = Recessive homozygous female	Daughters—100% carriers
	Sons—100% affected
Affected male = Normal female	Daughters—100% carriers
	Sons—100% normal
Affected Male = Recessive heterozygous female	Daughters—50% normal 50% carriers
	Sons—50% normal 50% affected
Affected male = Recessive homozygous female	All affected

Characteristics
1. The phenotypic presentation occurs only in homozygotes who have received the recessive gene from both parents. Affected persons have carrier parents.
2. The trait characteristically appears (often unexpectedly) in siblings but not in the parents.
3. The risk of the trait occurring in the siblings of the proband is 1 in 4; that is, there is a 25 percent risk.
4. There is no sexual predilection for transfer of the trait; i.e., males and females are equally affected.
5. The parents of an affected child may be consanguineous; i.e., blood line relatives.

Typical Pedigree

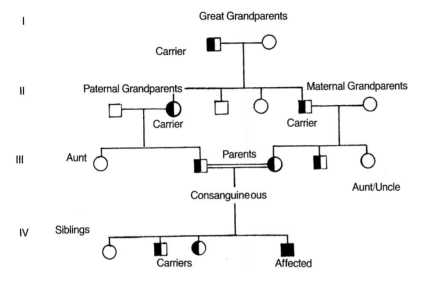

A

Predicting the Offspring of AR Affected

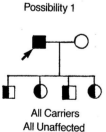
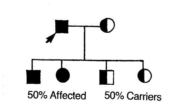

Ocular Problems Suspected of AR Inheritance

Choroidal Sclerosis
CONGENITAL CONE DYSFUNCTION
CONE-RODE DYSTROPHY
Corneal Dystrophy
FUNDUS FLAVIMACULATUS

GYRATE ATROPHY
LAURENCE-MOON-BIEDL
Oguchi Disease
RETINITIS PIGMENTOSA
STARGARDT'S
USHER'S SYNDROME

Figure 7–5. A. Characteristics of AR inheritance patterns. **B.** Predicting the offspring of AR affected and ocular problems suspected of AR inheritance.

B

Characteristics

1. The trait appears in every generation. Exceptions arise because of mutations and/or variability of expression or penetrance.
2. The children of an affected person have a 50 percent risk of inheriting the trait.
3. Unaffected family members will not transmit the trait through family lines.
4. There is no sexual predilection for transfer of the trait; i.e., males and females are affected equally.

Ocular Problems Suspected of AD Inheritance

Amyloidosis
Aniridia
Axenfeld Syndrome
Angiomatosis Retinae
CENTRAL AREOLAR CHOROIDAL DYSTROPHY
Corneal Dystrophies
CONE-ROD DYSTROPHIES
DOMINANT DRUSEN
Marfan Syndrome
Neurofibromatosis
NIGHT BLINDNESS (Congenital Stationary)
RETINOBLASTOMA
RETINITIS PIGMENTOSA
STARGARDT'S
VITELLIFORM DYSTROPHY

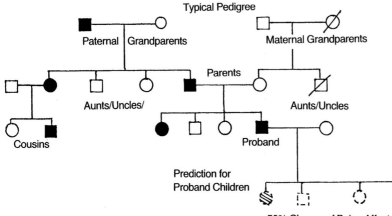

Figure 7–6. Characteristics of AD inheritance patterns.

Characteristics

1. Sex-linked inheritance may be related to X or Y but X-linked has the only clinical significance. The Y chromosome is essential for male sex determination.
   Male XY   Female XX
2. The incidence of the trait is higher in males than females.
3. The trait is never transmitted directly from father to son.
4. The trait is transmitted from an affected male through all his daughters (carriers) to 50 percent of their sons.
5. The trait may be transmitted through carrier females.
6. Carriers may show variable phenotypic expression of the trait.

Ocular Problems Suspected of X-Linked Inheritance

OCULAR ALBINISM
Juvenile Retinoschisis
Choroideremia
RETINITIS PIGMENTOSA
CONGENITAL CONE DYSFUNCTION

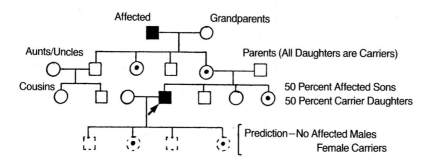

Figure 7–7. Characteristics of X-linked recessive inheritance patterns.

Characteristics
1. Affected males have no normal daughters.
2. Affected females are more common than affected males but they are heterozygous therefore have variable expression.
3. The trait is never transmitted directly from father to son.
4. Affected heterozygous females transmit the trait to 50 percent of children of either sex.
5. Affected homozygous females transmit the trait to all their children.
6. Heterozygous and homozygous females transmit the trait exactly like an autosomal dominant trait.
7. There are no "carriers."

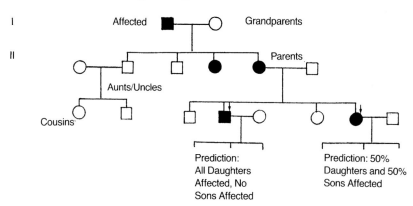

Typical Pedigree – X-Linked Dominant

Prediction:
All Daughters
Affected, No
Sons Affected

Prediction: 50%
Daughters and 50%
Sons Affected

Figure 7–8. Characteristics of X-linked dominant inheritance patterns.

HEREDITARY RETINAL–CHOROIDAL DYSTROPHIES

Hereditary retinal–choroidal diseases will be grouped according to affected peripheral or night vision and affected central vision or color vision. This concept makes application of low-vision devices a bit easier to understand. There are cases where crossover occurs, such as macular involvement in retinitis pigmentosa. The descriptions will be clinical and truncated, as the complexity of each process exceeds the boundaries of primary care.

DYSTROPHIES INITIALLY AFFECTING PERIPHERAL OR NIGHT VISION

Retinitis Pigmentosa Group

Introduction and Description. Retinitis pigmentosa (RP) is the most common of the hereditary retinal dystrophies (Figs. 7–9 and 7–10). RP is the term usually given to a group of hereditary conditions characterized by progressive visual field loss, night blindness, and abnormal electroretinograms. The majority of RP patients are also myopic, with the cone–rod variation typically being more myopic than the rod–cone variation. The cone–rod variant is actually an electroretinographic term used in describing the pattern occurring in RP patients with late-onset night blindness, less pigment deposition, better preservation of visual

fields, and more recordable ERG patterns than the patients with the rod–cone variant. It must be emphasized at this point that there is a tremendous variability in the presentation (Table 7–3), but the typical patient complains of night blindness (often not appearing in the cone–rod variety until the visual field constricts to 10 degrees) dating from the childhood

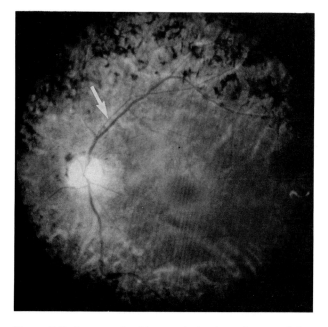

Figure 7–9. An example of bone-spicule pigment accumulation and arterial attenuation (*arrow*) in retinitis pigmentosa.

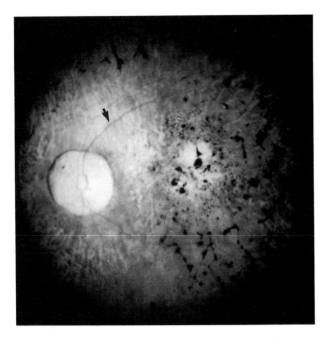

Figure 7–10. Example of the retinal and vascular changes associated with retinitis pigmentosa. The small arrow points to arterial attenuation.

years, with noticeable symptoms of loss of visual field presenting in the late 20s. The typical condition would progress to severe visual compromise with field constriction and severe night blindness in the 40s, and would have considerable loss of functional vision by the 60s. The patient with RP also often complains of variable vision; for example, vision in the morning is very good but becomes blurry as the day progresses. The later stages of the disease are characterized by flashes or waves of light. Development of cataracts usually occurs in about 50 percent of patients in the later stages. As with so many other ocular conditions, the "itis" suffix is misleading, as inflammation is not a consideration in this condition. The incidence of RP varies with the definition employed and study cited, but is considered to be between 0.25 per 1000 to 1 per 7000. A conservative estimate is put at 0.25 per 1000, or 2.5 percent of the general population. RP appears to respect no racial boundaries but does occur slightly more frequently in males.

Heredity plays an important role in RP, but many epidemiologic studies point to the difficulty of genealogic analysis. Reports also suggest that the traditional definition of RP as consisting of a group of simple Mendelian traits does not account for the true distribution of patients. Most clinicians do, however, continue to group RP patients into categories of autosomal recessive, autosomal dominant, and X-linked inheritance patterns. Unfortunately nature is not quite so simplistic, as over 50 percent of cases of RP are simplex (no family history) or are multiplex (affected siblings only). There is considerable disagreement regarding the sporadic appearance of RP, as many clinicians believe this to be a representation of the autosomal recessive form. The percentages of distribution of the various forms of RP hereditary patterns are useless, as there is tremendous variation reported in the literature. As a general rule, however, autosomal recessive forms are considered the most prevalent, followed by autosomal dominant and X-linked forms. There is also the suggestion that snowflake vitreoretinal degeneration is a variant of RP.

In general, hereditary dystrophies are secondary to defects in the genetic code that result in abnormal amino acid composition of specific proteins. Although yet unproven and somewhat controversial, it appears that the defect in RP is related to a disturbance in the disk membrane renewal process in the outer segments of the photoreceptor cells. The disk membranes are shed in the normal renewal process, and it is the responsibility of the RPE to mediate the disposal of the membranes. When this system is interrupted, the normal process is altered, allowing for accumulation of debris (lipofuscin) and alteration of photoreceptor

TABLE 7–3. VARIATIONS IN THE PRESENTATION OF RETINITIS PIGMENTOSA

Congenital Onset Variations

Leber's congenital amaurosis	Congenital RP with macular coloboma
Juvenile Leber's amaurosis	Autosomal dominant form

Rod–Cone Dystrophy Forms

Autosomal dominant	Autosomal recessive
X-linked recessive	Simplex
Multiplex	Retinitis punctata albescens

Cone–Rod Dystrophy Forms

Autosomal dominant	Autosomal recessive
X-linked recessive	Simplex
Multiplex	

TABLE 7–4. SYNDROMES ASSOCIATED WITH RETINITIS PIGMENTOSA

Syndrome	Inheritance	Associated Findings
Usher's	AR, AD	Hearing loss
Hallgren's	AR	Ataxia, mental retardation, nystagmus, deafness
Refsum's	AR	Ataxia, polyneuropathy, deafness
Laurence–Moon–Bardet–Biedl	AR	Obesity, mental retardation, polydactyly, syndactyly, hypogenitalism
Pelizaeus–Merzbacher	X-linked, AR, AD	Head tremors, nystagmus, ataxia, mental retardation
Bassen–Kornzweig	AR	Celiac disease (diarrhea), spinocerebellar ataxia

AR, autosomal recessive; AD, autosomal dominant.

TABLE 7–5. APPROXIMATE AGE OF ONSET FOR VARIOUS HEREDITARY FORMS OF RETINITIS PIGMENTOSA

	Autosomal Recessive	Autosomal Dominant	X-linked	Simplex	Multiplex
Mean age of onset	16 yr	19 yr	9 yr	20 yr	16 yr
Range in years	0–54 yr	0–57 yr	3–18 yr	0–71 yr	0–67 yr
95% symptomatic by age	40 yr	50 yr	18 yr		

function, as well as gliosis, neuronal loss, photoreceptor loss, choriocapillaris occlusion, and invasion of the retina to the internal limiting membrane by the RPE cells. RP can be considered a primary and a secondary process. The primary form is considered to be unassociated with systemic disease processes, whereas the secondary form is the result of systemic disease processes. Table 7–4 lists syndromes associated with RP. It appears that in addition to creating dysfunction of the photoreceptors, the RPE alteration creates an alteration of the blood–retinal barrier, leading to leakage and potential macular edema seen in the later stages of RP. Table 7–5 outlines "typical" ages of onset for the various forms of RP.

The ophthalmoscopic picture of RP is considered typical, but this author has observed many variations. Figure 7–11 illustrates the "typical" ocular changes associated with the evolution of retinitis pigmentosa.

Pigmentation. The earliest sign of RP is the generalized diffuse depigmentation of the RPE with granularity in the equatorial zone of the retina. Even at this stage, the ERG may be abnormal. Virtually all patients progress through this stage with little to no pigment deposition (retinitis pigmentosa sine pigmento); this stage may persist longer in some patients than in others. The pigmentary alterations that "typify" RP often take the form of clumps and strands of pigment most often in the retinal periphery and accumulated in the perivascular area secondary to pigment deposition in

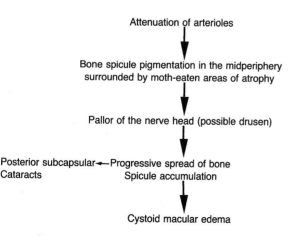

Figure 7–11. A flowchart illustrating the ocular changes associated with retinitis pigmentosa.

the vascular walls. The classically described bone spicule pigmentation occurs in the midperiphery, presenting early as fine pigment mottling surrounded by motheaten areas of atrophy. It should be noted, however, that small, irregular clumps and spots of pigment are seen as often as the bone corpuscle pattern. As the disease progresses there is a clumping of pigment with an affinity for perivascular accumulation. With further degeneration, there may be development of large areas of RPE mottling in the midperiphery, which take on a lobular pattern similar to that seen in fundus flavimaculatus. RPE loss may be severe enough that the choroidal vessels become very visible, simulating choroidal sclerosis. (*Note:* Variations in presentation occur, such as RP sine pigmento or without pigment.) **See color plate 112.**

Artery Attenuation. Among the first signs of RP is attenuation or narrowing of the arterioles and arteries, which becomes very pronounced in the posterior pole as the disease progresses. Arterial narrowing is thought to be almost omnipresent in all forms of RP. This is thought to be secondary to the retinal destruction necessitating less oxygenated blood, resulting in a normal response of arterial narrowing.

Wrinkling of the ILM and Optic Nerve Changes. At times the retina has an edematous appearance and may have an associated wrinkling of the internal limiting membrane. Also later in the process there is reported pallor of the nerve head secondary to poor vascular perfusion and gliosis as well as the development of beading or focal dilatations of capillaries on the nerve head. These vascular alterations are often more apparent on fluorescein angiography. The pallor may be located in the temporal nerve head in the cone–rod variant of RP. In general, patients with RP have smaller cup-to-disk ratios than the normal population. In the later stages, a thin white rim may present at the edge of the disc, representing circumpapillary loss of the RPE.

Hyaline bodies (buried drusen) are often associated with RP. These have been called astrocytic hamartomas by some, but are generally thought to be secondary to alterations in axoplasmic flow allowing for the deposition of the material. The drusen associated with RP are often very near the edge of the disc

Retinitis Pigmentosa Group

Characteristics

△ Actually a group of dystrophies characterized by progressive visual field loss, night blindness, myopia, photophobia, and abnormal electroretinograms

△ Night blindness in childhood years in rod–cone but often not until 10 degree visual fields in cone–rod variant

△ Complaint of variable vision throughout the day, flashes or waves of light in the later stages of the disease

△ Variable inheritance pattern—AR, AD, X-linked, simplex, multiplex—that is often difficult to elicit

△ Mean age of onset 9 to 19 years

△ Defect in genetic code of amino acids of specific proteins altering RPE metabolism

△ Secondary form may be associated with a number of systemic syndromes: Usher's, Hallgren's, Refsum's, Laurence–Moon–Biedl, Pelizaeus–Merzbacher, Bassen–Kornzweig, abetalipoproteinemia, Senior–Loken

△ Ophthalmoscopic appearance:
   RPE granularity in equatorial zone
   Clumps and strands of pigment near perivascular area
   Bone spicule pigment
   Motheaten retina often becoming lobular, simulating fundus flavimaculatus
   Arterial attenuation
   Wrinkling of internal limiting membrane
   Pallor of optic nerve, capillary changes on nerve
   Thin white rim around nerve head in late stages
   Optic nerve head drusen
   Cystoid macular edema late
   Pigment flecks in anterior vitreous, syneretic vitreous

△ Posterior subcapsular cataracts develop in about 50 percent

△ Unpredictable progressive field loss, starting in superior zone with scotomas coalescing in midperiphery

△ Abnormal electroretinography, abnormal dark adaptation, both of which worsen with progression

△ Fluorescein angiography demonstrates areas of atrophy and leakage associated with cystoid macular edema

Management

△ Pedigree analysis

△ Rule out associated systemic diseases:
   Family history
   Deafness or partial hearing impairment
   Heart problems
   Polydactyly
   Kidney disease
   Neurologic disease

△ Genetic counseling when indicated

△ Routine examinations with provision of best refraction, routine threshold visual fields, consideration of lenses that block short wavelengths, consideration of employment of oral antioxidant therapy
   Fundus photographs when indicated

△ Possible benefit of grid photocoagulation in the development of cystoid macular edema

△ Laser photocoagulation indicated in choroidal neovascular membrane development

△ Cataract extraction when indicated

△ Counseling regarding vocation, avocation, driving, depending on status of visual fields and visual acuity

△ Low-vision and mobility rehabilitation when necessary

△ Consider psychological counseling or peer groups to lessen the trauma of diagnosis or progression of the condition

and have a tendency to migrate out underneath the sensory retina.

Cystoid Macular Edema. There is also the potential of development of cystoid macular edema (CME). The appearance of cystoid macular edema is thought to be as high as 70 percent. Macular cysts (possibly a variation of a macular schisis) and bull's-eye-like RPE changes have also been reported in the macular area. Coincidental choroidal neovascularization is always a potential threat, especially as the patient ages.

Vitreous Changes. With careful slit-lamp examination, there are also flecks of pigment apparent in the anterior vitreous space accompanied by syneresis of the vitreous. The development of cataracts (often posterior subcapsular) is also a characteristic of the condition.

Visual Fields. Progression of visual field loss is a primary diagnostic sign of any variation of retinitis pigmentosa. Serial threshold visual field tests on either a patient suspected of having RP or a confirmed RP patient are an absolute necessity. Early visual field findings include a depression in the superior peripheral field accompanied by scotomas in the midequatorial zone. During progression the midequatorial scotomas coalesce to develop the classical ring scotoma. With further progression, the superior and nasal fields constrict, leaving a central island of vision. The rate of progression of visual field loss is highly variable, and in discussing the case with the patient, probabilities of degree of loss of visual field over time should be avoided. The visual field loss is usually relatively symmetrical and progresses in a fairly symmetrical fashion. Table 7–6 compares the visual field characteristics of cone–rod versus rod–cone RP dystrophy.

Electrodiagnostic testing demonstrates variability with the hereditary "type" of RP, but can be said to present an abnormal ERG and EOG. Dark adaptometry testing will as well demonstrate abnormalities.

In the later stages, fluorescein angiography will demonstrate areas of atrophy as well as an alteration of the blood–retinal barrier in the form of cystoid macular edema. There is an association of RP to myopia, and X-linked carriers often have the presence of astigmatism over 1.50 diopters.

Management. As with all hereditary dystrophies, the best management is the development of a pedigree and genetic counseling to advise of the risk and to attempt to prevent the occurrence. Routine eye examinations with the provision of the optimal prescription are necessary. A crucial aspect of each examination is the recording of a threshold visual field, both to give the patient an idea of the degree of progression and to advise regarding modifications in vocational and avocational pursuits. Activities such as driving may need to be modified, as patients with RP are documented to have more frequent motor vehicle accidents than non-RP patients. Fundus photographs may also be advisable in consideration of future follow-up for the patient.

Management of the symptoms is best achieved by low-vision consultation as well as appropriate rehabilitation. Low-vision management has evolved to a very sophisticated level. Provision of infrared-blocking sun lenses is recommended in spite of the fact that there is no concrete support that chronic exposure to sunlight has a deleterious effect on the disease. Information presented in Chapter 5, however, supports the fact that short-wavelength light does have a potentially damaging effect on the RPE and retina with age.

TABLE 7–6. COMPARISON OF VISUAL FIELD DEFECTS IN ROD–CONE VERSUS CONE–ROD DYSTROPHY

Rod–Cone Dystrophy

Superior visual field depression
Midequatorial scotomas
Enlargement of the blind spot
Shallow defects (sloping demarcation)
Ring scotoma (30 to 50 degrees)

Cone–Rod Dystrophy

Superior visual field depression
Midequatorial scotomas
Enlargement of the blind spot earlier than in rod–cone dystrophy
Ring scotoma closer to fixation than rod–cone dystrophy (5 to 30 degrees)
Pseudoaltitudinal field loss
Steep defects (definite demarcation)

Vitamin A palmitate, 15,000 IU per day, has been shown to be of benefit in the treatment of RP. Vitamine seems to have a negative effect. Side effects include headache, appetite and weight loss, vomiting, and hair loss. Blood chemistries with liver function tests may be considered during treatment. The potential toxicity must be remembered.

It is also imperative to assure that the RP is primary rather than secondary to a systemic-based disease. The medical history becomes invaluable in this aspect of management. Ask about family history, associated medical problems such as deafness or partial hearing loss, polydactyly, heart problems, kidney disease, and neurologic signs or symptoms.

One aspect of the disease, the appearance of cystoid macular edema, which is a direct threat to the remaining central vision, can be actively treated. It has been shown that grid photocoagulation may actually minimize the risk of severe vision loss over the short term in cystoid macular edema in RP. Laser is also of benefit when choroidal neovascularization complicates RP.

There has been some disagreement in the past regarding the advisability of cataract extraction in patients with RP. It has been shown, however, that cataract extraction or intraocular lens (IOL) implantation has no negative effect on prognosis when performed skillfully. Unfortunately, predicting prognosis for patients is as difficult as all other aspects of RP.

It appears that the AD patients with RP maintain excellent vision until after childbearing years, with a slow visual deterioration after that. AR patients maintain reasonable vision until their 30s, and a few have significant early central loss. The X-linked patients usually present an early rapid loss of acuity. Simplex varieties of RP are characterized by unpredictability, but many have good vision past childbearing years. Night blindness and eventual severity of RP are not well correlated. Because of the relatively slow progression of the disease, the patients are often able to adapt well to their handicap as the disease progresses. It has been suggested that once the best corrected visual acuity is 20/40 or poorer from macular changes, the visual acuity is unstable and will worsen over the next 6 years.

Because of the fact that people value the sense of sight more than any other sense, the diagnosis of RP is often devastating to patients. It is probably advisable in newly diagnosed or actively progressing cases to ask for a consultation for patients with a psychologist or a peer group, to help them accept the news and adapt to the potential changes in their lives. It is important to emphasize that vision is often maintained until later in life, and that low-vision rehabilitation will keep the patient active and contributing to society for years.

Retinitis Pigmentosa Variants

Retinitis pigmentosa variants include retinitis punctata albescens, retinitis pigmentosa sine pigmento, sector retinitis pigmentosa, inverse retinitis pigmentosa, and Leber's congenital amaurosis. These dystrophies are described in the following sections.

Retinitis Punctata Albescens (RPA)

Introduction and Description. Retinitis punctata albescens (RPA) is typically an AR progressive retinal dystrophy characterized by many punctate whitish-yellow spots radiating outward from the posterior pole. The spots are concentrated in the equatorial area and usually spare the macula. The spots usually remain stable, but a progression of RPE degeneration starts peripherally and encroaches toward the macula over the years. Advanced cases demonstrate pigmentary clumping and spicule formation in the equatorial retina, with disc atrophy and vessel attenuation similar to that found in typical RP. With advancement, the choroidal vessels become more visible, and this is reflected in fluorescein studies.

Symptoms parallel those of RP, including progressive loss of the visual fields, night blindness, eventual compromise of visual acuity, altered color vision, photophobia, early depression of the scotopic ERG, and abnormal ERG in the late stages. Dark adaptation testing is also altered.

The clinical signs and symptoms are similar to RP, but progress is slower, with maintenance of good vision into and beyond the fifth decade. Pedigree analysis and genetic counseling are important.

Management. Management of retinitis punctata albescens parallels that of retinitis pigmentosa. The primary care practitioner must attempt to generate a pedigree, consider genetic counseling, and provide the best possible visual correction. Routine eye examinations should include threshold visual field analysis. Low-vision rehabilitation as well as mobility rehabilitation may become necessary. Consideration should be given to blocking short-wavelength light and prescription of oral antioxidants. Counseling should be provided regarding vocation, avocation, and driving based on clinical findings and visual fields. Psychological counseling and/or peer group interaction may be indicated to minimize the trauma of the condition.

Pearls

Retinitis Punctata Albescens

Characteristics

Δ Usually AR progressive dystrophy

Δ Multiple punctate whitish yellow spots that remain stable, radiating out from the posterior pole but concentrated in the equatorial area

Δ RPE degeneration starts peripherally and encroaches toward the macula over the years, eventually depositing clumps or spicules of pigment similar to RP

Δ Disc atrophy and arterial attenuation occurs similar to RP

Δ Symptoms parallel RP—night blindness, field constriction, loss of vision, altered color vision, photophobia, altered ERG, altered dark adaptation—but slower progression than RP

Management

Δ Pedigree analysis

Δ Genetic counseling when indicated

Δ Routine examinations with provision of best refraction, routine threshold visual fields, consideration of lenses that block short wavelengths, consideration of employment of oral antioxidant therapy
  Fundus photographs when indicated

Δ Counseling regarding vocation, avocation, driving, depending on status of visual fields and visual acuity

Δ Low-vision and mobility rehabilitation when necessary

Δ Consider psychological counseling or peer groups to lessen the trauma of diagnosis or progression of the condition

---

■ ■ ■ ■ ■ ■

Clinical Notes: Fundus Albipunctatus

Fundus albipunctatus degeneration presents as dull white dots scattered throughout the retina but concentrated in the midperiphery and perimacular zone. The fundus appearance is similar to RPA but lacks the RPE degeneration. Vessels are not attenuated, and the optic disc is normal. Nonprogressive night blindness is characteristic and is often the only symptom. Vision is usually excellent. These patients often have alterations in dark adaptation but improve in the dark with prolonged adaptation. Minimally abnormal ERGs may be present. Pedigree analysis and genetic counseling are indicated. Fundus albipunctatus degeneration is usually AR (see Table 7–7).

Retinitis Pigmentosa Sine Pigmento

Although often recognized as a distinct entity, retinitis pigmentosa sine pigmento is probably a variation of RP in which the alterations of the RPE are so subtle that they are clinically unrecognizable. It has been suggested that virtually every RP patient progresses through this stage, with some just remaining at this

TABLE 7–7. COMPARISON OF HEREDITARY WHITE-DOTS-IN-THE-RETINA SYNDROMES

	Heredity	Symptoms	Fundus Picture	ERG	EOG	Progression/Final Visual Acuity
Progressive albipuncate dystrophy (RP-like)	AR	Night blindness, field constriction	Small white dots concentrated in posterior pole but also into periphery, nonconfluent	Abnormal	Abnormal	Maintains visual acuity until fifth decade, but is slowly progressive
Fundus albipunctatus degeneration	AR	Night blindness	Dull white dots concentrated in midperiphery and perimacular zone	Normal to abnormal	Normal to abnormal	Nonprogressive with good final visual acuity
Dominant drusen	AD	Metamorphopsia and decreased central vision	White dots in or near macula that increase in size and become confluent, leading to a macular plaque or wet maculopathy	Normal to abnormal	Abnormal in late stages	Progressive, leading to variable acuity reduction
Fundus flavimaculatus	AR	None to mild vision reduction	Yellow-white fishtail flecks in posterior pole; progression toward macula	Normal to abnormal	Normal to abnormal	Mild progression, but macula may become atrophic
Stargardt's disease	AR	Vision loss, color vision loss	Slimed oval macular zone leading to beaten bronze; surround of fundus flavimaculatus	Normal to abnormal	Normal to abnormal	Severe progression

AR, autosomal recessive; AD, autosomal dominant.

stage a bit longer. This may actually just be an early stage in the full-blown development of RP, as longitudinal observations will often present development of the classical picture. The standard symptoms and clinical signs are present, with prognosis and management similar to RP. **See color plate 76.**

Sector Retinitis Pigmentosa

Sector RP is a variant of RP that is usually bilateral and symmetrical, involving both inferior quadrants, more often the inferior nasal quadrant. The remainder of the retina appears normal but actually has RPE changes demonstrable with fluorescein angiography. The pigmentary retinopathy is well demarcated from the normal retina and the vessels are attenuated in the affected area. The most common complaint is night blindness, which is usually late onset similar to cone–rod RP. Threshold visual field loss is usually superior corresponding to the RPE changes. A pseudo-altitudinal defect respecting the horizontal raphe may present similar, again to cone–rod RP and mimicking the field loss associated with pituitary adenoma. The ERG is usually subnormal, but not as altered as the ERG in circumferential RP. Progression of sector RP is slow, with function remaining intact until the ages of 50 to 60 years and some patients actually remaining stable. Sector RP has been reported as AR and AD, the

Pearls

Sector Retinitis Pigmentosa

Characteristics

Δ Usually AD but may be AR
Δ Usually bilateral and symmetrical affecting the inferior quadrants; nasal more often than temporal
Δ The pigmentary changes are well demarcated from the normal retina, with the arteries attenuated within the affected area
Δ Late-onset complaints of night blindness
Δ Superior threshold visual field defects that are often pseudo-altitudinal, simulating fields associated with pituitary adenoma
Δ Subnormal ERG is present but variable
Δ Stability to slow progression is characteristic
Δ Localized retinal trauma and inflammation can mimic sector RP

Management

Δ Pedigree generation and genetic counseling are recommended
Δ Provision of best possible prescription
Δ Consideration of a prescription to block shorter wavelengths and consideration of prescription of oral antioxidants
Δ Routinely monitor threshold visual fields
Δ Provide low-vision rehabilitation if and when necessary

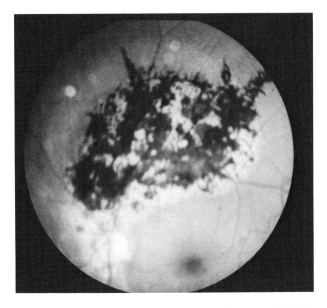

Figure 7–12. An example of a misdiagnosis of sector retinitis pigmentosa. This is an example of reactive RPE hyperplasia secondary to trauma.

most frequent being AD. Sector RP has also been reported to be associated with a family that also had chronic angle-closure glaucoma. Retinal trauma and inflammation can mimic sector RP because of reactive RPE hyperplasia occurring in the affected areas (Fig. 7–12). **See color plate 113.**

Sector retinitis pigmentosa should be managed as other forms of the disease with intervention depending on the extent of retinal and vision compromise. Certainly generation of a pedigree and genetic counseling must be provided.

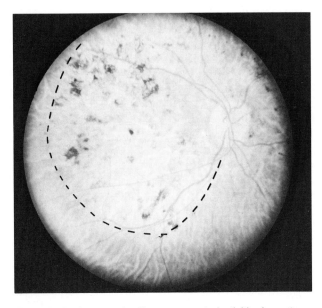

Figure 7–13. An example of inverse or central retinitis pigmentosa. The dotted line outlines the RPE clumping in the macular area.

Inverse Retinitis Pigmentosa

Inverse RP (Fig. 7–13) is thought to occur in an AR inheritance pattern. Inverse or central RP is manifested by clumped or spiderlike pigmentary changes around the macular area rather than the periphery. Night blindness is a common early finding. Visual function is compromised, as it is in typical RP, with central vision loss often the result. Arterial attenuation and disc pallor occur. Choroidal atrophy occurs and is obvious on fluorescein angiography. Color vision loss and central scotomas are the rule, and the ERG photopic wave is altered. The findings are very similar to a form of cone dystrophy. Prognosis is poor because of severe central vision loss. Effective treatment modalities are currently unavailable. Pedigree generation and genetic counseling are absolutely necessary. **See color plate 114.**

Leber's Congenital Amaurosis (Congenital Pigmentary Dystrophy)

Leber's congenital amaurosis (LCA) is a cause of blindness in the first year of life. The condition is usually AR. The child presents with profound visual impairment; coarse, searching nystagmus; extinguished ERG; and at times, photophobia in the first year. The patient also has a tendency to poke at the eyes (digito-ocular sign), which is often associated with an increased prevalence of keratoconus. Pupils are poorly reactive, and the retina eventually develops pigmentary and degenerative changes with optic atrophy. The pigmentary changes may not develop until later in childhood, with a variation from yellow flecks in the midperiphery to pigmentary deposition. Cataract formation typically starts prior to age 10 years. There is a variation of LCA associated with the presentation of a hereditary macular pseudocoloboma.

The patient often has accompanying neurologic disorders, mental retardation, and other ocular findings. The uncomplicated form of LCA is characterized by congenital blindness, an extinguished ERG, searching nystagmus, hyperopia exceeding 5 diopters, and the absence of systemic abnormalities. The complicated form of LCA has associated systemic problems, which may include cerebrohepatorenal syndrome of Zellweger, Moore–Taylor syndrome, Senior–Loken syndrome, and Saldino–Mainzer syndrome. Juvenile LCA is characterized by signs of visual alteration in the first several years of life with the onset of retinal degeneration by age 6 years. Juvenile LCA patients do not have nystagmus and retain good central vision in spite of severe visual field constriction. There is also the variation of LCA referred to as early-onset RP with night vision problems by age 6 years, minor visual field alterations, and visual acuity in the 20/50 to 20/80 range.

Leber's Congenital Amaurosis

Characteristics

Δ Cause of blindness at birth

Δ Classical LCA has profound visual impairment, coarse searching nystagmus, extinguished ERG

Δ Pigmentary changes in the retina may not develop until later in childhood

Δ Strong association of cataract formation by age 10 years

Δ Variation that presents with a macular pseudo-coloboma

Δ Variations include:

Uncomplicated form with no associated systemic disease but hyperopia exceeding 5 diopters

Complicated form associated with several syndromes

Juvenile LCA with no nystagmus, maintenance of central vision, but severe field constriction

Early-onset RP with vision at 20/50 to 20/80, minor visual field loss, and night vision problems by age 6 years

Management

Δ Pedigree analysis and genetic counseling are important

Δ Must rule out potential associated systemic diseases

Δ Provide maximum prescription, consider blocking short wavelengths, consider antioxidant therapy

Δ Provide low-vision rehabilitation when possible

The ERG is either minimally present or non-recordable in the patient and affords an excellent method for differential diagnosis from other conditions that may cause blindness in childhood. Prognosis is poor. Pedigree analysis and genetic counseling are crucial as well as a search for the possibility of associated systemic conditions. Routine eye examinations are important including provision of best possible prescription, consideration of blocking the shorter wavelengths and minimizing photophobia, and consideration of antioxidant therapy. Low-vision rehabilitation should be provided when appropriate.

Mimickers of Retinitis Pigmentosa

Mimickers of retinitis pigmentosa include unilateral pigmentary retinopathy, pigmented paravenous retinochoroidal atrophy, syphilitic chorioretinitis, and rubella retinopathy. These dystrophies are described in the following sections.

Unilateral Pigmentary Retinopathy

Unilateral retinitis pigmentosa is probably extremely rare, having never been reported as a hereditary form; it is therefore referred to here as unilateral pigmentary retinopathy. The appearance is usually a manifestation of blunt trauma, retained intraocular foreign bodies, resolved retinal detachment, choroidal vascular occlusions, or inflammation. When there is a bona fide case of unilateral RP, the patient is often asymptomatic until the macula becomes involved. Prognosis is similar to bilateral RP, but management problems are minimized. Genetic counseling is necessary if the rare case is uncovered.

When unilateral RP is suspected, it probably is unilateral pigmentary retinopathy, and another cause should be investigated.

Pigmented Paravenous Retinochoroidal Atrophy (PPRA)

Introduction and Description. Pigmented paravenous retinochoroidal atrophy (PPRA) was at one time considered a rare occurrence. Many case reports have surfaced lately, and the author has personally seen several cases. The age range for presentation of PPRA has been reported as 4 to 70 years, although one report suggests a congenital onset. The majority of reported cases are males, which suggests a hereditary nature. The author has seen both males and females with PPRA. The disease has also been reported to be passed from mother to son. The presentation of the condition is extremely variable, which suggests that if it is hereditary in nature, there is variable penetrance. There appears to be no racial predilection.

Cases of PPRA have been reported to be associated with measles, which suggests that an infectious process cannot be ruled out. There have been suggestions that PPRA is an incomplete, self-limited form of retinitis pigmentosa. There is, however, no firm basis for this deduction.

In spite of the dramatic ophthalmoscopic presentation, PPRA is considered to be a relatively benign process that rarely affects macular vision in spite of the fact that it may be progressive. PPRA is usually bilateral and symmetrical, but unilateral cases have been reported.

The origin of this condition seems to be in the retinal pigment epithelium. There appears to be atrophy of the RPE surrounding the optic nerve head and the veins. These corridors of RPE atrophy hyperfluoresce on fluorescein angiography but do not leak. There is marked bone-spicule cuffing of pigment surrounding the retinal veins. However, as the disease is highly variable, many variations of the classical picture can present.

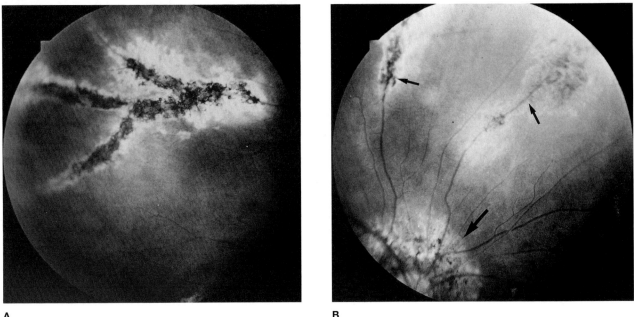

Figure 7–14. A. Significant paravenous pigment associated with PPRA. **B.** The arrows point to circumpapillary and paravenous changes associated with PPRA.

The ophthalmoscopic signs rarely progress to involve the macula in PPRA (Fig. 7–14). It does seem that changes start to invade the clinical posterior pole with time and may even resemble gyrate atrophy. Should progression occur to the stage of resembling the scalloping of gyrate atrophy, serum and urine ornithine levels will help in the differential diagnosis. Serum and urine ornithine levels are elevated in gyrate atrophy.

PPRA is usually asymptomatic. PPRA is usually found during a routine ophthalmoscopic examination. Visual field defects correspond to the areas of RPE atrophy and may demonstrate overall constriction or a ring scotoma. Dark adaptation and electroretinography may be normal or abnormal. Electrooculograms are usually abnormal but have also been reported as normal. There does not appear to be any strong relationship to positive findings on routine laboratory diagnostic tests.

Management. Visual acuity is usually unaffected in PPRA, even in cases judged to be severe by ophthalmoscopy. There is, however, a progressive constriction of visual fields in some cases associated with progressive fundus changes. Serial visual fields should be performed to keep the patient aware of any potential compromise that may affect activities of daily life.

Some reported cases of PPRA have a severe, progressive loss of vision. As such it would be prudent in cases of suspected PPRA to (1) establish a pedigree, (2) perform visual field tests, (3) obtain retinal photographs, (4) perform electrodiagnostic testing to rule out other similar conditions, and (5) follow the patient on routine intervals.

Syphilitic (Leutic) Chorioretinitis

Introduction and Description. Numerous treponemal and viral infections may produce pigmentary retinopathies and as such must always be a consider-

Pigmented Paravenous Retinochoroidal Atrophy (PPRA)

Characteristics

△ Broad range of age presentation
△ Suggestions of a hereditary basis but no strong evidence
△ Usually bilateral, symmetrical atrophy and migration of the RPE surrounding the optic nerve head and corridors along the veins
△ Bone-spicule cuffing of veins
△ May progress toward macula but rarely affects vision
△ Usually asymptomatic but affected areas will demonstrate field compromise
△ Electrodiagnosis is normal to abnormal

Management

△ Establish a pedigree
△ Educate the patient regarding the condition
△ Perform serial visual fields to keep patient aware of potential for compromise of activities of daily life
△ Monitor on routine intervals

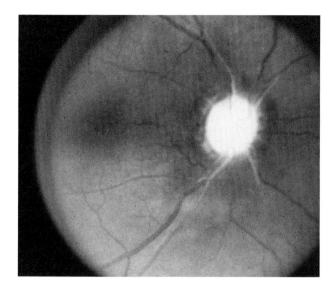
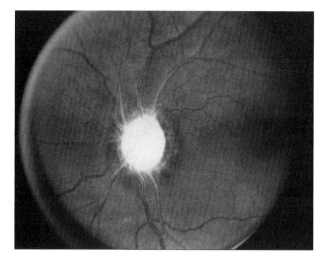

Figure 7–15. Example of bilateral syphilitic optic neuropathy with no evidence of any other retinal or optic nerve head changes.

ation in the differential diagnosis of RP. Congenital syphilis often has a diffuse salt-and-pepper pigmentary retinal pattern with severely affected visual fields that are often asymmetrical. Usually the patient with congenital syphilis presents in the first or second decade with infiltration and vascularization of the cornea in the form of interstitial keratopathy. With resolution, the cornea thins and scars. There may also be anterior uveitis. The systemic signs include widely spaced peg teeth (Hutchinson's teeth), depressed nasal bridge, deafness, arthropathy, mental retardation, and frontal bossing. Differential diagnosis is through blood tests, which may include RPR, VDRL, FTA-ABS, or MHA-TP. All tests may be positive in an infant without syphilis born to a mother with syphilis, but all convert back to negative within 6 months. An IgM-FTA-ABS that is positive in an infant is strongly suggestive of active syphilis.

Some patients with acquired syphilitic chorioretinitis have a fundus that appears similar to choroidal sclerosis with scattered clumps of pigment or bone spicules, but again with asymmetrical constricted visual fields. The chorioretinitis has also been reported to mimic RP. The chorioretinitis usually appears in the secondary stage of the disease. Systemic signs of acquired syphilis include the following.

1. *Primary stage:* The chancre, lymphadenopathy.
2. *Secondary stage:* Skin and mucous membrane lesions, lymphadenopathy, sore throat, fever, uveitis, optic neuritis, retinal vasculitis, conjunctivitis, dacryoadenitis, dacryocystitis, episcleritis, scleritis, interstitial keratopathy, and perhaps meningitis.

3. *Latent stage:* No observable signs.
4. *Tertiary stage:* CNS disease, optic atrophy, chronic anterior uveitis, Argyll Robertson pupil, and cardiovascular disease (Figs. 7–15 and 7–16).

The VDRL or RPR reflects active disease. The differential diagnostic test to perform is the FTA-ABS or MHA-TP, which are very sensitive to all stages and do not revert back to normal, as do the RPR or VDRL. It is important to realize that patients with previously treated syphilis or the neurologic form may pass the VDRL. Screening for HIV is also advised because of the commonality of the two disease processes.

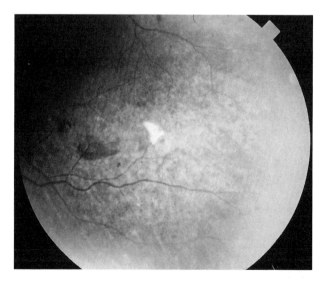

Figure 7–16. Peripheral salt-and-pepper chorioretinal lesions associated with syphilitic retinopathy.

Syphilitic (Leutic) Chorioretinitis

Characteristics

Δ Congenital

Diffuse salt and pepper pigmentary retinal pattern

Severely affected asymmetrical visual fields

Interstitial keratopathy in first or second decade

Systemic signs

Hutchinson's teeth

Depressed nasal bridge

Deafness

Arthropathy

Mental retardation

IgM-FTA-ABS diagnostic in infant

FTA-ABS or MHA-TP diagnostic after 6 months

Δ Acquired

Salt-and-pepper fundus that may develop choroidal sclerosis appearance with pigment clumps

Asymmetrical constricted visual fields

Systemic signs

Primary stage: chancre, lymphadenopathy

Secondary stage: skin and mucous membrane lesions, lymphadenopathy, sore throat, fever, uveitis, optic neuritis, vasculitis, conjunctivitis, dacryoadenitis, dacryocystitis, episcleritis, scleritis, interstitial keratopathy, meningitis

Latent stage: no observable signs or symptoms

Tertiary stage: CNS disease, optic atrophy, chronic anterior uveitis, Argyll Robertson pupil, cardiovascular disease

VDRL or RPR reflect active disease

FTA-ABS or MHA-TP sensitive to all stages

Include test for HIV

Management

Δ Use of aqueous penicillin

Δ Treat anterior segment with cycloplegia and steroids

Δ Follow-up dependent on status of disease process

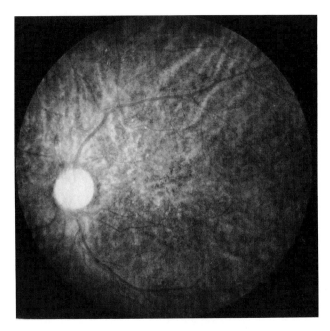

Figure 7–17. Example of retinal changes associated with rubella.

pepper pigmentation. The pigment may at times even have the appearance of bone spicules (Fig. 7–17). In contrast with RP, the vessels are usually of normal caliber. Other characteristics of the patient with rubella retinopathy include partial to full hearing impairment

Management. Management of active forms of syphilis is somewhat complex but is usually accomplished by variations in dosage of aqeous penicillin. Anterior segment manifestations should be treated with a combination of cycloplegia and steroids. Follow-up should depend on the status of the disease process.

Rubella Retinopathy

Introduction and Description. Patients with rubella retinopathy simulate RP as they often have scattered pigmentary deposits, pigment clumps, or salt-and-

Rubella Retinopathy

Characteristics

Δ The result of maternal infection with the rubella virus in the first trimester of pregnancy

Δ Scattered salt-and-pepper pigmentation in the periphery that may simulate RP

Δ Normal vessel caliber

Δ Possibility of hearing deficit, cardiac anomalies, and other systemic problems associated with congenital rubella

Δ Typically, visual acuity is normal to a mild reduction and visual fields are nonprogressive

Δ Usually normal ERG

Δ May progress as RPE degeneration, may develop cataracts, glaucoma, optic atrophy, and transillumination. Microphthalmos has been reported

Management

Δ Differential diagnosis from RP by ERG, serial visual fields, and dark adaptation

Δ An elevated antirubella antibody titer may assist in the diagnosis

Δ Routine eye examinations are indicated with best possible prescription and monitoring for progress (differential in Usher's syndrome and RP) as well as the knowledge that the mother had been infected in the first trimester with the rubella virus. Visual acuity may be reduced to the 20/50 level or may be unaffected. There may be visual field loss at threshold, but it is typically nonprogressive to differentiate it from RP. If progression occurs, there is usually no alteration of the peripheral salt-and-pepper appearance but rather a progressive alteration of the RPE. There may be an association with early cataract development, glaucoma, microphthalmos, optic atrophy, and iris transillumination. Choroidal neovascularization has been reported as a potential complication in the areas of RPE/Bruch's compromise. It is believed that the ERG in patients with rubella retinopathy is usually normal to borderline.

Management. Management of rubella retinopathy primarily revolves around making the correct diagnosis. Although often a diagnosis of exclusion, an elevated antirubella antibody titer can usually be shown. Differentiation from RP can be accomplished by a combination of serial visual field evaluation, ERG, and dark adaptation. Routine ocular evaluations with provision of the maximal refractive correction and monitoring for progress are both indicated.

If not previously performed, the patient should also be evaluated for cardiac, hearing, and other anomalies associated with congenital rubella.

Congenital Stationary Night Blindness (CSNB)

Introduction and Description. Congenital stationary night blindness (CSNB) may be transmitted in AR, AD, or X-linked forms. X-linked CSNB is characterized by night blindness, mild acuity reduction, high myopia, tilted optic nerve heads, and a normal retina. In general, CSNB is characterized by moderate night blindness, possible acuity reduction, myopia, and a normal appearing retina. As the name implies, the night blindness—although severe at times—is stationary.

The retina appears essentially normal, but the macular reflex is lost if and when the vision is reduced. Most patients with CSNB maintain 20/40 or better visual acuity. It has been proposed that the defect involves the light-activated enzymatic processes involved in normal rod functioning or a defect in the synaptic transfer of the message. Reflectance densitometry studies have shown that the rhodopsin content of the rods is normal in this condition.

Night blindness is the primary symptom. When AR or X-linked, vision may be reduced to 20/30 to 20/50. Nystagmus and severely reduced acuity may also present. Myopia is omnipresent in AR and X-linked forms. There appear to be two distinctive

Congenital Stationary Night Blindness

Characteristics

- △ Variable inheritance pattern: AR, AD, X–linked
- △ Normal-appearing retina but loss of foveal reflex if and when visual acuity drops
- △ Night blindness, myopia, usually not worse than 20/40, possible nystagmus if severe vision reduction
- △ Variable electrodiagnostic findings but usually reduction in scotopic conditions, field constriction in low light but normal in photopic conditions
- △ Dark adaptation is affected

Management

- △ Pedigree analysis is important
- △ Genetic counseling is recommended in spite of the fact that severe vision loss is not the rule
- △ Low-vision rehabilitation and mobility instruction when necessary
- △ Routine eye examinations are indicated with provision of the best possible prescription

patient responses to electrodiagnostic testing. In one form there is a markedly reduced-to-absent rod response in scotopic conditions, similar implicit times for scotopic and photopic b-waves, and an abnormal EOG. In another form there is a normal scotopic a-wave and a severely reduced b-wave, while the photopic ERG and EOG are normal. Color vision is usually normal, and visual fields are constricted in mesopic conditions but are usually normal in photopic situations. Dark adaptation is also affected.

Management. Congenital stationary night blindness is considered to be a stable condition in most instances. In the AR and X-linked forms, central vision may be affected but not severely reduced. Pedigree analysis and genetic counseling are important in CSNB. Routine eye examinations are indicated for the patient with CSNB with the provision of the best possible prescription. Support through low-vision consultation is important when indicated. Mobility consultation may be a consideration if the patient is having particular problems at night.

■ ■ ■ ■ ■ ■

Clinical Note: Oguchi's Disease— A Variation of CSNB

Oguchi's disease is a variety of CSNB associated with discoloration of the retina that is reversed to normalcy by 2 to 3 hours of dark adaptation (Mizuo's sign). There are varieties of the condition reported in the literature that do not adhere to the characteristic of Mizuo's sign. Under light adaptation the retina has a yellow-gray tint that may extend to the equator. Retinal and choroidal vessels are difficult to differentiate, as their color is altered. Clinical findings are similar to CSNB, with only mild reduction of acuity (20/40) likely. Fluorescein angiography demonstrates hyperfluorescence under light adaptation. The condition appears to be secondary to structural alterations between the retina and RPE and within the outer segments of the rods and cones. The condition is inherited in an AR fashion, with consanguinity common. Genetic counseling is in order.

Choroideremia

Introduction and Description. Choroideremia (Figs. 7–18 and 7–19) is an X–linked recessive dystrophy characterized by progressive degeneration of the RPE and secondarily by degeneration of the choriocapillaris with initial symptoms of night blindness presenting in the first to second decades. This disease is usually manifest as diffuse atrophy of the entire choroid and RPE in males in the end stage, and as aborted atrophy characterized by retinal granularity that is usually stationary in female carriers. Choroideremia has all of the characteristics of retinitis pigmentosa except for the fundus appearance. There is even one report of the association of choroideremia and congenital deafness.

The first changes in the retinal appearance **(see color plate 115)** consist of a generalized loss of the RPE appearing as a fine stippling or a blond fundus in the midperiphery (equatorial zone) in the affected male

(ages 3 months to 15 years). The RPE disorganization then spreads in both directions, with the oldest areas developing choriocapillaris and choroidal atrophy in a scalloped fashion simulating gyrate atrophy (ages 15 to 45 years). Usually by age 30 there is also fibrillary degeneration of the vitreous and there may be pigmentary dispersion in the anterior chamber. Eventually bare sclera shows through and simulates gyrate atrophy but usually spares the macular area until the later stages (45+ years) of the disease. In the later stages optic atrophy and vessel attenuation may occur. Three specific fundus appearances have been identified: (1) light-complexion males with RPE and choroidal pigmentation loss leaving bare sclera and large choroidal vessels, (2) darker-complexion males with complete

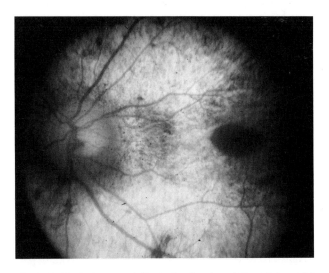

Figure 7–18. A photograph illustrating the devastation of choroidal structure in choroideremia.

Choroideremia

Characteristics

△ All of the characteristics of RP except the fundus appearance

△ Inherited as X-linked, males affected and females are carriers

△ Starts as RPE stippling and blond fundus appearance in midperiphery (ages 3 months to 15 years), followed by choriocapillaris/choroidal atrophy in these areas (ages 15 to 45 years), which spreads with age

△ Loss of macular function occurs in the older patient

△ Posterior subcapsular cataracts, temporal optic atrophy, optic nerve head telangiectasia, fibrillary vitreous degeneration, and pigment in the anterior chamber may also occur

△ Night blindness, progressive field constriction, loss of central vision, and altered electrodiagnosis are all characteristics

△ Fluorescein angiography shows hypofluorescence in scalloped areas and hyperfluorescence of larger choroidal vessels and areas of granularity

△ Female carriers often show areas of RPE granularity in the equatorial zone that may even simulate RP.

△ Carriers usually are stable but may degenerate with age

Management

△ Pedigree analysis is imperative

△ Genetic counseling is the only treatment, as prevention is crucial

△ Low-vision rehabilitation and psychological counseling when appropriate

△ Routine eye examinations with provision of best possible refraction

△ There should be consideration of blocking short-wavelength light and provision of oral antioxidants

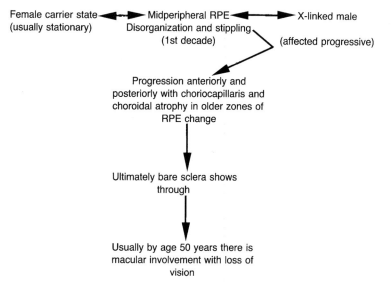

Figure 7–19. A flowchart depicting the ocular changes associated with the progression of choroideremia.

loss of RPE pigmentation but maintenance of choroidal pigment, and (3) overall pink-orange pigmentation with patches of black pigmentation throughout the area. Posterior subcapsular cataracts and temporal atrophy of the optic nerve head and telangiectatic vessel formation on the optic nerve head have also been reported.

Female carriers will often show areas of RPE disorganization and granularity in the midperiphery and at times in the macular area. Some carriers may even have changes simulating RP. Carriers may have some fundus changes associated with aging that may actually create functional vision and visual field compromise. The ERG in the carrier is usually only borderline if affected at all.

Although genetic mapping has been accomplished, the underlying biochemical/structural retinal choroidal alteration has not been elucidated. Both histologic and clinical studies suggest, however, that the RPE is altered first, with subsequent affectation of the choriocapillaris soon after.

In the first to second decades the affected male patient presents with night blindness (preschool) and peripheral field constrictions (usually teenage years). The erosion of the visual field progresses through life, with central vision often affected by ages 50 to 60 years. The field changes usually start in the midperiphery (25 to 45 degrees), eventually coalescing into a ring scotoma that insidiously encroaches into the central zone with time. As in other progressive choroidal dystrophies, visual fields, electrodiagnostic testing, and dark adaptation are altered. The ERGs of patients with choroideremia are consistent with a rod–cone dystrophic pattern. Fluorescein angiography is the best possible study to order for differential diagnosis in choroideremia. The scalloped areas of

RPE loss and choriocapillaris atrophy hyperfluoresce, whereas the larger choroidal vessels and other areas of RPE granularity hypofluoresce.

Management. Prognosis for males affected with choroideremia is grim. Loss of central vision is almost inevitable in later life. The affected male should be counseled regarding the potential loss of vision and should receive regular eye examinations, routine threshold visual field tests, and the best possible prescription. Psychological counseling may be in order during the evolutionary process of vision loss. Again, with the implication of short-wavelength light and antioxidant action at the level of the RPE, consideration of blocking short-wavelength light and provision of oral antioxidants may be considered. Female carriers usually have an excellent prognosis, but there are reports of progressive degeneration of the RPE with age.

Fortunately, affected males have a slow progression of choroideremia and as such are usually prepared for the loss of central vision. Rehabilitation with low-vision aids is difficult at this stage, as central and peripheral vision are both compromised. Genetic counseling after pedigree generation is imperative, as prevention is the only known cure. It can be expected that 100 percent of female children of those affected will be carriers.

Gyrate Dystrophy of the Choroid and Retina

Introduction and Description. Gyrate dystrophy of the choroid and retina (Figs. 7–20 and 7–21) is an autosomal recessive, progressive dystrophy usually associated with hyperornithinemia and deficient ornithine ketoacid aminotransferase (OAT), which converts ornithine to proline. The enzyme levels in af-

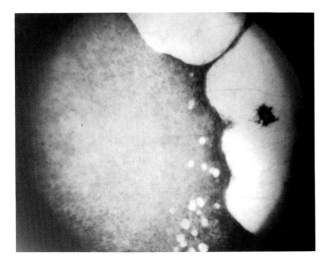

Figure 7–20. A photograph illustrating the destruction of the RPE and choroid with scalloped borders associated with gyrate dystrophy. (*Photo courtesy of R. Nowakowski.*)

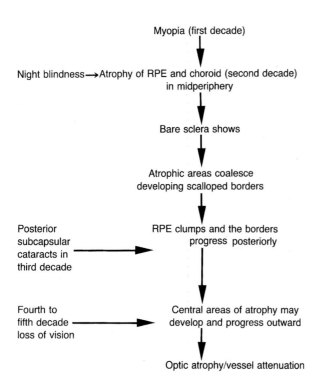

Figure 7–21. A flowchart illustrating the progression of ocular changes associated with gyrate dystrophy.

fected individuals are very low to absent and are reduced in carriers. This association is not absolute but is typical. Serum lysine levels are usually low. Plasma ornithine levels are often 10 to 20 times elevated over normal levels. Age of onset is typically in childhood, but symptoms start to appear at ages 15 to 45 years, with progression to legal blindness often by midlife.

Initial fundus changes occur in the midperiphery in early childhood **(see color plate 116).** There is atrophy of the RPE and choroid in the mid to far peripheral retina with bare sclera showing through. The retina next to the areas of atrophy is often hyperpigmented and has been reported to have crystal deposition in some cases. The areas of atrophy coalesce and assume scalloped borders. The RPE clumps, and the borders progress posteriorly. At times, central zones of atrophy may develop and expand to meet the peripheral zone. The transition between the atrophic zones and the normal islands of retina are abrupt, contrasting with the appearance of choroideremia. Late in the disease, optic atrophy and vessel attenuation occur.

Moderate to very progressive myopia is present in the first decade in 80 percent to 100 percent of cases of gyrate dystrophy, with variable night blindness occurring with the presentation of midperipheral RPE changes in the second decade. Peripheral field loss occurs with progression of atrophy. Posterior subcapsular cataracts occur at an early age in about 40 percent of cases, requiring extraction by the third to fourth decades. Visual acuity may be reduced secondary to cataracts, CME, preretinal macular fibrosis, or degenerative maculopathy. Macular changes result in loss of central vision in the fourth to fifth decades. Electrodiagnostic testing and dark adaptometry show abnormalities consistent with the degree of destruction, but these tests are not as severely affected in patients who are vitamin B_6 responsive. The ERG and EOG are often profoundly affected. Color vision loss also occurs when visual acuity reaches 20/40. Fluorescein angiography shows hyperfluorescence in the area of the gyrate lesions with leakage at the margins of the healthy-appearing retina. In all cases, vitamin B_6 responsive patients appear to have a milder form of the disease.

Neurologic signs may occur in the form of seizure disorders. Mental retardation, language development delays, and abnormal IQ levels have also been reported. Muscle weakness, as demonstrated by abnormal electromyography, may also be present.

Management. Because gyrate dystrophy is related to accumulation of serum ornithine levels, it is thought that reductions in these levels may positively affect outcome. These levels can be modified by protein-restriction diets. Protein-restriction diets can result in significant systemic side effects and should only be recommended when supervised by a nutritionist who

Gyrate Dystrophy

Characteristics

△ Inherited as AR

△ Associated with hyperornithinemia and deficient ornithine aminotransferase (OAT) and reduced serum lysine levels

△ Age of onset in childhood with legal blindness by midlife

△ Starts as RPE atrophy and choroidal atrophy in midperiphery in childhood; these areas coalesce and have scalloped borders that progress inward and outward

△ Retinal areas next to atrophy are hyperpigmented and may have crystal deposition

△ Development of central zones of atrophy, optic atrophy, early-onset cataracts (extraction by ages 30 to 40 years); variable night blindness and peripheral field loss usually occur with age

△ Moderate to progressive myopia is the rule

△ Electrodiagnostic testing is consistent with the degree of the disease

△ Color vision compromise when vision drops below 20/40

△ Fluorescein angiography shows hyperfluorescence in the area of the gyrate lesions with leakage at the borders

△ Systemic signs:
Seizure disorders
Mental retardation
Delayed language development
Abnormal IQ levels
Muscle weakness

Management

△ Pedigree analysis

△ Genetic counseling

△ Protein restriction diets limiting protein intake to 0.2 g/kg per day with supplementation of normal metabolic needs

△ Oral vitamin B_6 at 20 to 500 mg/day to reduce serum ornithine levels and stabilize lysine levels in responsive individuals

△ Proline supplementation at 3 mg/day may hold retinal progression in check

△ Low–vision rehabilitation may be coupled with psychological counseling when indicated

△ Rule out associated systemic disorders

△ Routine eye examinations with serial visual field tests and provision of the best possible prescription.

△ Nutritional supplementation is definitely a part of the management of this condition

maintains normal metabolic needs. Arginine-deficient diets consisting of limiting protein intake to 0.2 g/kg per day may reduce serum ornithine levels. Oral pyridoxine (vitamin B_6) at 20 to 500 mg/day may also reduce serum ornithine levels and normalize serum lysine levels in certain responsive individuals. Later studies have shown that 15 to 20 mg of pyridoxine is as effective as larger doses. Pyridoxine may result in a 50 percent lowering of serum ornithine levels. Proline supplementation at 3 mg/day has also been reported to hold the retinal progression in check. There is some evidence that if serum ornithine levels are maintained between 55 and 355 μm, the dystrophy does not progress as fast but will not regress. Genetic counseling is mandatory in cases of gyrate dystrophy. Psychological counseling may be necessary for the patient facing severe vision loss. Routine eye examinations with threshold visual field tests are recommended. Low-vision rehabilitation is difficult once central vision is compromised, but must be considered. Once the patient has severe vision compromise, nonsighted rehabilitation should be recommended. It is also recommended that the practitioner should rule out any potential associated systemic anomalies.

Table 7–8 summarizes the characteristics of hereditary choroidal/retinal disease primarily affecting peripheral and night vision.

Retinal Dystrophies Associated With Storage Diseases

Introduction and Description. Gyrate dystrophy represents a retinal dystrophy that develops as a result of genetically determined abnormal enzymatic function. There are approximately 100 metabolic disorders of carbohydrate, lipid, and protein metabolism that are currently known. In these conditions, the retinal dystrophies that develop are apparently associated with abnormal enzymatic function. Two major categories will be discussed here, not in detail but in a manner sufficient for the primary care practitioner to be alerted to the disorders because of the associated morbidity and mortality.

Alterations in Carbohydrate Metabolism. Mucopolysaccharidosis (MPS) results from a deficiency of enzymes and affects the connective tissues, creating a variety of clinical features. Skeletal deformities, distorted facial characteristics, deafness, cardiac disease, mental deficiency, corneal clouding, optic atrophy, and retinal pigment dystrophies are characteristic. All of the associated disorders are inherited as autosomal recessive except for Hunter's syndrome, which is X-linked recessive. The characteristics of the more common mucopolysaccharidoses follow.

TABLE 7-8. HEREDITARY RETINAL/CHOROIDAL DISEASE PRIMARILY AFFECTING PERIPHERAL AND NIGHT VISION

	Heredity	Mean Age Onset	Progressive/ Stationary	Signs/ Symptoms	ERG	EOG	Fundus Appearance	Visual Fields
RP	AR, AD, X-linked, simplex, multiplex	9–19 years	Progressive but variable	Night blind, restricted fields, loss of central vision possible, photophobia	Abnormal	Abnormal	Attenuation of arterioles, midperipheral motheaten appearance, midperipheral bone spicules, disc pallor, cystoid macular edema (variations exist)	Spreading ring scotomas from 30–50°
CSNB	AR, AD, X-linked	Congenital	Stationary	Night blind, possible mild vision reduction, possible nystagmus	Variable but often abnormal	Variable but often abnormal	Normal, but may have loss of foveal reflex	Constricted in mesopic conditions
Choroideremia	X-linked males	First to second decade	Slowly progressive	Night blind, eventual loss of central vision	Altered	Altered	RPE stippling in midperiphery spreading, eventual choriocapillaris/ choroid atrophy in areas of stippling, macular atrophy	Peripheral field constriction
Gyrate dystrophy	AR	First to second decade	Progressive	Night blind, loss of central vision, myopia	Abnormal	Abnormal	RPE atrophy and choroidal atrophy in midperiphery with scalloped borders progressing anteriorly and posteriorly, possible central atrophy	Peripheral field constriction

ERG, electroretinogram; EDG, electro-oculogram; AR, autosomal recessive; AD, autosomal dominant.

Hurler's Syndrome, MPS I-H

- Normalcy in infancy, with dwarfism appearing at age 2 to 3 years
- Large head, grotesque facial features, mental deficiencies, stiff joints, deafness
- Corneal clouding by age 1 to 3 years and photophobia
- Bone spicule pigmentary retinopathy and vessel attenuation with associated night blindness, abnormal ERG
- Optic disc edema and late optic atrophy
- Often death before age 10 years

Scheie's Syndrome, MPS I-S

- Age of onset at 5 to 7 years
- Nearly normal stature, mild facial characteristics, stiff joints, hand deformity, aortic valve disease, hernias, deafness
- Diffuse corneal clouding after age 4 years
- Possible glaucoma
- Bone spicule pigmentary retinopathy in the teens with night blindness in the 20s to 30s, vessel attenuation, abnormal ERG
- Possible optic disc edema and optic atrophy
- May have normal lifespan

Hurler–Scheie Syndrome, MPS I-H-S

- Onset usually ages 2 to 4 years
- Dwarfism, moderate retardation, stiff joints, deafness, hirsutism, heart disease, receding chin
- Severe arachnoid cysts/papilledema and optic atrophy
- Diffuse progressive corneal clouding
- Bone spicule pigmentary retinopathy, associated night blindness, vessel attenuation, abnormal ERG
- Often death at ages 20 to 30 years

Hunter's Syndrome, MPS II-A

- X-linked recessive
- Symptoms prior to age 1 year
- Phenotype resembling Hurler's syndrome but less severe
- Hoarse voice and nodular skin lesions
- Bone spicule pigmentary retinopathy, night blindness, vessel attenuation, abnormal ERG
- Optic disc edema and optic atrophy
- Cornea is clear
- Death often by age 15 years
- MPS II-B has onset around age 4 years, normal mental function, and survival to age 60 years plus, but all of the retinal characteristics

Sanfilippo's Syndrome, MPS III-A,B,C,D

- Age at onset is 2 to 6 years
- Absence of corneal clouding, optic disc edema, and optic atrophy
- Severe progressive retardation, moderate dwarfism, stiff joints, hirsutism, altered facial characteristics, behavioral problems, speech loss
- Bone spicule pigmentary retinopathy, vessel attenuation, night blindness, altered ERG
- Death typically prior to age 30 years

Clinical laboratory tests are available to diagnose the mucopolysaccharidoses both prenatally and postnatally.

Abnormal Lipid Metabolism. Alteration in lipid metabolism (mucolipidoses and ceroid lipofuscinoses) may likewise create significant systemic and ocular conditions. There are some similarities with the mucopolysaccharidoses and many differences. A synopsis of the more common conditions follows.

Mucolipidosis IV

- Autosomal recessive
- Corneal clouding
- Progressive psychomotor retardation within the first year
- Strabismus is common
- Pigmentary clumping in the retina, vessel attenuation, and optic atrophy
- Death by age 30 years

Fucosidosis

- Autosomal recessive
- Onset in first year of life
- Features develop similar to Hurler's syndrome
- Variable corneal opacities and possible strabismus
- Bull's-eye macular appearance and tortuous vessels
- Death common in first 3 to 5 years

Ceroid Lipofuscinoses, Haltia–Santavuori Syndrome

- Onset at 8 to 18 months
- Strabismus
- Early optic atrophy
- Pigment granularity of the macula and periphery with vessel attentuation
- Loss of vision begins at ages 2 to 3 months, with blindness at 2 years
- Death by age 5 to 7 years

Ceroid Lipofuscinoses, Jansky–Bielschowsky Syndrome

- Onset 2 to 4 years
- Strabismus
- Late optic atrophy
- Pigment granularity of the macula and periphery, with bull's-eye macula and vessel attenuation
- Loss of vision begins at 4 to 7 years of age, with blindness at ages 7 to 10 years
- Death by age 10 years

Ceroid Lipofuscinoses, Batten's Syndrome

- Onset at 4 to 8 years
- Strabismus
- Late optic atrophy
- Pigment granularity of macula, bone spicule, and salt-and-pepper appearance with vessel attenuation
- Loss of vision begins at 5 to 8 years, with blindness at 8 to 10 years
- Death by ages 15 to 25 years

Management. Although the prognosis for vision and life is fairly grim for the majority of the lipid storage diseases, it is important for the primary practitioner to recognize the potential abnormalities in the infant or child and ask for appropriate consultation for differential diagnosis. Storage diseases can be differentially diagnosed by a combination of laboratory tests as well as biopsy in some cases. The important aspect of this group of diseases is the development of a differential diagnosis from some of the other less ma-

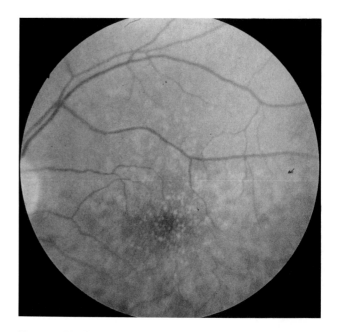

Figure 7–23. Pisciform RPE lesions characteristic of fundus flavimaculatus with early macular changes.

lignant pigmentary retinopathies. Low-vision rehabilitation may be attempted as well as keratoplasty in some of the cases.

DYSTROPHIES INITIALLY AFFECTING CENTRAL VISION AND COLOR VISION

Fundus Flavimaculatus (With Stargardt's Dystrophy)

Introduction and Description. Fundus flavimaculatus is a bilateral progressive autosomal recessive disorder characterized by subretinal yellow flecks, and is often associated with macular degeneration known as Stargardt's dystrophy (Figs. 7–22 to 7–28). There are a few reported cases of autosomal dominant forms of the dystrophy. Although there are still those that distinguish between fundus flavimaculatus and Stargardt's dystrophy, it is accepted that the end stages of both processes are the same from the standpoint of appearance, genetic characteristics, fluorescein angiography findings, and electrodiagnostic characteristics. Prevalence of the disorder is estimated at 1 in 8000 to 1 in 10,000. The ophthalmoscopic picture can be so varied that often fundus flavimaculatus becomes a diagnosis by exclusion of other ocular disorders.

The ophthalmoscopic presentation of fundus flavimaculatus is so varied that classification systems have been developed. The most typical finding is yellow pigment epithelial flecks that are described as fish-form or pisciform that surround the macula or are scattered throughout the posterior pole. Peripheral

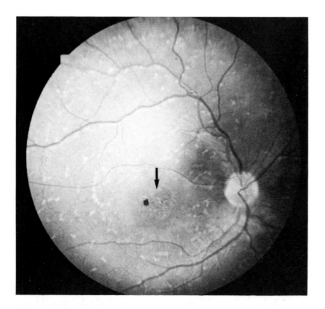

Figure 7–22. A patient with the characteristic fishtail flecks of fundus flavimaculatus surrounding the early macular changes (*arrow*) of Stargardt's disease.

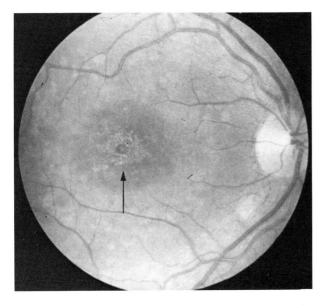

Figure 7–24. A patient with mild fundus flavimaculatus changes surrounding the pigmentary changes in the macula (*arrow*) in Stargardt's disease.

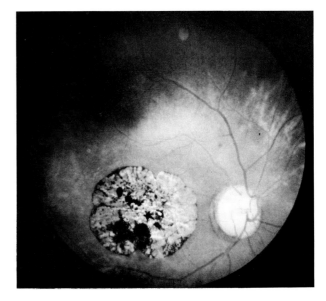

Figure 7–26. An illustration of severe atrophy of the macular area in Stargardt's disease with minimal fundus flavimaculatus changes.

changes may also include a reticular pattern of flecks and/or atrophy, pigment clumps or spicule formation, and punched out areas of atrophy simulating POHS. Vessels are usually not attenuated, but temporal optic atrophy occurs when the macular is significantly affected. The peripheral changes often increase when the macular function is affected. In spite of peripheral changes, the peripheral vision function remains intact even late into the process. Ultimately, loss of vision occurs associated with atrophic macular changes. **See color plates 117 and 119 to 123.**

The classification of the fundus appearance varies with different authors but is approximately as follows:

- *Group 1:* Macular degeneration without flecks
- *Group 2:* Macular degeneration with flecks
- *Group 3:* Macular degeneration with diffuse flecks
- *Group 4:* Diffuse flecks without degeneration

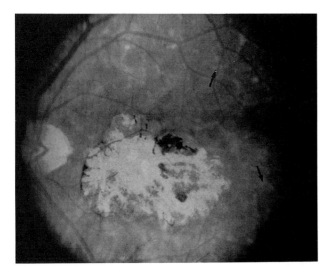

Figure 7–25. An example of a variation of Stargardt's disease with severe macular alterations and the small black arrows pointing to the pisciform lesions of fundus flavimaculatus.

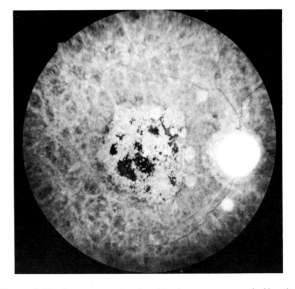

Figure 7–27. Severe macular atrophic changes surrounded by significant RPE changes associated with fundus flavimaculatus.

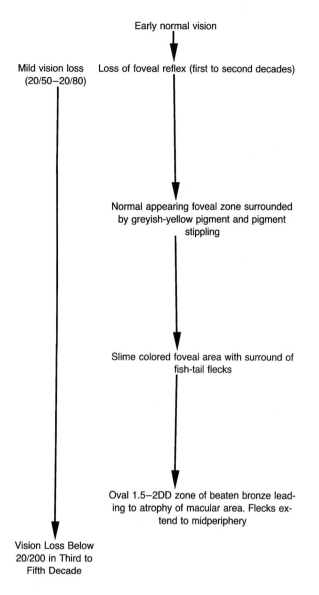

Early normal vision

Loss of foveal reflex (first to second decades)

Mild vision loss
(20/50–20/80)

Normal appearing foveal zone surrounded
by greyish-yellow pigment and pigment
stippling

Slime colored foveal area with surround of
fish-tail flecks

Oval 1.5–2DD zone of beaten bronze leading to atrophy of macular area. Flecks extend to midperiphery

Vision Loss Below
20/200 in Third to
Fifth Decade

Figure 7–28. A flowchart illustrating the progression of Stargardt's disease and fundus flavimaculatus.

In the initial stages of Stargardt's dystrophy there are minimal fundus changes, in spite of vision reduction. The first fundus sign is loss of the foveal reflex and a fine granularity to the RPE. At this stage, fluorescein angiography will demonstrate a faint "bulls-eye" appearance. In one of the groups, this may progress to an area of normal-appearing central retina surrounded by a zone of grayish yellow depigmentation and pigment stippling. The foveal area then progresses to develop a slime-covered appearance with yellow flecks (called pisciform or fishtail) developing deep in the retina peripheral to the macula. Eventually a horizontal oval area (2 by 1.5 disc diameters) of

atrophic RPE appears as "beaten bronze" or metallic in nature, surrounded by flecks. As the lesion continues to develop, further atrophy of the macular area occurs, and the flecks extend to the midperiphery. It is of interest that the flecks may precede, be coincident with, or follow the macular atrophy. From a clinicopathologic standpoint, there is an enlargement of RPE cells thought to be secondary to excessive lipofuscin deposition in the zones of the flecks with a total disappearance of the cones, rods, and RPE cells in the circumfoveal zone.

Blurring of central vision usually presents in the first to second decades (average age of onset in the 20s) in a patient with prior normal vision and is often the presenting symptom of the disease. Best corrected vision at the first examination ranges from 20/20 to 5/200 but averages around 20/100. The average time for reduction from 20/40 to the 20/120 range is 4 to 5 years. Myopia also seems to be a characteristic of fundus flavimaculatus. The condition may be mistaken for a conversion reaction in the young because vision is reduced without dramatic fundus changes. Night blindness is usually not a complaint. Photophobia is rare as an early complaint, but the patients reportedly prefer subdued lighting. As the condition progresses, vision drops significantly.

Color vision defects are not a characteristic until late in the macular atrophy, but do serve as a differential diagnostic basis to distinguish this condition from cone dystrophies. The ERG is usually normal to slightly abnormal, and the EOG is variable but is often abnormal, depending on the extent of fleck formation resulting from RPE disease. Dark adaptation is usually normal but it takes much longer to achieve threshold. Visual fields demonstrate central scotomas when macular atrophy occurs, but there is maintenance of peripheral vision even late in the process.

Fluorescein angiography is crucial in the differential diagnosis of fundus flavimaculatus. The RPE cells are thought to accumulate lipofuscin, which effectively blocks fluorescein visibility. As such, the absence of choroidal fluorescence occurs in up to 90 percent of cases, especially in the early stages of the disease. This diffuse blocked choroidal fluorescence (often referred to as a dark or silent choroid) is accompanied by the fact that the flecks do not fluoresce. The atrophic macular area does fluoresce throughout the course of the study.

Associated systemic conditions include pigmentary retinopathy that simulates RP and the Laurence–Moon–Bardet–Biedl syndrome (LMBB). LMBB is characterized by obesity, hypogenitalism, mental retardation, pigmentary retinopathy, and polydactyly.

Choroidal neovascularization may be a secondary complication of fundus flavimaculatus.

Pearls

Fundus Flavimaculatus (With Stargardt's Dystrophy)

Characteristics

△ Bilateral progressive AR disorder with multiple ophthalmic presentations but characterized by subretinal yellow flecks

△ End stage of fundus flavimaculatus and Stargardt's dystrophy are the same from the standpoint of appearance, genetics, fluorescein findings, and electrodiagnosis

△ Variable fundus presentation including:

Macular degeneration may occur with or without flecks

Flecks may occur without macular degeneration

Peripheral changes may include reticular flecks, pigment clumps, spicule formation, punched-out atrophic areas

Vessels are normal but may have temporal optic atrophy when macula is compromised

△ Macular involvement includes:

Fine granularity to RPE in fovea and loss of reflex

Faint bull's-eye on fluorescein early in process

Possible gray-yellow surrounding of central retina

Possible "sliming" of the macular area

Possible 2-DD oval beaten bronze area in macula

Further development of macular atrophy with coincidental progression of peripheral flecks

△ Blurring of central vision in the 20s (best corrected) to 20/50 to 5/200 is first sign

△ Characteristic of myopia

△ Patients typically prefer subdued light but do not complain of photophobia

△ Electrodiagnostic characteristics dependent on degree of progression

△ Dark adaptation normal but delay to threshold

△ Maintenance of peripheral vision but central scotomas when macula involved

△ Color vision loss occurs late when macula atrophies

△ Fluorescein angiography is diagnostic

Early dark or silent choroid—blockage of choroidal fluorescence

Fluorescence of atrophic macular area throughout study

△ Laurence–Moon–Bardet–Biedl syndrome may be associated as well as pigmentary retinopathy simulating RP

△ Secondary choroidal neovascularization may occur

Management

△ Vision loss is eventually inevitable, but the best possible correction should always be provided with consideration of blocking short-wavelength light

△ Pedigree analysis is of assistance in diagnosis and counseling

△ Genetic counseling is in order in spite of the fact that many reported cases are sporadic

△ Low-vision rehabilitation is necessary when appropriate

△ Psychological counseling may be necessary to assist in trauma of vision loss

---

Management. The diagnosis of fundus flavimaculatus is complex, often requiring that all other possibilities be eliminated.

The probability of maintaining vision of 20/40 in at least one eye in fundus flavimaculatus is over 50 percent by the age of 19 years, over 30 percent by the age of 29 years, and over 20 percent by the age of 39 years. Once acuity drops below 20/40, it appears that vision then deteriorates rapidly to 20/200. Routine eye examinations are indicated, with provision of the best possible prescription and consideration of recommending use of lenses to block short wavelengths to minimize retinal photo-oxidative trauma. Routine evaluations can offer information regarding avocation, vocation, and other pursuits. Psychological counseling may be in order to assist in the trauma of vision reduction.

Low-vision rehabilitation can offer help to the patient with fundus flavimaculatus, and genetic counseling is an absolute necessity. LMBB must be ruled out as an associated systemic condition. Should choroidal neovascularization occur, laser intervention may be of benefit.

Patterned Anomalies of the Retinal Pigment Epithelium

Introduction and Description. Patterned anomalies of the RPE are probably RPE dystrophies, but there is controversy as to the exact etiology. These anomalies appear as variations of (1) Sjögren's RPE dystrophy, (2) macroreticular pattern dystrophy, (3) butterfly dystrophy, and (4) a few other known by other names. In general, they can be categorized as macular pigment epithelial dystrophies. These dystrophies affect the macular area and are usually inherited in an AD pattern. The onset of signs is usually in the first to third decades. The initial changes usually appear in the macular area at ages 10 to 12 years of age, but later onset has been reported. The signs are usually bilateral and somewhat symmetrical.

See color plate 124. In the reticular form of patterned anomalies of the macula, pigmented lines form that radiate from the fovea. This may be preceded by fine granular pigment dispersed in the macular area. The lines join to form a "fishnet" appearance with "knots" at points of overlap. The fishnet extends to the

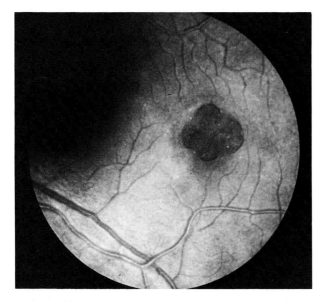

Figure 7–29. An example of a patterned anomaly of the RPE. The shape is often in the form of butterfly wings or an iron cross.

equator. In the butterfly form (Fig. 7–29), the pigmentary changes are more solid and appear as butterfly wings or as an iron cross overlying the macula. The macroreticular form is a variation of the fishnet form. The remainder of the retina usually appears normal.

Patterned Dystrophies of the RPE

Characteristics

△ Inherited as autosomal dominant; a pedigree is crucial in determining the differential diagnosis

△ Reticular, macroreticular, butterfly types—bilateral and symmetrical

△ Reticular—fishnet of pigment with knots at crossings to equator

△ Butterfly—solid RPE changes at macula as butterfly wings

△ Earliest changes appear in macular area at ages 10 to 12 years, but have been reported later in life

△ Mild reduction in acuity usually, but may be severe

△ Remote possibility of the development of choroidal neovascularization

Management

△ Pedigree analysis is crucial in diagnosis

△ Genetic counseling is advised in spite of the limited damage characteristic of the condition

△ Provision of best possible prescription is necessary

△ Routine eye examinations are recommended

Many variations of the dystrophies exist. The diagnosis is made by establishing a pedigree and performing an electro-oculogram, which is usually depressed. Different members in the pedigree may present totally different fundus pictures. Patients usually have minimal acuity loss in most cases in spite of a dramatic macular picture. Long-term prognosis for vision is favorable in most cases. There is a remote possibility for the development of choroidal neovascularization in cases of macular pigment epithelial dystrophy.

One case has been reported (Giaffrie et al, 1986) in which the patient had butterfly dystrophy in one eye and vitelliform in the other, suggesting a common etiopathogenesis, although this report must be questioned.

Symptoms usually do not match the appearance of the macula. Visual acuity is usually in the 20/20 to 20/50 range, although scant reports show visual reduction to be severe. Color vision and central scotomas are consistent with acuity reduction. Fluorescein angiography demonstrates hypofluorescence in areas of increased pigmentation and hyperfluorescence in areas of RPE atrophy. The ERG is normal, but the EOG is variable but usually depressed, depending on RPE dysfunction. The differential diagnosis is aided by examining other family members.

Management. Prognosis is good, with most cases having vision loss limited to the 20/50 level. The best refraction should be provided along with routine eye examinations, and genetic counseling is advised. In cases with associated late-stage atrophic stages, vision may be reduced, necessitating low-vision rehabilitation.

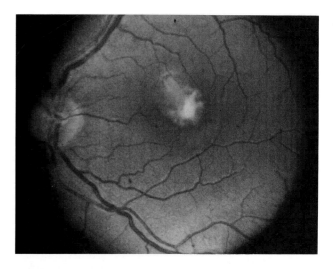

Figure 7–30. The "egg yolk" pattern in the macula associated with vitelliform dystrophy.

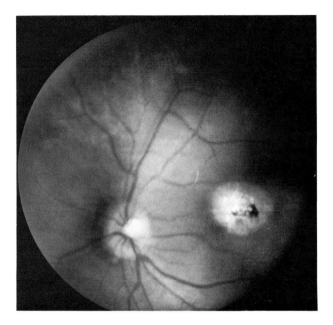

Figure 7–31. The "egg yolk" pattern has been scrambled, resulting in vision reduction in this case of vitelliform dystrophy.

Vitelliform Dystrophy (Best's Disease)

Introduction and Description. Best's vitelliform dystrophy is an AD inherited macular disorder characterized by an early-onset "egg yolk" appearance in the foveal area (Figs. 7–30 to 7–32). Vitelliform dystrophy is considered to be autosomal dominant, with variable penetrance and variable phenotypic expressivity, and as such appearance in another family member is important in the differential diagnosis. The EOG is the differential diagnostic test to order, as even heterozygous carriers (no penetrance) can be detected by an abnormal EOG. Presentation of the lesion is usually between the ages of 4 to 10 years, with minimal reduction in acuity initially. The lesion has been reported in some cases at birth.

Stages of progression characterize the fundus appearance of vitelliform dystrophy **(see color plates 125 and 126).** Even before there is any fundus change, an abnormal EOG may be recorded. The disease is usually bilateral, but there is often asymmetry. The previtelliform stage is characterized by fine yellow pigment disturbances under the central fovea at a very young age. The classically described "egg yolk" (Fig. 7–30) usually appears between the ages of 4 and 10 years. The "egg yolk" is a yellow mound surrounded by a darker border, and is thought to be the result of an abnormal accumulation of lipofuscin materials in the RPE cells. The vitelliform lesion is usually centered on the fovea and is often one-half to 5 DD in size. Variations of centricity will occur. Tremendous variation occurs in the actual presentation of the yellow deposits and can make recognition difficult. The "egg yolk" often remains stable for years, with only a mild reduction in visual acuity (20/30 to 20/50), even into midlife. With age the yolk may disappear, leaving an indistinct area of RPE atrophy, only to reappear at a later date. This area of RPE atrophy offers the opportunity for the development of choroidal neovascularization, which often occurs in these cases at a very young age. The yolk material may also disintegrate,

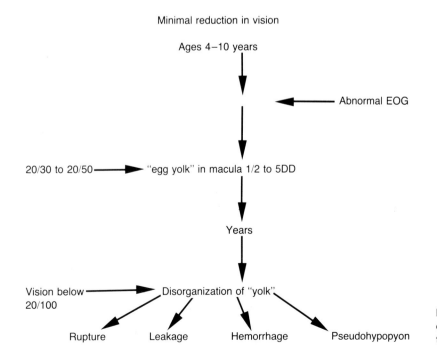

Figure 7–32. A flowchart illustrating the development of ocular changes in vitelliform dystrophy.

leaving a "scrambled egg" appearance (Fig. 7–31). Leakage, rupture, or hemorrhage may occur, resulting in vision loss. The cyst may also liquefy at the later stage, resulting in a layering effect within the cyst, giving what is described as the pseudohypopyon stage. In the pseudohypopyon stage, movement within the cyst may be seen when the patient alters head position. With rupture of the "egg yolk" cyst, there is retinal infiltration and scarring, resulting in vision reduction below 20/100. It is important to understand that up to 75 percent of patients with Best's vitelliform dystrophy maintain visual acuity at better than 20/40 in spite of the dramatic fundus appearance.

From a clinicopathologic standpoint, it is thought that the RPE is the focus of the disease process. Material (possibly lipofusion) accumulates in the RPE cells, resulting in malfunction, atrophy, and eventual loss of photoreceptor function. The abnormal EOG characteristic of vitelliform dystrophy supports the hypothesis of a widespread RPE disease even though funduscopic changes are often not visible in the retinal periphery.

Vitelliform dystrophy is a disease that has a fundus appearance much more dramatic than the resultant acuity loss until the later stages. Fundus changes occur in the first to second decades, with only a slight reduction in acuity. Vision is usually maintained at a fairly good level until later life.

Fluorescein angiography demonstrates hypofluorescence early within the areas of yellow material accumulation. As the RPE breaks down, hyperfluorescence will occur in those zones. Should leakage or neovascularization occur, fluorescein angiography will reflect these changes. The ERG will be normal to minimally abnormal, while the EOG is always abnormal. The EOG is the definitive test even in heterozygous carriers. An abnormal EOG in the presence of a normal ERG is virtually pathognomonic of vitelliform dystrophy. Color vision will be compromised concordant with vision loss but is classically normal. Central scotomas will vary depending on the stage of the disease.

Management. Visual acuity remains in the minimally compromised zone (20/30 to 20/50) for many years, with degeneration of the vitelliform lesion, vision drops to below 20/100. The omnipresent threat of choroidal neovascularization demands routine eye examinations. Provision of the best possible prescription is in order. As the disease is thought to be the result of abnormal accumulation of lipofuscin in the RPE or retina, blockage of short-wavelength light may be of benefit. Likewise, use of oral antioxidants may prove to be of benefit. Complications such as hemorrhage and neovascularization can also result in decreased visual acuity. Should choroidal neovascularization present, laser intervention may be of benefit.

Pearls

Vitelliform Dystrophy (Best's Disease)

Characteristics

Δ Inherited as autosomal dominant with phenotypic variability

Δ Thought to be an abnormal accumulation of lipofuscin in the RPE

Δ Previtelliform signs usually in early childhood as fine yellow pigment disturbances in the central fovea

Δ Fundus signs usually start at ages 4 to 10 years as a ½- to 5-DD elevated "egg yolk" lesion in macula that may remain stable for a long period of time. Usually symmetrical

Δ At this stage there is usually only a mild reduction in visual acuity to the 20/30 to 20/50 level

Δ With time, the yolk may rupture, leak, hemorrhage, or create a pseudohypopyon that moves with head movements

Δ RPE degeneration and choriocapillaris atrophy may occur in the foveal area

Δ Strong chance for early development of choroidal neovascularization

Δ Key sign is abnormal EOG even before vision loss with EOG abnormalities even in the carrier state. Normal ERG and abnormal EOG are pathognomonic of vitelliform dystrophy

Δ Vision loss may occur later with central scotoma but up to 75 percent of patients maintain 20/40 vision or better

Δ Fluorescein angiography demonstrates hyperfluorescence in areas of RPE atrophy but hypofluorescence in areas where there is accumulation of yellow lipofuscin

Management

Δ Pedigree analysis is crucial for differential diagnosis with subsequent utilization of EOG in family members

Δ Genetic counseling is in order in spite of the fact that in many instances the condition is not totally visually devastating

Δ Low-vision rehabilitation should be considered when appropriate

Δ Routine eye examinations documenting progression with provision of the best possible prescription are necessary

Δ Lenses to block short-wavelength light and oral antioxidants may prove to be of benefit in this disease process

Δ Rule out pseudovitelliform dystrophy

Pedigree analysis and genetic counseling are important in this autosomal dominant disease. This is one condition in which a heterozygous carrier can be determined by EOG in spite of the lack of funduscopic changes.

It is important to rule out pseudovitelliform dystrophy and other variants.

■ ■ ■ ■ ■ ■

Clinical Note: Pseudovitelliform Macular Dystrophy (Foveomacular Vitelliform Dystrophy, Adult Type)

Pseudovitelliform macular dystrophy is an AD disease usually presenting after age 30 years with mild decreased visual acuity (20/30 to 20/40) and possibly metamorphopsia. There are reports, however, of presentation at a younger age. An elevated vitelliform-like lesion one-fourth to one-third DD presents in the foveal area with a surrounding of a white or gray depigmented area and possibly a central hyperpigmented spot. Color vision and electrodiagnostic testing are entirely normal. The fluorescein angiography demonstrates hyperfluorescence in the depigmented area and hypofluorescence in the hyperpigmented area. Vision is usually stable but can progress in some cases to legal blindness. Choroidal neovascularization is a distinct possibility because of the compromise in the RPE/Bruch's barrier. Treatment for choroidal neovascularization is indicated.

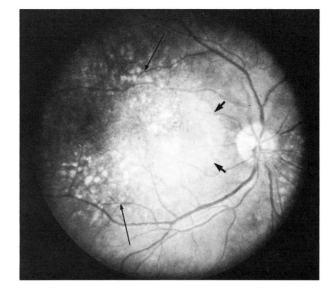

Figure 7–33. In this photograph the broad arrows outline the area of RPE degeneration in the macular area associated with dominant drusen. The thin arrows point to the large dominant drusen.

Dominant Drusen (Doyne's Honeycomb Dystrophy)

Introduction and Description. Dominant drusen (Doyne's honeycomb dystrophy) is a condition that is inherited in an autosomal dominant pattern with variable penetrance and variable expressivity. The drusen usually present in the posterior pole and are contrasted with "senile type" drusen that result from age-related degeneration of the RPE by the age of onset. Dominant drusen present within the first 3 decades and progress to include the macular area, resulting in decreased vision by the fifth to sixth decade.

Initially, the dominant drusen appear as irregular white dots in or near the macula at the layer of the RPE (Figs. 7–33 and 7–34). With age, the drusen increase in number and enlarge. The drusen decrease in size as they become more remote to the macula. In addition to enlarging, the drusen become more confluent and often develop associated RPE hyperplasia. Eventually the drusen calcify, and the RPE atrophies, resulting in a white plaque in the macular zone. **See color plate 118.**

As the RPE/Bruch's barrier is compromised, there is the strong possibility of the development of sensory retina or RPE detachments, choroidal neovascularization, or disciform maculopathy.

From a clinicopathologic standpoint, dominant drusen result from a faulty RPE. There appears to be an inherited faulty metabolic process in the RPE. Deposition of acid mucopolysaccharide and cerebroside

Pearls

Dominant Drusen

Characteristics

△ Inherited as autosomal dominant with variability in both penetration and expressivity

△ White dots in or near macula within the first 3 decades of life that enlarge, become more confluent, and may form a plaque in macula

△ May also have the development of associated choroidal neovascularization

△ Variable visual acuity reduction, variable color vision compromise, central scotomas, and metamorphopsia that usually does not present until the fourth decade of life

△ Fluorescein angiography demonstrates the RPE compromise well

△ The photopic ERG is normal to abnormal depending on the stage of progression

Management

△ Pedigree analysis is indicated

△ Genetic counseling is advisable as symptoms usually do not appear until after childbearing years

△ Low-vision rehabilitation should be considered when appropriate

△ Laser intervention in "wet" maculopathies may be beneficial, although the RPE/Bruch's membrane barrier is severely compromised

△ Routine eye examinations are in order to document progress and to assure the best possible prescription

△ Possible benefit for providing glasses that block short wavelengths of light

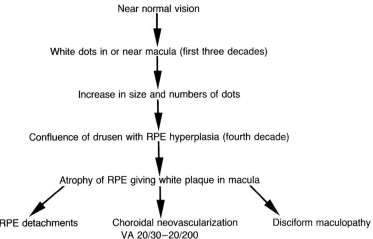

Near normal vision

↓

White dots in or near macula (first three decades)

↓

Increase in size and numbers of dots

↓

Confluence of drusen with RPE hyperplasia (fourth decade)

↓

Atrophy of RPE giving white plaque in macula

Sensory or RPE detachments   Choroidal neovascularization   Disciform maculopathy
                                        VA 20/30–20/200

Figure 7–34. A flowchart illustrating the stages of development in dominant drusen.

develops as the result of the RPE dystrophy. The RPE cells then become grossly abnormal, creating compromise of the blood–retinal barrier and the overlying photoreceptors.

The symptoms of dominant drusen are metamorphopsia and loss of central vision and usually do not present until after the fourth decade. Final acuity can vary between 20/30 to worse than 20/200. Color vision is variably affected, and central scotomas present as drusen accumulate and coalesce. Fluorescein angiography best demonstrates the loss of RPE by gross areas of hyperfluorescence. The ERG is normal to minimally abnormal, and the EOG is subnormal in the later stages but not as dramatic as in vitelliform dystrophy. Should choroidal neovascularization occur, signs and symptoms associated with that process will present.

Management. Final visual acuity is unpredictable in cases of dominant drusen because of incomplete penetrance and variable expressivity. Should choroidal neovascularization develop, prognosis becomes more grim. At this point intervention with laser photocoagulation should be considered.

Pedigree analysis, genetic counseling, and low-vision consultation when appropriate are indicated in patients with dominant drusen. Routine eye examinations are important to document any progression as well as to assure early detection of choroidal neovascularization. Provision of glasses to block short-wavelength light may be of value.

Central Areolar Choroidal Dystrophy (CACD)

Introduction and Description. Central areolar choroidal dystrophy (CACD) has been described as having AD and AR inheritance patterns as well as sporadic cases. There is considerable confusion regarding this condition, as clinical presentation is dramatically variable. At times, only the choriocapillaris is involved, whereas other cases show involvement deep into the choroid. CACD rarely occurs before the age of 30 years and usually presents after the age of 40 years.

The earliest fundus changes that present in CACD are bilateral areas of RPE stippling in and around the macula (Figs. 7–35 to 7–37). These areas progress to atrophy of the RPE and choriocapillaris in a sharply outlined zone in the fovea or around it. The RPE may clump, but this is rare. The further atrophy of the deeper vessels may occur, and the lesion may enlarge and expand with time, but usually stays confined to the region surrounding the fovea. The at-

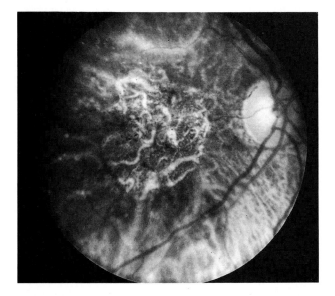

Figure 7–35. A photograph illustrating one stage in the development of CACD. Note atrophy of the RPE, choriocapillaris, and choroid in the macular area.

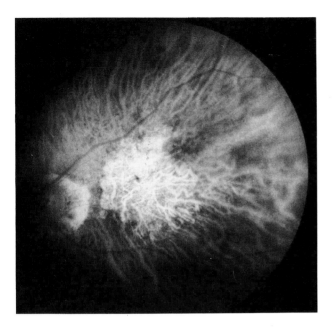

Figure 7–36. Example of central areolar choroidal dystrophy with an excavated zone in the macular area and an increase in the visibility of the choroidal system.

rophic area is excavated with stereoscopic observation. Optic disc atrophy and vessel attenuation have been reported but only in isolated cases. The fundus appearance is usually bilateral and symmetrical. From a clinicopathologic standpoint, it appears that choriocapillaris atrophy exists with subsequent RPE loss and sensory retinal atrophy. **See color plate 128.**

The primary symptom of CACD is reduced vision presenting from age 30 to 40 years, with a slow progression to 20/200 or below with further aging. Color vision loss and central scotomas are related to degree of destruction. Peripheral vision is usually nor-

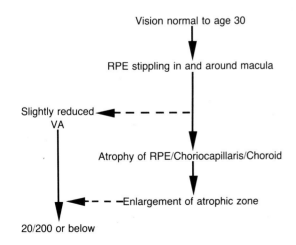

Figure 7–37. A flowchart illustrating the stages of development of CACD.

Central Areolar Choroidal Dystrophy

Pearls

Characteristics

△ Inherited as AD and AR but also reported sporadically

△ Usually presents as vision reduction between ages 30 and 50 years, but progresses to 20/200 or worse with age

△ Starts as bilateral RPE stippling in and around macula, with continued atrophy of RPE/choriocapillaris/choroid resulting in visible white choroidal vessels

△ The lesion usually spreads slightly but remains confined to the macular area

△ The late stage is actually excavated on stereoscopic evaluation

△ Only rare associated pigmentary clumping

△ Pericentral and central scotomas and color vision compromise are common with retention of peripheral visual fields and no complaints of night blindness or photophobia

△ Peripapillary choroidal dystrophy is a variation that presents in young adult life in the posterior pole with development of white choroidal vessels surrounding the optic nerve head and often spreading into the macula

△ Generalized choroidal dystrophy may also simulate CACD, but the white choroidal vessel atrophy involves the entire fundus, causing decreased vision, visual field compromise in the periphery, and dark adaptation problems

Management

△ Pedigree analysis is necessary for diagnosis and counseling

△ Genetic counseling is in order, but unfortunately the patient has usually passed through childbearing years prior to initial symptoms

△ Low-vision rehabilitation should be considered when appropriate

△ The loss of vision is usually insidious, giving the patient the time necessary to adapt to the psychological trauma

mal and there is no complaint of night blindness or photophobia. Fluorescein angiography shows hyperfluorescence early in the disease, with eventual loss of choriocapillaris flow but no obvious leakage. The ERG and EOG are normal to minimally abnormal.

With the absence of a viable choriocapillaris or choroidal vascular system, the likelihood of choroidal neovascularization is extremely remote.

A variation of choroidal atrophy in the posterior pole that can simulate CACD is **peripapillary choroidal dystrophy (PCD).** This condition presents not only in the macular area but also emanates outward from the optic nerve head in the same pattern as geographic helicoid peripapillary choroidopathy. PCD starts in young adult life in the posterior pole, not necessarily centered on the macula as with CACD. The choroidal atrophy shows a pattern of whitish development that spreads slowly in unpredictable directions. The alteration of visual function depends on extent of fundus involvement and macular damage. There have been reports of AR, AD, and sporadic appearance of PCD. Management of PCD is similar to CACD.

Generalized choroidal dystrophy may also simulate CACD. In generalized choroidal dystrophy, there is the whitish appearance of the atrophic choroidal vessels spread throughout the entire fundus. The generalized loss usually does not present until later in life. There may be some associated pigmentary clumping without vascular attenuation. The visual fields, dark adaptation, and electroretinographic findings vary according to degree of affectation of the retina and choroid. Both AD and X-linked patterns have been described. Management of total choroidal dystrophy becomes a challenge because of both central and peripheral visual compromise.

Management. The patient with CACD has a poor prognosis for visual acuity, as eventually acuity drops to below 20/200. The peripheral vision is, however, retained, which improves the changes of rehabilitation with low-vision devices. Pedigree generation and genetic counseling is again in order. The loss of vision is usually insidious, giving the patient time to prepare vocationally, avocationally, and psychologically for the inevitable. Peripapillary choroidal dystrophy may simulate CACD, but the management is similar in both instances.

■　■　■　■　■　■

Clinical Note: Total Choroidal Vascular Atrophy (TVCA)

Total choroidal vascular atrophy (TVCA) is inherited in an AD manner. TVCA begins at birth with a large area of choroidal atrophy in the temporal retina. Over the next 10 to 15 years the lesion enlarges, with finger projections to the equator. Next, the process begins in the nasal retina until the entire fundus is involved to the equator. The entire retina to the equator, except for small strips extending inferior and superior from the disc, is involved by the third or fourth decades of life. Because the condition begins at birth, nystagmus may be a sign. Genetic counseling is in order, and low-vision rehabilitation has minimal success.

Rod Monochromatism (Stationary Congenital Cone Dystrophy; Complete Achromatopsia)

Introduction and Description. Rod monochromatism is the most common and most visually debilitating of the stationary congenital cone dystrophies. The condition is inherited in an AR manner, with an incidence of about 3 per 100,000. Rod monochromatism is also known as complete achromatopsia.

The fundus is usually normal in appearance (Fig. 7–38). Foveal reflexes may be absent, and mild macular pigment stippling may occur. This is a disease in which there is either a congenital absence of cones or the presence of abnormal photoreceptors.

Signs and symptoms are the key to the diagnosis in rod monochromatism. Photophobia is a key symptom but aversion to light is a more descriptive symptom. Pendular nystagmus is present associated with decreased visual acuity. Acuity is variable, but is usually reduced to below 20/200, which corresponds with "normal" scotopic acuity levels. Color vision tests are abnormal, and the photopic ERG corresponding to the cone function is decreased. The scotopic ERG is normal to only slightly abnormal. Fluorescein angiography is normal, and visual fields are often unattainable because of the nystagmus.

Management. Symptoms improve with age, and nystagmus may often minimize. The condition is typically stationary. Provision of the best possible pre-

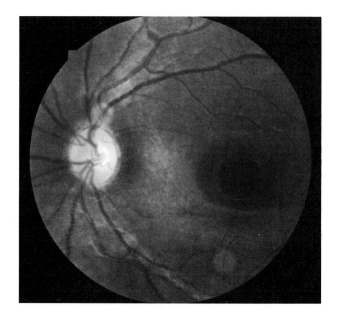

Figure 7–38. A photograph of the fundus of a patient known to have rod monochromatism. This photo illustrates that there are no readily demonstrable retinal/choroidal changes by ophthalmoscopy.

Rod Monochromatism (Complete Achromatopsia)

Characteristics

△ Inherited as AR

△ Typically the fundus appears normal with loss of foveal reflex and perhaps mild pigmentary mottling in the macula

△ Photophobia or aversion to light is the key symptom; others include vision reduction to 20/200, nystagmus, and color vision loss

△ The photopic ERG is abnormal

△ Fluorescein angiography is typically normal

Management

△ Pedigree analysis is indicated

△ Genetic counseling is the only definitive method of prevention

△ Sun lenses may help to minimize the associated photophobia

△ Low-vision rehabilitation should be considered when appropriate

△ Routine examinations with provision of the best possible prescription are in order

scription and routine eye examinations are in order. Low-vision rehabilitation is indicated, and dark glasses may be prescribed to minimize the aversion to light. Pedigree analysis and genetic counseling are recommended.

■ ■ ■ ■ ■ ■

Clinical Note: Incomplete Rod Monochromatism

In incomplete rod monochromatism, visual acuity is in the 20/40 to 20/100 range, with less severe photophobia and a variable presentation of nystagmus. The status of the color vision defect is also variable. The most common variety is blue cone monochromacy or X-linked recessive incomplete achromatopsia. The ERG may demonstrate a minimal waveform.

Progressive Cone Dystrophies (Progressive Cone Degeneration)

Introduction and Description. Heredity is considered AD, but recessive and X-linked forms have also been reported. Progressive cone dystrophy is considered to be congenital. The progressive cone dystrophies or cone–rod dystrophies are typically di-

vided into categories by the variability in the ERG response.

At first presentation, patients with cone dystrophies often have no abnormal findings on fundus evaluation. There are three types of fundus lesions that occur associated with cone dystrophy: (1) the "bulls-eye" lesion, (2) patchy central RPE defects, and (3) localized central RPE and choriocapillaris atrophy.

The most common type of fundus lesion is the "bull's-eye" zone of atrophic RPE surrounding a central homogenous darker zone in the macula (Figs. 7–39 and 7–40). Fluorescein angiography greatly enhances the visibility of the bull's-eye in the early stages of development (Fig. 7–41). Visual acuity is most variable in the "bull's-eye" variety because of the retained central pigment. This type of cone dystrophy simulates chloroquine retinopathy.

In some varieties (most thought to be AR) there may be a diffuse pigment stippling in the posterior pole with pigment clumps. This may be associated with a loss of foveal reflex. With fluorescein angiography, there are diffuse patchy RPE transmission defects over an area that is larger than expected from the ophthalmoscopic view. Vision is compromised in this variety earlier in the disease process and usually is more significantly reduced.

In the third variation, the RPE atrophies along with the choroid. This presentation of cone dystrophy is associated with early onset and severe vision loss. Optic atrophy and vessel attenuation are also findings in this condition. As with other hereditary retinal and choroidal problems, temporal optic atrophy and telangiectatic vessels on the optic disc may be associated findings.

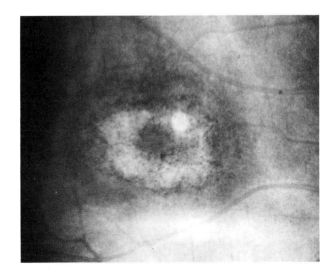

Figure 7–39. A "bull's-eye" lesion associated with a cone dystrophy.

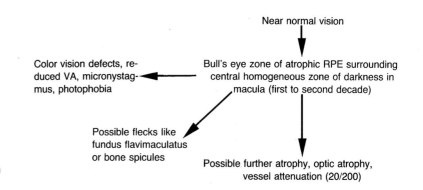

Figure 7–40. A flowchart illustrating the stages in the development of progressive cone dystrophy.

Retinal changes may occur away from the macula in the form of flecks similar to fundus flavimaculatus or bone-spicule clumping similar to RP. A tapetal sheen most prominent temporal to the macula with round, red lesions deep within is also a reported finding. Attenuation of retinal vessels and pigment clumping may occur late in the development of cone dystrophies.

Clinicopathologic findings in progressive cone dystrophy are rarely reported. It appears that there is a loss of the outer nuclear layer of rods and cones with RPE changes.

Patients with progressive cone dystrophy usually have vision reduced to 20/60 to 20/100 in the first to second decades of life with a prior history of "near normal" vision. The patient typically presents for an eye examination complaining of blurred vision. Over

time the vision reduction progresses to a 20/400 to 10/400 level, especially with atrophy of the RPE and choriocapillaris in the macular zone. Photophobia is often severe, with glare producing a noticeable reduction in central acuity levels. A fine micronystagmus that is often acquired may be present that is only visible with slit lamp or by fine oscillations of the fundus view with direct ophthalmoscopy. When central vision falls to 20/40 to 20/60, marked color-vision abnormalities occur. Central or pericentral scotomas are invariable with reduction in acuity. Myopia and astigmatism also appear to be common findings. Night vision is rarely affected.

The fluorescein angiography demonstrates a classical "bull's-eye" hyperfluorescent ring that may actually demonstrate some fine areas of leakage. The photopic ERG is abnormal, and the scotopic ERG is normal to slightly abnormal. The photopic ERG is only mildly subnormal in the bull's-eye variant, with more flattening as the condition progresses or with diffuse pigmentary changes and choriocapillaris atrophy. In a certain subgroup there is a supernormal scotopic ERG that occurs with a flash of moderate intensity. The EOG may be abnormal if midperipheral RPE demonstrates dystrophic changes. It should be noted that the detection of a photopic ERG, however small, is a sign that dysfunction is incomplete and that the prognosis is slightly improved.

Management. In progressive cone dystrophies, vision usually decreases to 20/200 or worse over several years, and then stabilizes. Photophobia is a problem that can be managed by dark glasses. Low-vision rehabilitation is very useful in progressive cone dystrophy. Pedigree analysis and genetic counseling are of utmost importance. The patient should receive routine examinations and be provided with the best possible prescription.

Table 7–9 summarizes the characteristics of hereditary retinal/choroidal disease primarily affecting central and color vision.

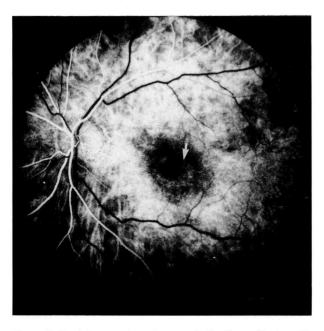

Figure 7–41. A fluorescein angiogram of a "bull's-eye" lesion with the arrow pointing to the hyperflourescent zone.

TABLE 7–9. HEREDITARY RETINAL/CHOROIDAL DISEASE PRIMARILY AFFECTING CENTRAL AND COLOR VISION

	Heredity	Mean Age Onset	Progressive/ Stationary	Signs/ Symptoms	ERG	EOG	Fundus Appearance	Visual Fields
Stargardt's disease	AR	First to second decades	Progressive	Color vision loss, vision loss	Normal to abnormal	Normal to abnormal	Loss of foveal reflex, then zone of normal retina surrounded by RPE changes; slimed fovea then progresses to 2-DD oval beaten bronze, fundus flavimaculatus surrounds macula	Central scotoma
Vitelliform dystrophy (Best's disease)	AD with variability	First decade	Progressive	Color vision loss, vision loss	Normal to abnormal	Abnormal[a]	½–5 DD "egg yolk" in macula; may scramble, giving rupture, hemorrhage, pseudohypopyon	Central scotoma
Dominant drusen (Doyne's syndrome)	AD with variability	First three decades	Progressive	Vision loss, metamorphopsia	Normal to abnormal	Abnormal in late stages	White dots in or near macula that increase in size and become confluent; macular plaque or wet maculopathy	Central scotoma
CACD	AD, AR	Third to fifth decades	Progressive	Vision loss	Normal to abnormal	Normal to abnormal	RPE stippling in and around macula, then atrophy of RPE/choriocapillaris in macula	Pericentral and central scotomas
Rod monochromatism	AR	Congenital	Stationary	Photophobia, nystagmus, vision loss, color vision loss	Abnormal	Normal to abnormal	Normal fundus with possible loss of foveal reflex	N/A
Progressive cone dystrophy	AD, possible AR, X-linked	First to second decade	Progressive	Photophobia, micronystagmus, color vision loss, reduced VA	Abnormal	Normal to abnormal	Bull's-eye zone of RPE atrophy surrounding dark macula, possible disc pallor and vessel attenuation and further macular atrophy	N/A

ERG, electroretinogram; EOG, electro-oculogram; AR, autosomal recessive; AD, autosomal dominant; CACD, control areolar choroidal dystrophy; VA, visual acuity.
[a]Definitive diagnostic test.

Progressive Cone Dystrophies (Degenerations)

Characteristics

Δ Inherited as AD but possible AR and X–linked

Δ First presentation usually has reduced acuity, but often no fundus signs

Δ Fundus signs consist of three variations:

Bull's-eye zone of atrophic RPE surrounding central homogeneous dark macula with variable vision and characteristic fluorescein angiography

Diffuse pigment stippling and clumping that may have associated loss of foveal reflex and areas of fluorescein transmission greater than that observed ophthalmoscopically. Usually more reduced vision

RPE and choriocapillaris atrophy with more early onset and severe vision loss

Δ Possible further macular atrophy, optic atrophy, vessel attenuation, possible midperiphery flecks/spicules, and a tapetal sheen temporal to the macula with indwelling deep red spots

Δ Photophobia, micronystagmus that is acquired, color vision reduction related to variable reduced vision, altered electrodiagnosis depending on extent of affectation

Δ Visual acuity reduction in first to second decades at 20/60 to 20/100 that progresses

Management

Δ Pedigree analysis is indicated

Δ Genetic counseling is of value, as this is the only means of prevention

Δ Low-vision rehabilitation should be considered when appropriate

Δ Sun lenses for photophobia should be provided

Δ Routine examinations to provide the best possible prescription are indicated

■ ■ ■ ■ ■ ■

Clinical Note: Benign Concentric Annular Macular Dystrophy (BCAMD)

Benign concentric annular macular dystrophy (BCAMD) consists of a depigmented ring around an intact macular/foveal region. Acuity ranges from 20/20 to 20/60, with mild to moderate color vision defects. On threshold visual field testing, there are paracentral scotomas. Electrodiagnosis may be slightly altered to normal. Usually this condition is asymptomatic and does not progress.

Albinism

Albinism is a broad term used to describe a group of genetically determined disorders of the melanin pigmentary system. Albinism can be separated into several different categories, but even this is an oversimplification. Ocular characteristics of ocular albinism and oculocutaneous albinism include nystagmus, foveal hypoplasia, photophobia, and reduced visual acuity. Classical definitions include the terms albinoidism, oculocutaneous albinism, and ocular albinism. Albinoidism (cutaneous hypopigmentation) refers to conditions of hypopigmentation with normal visual acuity and no nystagmus. Oculocutaneous albinism is characterized by hypopigmentation of the hair, skin, and eyes, and is inherited as AR in all but one AD form. Ocular albinism is characterized by hypopigmentation (Figs. 7–42 and 7–43) limited to ocular structures and inherited in an X–linked and AR manner. These variants of albinism are described in the following sections.

Oculocutaneous Albinism (OCA)

Introduction and Description. The genesis of the basic defects surround a defect in melanogenesis before birth. Oculocutaneous albinism (OCA) is recognized as an autosomal recessive condition. This appears to be related to an abnormality in tyrosinase, which is a copper-containing enzyme. Tyrosinase-negative patients' hair bulbs have no reaction when incubated in tyrosine,

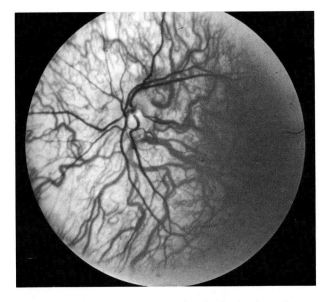

Figure 7–42. A photograph illustrating the fundus hypopigmentation characteristics of albinism and its effects on the ocular system.

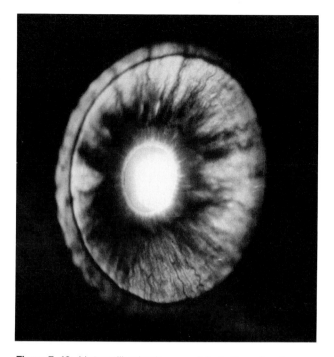

Figure 7–43. Iris transillumination associated with oculocutaneous albinism.

whereas tyrosinase-positive patients' hair bulbs darken when incubated in tyrosine. Tyrosinase-negative patients maintain the same degree of depigmentation throughout life, whereas tyrosinase-positive patients may experience pigmentary changes in the hair and skin. Without the presence of melanin in the pigment cells, an anomalous routing of neurons develops to the brain from the eye as well as an anomaly in the development of the fovea (foveal hypoplasia). Similar developmental anomalies occur in the auditory system. With foveal hypoplasia, there is reduced vision and nystagmus. In most humans, 45 to 50 percent of optic nerve fibers remain uncrossed at the chiasm—that is, temporal retinal nerve fibers remain uncrossed. In the albino the majority of nerve fibers originating in the temporal retina decussate at the chiasm, resulting in a transfer of abnormal field representations to the visual cortex. This crossing results in abnormal hemifield VEP responses and creates a situation in which there is a poor anatomic substrate for the development of efficient binocular vision. Even with surgical correction of strabismus, recovery of functional binocular vision is highly unlikely. This decussation of temporal fibers does not appear to occur in patients without nystagmus.

Appearances of the types of OCA and ocular albinism vary considerably; **see color plate 127,** Table 7–10, and Table 7–11. Characteristics common in tyrosinase-negative OCA forms of albinism include (1)

snow-white hair, (2) pink to white skin, (3) gray to blue-gray irides, (4) visual acuity reduced below 20/100, (5) iris transillumination, (6) nystagmus present at birth that may lessen as the child grows older, (7) foveal hypoplasia (absence of foveal reflex), (8) fundus hypopigmentation resulting in increased visibility of choroidal vasculature, (9) a high incidence of strabismus, (10) normal color vision, (11) photophobia, (12) tendencies toward cancerous and precancerous skin lesions, (13) high refractive errors, and (14) supernormal ERG and EOG due to light scatter.

Characteristics common in tyrosinase-positive OCA include (1) variable pigmentation of the skin and eyes; (2) a relationship to multiple syndromes including Cross syndrome, Hermansky–Pudlak syndrome (increased bleedability) primarily in patients of Puerto Rican descent, and Chédiak–Higashi syndrome (increased rates of systemic infection with decreased life expectancy); (3) darkening of skin, hair, and iris over the years; (4) better vision (20/40 to 20/200) than with tyrosinase-negative albinism and less nystagmus; (5) iris transillumination; (6) poor foveal reflex; and (7) an increased rate of strabismus.

Management. Because OCA is congenital, resulting in nystagmus, the clinician must deal with reduced vision from the onset. The nystagmus and reduced vision tend to improve with age, but the basic problem of a visual handicap always exists.

The clinician is responsible for providing the best possible refraction. It should be emphasized that near vision is often better than distance vision because of the convergence-induced reduction of nystagmus. As with many patients with nystagmus, the use of a reading addition at all ages may improve performance. The photophobia accompanying OCA may be managed by using tinted sun lenses or prescription sun lenses.

From a systemic standpoint, it is important to advise the patient regarding dermatologic protection against cancerous and precancerous ultraviolet-light-induced lesions as well as to remain alert to life-threatening syndromes that may be associated with albinism. Ask questions about ease of bruisability (Hermansky–Pudlak syndrome), frequent nosebleeds, and frequent infections (Chédiak–Higashi syndrome). It is also important that the patient with albinism understand the importance of obtaining bleeding times prior to any surgical technique. Pedigree analysis and genetic counseling are also indicated in all cases of albinism.

Ocular Albinism (OA)

Introduction and Description. There are three forms of ocular albinism (OA) that are classically described: Nettleship–Falls, Forsius–Eriksson, and au-

TABLE 7-10. VARIATIONS IN OCULOTANEOUS ALBINISM (OCA)

	Inheritance	Skin	Hair	Eyes	Vision	Eye Signs/Symptoms	Systemic Problems
Tyrosinase-negative OCA	AR	Pink, no freckles	Snow white	Iris translucency, foveal hypoplasia	20/200	Severe photophobia, nystagmus, strabismus	
Platinum OCA	AR	Pink	Cream/platinum	Iris translucency, foveal hypoplasia, possible small amount pigment in iris	20/200–20/400	Photophobia, nystagmus, strabismus	
Yellow mutant OCA	AR	Whites—cream to yellow with capacity to tan; blacks—dark cream with nevi	Whites—yellow to red hair; blacks—dark yellow to red hair	Early iris translucency with pigment accumulation in a cartwheel by age 3 years, foveal hypoplasia, reduced fundus pigment	Improves with age but still reduced 20/200	Mild photophobia, mild nystagmus	
Tyrosinase-positive OCA, pigment, accumulates with age	AR	Pink at birth but freckles, nevi, and tanning with age	White at birth but yellow to tan with age	Iris translucency is variable with cartwheel pattern, foveal hypoplasia, reduced fundus pigment	20/60–20/120	Mild photophobia, mild nystagmus	
Hermansky–Pudlak syndrome	AR—Puerto Ricans	Variable	Variable	Iris translucency, foveal hypoplasia	20/100–20/300	Nystagmus, photophobia	Hemorrhagic diathesis, lung disease
Chédiak–Higashi syndrome	AR	Creamy white with patches of slate gray	Light brown with metallic sheen	Variable with reduced pigment, foveal hypoplasia	Variable reduction	Variable nystagmus and photophobia	Susceptibility to gram-positive infection, malignancies
Rufous (red) OCA	AR	Red	White to black	Mild to absent iris translucency, fovea, hypoplasia	Variable reduction	Nystagmus (66%), photophobia	
AD OCA	AD	Pink but variable	White but variable	Marked iris translucency, foveal hypoplasia	Variable reduction	Nystagmus, photophobia	

AR, autosomal recessive; AD, autosomal dominant.

TABLE 7–11. VARIATIONS IN OCULAR ALBINISM (OA)

	Inheritance	Skin	Hair	Eyes	Vision	Eye Signs/Symptoms	Systemic Problems
X-linked OA	X-linked affected males	Normal but lighter than sibs, spots of hypopigment	Normal but lighter than sibs	Iris translucency, foveal hypoplasia, reduced fundus pigment, not apparent in blacks	20/80 or less	Photophobia, nystagmus strabismus	
	Heterozygous females	Normal	Normal	Hypopigmented and hyperpigmented spots in fundus, iris translucency	Usually normal	Usually none	
Forsius–Eriksson syndrome	X-linked affected males	Normal	Normal	Iris translucency, foveal hypoplasia, reduced fundus pigment	Reduced but variable	Protan color blind, nystagmus, astigmatism, axial myopia, photophobia	
AR OA	AR	Normal but lighter than sibs	Normal but lighter than sibs	Iris translucency, foveal hypoplasia, reduced fundus pigment	Reduced but variable	Nystagmus, photophobia	
OA–lentigenes—deafness	AD	Normal	Normal	Iris translucency, foveal hypoplasia, reduced fundus pigment	Reduced	Nystagmus, photophobia	Cutaneous lentigenes, deafness, imbalance

AR, autosomal recessive; AD, autosomal dominant.

Albinism

Characteristics

Δ Oculocutaneous albinism (OCA)

Tyrosinase negative never develop pigment
1. Snow-white hair
2. Pink to white skin
3. Gray to blue-gray irides
4. Visual acuity below 20/100
5. Iris transillumination
6. Nystagmus at birth
7. Foveal hypoplasia
8. Fundus hypopigmentation
9. Congenital strabismus
10. Abnormal crossing of temporal fibers at chiasm
11. Tendencies toward cancerous skin lesions
12. Normal color vision but photophobia
13. Supernormal electrodiagnostic tests
14. Autosomal recessive
15. High refractive errors

Tyrosinase positive develop variable pigmentation throughout life
1. Variable pigmentation of skin and eyes
2. Vision reduced to 20/40 to 20/200
3. Iris transillumination
4. Poor foveal reflex
5. Often strabismus
6. Strong relationship to systemic syndromes that may be life threatening
7. Autosomal recessive

Δ Ocular albinism (OA)

Nettleship–Falls albinism
1. Decreased visual acuity
2. Nystagmus
3. Fundus hypopigmentation in caucasians
4. Iris transillumination in caucasians
5. Absence of foveal reflex
6. Strabismus
7. X-linked inheritance
8. Female carriers have equatorial fundus hypopigmentation and patches of skin hypopigmentation

Forsius–Eriksson albinism
1. Decreased visual acuity
2. Nystagmus
3. Fundus hypopigmentation
4. High myopia
5. Color vision defects
6. X-linked inheritance
7. Female carriers without fundus changes but they have nystagmus

Δ Albinoidism (cutaneous hypopigmentation) refers to hypopigmentation of skin or skin and eyes without foveal hypoplasia or reduced vision but with an association to deafness in some cases

Management

Δ Pedigree analysis is crucial

Δ Genetic counseling is indicated in cases of albinism

Δ Provision of best prescription as early as possible in OCA to assist in the development of the best possible vision

Δ A reading addition in all cases of congenital nystagmus may be of functional benefit to the patient

Δ Consider tinted lenses because of the associated photophobia

Δ Low-vision rehabilitation should be considered when appropriate

Δ Urge the patient to protect against skin cancer, as there is an increased incidence associated with hypopigmentation

Δ Rule out associated systemic diseases with OCA
Question frequent bruising, increased bleed-ability
Question frequency of infections
Advise to obtain bleeding times prior to surgical techniques

Δ Advise routine eye examinations

tosomal recessive OA. Nettleship–Falls OA presents many clinical pictures, but all patients have decreased visual acuity, nystagmus, pale fundi in caucasians, iris transillumination in caucasians, and absence of foveal reflexes. The absence of iris transillumination and fundus hypopigmentation in patients with a dark complexion may make the diagnosis more difficult. Many of these patients present with congenital strabismus, and female carriers of this condition have irregular areas of retinal hypopigmentation scattered throughout the retinal equatorial area as well as patches of skin hypopigmentation. Nettleship–Falls OA is inherited in an X-linked pattern.

Forsius–Eriksson OA is also X-linked, presenting with decreased visual acuity, nystagmus, high myopia, pale fundi, absence of foveal reflex, and color vision defects. Carrier females of this condition may show nystagmus but have no fundus pigment changes in the equatorial zone that are characteristic of Nettleship–Falls OA.

The autosomal recessive form of OA presents wih light pigmentation at birth that increases with age. The patients have decreased visual acuity, iris transillumination, photophobia, congenital nystagmus, and strabismus.

Management. The clinician is responsible for providing the best possible refraction. It should be emphasized that near vision is often better than distance vision because of the convergence-induced reduction of nystagmus. As with many patients with nystagmus, the use of a reading addition at all ages may improve performance. The photophobia occasionally accompanying OA may be managed by using tinted sun lenses or prescription sun lenses. Pedigree analysis and genetic counseling are also indicated in all cases of albinism. The abnormal crossing of temporal nerve fibers also exists in OA, precluding maximizing of binocular vision function.

Cutaneous Hypopigmentation (Albinoidism)

Introduction and Description. Cutaneous hypopigmentation or albinoidism is differentiated from oculocutaneous albinism and ocular albinism by the absence of nystagmus and photophobia and usually by the lack of reduced vision. There is a generalized hypopigmentation of the skin or skin and eyes, without the foveal hypoplasia. Albinoidism is often associated with deafness. Cutaneous hypopigmentation with deafness is a characteristic of many syndromes.

Management. The responsibility of primary eyecare practitioners in patients with cutaneous pigmentation is the recognition that the condition may be associated with deafness and that there are many syndromes that present the characteristic skin hypopigmentation. There is always the increased risk of skin cancer with lightly pigmented individuals, and the associated possible systemic risks must be addressed.

Provision of the best possible refraction with routine follow-up examinations is indicated in patients with albinoidism.

REFERENCES

Retinitis Pigmentosa

Albert DM, et al. Transmission microscopic observations of vitreous abnormalities in retinitis pigmentosa. *Am J Ophthalmol.* 1986;101:665–672.

Berson EL, et al. Course of retinitis pigmentosa over a three-year interval. *Am J Ophthalmol.* 1985;99:240–251.

Berson EL, et al. A randomized trial of vitamine supplementation for retinitis pigmentosa. *Arch Ophthalmol.* 1993;111:761–772.

Bloome MA, Garcia CA. *Manual of Retinal and Choroidal Dystrophies.* New York: Appleton-Century-Crofts; 1982.

Carr RE, Siegel IM. *Visual Electrodiagnostic Testing. A Practical Guide for the Clinician.* Baltimore: Williams & Wilkins; 1972.

Fagerholm PP, Philipson BT. Cataract in retinitis pigmentosa. An analysis of cataract surgery results and pathological changes. *Acta Ophthalmol.* 1985;89:883–884.

Fishman GA, et al. Driving performance of retinitis pigmentosa. *Br J Ophthalmol.* 1981;65:122–126.

Fishman GA, et al. X–linked recessive retinitis pigmentosa. Clinical characteristics of carriers. *Arch Ophthalmol.* 1986;104:1329–1335.

Foxman SG, et al. Classification of congenital and early onset retinitis pigmentosa. *Arch Ophthalmol.* 1985;103:1502–1506.

Franceschetti A, et al. *Chorioretinal Heredodegenerations.* Springfield, IL: Thomas; 1974.

Francois J, et al. Visual functions in pericentral and central pigmentary retinopathies. *Ophthalmologica.* 1972;165:38–61.

Goldberg MF. *Genetic and Metabolic Eye Disease.* Boston: Little, Brown; 1974.

Heckenlively JR. *Retinitis Pigmentosa.* Philadelphia: Lippincott; 1988.

Heckenlively JR. The frequency of posterior subcapsular cataract in the hereditary retinal degenerations. *Am J Ophthalmol.* 1982;93:733–738.

Heckenlively JR, et al. Autoimmunity in hereditary retinal degenerations, II. Clinical studies: Antiretinal antibodies and fluorescein angiogram findings. *Br J Ophthalmol.* 1985;69:758–764.

Heckenlively JR, et al. Telangiectasia and optic atrophy in cone–rod degenerations. *Arch Ophthalmol.* 1981;99:1981–1991.

Hyvarinen L, et al. Fluorescein angiographic findings in retinitis pigmentosa. *Am J Ophthalmol.* 1971;71:17–26.

Krauss HR, Heckenlively JR. Visual field changes in cone–rod degenerations. *Arch Ophthalmol.* 1982;100:1784–1790.

Krill AE, et al. Sector retinitis pigmentosa. *Am J Ophthalmol.* 1970;69:677–687.

Krill AE. *Hereditary Retinal and Choroidal Diseases.* Hagerstown, MD: Harper & Row; 1977;2:355.

Krill AE. *Hereditary Retinal and Choroidal Diseases.* Hagerstown, MD: Harper & Row; 1972;1:1.

Krill AE. Retinitis pigmentosa: A review. *Sightsav Rev.* 1972;42:21–28.

Krill AE, Archer D. Classification of the choroidal atrophies. *Am J Ophthalmol.* 1971;72:562–583.

Krill AE, Fold MR. Retinitis punctata albescens. *Am J Ophthalmol.* 1962;53:450–454.

LaVail MM, et al. *Retinal Degeneration. Experimental and Clinical Studies.* New York: Liss; 1985.

Marmor MF. Visual loss in retinitis pigmentosa. *Am J Ophthalmol.* 1980;89:692–698.

Marmor MF, et al. Retinitis pigmentosa: A symposium on terminology and methods of examination. *Ophthalmology.* 1983;90:126–131.

Massof RW, Finkelstein D. Vision threshold profiles in X-linked retinitis pigmentosa. *Invest Ophthalmol.* 1979;18:426–429.

Massof RW, et al. Bilateral symmetry of vision disorders in typical retinitis pigmentosa. *Br J Ophthalmol.* 1979;63:90–96.

Newsome DA. Retinal fluorescein leakage in retinitis pigmentosa. *Am J Ophthalmol.* 1986;101:354–360.

Newsome DA, Blacharski PA. Grid photocoagulation for macular edema in patients with retinitis pigmentosa. *Am J Ophthalmol.* 1987;103:161–166.

Newsome DA, et al. Cataract extraction and intraocular lens implantation in patients with retinitis pigmentosa or Usher's syndrome. *Arch Ophthalmol.* 1986;104:852–854.

Noble KC, Carr RE. Leber's congenital amaurosis. *Arch Ophthalmol.* 1978;96:818–821.

Novack RL, Foos RY. Drusen of the optic disk in retinitis pigmentosa. *Am J Ophthalmol.* 1987;103:44–47.

Pillai S, et al. Optic disc hamartoma associated with retinitis pigmentosa. *Retina.* 1983;3:24–26.

Pruett RC. Retinitis pigmentosa: A biomicroscopical study of vitreous abnormalities. *Arch Ophthalmol.* 1975;93: 603–608.

Rabin J. Visual function in retinitis pigmentosa. *J Am Optom Assoc.* 1986;57:840–842.

Rodrigues MM, et al. Retinitis pigmentosa with segmental massive retinal gliosis. An immunohistochemical, biochemical, and ultrastructural study. *Ophthalmology.* 1987;94:180–186.

Rodrigues MM, et al. Dominantly inherited retinitis pigmentosa. Ultrastructure and biochemical analysis. *Ophthalmology.* 1985;92:1165–1172.

Ross DF, et al. Variability of visual field measurements in normal subjects and patients with retinitis pigmentosa. *Arch Ophthalmol.* 1984;102:1004–1010.

Sheffield JB, Hilfer SR. *Hereditary and Visual Development.* New York: Springer-Verlag, 1985.

Sieving PA, Fishman GA. Refractive errors in retinitis pigmentosa patients. *Br J Ophthalmol.* 1978;62:163–167.

Spencer WH. Drusen of the optic disc and aberrant axoplasmic transport. *Ophthalmology.* 1978;85:21–38.

Thompson JS, Thompson MW. Genetics in Medicine. 4th ed. Philadelphia: Saunders; 1986.

Uliss AE, et al. Retinitis pigmentosa and retinal neovascularization. *Ophthalmology.* 1986;93:1599–1603.

Retinitis Punctata Albescens

Bloome MA, Garcia CA. *Manual of Retinal and Choroidal Dystrophies.* New York: Appleton-Century-Crofts; 1982.

Ellis D, Heckenlively J. Retinitis punctata albescens. Fundus appearance and functional abnormalities. *Retina.* 1983;3: 27–31.

Franceschetti A, et al. *Chorioretinal Heredodegenerations.* Springfield, IL: Thomas; 1974.

Goldberg MF. *Genetic and Metabolic Eye Disease.* Boston: Little, Brown; 1974.

Heckenlively JR. *Retinitis Pigmentosa.* Philadelphia: Lippincott; 1988.

Krill AE. *Hereditary Retinal and Choroidal Diseases.* Hagerstown, MD: Harper & Row; 1977;2:355.

Krill AE. *Hereditary Retinal and Choroidal Diseases.* Hagerstown, MD: Harper & Row; 1972;1:1.

Krill AE, Fold MR. Retinitis punctata albescens. *Am J Ophthalmol.* 1962;53:450–454.

Marmor MF. Defining fundus albipunctatus. *Doc Ophthalmologica Proc Ser.* 1977;13:227–234.

Sheffield JB, Hilfer SR. *Hereditary and Visual Development.* New York: Springer-Verlag; 1985.

Smith BF, et al. Retinitis punctata albescens. A functional and diagnostic evaluation. *Arch Ophthalmol.* 1959;61: 93–101.

Thompson JS, Thompson MW. *Genetics in Medicine.* 4th ed. Philadelphia: Saunders; 1986.

Sector Retinitis Pigmentosa

Heckenlively JR. *Retinitis Pigmentosa.* Philadelphia: Lippincott; 1988.

Hellner KA, Rickers J. Familiary bilateral segmental retinopathia pigmentosa. *Ophthalmologica.* 1973;166: 327–341.

Krill AE, et al. Sector retinitis pigmentosa. *Am J Ophthalmol.* 1970;69:977–987.

Omphroy CA. Sector retinitis pigmentosa and chronic angle-closure glaucoma: A new association. *Ophthalmologica.* 1984;189:12–20.

Inverse Retinitis Pigmentosa

Bloome MA, Garcia CA. *Manual of Retinal and Choroidal Dystrophies.* New York: Appleton-Century-Crofts; 1982.

Franceschetti A, et al. *Chorioretinal Heredodegenerations.* Springfield, IL: Thomas; 1974.

Francois J, et al. Visual functions in pericentral and central pigmentary retinopathies. *Ophthalmologica.* 1972;165: 38–61.

Goldberg MF. *Genetic and Metabolic Eye Disease.* Boston: Little, Brown; 1974.

Heckenlively JR. *Retinitis Pigmentosa.* Philadelphia: Lippincott; 1988.

Krill AE. *Hereditary Retinal and Choroidal Diseases.* Hagerstown, MD: Harper & Row; 1977;2:355.

Krill AE. *Hereditary Retinal and Choroidal Diseases.* Hagerstown, MD: Harper & Row; 1972;1:1.

Krill AE. Retinitis pigmentosa: A review. *Sightsav Rev.* 1972;42:21–28.

Newsome DA. *Retinal Dystrophies and Degenerations.* New York: Raven; 1988;155.

Leber's Congenital Amaurosis

Chew E, et al. Yellowish flecks in Leber's congenital amaurosis. *Br J Ophthalmol.* 1984;68:727–731.

Foxman SG, et al. A classification of congenital and early-onset retinitis pigmentosa. *Arch Ophthalmol.* 1985;108: 1502–1506.

Godel V, et al. Congenital Leber amaurosis, keratoconus, and mental retardation in familial juvenile nephronophthsis. *J Pediatr Ophthalmol Strabismus.* 1978;15:81–91.

Heckenlively JR. *Retinitis Pigmentosa.* Philadelphia: Lippincott; 1988.

Hussels IE. Leber's congenital amaurosis and mental retardation. *Birth Defects.* 1971;7:198.

Karel I. Keratoconus in congenital diffuse tapetoretinal degeneration. *Ophthalmologica.* 1968;155:8–15.

Linstone F, Heckenlively J. Autosomal dominant Leber's amaurosis congenita. *Invest Ophthalmol Vis Sci.* 1983; 24(suppl):293.

Margolis S, et al. Macular colobomas in Leber's congenital amaurosis. *Am J Ophthalmol.* 1977;83:27–31.

Mizuno KI, et al. Leber's congenital amaurosis. *Am J Ophthalmol.* 1977;83:32–42.

Rajacich GM, et al. The usefulness of refractive error in diagnosing RP subtypes. *Invest Ophthalmol.* 1983;24(suppl): 294.

Vaizey MJ, et al. Neurological abnormalities in congenital amaurosis of Leber. *Arch Dis Child.* 1977;52:399–402.

Unilateral Pigmentary Retinopathy

Bastek JV, et al. Traumatic pigmentary retinopathy. *Am J Ophthalmol.* 1981;92:621–624.

Cogan DG. Pseudoretinitis pigmentosa. *Arch Ophthalmol.* 1969;81:45–53.

Heckenlively JR. *Retinitis Pigmentosa.* Philadelphia: Lippincott; 1988.

Kandori T, et al. Unilateral pigmentary degeneration of the retina. *Am J Ophthalmol.* 1968;66:1091–1101.

Pigmented Paravenous Retinochoroidal Atrophy

Brooks DN, et al. Pigmented paravenous retinochoroidal atrophy. *J Am Optom Assoc.* 1980;51:1097–1101.

Miller SA, et al. Pigmented paravenous retinochoroidal atrophy. *Ann Ophthalmol.* 1978;10:867–871.

Noble KG, Carr RE. Pigmented paravenous chorioretinal atrophy. *Am J Ophthalmol.* 1983;96:338–344.

Peduzzi M, et al. Bilateral pigmented paravenous retinochoroidal degeneration following measles. *Int Ophthalmol.* 1984;7:11–14.

Traboulsi EI, Maumenee IH. Hereditary pigmented paravenous chorioretinal atrophy. *Arch Ophthalmol.* 1986;104:1636–1640.

Syphilitic Chorioretinitis

Blodi FC, Hervouet F. Syphilitic chorioretinitis. *Arch Ophthalmol.* 1968;79:294–296.

Folk JC, et al. Syphilitic neuroretinitis. *Am J Ophthalmol.* 1983;95:480–486.

Heckenlively JR. *Retinitis Pigmentosa.* Philadelphia: Lippincott; 1988.

Heckenlively JR. Secondary retinitis pigmentosa (syphilis). *Doc Ophthalmol Proc Ser.* 1976;13:245–255.

Rakel RE, ed. *Conn's Current Therapy.* 39th ed. Philadelphia: Saunders; 1987;594.

Tramont EC. Persistence of *Treponema pallidum* following penicillin G therapy. *JAMA.* 1976;236:2206–2207.

Rubella Retinopathy

Deutman AF, Grizzard WS. Rubella retinopathy and subretinal neovascularization. *Am J Ophthalmol.* 1978;85:82–87.

Heckenlively JR. *Retinitis Pigmentosa.* Philadelphia: Lippincott; 1988.

Metz HS, Harkey ME. Pigmentary retinopathy following maternal measles (morbilli) infection. *Am J Ophthalmol.* 1968;66:1107–1110.

Newsome DA. *Retinal Dystrophies and Degenerations.* New York: Raven; 1988;215.

Obenour LC. The electroretinogram in rubella retinopathy. *Int Ophthalmol Clin.* 1972;12:105–110.

Wolff SM. The ocular manifestations of congenital rubella. A prospective study of 328 cases of congenital rubella. *J Pediatr Ophthalmol.* 1978;10:101–107.

Zimmerman LE. Histopathologic basis for ocular manifestations of congenital rubella syndrome. The eighth William Hamlin Wilder memorial lecture. *Am J Ophthalmol.* 1968;86:106–109.

Congenital Stationary Night Blindness

Bloome MA, Garcia CA. *Manual of Retinal and Choroidal Dystrophies.* New York: Appleton-Century-Crofts; 1982.

Carr RE. Congenital stationary night blindness. *Trans Am Ophthalmol Soc.* 1974;72:448–487.

Cotlier E, et al. *Genetic Eye Diseases. Retinitis Pigmentosa and Other Inherited Eye Disorders.* New York: Liss; 1982.

Franceschetti A, et al. *Chorioretinal Heredodegenerations.* Springfield, IL: Thomas; 1974.

Heckenlively JR, et al. Loss of electroretinographic oscillatory potentials, optic atrophy, and dysplasia in congenital stationary night blindness. *Am J Ophthalmol.* 1983;96:526–534.

Krill AE. *Hereditary Retinal and Choroidal Diseases.* Hagerstown, MD: Harper & Row; 1977;2:355.

Krill AE. *Hereditary Retinal and Choroidal Diseases.* Hagerstown, MD: Harper & Row; 1972;1:1.

Kubota Y. The ERG in Oguchi's disease and retinitis punctata albescens. *Acta Soc Ophthalmol Jpn.* 1965;69:19–25.

Kuwabara T, et al. Histopathological and electron-microscope studies of the retina in Oguchi's disease. *Acta Soc Ophthalmol Jpn.* 1963;64:1323–1351.

Newsome DA. *Retinal Dystrophies and Degenerations.* New York: Raven; 1988;178–179.

Choroideremia

Ayazi S. Choroideremia, obesity, and congenital deafness. *Am J Ophthalmol.* 1981;92:63–69.

Bloome MA, Garcia CA. *Manual of Retinal and Choroidal Dystrophies.* New York: Appleton-Century-Crofts; 1982.

Carr RE, Siegel IM. *Visual Electrodiagnostic Testing. A Practical Guide for the Clinician.* Baltimore: Williams & Wilkins; 1972.

Cotlier E, et al. *Genetic Eye Diseases. Retinitis Pigmentosa and Other Inherited Eye Disorders.* New York: Liss; 1982.

Franceschetti A, et al. *Chorioretinal Heredodegenerations.* Springfield, IL: Thomas; 1974.

Francois J, et al. Visual functions in pericentral and central pigmentary retinopathies. *Ophthalmologica.* 1972;165:38–61.

Goldberg MF. *Genetic and Metabolic Eye Disease.* Boston: Little, Brown; 1974.

Harris GS, Miller JR. Choroideremia. Visual defects in a heterozygote. *Arch Ophthalmol.* 1968;80:423–429.

Heckenlively JR. *Retinitis Pigmentosa.* Philadelphia: Lippincott; 1988.

Krill AE. *Hereditary Retinal and Choroidal Diseases.* Hagerstown, MD: Harper & Row; 1977;2:355.

Krill AE. *Hereditary Retinal and Choroidal Diseases.* Hagerstown, MD: Harper & Row; 1972;1:1.

Krill AE, Archer D. Classification of the choroidal atrophies. *Am J Ophthalmol.* 1971;72:562–583.

Kurstjens JH. Choroideremia and gyrate atrophy of the choroid and retina. *Doc Ophthalmol.* 1965;19:1–122.

LaVail MM, et al. *Retinal Degeneration. Experimental and Clinical Studies.* New York: Liss; 1985.

Lesko JG, et al. Multipoint linkage analysis of loci in the proximal long arm of the human x-chromosome: Application to mapping the choroideremia locus. *Am J Hum Genet.* 1987;40:303–311.

McCulloch C. Choroideremia and other choroidal atrophies. In: Newsome DA, ed. *Retinal Dystrophies and Degenerations.* New York: Raven; 1988;285–295.

Sieving PA, et al. Electroretinographic findings in selected pedigrees with choroideremia. *Am J Ophthalmol.* 1986;101: 361–367.

Takki K. Differential diagnosis between primary choroidal vascular atrophies. *Br J Ophthalmol.* 1974;58:24–35.

Thompson JS, Thompson MW. *Genetics in Medicine.* 4th ed. Philadelphia: Saunders; 1986.

Gyrate Dystrophy

Bell L, et al. Dietary treatment of hyperornithinemia in gyrate atrophy. *J Am Diet Assoc.* 1981;79:139–145.

Berson EL, et al. A two-year trial of low protein, low arginine diets or vitamin B_6 for patients with gyrate atrophy. *Birth Defects.* 1982;18:209–218.

Berson EL, et al. Ocular findings in patients with gyrate atrophy on pyridoxine and low-protein, low-arginine diets. *Ophthalmology.* 1981;88:311–315.

Berson EL, et al. Ocular and biochemical abnormalities in gyrate atrophy of the choroid and retina. *Ophthalmology.* 1978;85:1018–1027.

Bloome MA, Garcia CA. *Manual of Retinal and Choroidal Dystrophies.* New York: Appleton-Century-Crofts; 1982.

Cotlier E, et al. *Genetic Eye Diseases. Retinitis Pigmentosa and Other Inherited Eye Disorders.* New York: Liss; 1982.

Francois J. Metabolic tapetoretinal degenerations. *Surv Ophthalmol.* 1982;26:293–333.

Giordano C, et al. Lysine in treatment of hyperornithinemia. *Nephron.* 1978;22:97–106.

Goldberg MF. *Genetic and Metabolic Eye Disease.* Boston: Little, Brown; 1974.

Hayasaka S, et al. Gyrate atrophy with hyperornithinemia: Different types of responsiveness to vitamin B_6. *Br J Ophthalmol.* 1981;65:478–483.

Heckenlively JR. *Retinitis Pigmentosa.* Philadelphia: Lippincott; 1988.

Kaiser-Kupfer MI, et al. Gyrate atrophy of the choroid and retina: Early findings. *Ophthalmology.* 1985;92:394–410.

Kaiser-Kupfer MI, et al. Cataract in gyrate atrophy: Clinical and morphologic studies. *Invest Ophthalmol Vis Sci.* 1983; 24:432–436.

Kaiser-Kupfer MI, et al. Systematic manifestations of gyrate atrophy of the choroid and retina. *Ophthalmology.* 1981;88: 302–306.

Kaiser-Kupfer MI, et al. Gyrate atrophy of the choroid and retina: Improved visual function following reduction of plasma ornithine by diet. *Science.* 1980;210:1128–1131.

Kaiser-Kupfer MI, et al. A specific enzyme defect in gyrate atrophy. *Am J Ophthalmol.* 1978;85:200–204.

Krill AE. *Hereditary Retinal and Choroidal Diseases.* Hagerstown, MD: Harper & Row; 1977;2:355.

Krill AE. *Hereditary Retinal and Choroidal Diseases.* Hagerstown, MD: Harper & Row; 1972;1:1.

Krill AE, Archer D. Classification of the choroidal atrophies. *Am J Ophthalmol.* 1971;72:562–583.

Kurstjens JH. Choroideremia and gyrate atrophy of the choroid and retina. *Doc Ophthalmol.* 1965;19:1–122.

LaVail MM, et al. *Retinal Degeneration. Experimental and Clinical Studies.* New York: Liss; 1985.

McInnes RR, et al. Hyperornithemia and gyrate atrophy of the retina: Improvement of vision during treatment with a low-arginine diet. *Lancet.* 1981;1:513–517.

Sheffield JB, Hilfer SR. *Hereditary and Visual Development.* New York: Springer-Verlag; 1985.

Sipila I, et al. Supplementary creatine as a treatment for gyrate atrophy of the choroid and retina. *N Engl J Med.* 1981; 304:867–870.

Takki K. Differential diagnosis between primary choroidal vascular atrophies. *Br J Ophthalmol.* 1974;58:24–35.

Takki K. Gyrate atrophy of the choroid and retina associated with hyperornithaemia. *Br J Ophthalmol.* 1974;58:3–23.

Thompson JS, Thompson MW. *Genetics in Medicine.* 4th ed. Philadelphia: Saunders; 1986.

Vannas-Sulonen K, et al. Gyrate atrophy of the choroid and retina. A five year follow-up of creatine supplementation. *Ophthalmology.* 1985;92:1719–1721.

Weleber RG, et al. Gyrate atrophy of the choroid and retina: Clinical and biochemical heterogeneity and response to vitamin B_6. *Birth Defects.* 1982;18:219–230.

Weleber RG, Kennaway NG. Clinical trial of vitamin B_6 for gyrate atrophy of the choroid and retina. *Ophthalmology.* 1981;88:316–324.

Wirtz MK, et al. Heterogeneity and complementation analysis of vitamin B_6 responsive and non-responsive patients with gyrate atrophy of the choroid and retina. *J Inher Metab Dis.* 1985;8:71–74.

Retinal Dystrophies Associated With Storage Diseases

DelMonte MA, et al. Histopathology of Sanfilippo's syndrome. *Arch Ophthalmol.* 1983;101:1255–1262.

Hall CW, et al. Enzymic diagnosis of the genetic mucopolysaccharide storage disorders. *Methods Enzymol.* 1978;50:539.

Jensen OA, et al. Hurler/Scheie phenotype. Report of an inbred sibship with tapeto-retinal degeneration and electron-microscopic examination of the conjunctiva. *Ophthalmologica.* 1978;176:194–204.

Kenyon KR, et al. Mucolipidosis IV. Histopathology of conjunctiva, cornea and skin. *Arch Ophthalmol.* 1979;97: 1106–1111.

Lake BD, et al. A mild variant of mucolipidosis type IV (MLA). *Birth Defects.* 1982;18:391–404.

Lang GE, Maumenee IH. Retinal dystrophies associated with storage diseases. In: Newsome DA, ed. *Retinal Dystrophies and Degenerations.* New York: Raven; 1988; 319–340.

Maumenee IH, DelMonte MA. Diseases of the retinal pigment epithelium. *Birth Defects.* 1980;16:315–326.

McKusick VA. *Mendelian Inheritance in Man.* 7th ed. Baltimore: Johns Hopkins; 1986.

Merin S, et al. Mucolipidosis IV: Ocular, systemic, and ultrastructural findings. *Invest Ophthalmol.* 1973;14:437–448.

Newell FW, et al. A new mucolipidosis with psychomotor retardation, corneal clouding, and retinal degeneration. *Am J Ophthalmol.* 1975;80:440–449.

Riedel KG, et al. Ocular abnormalities in mucolipidosis IV. *Am J Ophthalmol.* 1985;99:125–136.

Sanfilippo SJ, et al. Mental retardation associated with acid mucopolysacchariduria (heparitin sulfate type). *J Pediatr.* 1963;63:837–842.

Santavuori P, et al. Infantile type of so-called neuronal ceroid lipofuscinosis, I. A clinical study of 15 patients. *J Neurol Sci.* 1973;18:257–267.

Scheie HG, et al. A newly recognized forme fruste of Hurler's disease (gargoylism). *Am J Ophthalmol.* 1962;53: 753–769.

Schochet SS, et al. Jansky–Bielchowsky form of neuronal ceroid-lipofuscinosis. *Arch Ophthalmol.* 1980;98:1083–1088.

Snodgrass MB. Ocular findings in a case of fucosidosis. *Br J Ophthalmol.* 1976;60:508–511.

Tonnesen T, et al. Reliability of the use of fructose 1-phosphate to detect Hunter cells in fibroblast-cultures of obligate carriers of the Hunter syndrome. *Hum Genet.* 1983; 64:371–375.

Wolfe LS, Kin NM. Batten disease: New research findings on the biochemical defect. *Birth Defects.* 1982;18:233–239.

Wolter JR, Allen RJ. Retinal neuropathology of late infantile amaurotic idiocy. *Br J Ophthalmol.* 1964;48:277–284.

Zwaan J, Kenyon KR. Two brothers with presumed mucolipidosis IV. *Birth Defects.* 1982;18:381–390.

Fundus Flavimaculatus (With Stargardt's Dystrophy)

Anmarkrud N. Fundus fluorescein angiography in fundus flavimaculatus and Stargardt's disease. *Acta Ophthalmol.* 1979;57:172–182.

Blacharski P. Fundus flavimaculatus. In: Newsome DA, ed. *Retinal Dystrophies and Degenerations.* New York: Raven; 1988;135–159.

Bloome MA, Garcia CA. *Manual of Retinal and Choroidal Dystrophies.* New York: Appleton-Century-Crofts; 1982.

Charney RE, et al. Stargardt's type macular dystrophy associated with retinitis pigmentosa. *Ann Ophthalmol.* 1982;14:118–119.

Cibis GW, et al. Dominantly inherited macular dystrophy with flecks (Stargardt's). *Arch Ophthalmol.* 1980;98: 1785–1789.

Colle CM, et al. Visual improvement with low vision aids in Stargardt's disease. *Ophthalmology.* 1985;92:1657–1659.

Doka DS, et al. Refractive errors in patients with fundus flavimaculatus. *Br J Ophthalmol.* 1982;66:227–229.

Eagle RC. Fundus flavimaculatus: Light and electron microscopic findings. *Ophthalmic Forum.* 1982;1:51–54.

Eagle RC, et al. Retinal pigment epithelial abnormalities in fundus flavimaculatus. *Ophthalmology.* 1980;81:1189–1200.

Fishman GA. Fundus flavimaculatus: A clinical classification. *Arch Ophthalmol.* 1976;94:2061–2067.

Fishman GA, et al. Visual acuity loss in patients with Stargardt's macular dystrophy. *Ophthalmology.* 1987;94: 809–814.

Fishman GA, et al. Blood–retinal barrier function in patients with cone or cone–rod dystrophy. *Arch Ophthalmol.* 1986; 104:545–548.

Francois J, et al. Visual functions in pericentral and central pigmentary retinopathies. *Ophthalmologica.* 1972;165: 38–61.

Goldberg MF. *Genetic and Metabolic Eye Disease.* Boston: Little, Brown; 1974.

Hadden OB, Gass JDM. Fundus flavimaculatus and Stargardt's disease. *Am J Ophthalmol.* 1976;82:527–539.

Klein R, et al. Subretinal neovascularization associated with fundus flavimaculatus. *Arch Ophthalmol.* 1978;96: 2054–2057.

Krill AE. *Hereditary Retinal and Choroidal Diseases.* Hagerstown, MD: Harper & Row; 1977;2:355.

Krill AE. *Hereditary Retinal and Choroidal Diseases.* Hagerstown, MD: Harper & Row; 1972;1:1.

LaVail MM, et al. *Retinal Degeneration. Experimental and Clinical Studies.* New York: Liss; 1985.

Leveille S, et al. Fundus flavimaculatus and subretinal neovascularization. *Ann Ophthalmol.* 1982;14:331–334.

Maloney JBM, et al. Retinal function in Stargardt's disease and fundus flavimaculatus. *Am J Ophthalmol.* 1983;96: 57–65.

McDonnell PJ, et al. Fundus flavimaculatas without maculopathy. A clinicopathologic study. *Ophthalmology.* 1986; 93:116–119.

Rabb MF, et al. Cone–rod dystrophy. A clinical and histopathologic report. *Ophthalmology.* 1986;93:1443–1451.

Sheffield JB, Hilfer SR. *Hereditary and Visual Development.* New York: Springer-Verlag; 1985.

Thompson JS, Thompson MW. *Genetics in Medicine.* 4th ed. Philadelphia: Saunders; 1986.

Patterned Dystrophies

Bloome MA, Garcia CA. *Manual of Retinal and Choroidal Dystrophies.* New York: Appleton-Century-Crofts; 1982.

Burgess D. Subretinal neovascularization in a pattern dystrophy of the retinal pigment epithelium. *Retina.* 1981; 1:151–155.

Chopdar A. Reticular dystrophy of retina. *Br J Ophthalmol.* 1976;60:342–344.

Cortin P, et al. Patterned macular dystrophy with yellow plaques and atrophic changes. *Br J Ophthalmol.* 1980;64: 127–134.

Cotlier E, et al. *Genetic Eye Diseases. Retinitis Pigmentosa and Other Inherited Eye Disorders.* New York: Liss; 1982.

Deutman AF. Dominant macular dystrophies. *Doc Ophthalmol.* 1976;9:415–430.

Deutman AF, et al. Butterfly-shaped pigment dystrophy of the fovea. *Arch Ophthalmol.* 1970;83:558–569.

Eagle RC, et al. Retinal pigment epithelial abnormalities in fundus flavimaculatus. *Ophthalmology.* 1980;81:1189–1200.

Franceschetti A, et al. *Chorioretinal Heredodegenerations.* Springfield, IL: Thomas; 1974.

Giuffrie G, Lodato G. Vitelliform dystrophy and pattern dystrophy of the retinal pigment epithelium. *Br J Ophthalmol.* 1986;70:526–532.

Goldberg MF. *Genetic and Metabolic Eye Disease.* Boston: Little, Brown; 1974.

Gutman I, et al. Vitelliform macular dystrophy and butterfly-shaped epithelial dystrophy: A continuum? *Br J Ophthalmol.* 1982;66:170–173.

Hsieh RC, et al. Patterned dystrophies of the retinal pigment epithelium. *Arch Ophthalmol.* 1977;95:429–435.

Krill AE. *Hereditary Retinal and Choroidal Diseases.* Hagerstown, MD: Harper & Row, 1977;2:355.

Krill AE. *Hereditary Retinal and Choroidal Diseases.* Hagerstown, MD: Harper & Row; 1972;1:1.

LaVail MM, et al. *Retinal Degeneration. Experimental and Clinical Studies.* New York: Liss; 1985.

Marmor MF, Byers B. Pattern dystrophy of the pigment epithelium. *Am J Ophthalmol.* 1977;84:32–44.

O'Donnell FE, et al. Autosomal dominant dystrophy of the retinal pigment epithelium. *Arch Ophthalmol.* 1979;97: 680–683.

Pinckers A, Craysberg JR. Pattern dystrophy of the retinal pigment epithelium. *Ophthalmic Paediatr Genet.* 1986;7: 35–43.

Prensky JG, Bresnick GH. Butterfly-shaped macular dystrophy in four generations. *Arch Ophthalmol.* 1983;101: 1198–1203.

Thompson JS, Thompson MW. *Genetics in Medicine.* 4th ed. Philadelphia: Saunders; 1986.

Watzke RC, et al. Pattern dystrophy of the retinal pigment epithelium. *Ophthalmology.* 1982;89:1400–1406.

Vitelliform Dystrophy

Alexander KR, Fishman GA. Supernormal scotopic ERG in cone dystrophy. *Br J Ophthalmol.* 1984; 68:69–78.

Barricks ME. Vitelliform lesions developing in normal fundi. *Am J Ophthalmol.* 1977;83:324–327.

Bloome MA, Garcia CA. *Manual of Retinal and Choroidal Dystrophies.* New York: Appleton-Century-Crofts; 1982.

Clemett R, Butt S. Vitelliform macular disease. *Trans Ophthalmol Soc NZ.* 1983;35:63–67.

Cotlier E, et al. *Genetic Eye Diseases. Retinitis Pigmentosa and Other Inherited Eye Disorders.* New York: Liss; 1982.

Deutman AF. Electro-oculography in families with vitelliform dystrophy of the fovea. *Arch Ophthalmol.* 1969;81: 305–316.

Epstein GA, Rabb MF. Adult vitelliform macular degeneration. *Br J Ophthalmol.* 1980;64:733–740.

Fishman GA, et al. Blood–retinal barrier function in patients with cone or cone–rod dystrophy. *Arch Ophthalmol.* 1986;104:545–548.

Fishman GA, et al. Pseudovitelliform macular degeneration. *Arch Ophthalmol.* 1977;95:73–76.

Francois J, et al. Visual functions in pericentral and central pigmentary retinopathies. *Ophthalmologica.* 1972;165: 38–61.

Frangieh GT, et al. A histopathologic study of Best's vitelliform dystrophy. *Arch Ophthalmol.* 1982;100:1115–1121.

Galinos SO, et al. Multifocal Best's disease and sickle cell trait. *Ann Ophthalmol.* 1981;13:1181–1183.

Giuffrie G, Lodato G. Vitelliform dystrophy and pattern dystrophy of the retinal pigment epithelium. *Br J Ophthalmol.* 1986;70:526–532.

Goldberg MF. *Genetic and Metabolic Eye Disease.* Boston: Little, Brown; 1974.

Gutman I, et al. Vitelliform macular dystrophy and butterfly-shaped epithelial dystrophy: A continuum? *Br J Ophthalmol.* 1982;66:170–173.

Hodes BL, et al. Progression of pseudovitelliform macular dystrophy. *Arch Ophthalmol.* 1984;102:381–383.

Kraushar MF, et al. Pseudohypopyon in Best's vitelliform macular dystrophy. *Am J Ophthalmol.* 1982;94:30–37.

Krill AE. *Hereditary Retinal and Choroidal Diseases.* Hagerstown, MD: Harper & Row; 1977;2:355.

Krill AE. *Hereditary Retinal and Choroidal Diseases.* Hagerstown, MD: Harper & Row; 1972;1:1.

LaVail MM, et al. *Retinal Degeneration. Experimental and Clinical Studies.* New York: Liss; 1985.

Marmor MF. "Vitelliform" lesions in adults. *Ann Ophthalmol.* 1979;11:1705–1712.

Miller SA, et al. Choroidal neovascular membrane in Best's vitelliform macular dystrophy. *Am J Ophthalmol.* 1976;82: 252–255.

Mohler CW, Fine SL. Long-term evaluation of patients with Best's vitelliform dystrophy. *Ophthalmology.* 1981;88: 688–692.

Patrinely JR, et al. Foveomacular vitelliform dystrophy, adult type. A clinicopathologic study including electron microscopic observations. *Ophthalmology.* 1985;92:1712–1718.

Sabates R, et al. Pseudovitelliform macular degeneration. *Retina.* 1982;2:197–205.

Schachat AP, et al. Macular hole and retinal detachment in Best's disease. *Retina.* 1985;1:22–25.

Sheffield JB, Hilfer SR. *Hereditary and Visual Development.* New York: Springer-Verlag; 1985.

Thompson JS, Thompson MW. *Genetics in Medicine.* 4th ed. Philadelphia: Saunders; 1986.

Vine AK, Schatz H. Adult-onset foveomacular pigment epithelial dystrophy. *Am J Ophthalmol.* 1980;89:680–691.

Weingeist TA, et al. Histopathology of Best's macular dystrophy. *Arch Ophthalmol.* 1982;100:1108–1114.

Dominant Drusen

Bloome MA, Garcia CA. *Manual of Retinal and Choroidal Dystrophies.* New York: Appleton-Century-Crofts; 1982.

Cotlier E, et al. *Genetic Eye Diseases. Retinitis Pigmentosa and Other Inherited Eye Disorders.* New York: Liss; 1982.

Deutman AF, Jensen LM. Dominantly inherited drusen of Bruch's membrane. *Br J Ophthalmol.* 1970;54:373–381.

Franceschetti A, et al. *Chorioretinal Heredodegenerations.* Springfield, IL: Thomas; 1974.

Goldberg MF. *Genetic and Metabolic Eye Disease.* Boston: Little, Brown; 1974.

Krill AE. *Hereditary Retinal and Choroidal Diseases.* Hagerstown, MD: Harper & Row; 1977;2:355.

Krill AE. *Hereditary Retinal and Choroidal Diseases.* Hagerstown, MD: Harper & Row; 1972;1:1.

Thompson JS, Thompson MW. *Genetics in Medicine.* 4th ed. Philadelphia: Saunders; 1986.

Central Areolar Choroidal Dystrophy

Bloome MA, Garcia CA. *Manual of Retinal and Choroidal Dystrophies.* New York: Appleton-Century-Crofts; 1982.

Burn RA. Further cases of a fundus dystrophy with unusual features. *Br J Ophthalmol.* 1950;34:393–395.

Carr RE. Central areolar choroidal dystrophy. *Arch Ophthalmol.* 1965;73:32–36.

Cotlier E, et al. *Genetic Eye Diseases. Retinitis Pigmentosa and Other Inherited Eye Disorders.* New York: Liss; 1982.

Fetkenhour CL, et al. Central areolar pigment epithelial dystrophy. *Am J Ophthalmol.* 1976;81:745–753.

Fraser HB, Wallace DC. Sorsby's familial pseudoinflammatory macular dystrophy. *Am J Ophthalmol.* 1971;71: 1216–1220.

Howard GM, Wolf E. Central choroidal sclerosis: A clinical

and pathological study. *Trans Am Acad Ophthalmol*. 1964; 68:674–676.

Krill AE. *Hereditary Retinal and Choroidal Diseases*. Hagerstown, MD: Harper & Row; 1977;2:355.

Krill AE. *Hereditary Retinal and Choroidal Diseases*. Hagerstown, MD: Harper & Row; 1972;1:1.

Krill AE, Archer D. Classification of the choroidal atrophies. *Am J Ophthalmol*. 1971;72:562–570.

LaVail MM, et al. *Retinal Degeneration. Experimental and Clinical Studies*. New York: Liss; 1985.

McCulloch C. Choroideremia and other choroidal atrophies. In: Newsome DA, ed. *Retinal Dystrophies and Degenerations*. New York: Raven; 1988;285–295.

Sheffield JB, Hilfer SR. *Hereditary and Visual Development*. New York: Springer-Verlag; 1985.

Takki K. Differential diagnosis between primary choroidal vascular atrophies. *Br J Ophthalmol*. 1974;58:24–35.

Thompson JS, Thompson MW. *Genetics in Medicine*. 4th ed. Philadelphia: Saunders; 1986.

Achromatopsias

Alexander KR, Fishman GA. Supernormal scotopic ERG in cone dystrophy. *Br J Ophthalmol*. 1984;68:69–78.

Auerbach E, Merin S. Achromatopsia with amblyopia. A clinical and electroretinographic study of 39 cases. *Doc Ophthalmol*. 1974;37:79–117.

Berson EL, et al. Progressive cone degeneration dominantly inherited. *Arch Ophthalmol*. 1968;80:77–83.

Berson EL, et al. Progressive cone–rod degeneration. *Arch Ophthalmol*. 1968;80:68–76.

Bloome MA, Garcia CA. *Manual of Retinal and Choroidal Dystrophies*. New York: Appleton-Century-Crofts; 1982.

Cotlier E, et al. *Genetic Eye Diseases. Retinitis Pigmentosa and Other Inherited Eye Disorders*. New York: Liss; 1982.

Daily MJ, Mets MB. Fenestrated macular dystrophy. *Arch Ophthalmol*. 1984;102:855–856.

Deutman AF. Benign concentric annual macular dystrophy. *Am J Ophthalmol*. 1974;78:384–396.

Franceschetti A, et al. *Chorioretinal Heredodegenerations*. Springfield, IL: Thomas; 1974.

Goldberg MF. *Genetic and Metabolic Eye Disease*. Boston: Little, Brown; 1974.

Heckenlively JR, et al. Telangiectasia and optic atrophy in cone–rod degenerations. *Arch Ophthalmol*. 1981;99:1983–1991.

Heckenlively JR, Weleber RG. X–linked recessive cone dystrophy with tapetal–like sheen. A newly recognized entity with Mizuo–Nakamura phenomenon. *Arch Ophthalmol*. 1986;104:1322–1328.

Krill AE. *Hereditary Retinal and Choroidal Diseases*. Hagerstown, MD: Harper & Row; 1977;2:355.

Krill AE. *Hereditary Retinal and Choroidal Diseases*. Hagerstown, MD: Harper & Row; 1972;1:1.

Krill AE, et al. The cone degenerations. *Doc Ophthalmol*. 1973;35:1–80.

LaVail MM, et al. *Retinal Degeneration. Experimental and Clinical Studies*. New York: Liss; 1985.

Pinckers A, Timmerman GJ. Sex-difference in progressive cone dystrophy, I. *Ophthalmic Paediatr Genet*. 1981;1:17–24.

Sheffield JB, Hilfer SR. *Hereditary and Visual Development*. New York: Springer-Verlag; 1985.

Thompson JS, Thompson MW. *Genetics in Medicine*. 4th ed. Philadelphia: Saunders; 1986.

Albinism

Ben Ezra D, et al. Chediak–Higashi syndrome: Ocular findings. *J Pediatr Ophthalmol Strabismus*. 1980;17:68–74.

Bergsma DR, Kaiser-Kupfer M. A new form of albinism. *Am J Ophthalmol*. 1974;77:837–844.

Bloome MA, Garcia CA. *Manual of Retinal and Choroidal Dystrophies*. New York: Appleton-Century-Crofts; 1982.

Cotlier E, et al. *Genetic Eye Diseases. Retinitis Pigmentosa and Other Inherited Eye Disorders*. New York: Liss; 1982.

Creel D, et al. Visual system anomalies in human ocular albinos. *Science*. 1978;201:931–933.

Eady RA, et al. Prenatal diagnosis of oculocutaneous albinism by electron microscopy of fetal skin. *J Invest Dermatol*. 1983;80:210–214.

Franceschetti A, et al. *Chorioretinal Heredodegenerations*. Springfield, IL: Thomas; 1974.

Goldberg MF. *Genetic and Metabolic Eye Disease*. Boston: Little, Brown; 1974.

Guillery RW, et al. Abnormal visual pathways in the brain of a human albino. *Brain Res*. 1975;96:373–377.

Kinnear PE, et al. Albinism. *Surv Ophthalmol*. 1968;66:1091–1101.

Krill AE. *Hereditary Retinal and Choroidal Diseases*. Hagerstown, MD: Harper & Row; 1977;2:355.

Krill AE. *Hereditary Retinal and Choroidal Diseases*. Hagerstown, MD: Harper & Row; 1972;1:1.

LaVail MM, et al. *Retinal Degeneration. Experimental and Clinical Studies*. New York: Liss; 1985.

McWilliams WG, Maumenee IH. Albinism. In: Newsome DA, ed. *Retinal Dystrophies and Degenerations*. New York: Raven; 1988;305–317.

O'Donnel FE, et al. Forsius–Eriksson syndrome: Its relation to the Nettleship–Falls X-linked ocular albinism. *Clin Genet*. 1980;17:403–408.

O'Donnel FE, et al. X-linked ocular albinism: An oculocutaneous macromelanosomal disorder. *Arch Ophthalmol*. 1976;94:1883–1892.

Piazza L, et al. Visual acuity loss in patients with Usher's syndrome. *Arch Ophthalmol*. 1986;104:1336–1339.

Sheffield JB, Hilfer SR. *Hereditary and Visual Development*. New York: Springer-Verlag; 1985.

Thompson JS, Thompson MW. *Genetics in Medicine*. 4th ed. Philadelphia: Saunders; 1986.

Appendix ■ ■ ■ ■ ■ ■

*I*CD Codes

Condition	ICD

CATARACTS

After cataract	366.50
Aphakia	379.31
Complicated	366.30
Cortical senile	366.14
Hypermature	366.18
Non-senile	366.00
Nuclear senile	366.16
Nuclear sclerosis	366.17
Posterior subcapsular	366.14
Pseudoexfoliation	366.11
Soemmerings/Elschnig	366.51
Subluxation	379.32
Traumatic	366.20

EXTERNAL

Abnormal pupil	379.40
Abrasion	918.10
Acute uveitis	364.00
Allergy	477.90
Arcus senilis	371.41
Arthritis, multiple sites	716.99
Blepharitis	373.00
Blepharochalasis	374.34
Blepharospasm	333.81
Blow out fracture	829.00
Bullous keratopathy	371.23
Burn eyes, unspecified	940.90
Chalazion	373.20
Concretion	374.56
Conjunctival hemorrhage	372.72
Conjunctivitis	
Allergic	372.14
EKC	077.10
Follicular	372.12
Gonococcal	098.40
Mucopurulent	372.03
Pharyngoconjunctival fever	077.20
Viral	077.90

Contusion	921.90
Corneal	
Dystrophy	371.50
Edema	371.20
Erosion	371.42
Neovascularization	370.61
Opacity	371.21
Scar	371.00
Ulcer	370.00
Dry eyes (Keratoconjunctivitis sicca)	375.15
Ecchymosis	921.00
Ectropion	374.10
Entropion	374.00
Epiphora	375.20
Episcleritis	379.00
Exophthalmos	376.30
Foreign body	
Corneal	930.00
Conjunctival	930.10
Eyelid	374.86
Fracture, unspecified	829.00
Herpes simplex	054.40
Dermatitis	054.41
Dendritic	054.42
Disciform	054.43
Iritis	054.44
Herpes zoster	053.20
Conjunctivitis	053.21
Iritis	053.22
Hordeolum, external	373.11
Hordeolum, internal (Meibomianitis)	373.12
Hyphema	364.41
Iridocyclitis	364.00
Iris synechiae	364.70
Keratitis	
Exposure	370.34
Filamentary	370.23
Interstitial	090.30
Sicca	370.33
Superficial punctuate	370.21
Keratoconus	371.60
Kruckenbergs' spindle	371.13
Laceration	871.40
Lacrimal disorder	371.60
Lagophthalmos	374.20

Myokimia	333.81
Photophobia	368.13
Pigmentary dispersion	364.53
Pinguecula	372.51
Pterygium	372.40
Ptosis	374.30
Punctal stenosis	375.54
Subconjunctival hemorrhage	372.72
Trauma	958.00
Thyroid disorder	242.00
Trichiasis	374.05
Verruca	078.10
Xanthelasma	374.51

GLAUCOMA

Glaucoma—acute angle closure	365.22
Glaucoma—low tension	365.12
Glaucoma—pigmentary	365.13
Pigmentary dispersion of iris	364.53
Glaucoma—primary open angle	365.11
Glaucoma—secondary to inflammation	365.22
Anterior uveitis	364.00
Peripheral anterior synechiae	364.71
Peripheral posterior synechiae	364.71
Glaucoma—secondary to pseudoexfoliation	365.52
Pseudoexfoliation	366.11
Glaucoma—steroid induced	365.31
Glaucoma—subacute angle closure	365.23
Glaucoma—suspect	365.00
Glaucoma—trauma	365.65
Iridodialysis	364.76
Hyphema	364.41
Angle recession	364.77
Contusion	921.30
Glaucoma—vascular	365.63
Rubeosis	364.42
Glaucomatocyclitic crisis	364.22

MACULA

APMPPE	363.15
Age-related maculopathy—dry	362.51
Age-related maculopathy—wet	362.52
Angioid streaks	363.43
Choroidal rupture	363.63
Choroidal sclerosis	363.40
Cystoid macular edema	362.53
Degenerative myopia	360.21
Drusen—retinal degenerative	362.57
ICSC	362.41
Macular hole	362.54
Toxic maculopathy	362.55

NEUROLOGICAL

Abnormal pupil	379.40
Amaurosis fugax	362.34
Anoxic brain damage	348.10
Post operative	997.00

Agnosia	368.16
Aphasia	784.30
Bell's palsy	351.00
Benign intracranial hypertension	348.20
Cerebral edema	348.50
Compression of brain	348.40
Cranial arteritis	446.50
Diplopia	368.20
Disorders	
Chiasmal	377.5_
Cortex	377.6_
Pathway	377.7_
Neoplasm .01	
Vascular .02	
Inflammatory .03	
Embolism	
Basilar artery occlusion	443.00
Cerebral	434.10
Esotropia	378.00
Exotropia	378.10
Dysphagia	784.50
Headache	784.00
Cluster	346.20
Migraine—classical	346.00
Migraine—common	346.10
Migraine—ophthalmic	346.80
Vascular	784.00
Hemorrhage	
Cerebral	431.00
Subarachnoid—non-trauma	430.00
Subarachnoid—trauma	852.00
Subdural—non-trauma	432.10
Subdural—trauma	852.30
Hydrocephalus	331.40
Aqueduct of sylvius stricture	742.30
Injury	
Trauma	958.00
Brain	854.10
Brain trauma	854.00
Cranial nerve III	951.00
Cranial nerve IV	951.10
Cranial nerve V	951.20
Cranial nerve VI	951.30
Cranial nerve VII	951.40
Optic nerve	950.00
Chiasm	950.10
Pathway	950.20
Cortex	950.30
Orbital fracture	829.00
Ischemia	459.90
Myasthenia gravis	358.00
Multiple sclerosis	340.00
Ocular/retinal ischemia	362.84
Paralysis	344.90
Hemiplegia	342.90
Paraplegia	344.10
Quadriplegia	344.00
Paralytic strabismus	378.50
Paresthesia	782.00
Stenosis	447.00
Basilar narrowing	433.00
Carotid narrowing	433.10

Stroke	436.00
Thrombus	437.90
Carotid	433.10
Cerebral	434.00
Unspecified condition of the brain	348.90
Unspecified condition of cranial nerves	352.90

OPTIC NERVE

Autosomal dominant optic atrophy	377.15
Coloboma, optic nerve	
Acquired	377.23
Congenital	743.57
Compression	377.49
Demyelinizing optic neuropathy	377.32
Drusen, optic nerve	377.21
Inflammatory optic neuropathy	377.31
Ischemic optic neuropathy	377.41
Megalopapilla	377.20
Oblique (tilted) disc	377.90
Optic atrophy	377.10
Papilledema	377.00
Pigmentation (Melanocytoma)	743.57
Pit	377.22
Pseudopapilledema	377.24
Toxic optic neuropathy	377.34

RETINA—GENERAL

Atrophic hole without detachment	361.31
Commotio retinae	921.30
Detachment	
With dialysis	361.04
With giant tear	361.03
Old and delimited	361.06
Rhegmatogenous with defect	361.00
Of RPE	362.42
Of RPE secondary to hemorrhage	362.43
Serous without defect	361.20
Traction	361.81
Horseshoe tear without detachment	361.32
Lattice degeneration	362.63
Melanoma	
Choroid—benign	224.60
Choroid—malignant	190.60
Retina—benign	224.50
Retina—malignant	190.50
Multiple retinal defects without detachment	361.33
Pavingstone degeneration	361.61
Peripheral retinal degeneration	362.60
Posterior staphyloma	379.12
Reticular degeneration	362.64
Retinal break	361.30
Retinal coloboma	743.56
Retinal pigment	
Acquired	362.74
Congenital	743.53
Retinoschisis	361.10
Flat	361.11
Bullous	361.12
Secondary vitreoretinal degeneration	362.66

RETINAL CHOROIDAL DYSTROPHIES

Achromatopsia	368.54
Albinism	270.20
Areolar choroidal dystrophy	363.53
Choroideremia	363.55
Dominant drusen	362.77
Fundus flavimaculatus	362.76
Geographic helicoid dystrophy	363.52
Gyrate dystrophy	363.54
Hereditary choroidal dystrophy, unspecified	363.50
Hereditary retinal dystrophy, unspecified	362.70
Juvenile (congenital) retinoschisis	362.73
Night blindness	368.60
Nystagmus, unspecified	370.50
Oguchi's disease	368.61
Progressive cone-rod dystrophy	362.75
Retinitis pigmentosa	362.74
Stargardt's disease	362.75
Vitelliform (Best's) dystrophy	362.76

RETINAL INFLAMMATORY DISEASE

Chorioretinal scars	363.30
Chorioretinitis	
Disseminated	363.10
Focal	363.00
Unspecified	363.20
Histoplasmosis	
Systemic	115.20
Choroidal neovascular net	362.16
Retinal pigment epithelial defect	362.42
Serous retinal detachment	361.20
Pars planitis	363.21
Sarcoidosis	
Systemic	135.00
Chorioretinitis	363.00
Iritis	364.00
Periphlebitis	362.18
Toxocariasis	
Systemic	128.00
Ocular	363.03
Toxoplasmosis	
Systemic	130.20
Chorioretinitis	363.00
Congenital	771.20
Iritis	364.00
Juxtapapillary	363.01
Optic nerve	377.30

RETINAL VASCULAR DISEASE

Angiomatosis retinae	
Ocular	362.17
Systemic	759.60
Blind hypotensive eye	360.41
Blind hypertensive eye	360.42
Behçet's disease	362.30
Branch retinal artery occlusion	362.32
Branch retinal vein occlusion	362.36

VISUAL FIELD/VISUAL DEFECTS

Visual Field Defects

Visual Defects

VITREOUS

*I*ndex

Page numbers followed by t refer to tables.
Page numbers followed by f refer to figures.